Brain Function Augmentation: Contemporary Clinical Neuroscience

Brain Function Augmentation: Contemporary Clinical Neuroscience

Editor: Benjamin Green

MURPHY & MOORE
www.murphy-moorepublishing.com

www.murphy-moorepublishing.com

MURPHY & MOORE

Cataloging-in-Publication Data

Brain function augmentation : contemporary clinical neuroscience / edited by Benjamin Green.
p. cm.
Includes bibliographical references and index.
ISBN 978-1-63987-082-0
1. Brain. 2. Brain--Physiology. 3. Neurosciences. 4. Neurology. 5. Brain--Localization of functions.
6. Neurophysiology. I. Green, Benjamin.
QP376 .B73 2022
612.82--dc23

Murphy & Moore Publishing,
1 Rockefeller Plaza,
New York City, NY 10020, USA

ISBN 978-1-63987-082-0 (Hardback)

Contents

Preface

The central nervous system of the human body is made up of the brain and the spinal cord. The brain is responsible for receiving and processing the information from the sense organs, taking decisions accordingly and sending directions to the rest of the body. There are various areas of the brain, each with a specialized function. The augmentation of brain functions involves enhancing the performance of the brain in healthy adults as well as people suffering from neurological disorders. Sensory, cognitive and motor functions are the three main areas which are targeted by this field. This augmentation can be done either through neurostimulation or through pharmacological means. This book includes some of the vital pieces of work being conducted across the world, on various topics related to brain functions. It presents researches and studies performed by experts across the globe. Scientists and students actively engaged in this field will find this book full of crucial and unexplored concepts.

After months of intensive research and writing, this book is the end result of all who devoted their time and efforts in the initiation and progress of this book. It will surely be a source of reference in enhancing the required knowledge of the new developments in the area. During the course of developing this book, certain measures such as accuracy, authenticity and research focused analytical studies were given preference in order to produce a comprehensive book in the area of study.

This book would not have been possible without the efforts of the authors and the publisher. I extend my sincere thanks to them. Secondly, I express my gratitude to my family and well-wishers. And most importantly, I thank my students for constantly expressing their willingness and curiosity in enhancing their knowledge in the field, which encourages me to take up further research projects for the advancement of the area.

Editor

1

Not all brains are created equal: the relevance of individual differences in responsiveness to transcranial electrical stimulation

Beatrix Krause* and Roi Cohen Kadosh

Department of Experimental Psychology, University of Oxford, Oxford, UK

Edited by:
Mikhail Lebedev, Duke University, USA

Reviewed by:
Peter B. Reiner, University of British Columbia, Canada
Marom Bikson, The City College of New York of The City University of New York, USA

***Correspondence:**
Beatrix Krause, Department of Experimental Psychology, University of Oxford, Tinbergen Building, 9 South Parks Road, Oxford, OX1 3UD, UK
e-mail: beatrix.krause@psy.ox.ac.uk

A current issue in the research of augmentation of brain functions using transcranial electrical stimulation (tES) is the diversity and inconsistency in outcome results. Similar studies often report different results, depending on the parameters and tasks used. Such inconsistencies have led to significant doubts about the efficacy of the method in the broader scientific community, despite its promising potential for patient recovery and treatment. Evidence on the large variability in individual cortical excitability and response to tES suggests that stimulation may affect individuals differently, depending on the subject's age, gender, brain state, hormonal levels, and pre-existing regional excitability. Certain factors might even lead to the reversal of polarity-dependent effects, and therefore have crucial implications for neurorehabilitation and cognitive enhancement. Research paradigms may have to be refined in the future to avoid the confounding effects of such factors.

Keywords: inhibition, excitation, transcranial electrical stimulation, individual, responsive, efficacy

INTRODUCTION

Transcranial electrical stimulation (tES) in its various forms (anodal vs. cathodal transcranial direct current stimulation (tDCS); transcranial random noise stimulation (tRNS); and transcranial alternating current stimulation (tACS)) has become a highly popular research tool to enhance a wide range of typical, as well as atypical cognitive patterns of behavior (Miniussi et al., 2008; Brasil-Neto, 2012; Cohen Kadosh, 2013; Krause and Cohen Kadosh, 2013). A multitude of studies include healthy participants, patients with behavioral and neuropsychiatric disorders, as well as brain damage or neurological conditions. The external modulation of cortical excitability aims to induce beneficial changes in cortical efficiency and functioning, and thereby enhance plasticity, which subsequently improves the outcome of the training or testing variable in question. The enhancement of synaptic plasticity in the stimulated area is thought to increase the area's processing efficiency, which supports learning and/or recovery (Cramer et al., 2011). However, the diversity of different interactions between deficits and functional systems in different individual populations, as well as the resulting potential individual differences in tES effects has not been disentangled yet. In fact, differences at the individual level of regional brain function and anatomy may lead to profoundly different outcomes. The current idea is that excitatory tES methods, such as anodal tDCS and tRNS enhance cortical excitability (Nitsche and Paulus, 2001; Terney et al., 2008), whereas cathodal tDCS decreases cortical excitation (Nitsche et al., 2003). However, while this might be a generally accepted idea, the real pattern seems more complex.

We have previously suggested that the optimal balance between cortical excitation and inhibition (E/I balance) differs between individual brain areas and subjects and therefore the application of, for instance, anodal tDCS may lead to fundamentally different results in an individual with high regional excitability (i.e., anodal tDCS will lead to overexcitation and non-optimal performance), whereas the same stimulation in a different brain regions with different E/I levels, or in an individual with lower excitation may be more beneficial (Krause et al., 2013). The optimal excitability level would then be at the tip of an inverted-U shaped function of excitation/inhibition and behavior. In line with this hypothesis, researchers have now discovered that experimental populations tDCS research can almost be split into two separate groups: responders and non-responders (López Alonso et al., 2014). The study was based on a previous study that used transcranial magnetic stimulation (TMS) to the motor cortex to investigate cortical excitability in the form of motor evoked potentials (MEPs) in a sample of 56 individuals at various different time points (Hamada et al., 2013). Instead of averaging across the whole group, as is most commonly done in brain stimulation research, Hamada et al. (2013) tracked the patterns of MEP amplitudes per subject across the eight time points. The result was that the individual responses were highly variable and when averaging across all subjects, the average result was nearly zero. More recently, López Alonso et al. (2014) observed a similar pattern using tDCS. A cluster analysis pointed to a subset of 55% of the subjects that not only failed to show an increase, but instead even a slight decrease in TMS-elicited MEP amplitudes in response to the stimulation, which was significantly distinguishable from the 45% of subjects that showed the expected increase. Similarly, another study has shown that increasing the level of excitation by increasing stimulation intensities of tRNS and tACS can reverse excitation to inhibition (Moliadze et al., 2012). There are methods to assess changes in cortical excitability, such as magnetic resonance spectroscopy (MRS) or TMS, but there are also methods to affect inhibition and excitation. For example, paired associative stimulation (PAS), deep brain stimulation (DBS) and direct current stimulation (DCS) in rodents, can improve the interpretation of data. In humans, MRS is an especially valuable research technique in this regard, as it is a noninvasive *in vivo* magnetic resonance imaging (MRI) method that reliably assesses total concentrations of GABA and glutamate in a predefined voxel (Mekle et al., 2009), typically between $1.5 \times 1.5 \times 1.5$ cm^3 and $3 \times 3 \times 3$ cm^3, which makes it possible to estimate E/I in the to-be-stimulated brain area. Such findings are highly relevant to the field of tES research and we will later discuss a variety of influences on cortical excitability that may be responsible for the drastic individual differences in responses to the stimulation previously described. The identification of such confounding variables may improve tES research and analysis strategies in the future and allow for better controlled design and application of tES in research and potentially in the future also in clinical settings.

NEUROTRANSMITTER BALANCES

The brain's main excitatory and inhibitory neurotransmitters, glutamate and GABA, respectively, are strongly involved in learning and experience-dependent plasticity (Trepel and Racine, 2000; Ge and Dani, 2005). For example, regional GABA levels decrease with learning in the domain associated with the stimulated brain region (e.g., motor learning in M1) (Floyer-Lea et al., 2006). Moreover, the higher the observed learning increment, the steeper the GABA decrease in response to anodal tDCS (Stagg et al., 2011). Such a reduction can in turn facilitate long-term potentiation (LTP), which allows for cortical reorganization (Hess and Donoghue, 1994) and the authors suggest that the responsiveness of an individual's regional GABA system to the stimulation is related to their learning capacity.

Assuming that an increase in cortical excitability is beneficial for learning, we should also be aware of some of its negative consequences. Overexcitation of the cortex (i.e., the excessive release of glutamate), leads to excitotoxicity and cell death (Faden et al., 1989; Belousov, 2012). Excessive GABAergic inhibition, however, prevents LTP and reduces neuronal output (Mcdonnell et al., 2007). Enhanced inhibition is therefore associated with higher network stability but also reduced cortical plasticity (Hess and Donoghue, 1996). Accordingly, a fine balance in the interaction between excitation and inhibition is required to optimize the efficiency of information transfer in the brain (Turrigiano and Nelson, 2000; Bavelier et al., 2010). For tES application, this means that there is a certain dose-response relationship that interacts with pre-existing baseline levels that are currently unknown to the experimenter. Besides other confounding factors in tES research that we will discuss later, this interaction could explain the observed individual differences in experimental outcomes and the large variability in the current literature.

So far, researchers have mainly been concerned with extreme abnormalities in excitability (for instance epileptic patterns of brain activity), and have used it as an exclusion criterion for tES experiments. It is important to note that other neurotransmitter systems also interact with cortical excitability and therefore abnormal neurotransmission in those may equally moderate the effects of tES and potentially the subjects' health. For instance, elevations in extracellular serotonin are associated with increased excitability induced by anodal, and surprisingly also by cathodal tDCS (Nitsche et al., 2009). Therefore, to avoid these confounds in experimental work, we generally recommend to exclude individuals with psychological or psychiatric problems, as well as individuals taking medication that influences hormone or neurotransmitter systems.

Individual differences in pre-existing neurotransmitter levels and in cortical efficiency are also reflected in brain activity, as measured by functional magnetic resonance imaging (fMRI), such that baseline levels of glutamate and GABA are associated with regional activity levels. For example, GABA concentrations measured by MRS correlate positively with γ oscillation frequency, which reflects inhibitory activity, and are inversely related with functional activity in the cortex (Muthukumaraswamy et al., 2009). This means that inhibition can be expressed in the strength of γ oscillations measured by electroencephalography (EEG) or magnetoencephalography (MEG), and that the task-related blood-oxygenated level dependent (BOLD) response decreases with elevated inhibition. Similarly, the baseline GABA concentration predicts the properties of the activation-dependent hemodynamic response function (HRF), such that higher baseline inhibition is related to lower activity (Muthukumaraswamy et al., 2012). Furthermore, task-dependent activity in several different cortical and subcortical areas is associated with glutamate levels in the brain area in question but also in remote areas that are heavily connected. However, the direction of the relationship between activity (low vs. high) and task demands is modulated by pre-existing glutamate levels (low vs. high) (Falkenberg et al., 2012).

These results demonstrate that common findings in brain activation studies can be reasonably well explained by local concentrations of baseline glutamate and GABA levels. Moreover, individual differences in pre-existing neurotransmitter levels cause research subjects to respond differently to external modulation of E/I. For example, a subject with high initial inhibition may never reach a similar level of regional cortical plasticity as a subject with low inhibition. In turn, with two different groups of individuals showing opposing effects in response to tES, the outcome effect will be reduced, or even regress the mean of the whole sample towards zero.

CURRENT APPLICATION

Given the large number of options available in the selection of tES parameters, the effects on the individual subject's cortical excitability and tissue may be very specific and extremely variable across a whole sample. For instance, there are sharp contrasts in outcomes observed using different current strengths, such that

1 and 2 mA of A-tDCS achieve different outcomes on cognitive tasks. One study reports reduced reaction times with prolonged but not shorter stimulation periods at 2 mA, whereas reaction times increased with longer stimulation times at 1 mA (Teo et al., 2011). Reaction times were therefore similarly low under short periods of 1 mA and longer periods of 2 mA. Similarly, 2 mA of C-tDCS over the motor cortex can even flip the intended inhibitory effect on MEPs achieved at 1 mA into cortical facilitation (Batsikadze et al., 2013). Such reversal effects suggest that more (in terms of both intensity and duration) is not necessarily better and there is a fine line between the optimal and accidentally impairing current application.

Several different variations of tES are available, whereby the underlying neurobiological mechanisms are better understood for some than for others. For instance, the user can decide whether to excite a region in one hemisphere and inhibit the same region in the other, or he can place one of the electrodes on an area with minimal or no interference (e.g., the vertex, forehead, cheek or arm). It is currently unclear, which option is ideal for which purpose (for a first step see Moliadze et al., 2010). One of the major reasons for this lies in the principle of interhemispheric inhibition. The two hemispheres work in concert to produce behavioral output and damage to an area in one hemisphere may unleash unprecedented activation of the same area in the other hemisphere (Cramer et al., 1997; Zimmerman and Hummel, in press). In the presence of brain damage or dysfunction for example, the contralateral hemisphere often tries to compensate for the loss and therefore responds with atypical patterns of activity (see Johnston, 2009). The particular pattern is known to the tES user, however, such that the prediction of tES effects is specific to the choice of parameters.

The effect of left anodal tDCS (cathode attached to the forehead) on resting state activity in a prefrontal network indeed demonstrated increases in functional connectivity to the same area in the right hemisphere, whereas connectivity to other areas within the same hemisphere was reduced (Park et al., 2013). The authors hypothesized that the behavioral results found in cognitive tES studies may be based on the changes in interhemispheric connectivity and that different placements of the cathode may have caused fundamentally different results. Such effects may be similar or different for different brain areas and between the two hemispheres. Additionally, different subject populations might respond differently to such effects, depending on the pre-existing interhemispheric connectivity patterns (e.g., see for elderly Cabeza, 2002). Given this fact, the question about the optimal stimulation method for a given purpose is critical.

In tACS the current alternates between the cathode and the anode at a fixed frequency (Zaghi et al., 2010) and it is known to modulate brain oscillations. Its beneficial effect on cognition or behavior has not yet been fully established, and has even been found to impair perceptual processes in certain cases (Brignani et al., 2013). From DBS we know that the stimulation frequency also leads to fundamental differences in the effectiveness of the treatment of for instance motor disorders, such as Parkinson's disease (PD) (see McConnell et al., 2012). Despite the fact that DBS (with its implanted electrodes) has a different mechanism of action, it demonstrates how varying the stimulation parameters can successfully direct the output effects of a stimulated cortical network. There is now also first evidence for the effectiveness of tACS in modulating Parkinson-related brain oscillations (Brittain et al., 2013). Similarly, the effect of the different stimulation frequencies used in tACS often depends on external factors, such as lighting conditions within the testing room (Kanai et al., 2008). In this case the same stimulation parameters in a well-lit room may differ from the ones in a room under darker conditions during perceptual processing. The authors point to an interaction between ongoing cortical oscillations in the cortex and the applied current frequency. Accordingly, the subject's current cortical excitability will interact with the stimulation. Where tACS has a variety of different frequencies that can be freely chosen (e.g., α, β and γ waves) tRNS also has different frequency settings, that are mostly split into full-spectrum, high-frequency (Hf-) and low-frequency (Lf-) tRNS. Under certain conditions, tACS has been shown to induce stronger excitability increases than full-spectrum tRNS (Moliadze et al., 2012), but when tRNS conditions are directly compared, Hf-tRNS induces stronger excitability than Lf-tRNS (Terney et al., 2008). Again, it is important to note that there are few experiments available that compare different parameters of tES within the same study and often the outcome measure is an excitability variable (mostly in the motor domain), rather than a cognitive or behavioral outcome. This means that the current knowledge might be restricted to very specific experimental conditions and it is unknown whether these effects are generalizable across domains and testing conditions.

There is a large variety of tES applications with its excitatory vs. inhibitory modulation (anodal and cathodal tDCS), excitation through noise induction (tRNS) and the modulation of cortical oscillations (tACS), as well as possible parameters including frequency range, current strength and electrode positioning interact with ongoing regional excitability of the cortex. The problem is that the experimenter is usually unaware of the excitability levels and these might differ under different experimental conditions and might be particularly sensitive in perceptual domains.

THE RESEARCH DESIGN

In addition to individual differences in biological substrates, variations in study design can have a striking impact on the outcomes of tES studies. For example, daily tDCS leads to greater excitability changes than second daily application (Alonzo et al., 2012) such that a more sensitive neural system may accumulate higher excitability over several sessions. In addition, it is crucial to assess long-term effects of improvements and potentially impairments, as these eventually determine the success of the intervention. Some have already demonstrated long-term positive effects (e.g., Reis et al., 2009; Cohen Kadosh et al., 2010b; Snowball et al., 2013), whereas most studies do not perform such follow-up testing. Another question is at what point in time an improvement in the testing variable will be visible. Many studies test and evaluate performance during the stimulation (e.g., Bolognini et al., 2010; Weiss and Lavidor, 2012), whereas others also compare pre- and post-measures (e.g., Dockery et al., 2009; Snowball et al., 2013). The quality of the effect may be different in such cases and before tES can be applied in clinical settings, the evolution of performance change should be monitored to find the optimal time for training assessments.

THE INITIAL BRAIN STATE

An important but hard to control factor in research is the brain state of the individual subject. Silvanto et al. (2007) point out the importance of subject factors, such as fatigue and wakefulness, attention, intoxication and the habituation to the presented task material. These and others can be potential confounders that can even flip polarity-dependent effects of tES into the opposite polarity. For example, state-dependent effects associated with baseline brain activity can be related to resting α-band power, which has been showed to modulate the threshold for excitability probed by TMS (Romei et al., 2008). Similarly, using tACS with its ability to entrain cortical oscillations, the stimulation frequency has been showed to interact with ongoing brain activity. The highest increase in motor cortical excitability at rest was achieved using β-tACS (20 Hz), whereas the highest excitability levels during motor imagery were observed during θ-tACS (5 Hz) (Feurra et al., 2013). The authors attribute the effect of θ-tACS to the underlying use of working memory processing during the imagery task, whereas β stimulation is thought to correspond to the natural cortical response during rest.

Using a neural adaptation paradigm, Silvanto et al. demonstrated that less active neuronal populations respond more strongly to TMS than more active ones (Silvanto et al., 2008). Further studies extended this finding to high-level cognition and the parietal lobes (Cohen Kadosh et al., 2010a). Furthermore, the experimental manipulation of cortical excitability responds in a similar way, such that preconditioning the cortex with A-tDCS causes repetitive TMS (rTMS) to be inhibitory, whereas C-tDCS preconditioning reverses subsequent rTMS effects to cortical excitation (Lang et al., 2004; Siebner et al., 2004). The effects of the initial brain state are even visible across different tasks. Motor cortical excitability could be reduced by A-tDCS, and increased by C-tDCS to M1 during a cognitive task, compared to the same stimulation during rest (Antal et al., 2007). However, cortical excitability was reduced by both A-tDCS and C-tDCS when engaging in a motor task, compared to during rest. In this study, A-tDCS therefore only increased cortical excitability during rest, but flipped the effect to inhibition during cognitive, and even more so during motor engagement. In contrast, C-tDCS led to a slight excitability decrease at rest but a sharp decrease during motor processing, while it increased excitability during cognitive processing. The authors concluded that areas that are not involved in the cognitive task at hand become deactivated, while the reduction in excitability during the motor task is more likely to be associated with muscle fatigue. It is therefore apparent that ongoing neuronal activation interacts with different types of stimulation to modulate cortical excitability and behavioral responses. The effects of experimentally uncontrolled influences on the brain seem so profound that they have the potential to even flip intended inhibition to excitation (and *vice versa*) and are therefore not consistent with the current idea of polarity-specific tDCS. Currently, such baseline cortical activity factors are unknown variables in tES research. Experimental instructions and procedures may bias the brain state of subjects to respond to the stimulation in a certain way, confounding the desired outcome.

THE INDIVIDUAL BRAIN

The situation is further complicated by individual variations in head and tissue morphology. Different head sizes and tissue thicknesses might cause different current distributions and require different current strengths to achieve the same current flow (Bikson et al., 2012). For example, depending on where on the head the electrodes are placed, the stimulation can be more focal than in other configurations, which may be related to the orientation of neurons and the current flow applied and how the current propagates along the tissue connections (Neuling et al., 2012). Individual morphologies of cortical gyri and sulci also affect the pattern of the current flow (Datta et al., 2012). The same stimulation design can therefore lead to large differences in the induced current and the resulting electric field, due to brain and body morphological differences (Datta et al., 2012; Truong et al., 2013). The resulting individual differences in the strength of the induced electric field effects on neuronal activity and E/I will therefore be fundamentally different. As observed in experiments applying different intensities of current (e.g., Batsikadze et al., 2013), an intended excitation can flip to inhibition in some subjects but not in others. This in turn will affect both physiological and behavioral effects negatively.

Furthermore, depending on the task applied under stimulation (especially using cognitive tasks), subjects may recruit different brain regions for the same task depending on their stage of brain and cognitive development and due to the individual strategy use (Rivera et al., 2005). The consequence of this is that one might stimulate an area that is currently not involved in the processing of the task (i.e., the "wrong" area for the task at hand based on previous fMRI studies in different populations), which will eventually not benefit the individual's abilities and add further noise to the experimental results.

Similarly, the interaction between brain areas might differ across individuals, e.g., due to differences in the strength and efficiency of network connections. Since tES has been found to affect whole networks rather than just the stimulated region in isolation (Keeser et al., 2011; Zheng et al., 2011), it is possible that by enhancing brain functioning at one point in the network, subsequent network areas might be negatively affected, such that the outcome is disadvantageous (Brem et al., 2014). For example, the increased cortical excitability may lead to reduced inhibition to a subsequent area, such that this area will produce excessive output and impair behavioral functioning. It has indeed been found that stimulation of frontal areas can improve certain cognitive aspects while interfering with others, while stimulating parietal areas reverses the pattern (Iuculano and Cohen Kadosh, 2013). Considering this possibility, individuals with certain neurological vulnerabilities, young and old individuals, as well as patients with brain abnormalities or damage can be expected to respond differently to the same type of stimulation. For instance, the behavioral effects of tES on elderly compared to younger participants seem to be reversed and hemisphere-dependent (Ross et al., 2010, 2011). The anticipation of tES effects should therefore never be generalized from one group to another, but should instead carefully explored to prevent a null result, or even an accidental induction of cognitive impairment.

THE DEVELOPING AND AGING BRAIN

The brain is not static. It changes continuously across the lifetime and, along with these changes, occur changes in behavior and how the individual responds to stimuli in the environment. During development, a certain relative balance between excitation and inhibition defining functional properties of the cortex is established and eventually maintained throughout later stages of life (Turrigiano and Nelson, 2004). However, evidence from animal research suggests that early experiences shape the coupling of excitatory and inhibitory neural activity and thereby affect cortical plasticity. Still, the initial interactive activity is subject to change and refinement across the course of postnatal development (Dorrn et al., 2010) and E/I balances may therefore guide the timing of developmental critical periods of plasticity for experience-dependent learning (Hensch and Bilimoria, 2012). Early experiences and E/I interactions may therefore determine the later responsiveness to tES.

Research using TMS demonstrated how age-related differences in cortical excitability affect the speed of signal transduction in motor pathways. Motor responses are slowed in elderly compared to younger adults (Smith et al., 2009), which is associated with age-related changes in intracortical inhibition. This leads to a decline in the functional modulation of corticospinal activity (Fujiyama et al., 2012). Similarly, the aging individual also has to face cognitive slowing, which has been associated with a weakening of white matter connections between different cortical areas but also a decline in structural gray matter, whereby the pace of change differs by the structure or area (Raz et al., 2005; Jackson et al., 2012).

Along with such changes in brain structure, regional neurotransmitter balances change as well, affecting experience-dependent plasticity (Hess and Donoghue, 1996). For example, GABAergic receptor distribution changes from early childhood to the early teenager years and then again during older age (Pinto et al., 2010). More specifically, there is an age-related decline in GABA levels that can be observed in the elderly brain using MRS (Gao et al., 2013). Glutamate availability has also been found to decrease in the aging brain in rodents (Mcentee and Crook, 1993). An observed loss in NMDA receptors (Wenk et al., 1991) (in rats and monkeys) may be responsible for such changes and may also impact the capacity to form LTP. With such changes and shifts in E/I, experience-dependent plasticity in the cortex changes across the lifetime (Hensch et al., 1998; for a comprehensive review on the role of spike timing-dependent plasticity in plasticity, see Caporale and Dan, 2008). Interestingly, the artificial reduction of GABAergic signaling can restore some of the age-related decline in learning in rodents (Lasarge et al., 2009). Therefore, the external modulation of GABA using tES may also lead to beneficial behavioral effects in the elderly but it is unclear how the type and dosage of the stimulation affects elderly individuals differently from younger age groups. The evidence on regional GABA and glutamate concentrations, as well as on the effects of tES in elderly populations is currently extremely scarce.

In summary, along with the continuous brain development and age-related changes in structure and function, we can expect changes in E/I balance across the lifespan, which are currently under-investigated. The interactions between tES and E/I balance are therefore even less predictable than in healthy young adults. This is due to the fact that the research on *in vivo* assessments of GABA and glutamate in developing and aging human samples and the use of tES in these groups is still in its infancy and there is little available evidence at this point.

CIRCADIAN RHYTHM

Circadian influences, such as sleep and time of the day have been found to affect cortical excitability, such that TMS-probed intracortical inhibition was found to decrease throughout the day (Lang et al., 2011). Moreover, with more time staying awake, especially after sleep deprivation, motor cortical excitability gradually increases along with an increase in EEG θ waves, which is commonly observed with prolonged wakefulness (Huber et al., 2013). This sleep-dependent increase in cortical excitability has critical implications for subjects' sleeping patterns prior to stimulation. Sleep deprivation may enhance the risk for seizure activity, especially in combination with repeated sessions of tES, which by itself increases excitability (Alonzo et al., 2012). Such combination could accumulate cortical excitability to potentially harmful levels in susceptible participants. A variety of different psychological and neuropsychiatric disorders involve abnormal circadian rhythms or deficient sleep patterns and some can already be distinguished on the basis of MRS-measured GABA and/or glutamate concentrations at a group level (e.g., Goto et al., 2009; Yoon et al., 2010; Rojas et al., 2013). Careful screening procedures should therefore be applied to monitor potential pre-existing abnormalities in E/I.

HORMONAL LEVELS

Another source of variation is related to hormonal levels, which fluctuate substantially more in women than men, such that some studies exclude females completely from their research on cortical excitability to reduce the noise (e.g., Alonzo et al., 2012). Two main phases in the menstrual cycle can be distinguished: the follicular phase, characterized by rising levels of estrogen and low levels of progesterone, and the luteal phase, which starts with ovulation and is associated with moderate levels of estrogen and high levels of progesterone. Cortical inhibition, as probed by TMS and measured by MEPs measured is enhanced and simultaneously excitability reduced, during periods of higher progesterone levels (i.e., the luteal phase) (Smith et al., 1999). Furthermore, cortical excitation is relatively low during the first half of the follicular phase (including the menstruation period), which is characterized by low levels of both progesterone and estradiol in particular, but then excitability increases in the second half of the follicular phase, when progesterone is still low but estradiol peaks (Smith et al., 2002). Excitation is then decreased again, and inhibition increased during the luteal phase, with rising progesterone and estradiol levels. Progesterone therefore seems to drive the increase in cortical inhibition, whereas estradiol increases excitability. This is supported by a study using MRS to assess GABA concentrations in the primary visual cortex, which appeared lower during the luteal than the follicular phase in healthy women and GABA was inversely related with both estradiol and progesterone levels (Epperson et al., 2002). However, since the study did not concurrently measure levels of glutamate, no inferences can be made on the E/I balance, as those might counteract or dominate GABA levels differentially during different phases of the cycle. Moreover, in the study that measured cortical excitability using TMS (Smith et al., 2002), the follicular phase was subdivided into an early and a late phase due to the peaking levels of estradiol in the second half, whereas the MRS study investigated the follicular phase as a whole, which may have failed to capture the measurement during the rising levels of estradiol. Instead, the researchers subdivided the luteal phase into early and late, the two halves of which show little difference in their respective estradiol and progesterone levels (Epperson et al., 2002). This might additionally have affected the interpretation of GABA levels throughout the cycle. For future studies it will be useful to subdivide both phases equally and inspect all four time points. In a different study, glutamate concentrations in the medial frontal cortex were found to be significantly lower during the luteal than the follicular phase (Batra et al., 2008). Since both studies investigated different brain areas, it is hard to draw conclusions but it is likely that assessments of the ratio of glutamate and GABA will confirm the findings of previous TMS studies that relative inhibition is increased during the luteal phase, and reduced during the follicular phase (see **Figure 1** for a summary of the current results in relationship with estrogens and progesterone).

For a more complete picture of global brain excitability, Harada and associates investigated three different brain areas (left frontal cortex, lentiform nuclei and cingulate cortex) using MRS and found that only in the lentiform nuclei and the left frontal cortex GABA levels were decreased during the luteal compared to the follicular phase but not in the anterior cingulate cortex (Harada et al., 2011). This means that E/I might additionally depend on the interaction between hormonal fluctuations and local brain regions. To make things more complex, smoking is another possible noise variable in E/I balance, as GABA levels have been found to differ across the menstrual cycle. Specifically, GABA is higher during the follicular than the luteal phase in nonsmoking women (Epperson et al., 2005). Furthermore, there was no difference between smoking and non-smoking men and their GABA levels were similar to women in the luteal phase. In contrast, smoking women in the follicular phase showed slightly but not significantly reduced levels of GABA, compared to all other groups. No differences in GABA concentrations were found after 48 h of abstinence in the smokers. Despite the fact that an individual's lifestyle may affect E/I and induce additional noise into tES experiments, long term smoking behavior in this case might even stabilize GABA concentrations (although causal inferences from these study results are not possible).

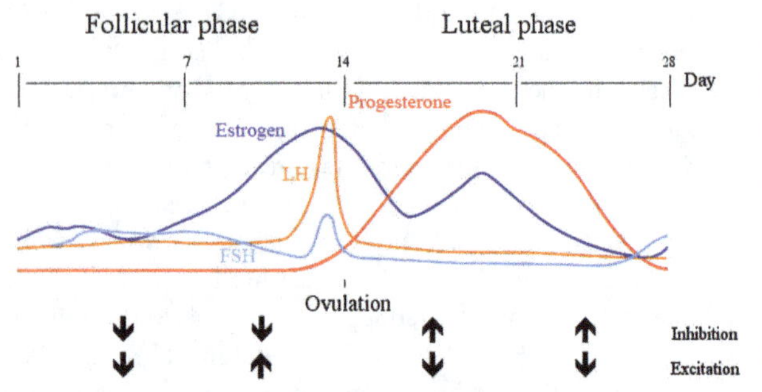

FIGURE 1 | Inhibition and excitation across the menstrual cycle. The early follicular phase (day 1 –the start of menstruation—until day 7) is characterized by low levels of estrogen and progesterone, during which both inhibition and excitation are low. With an increase in estrogen from day 7–14, luteinizing hormone (LH) and follicular stimulating hormone (FSH) peak and stimulate ovulation on day 14. During this late follicular phase inhibition is low and excitation high, which reverses in the following 14 days (early luteal phase). Estrogen, in particular estradiol is now moderately high but progesterone peaks.

A rapid change in E/I balance due to hormonal fluctuations has been associated with neurological conditions, which already serve as exclusion criteria and/or control variables in tES research. These are for instance migraine, epileptic seizures, but also premenstrual mood disorders (i.e., during periods of high cortical inhibition) (for a more detailed discussion on biological alterations, see Finocchi and Ferrari, 2011). Despite the increasing evidence on excitability differences due to hormonal changes, this type of information is not by itself informative about the efficiency of the information transfer in the brain and the degree of capacity for plastic changes.

DRIVING AND PREDICTING PLASTICITY

By transiently enhancing plasticity, we attempt to induce favorable long-lasting changes that allow for increased experience-dependent learning. However, there is also an optimal balance between plasticity (i.e., the flexibility of synaptic connections to change according to experience) and stability (keeping the system balanced). Critical periods of development are characterized by enhanced levels of brain plasticity because learning during such periods is crucial to shape the cortical networks for later efficient processing (stability). Stability is necessary to make the network cost-efficient in terms of energy expenditure and thereby provide constant and predictable patterns for the preferred output (Knudsen, 2004). Strengthening pathways in the "wrong" way during such a period of high plasticity levels can cause unwanted and irreversible (stable) changes during cortical development (Knudsen, 2004). Therefore, caution is needed when artificially enhancing plasticity, as behavioral changes in the wrong direction may be difficult to reverse.

Stability, in terms of long-term adaptation to plasticity-induced training effects may therefore be more crucial to tES than previously anticipated. This means that we should not aim for the maximum cortical excitability, but instead for the *optimal balance* between plasticity and stability in terms of E/I. Not only does the E/I balance determine the flexibility of a network and hence the functioning of the brain area (Knudsen, 2004; Murphy et al., 2005), but additional compensatory mechanisms also regulate the net output of the system. While Hebbian learning drives experience-dependent plasticity, compensatory mechanisms are required to maintain the stability in a homeostatic way and thereby maintain a fixed set point of firing rates (Turrigiano and Nelson, 2004). This process is called homeostatic plasticity. The previously discussed flip in excitatory and inhibitory effects after polarity-dependent tDCS is another example of homeostatic plasticity. Some authors have suggested that the cortex uses this flip to maintain a functionally useful range of cortical excitability, which subsequently affects the potential for plasticity (Lang et al., 2004; Siebner et al., 2004). They explain that pre-existing excitation and inhibition determine the net effect of TMS and whether its action is excitatory or inhibitory. Such pre-existing E/I levels may be directly related to differences in the state of the brain (e.g., alertness, attention or familiarity with a task and neuronal populations), and thereby interact with the applied stimulation (Silvanto et al., 2007). Therefore, in the presence of elevated levels of excitation, TMS or tES effects may be incapable of inducing further excitation and instead may suppress cortical activity. Neurorehabilitation would therefore be naturally limited.

Given a history of successful cognitive and clinically symptomatic improvements achieved by tES, the question is how strongly these homeostatic mechanisms are affected by the stimulation. This question has been neglected in tES research so far and is worth serious investigation. If tES is affected by homeostatic plasticity, there might be an upper level of improvement we cannot exceed and the question is whether excessive stimulation will lead to a ceiling effect or whether it reverses the effects to the worse. The latter possibility would reflect our previous hypothesis of an inverted-U shape of cortical excitability and behavioral outcome (Krause et al., 2013). Beyond a certain point the stimulation will start causing impairments rather than further improvements. Another question is if homeostatic set points differ across individuals and whether the range of possible plastic changes inducible by tES is similar in each individual. Furthermore, we also have to take into account that this set point may change with development and aging. Dose-response experiments monitoring changes, especially impairments in behavioral and cognitive outcomes, are therefore of high importance (e.g., Teo et al., 2011; Moliadze et al., 2012; Brignani et al., 2013).

In practice, these compensatory mechanisms are likely to occur over an extended period of time and may therefore not be immediately measurable in changes on behavioral tasks or symptom outcomes used during experiments. However, changes induced by homeostatic plasticity can even counteract Hebbian learning effects (Turrigiano and Nelson, 2004), which may moderate the effects of tES greatly. This again has important implications for rehabilitation, especially in epilepsy, where an unintended increase in excitability may have severe health effects.

HOW TO DEAL WITH THE VARIABILITY

The wide variety of options for tES parameters paired with the multitude of individual differences in pre-existing neurotransmitter levels makes the evaluation of tES research results as a whole difficult. Guleyupoglu et al. (2013) stress the importance of current dose for the outcome of the study. For example, they define tES dosage in terms of the parameters of the electrodes, including the size, number, shape, position and composition, as well as the waveform in terms of intensity and the general form of the waves administered, the pulse shape (wherever relevant), amplitude, width, polarity and repetition frequency of the current waves, the number of sessions and the inter-session interval. For research purposes, as well as for the generalization of results it is important to always report the exact parameters used, as the current flow and the resulting induced electric fields depends on these parameters (Peterchev et al., 2012). In severe clinical cases when the financial means are available, electrode shapes and sizes can even be custom designed to better control and enhance tES effects but this method requires structural brain scans (MRI) and neuronavigation for the production and fitting of the stimulation (Tecchio et al., 2013). Individualized tES with more focal effects (high-definition tDCS) may become more feasible in the future, with the development of more automated and less time-consuming methods for the prediction of current flow (Datta et al., 2012; Huang et al., 2012; Edwards et al., 2013).

One possible solution to specifically target the individual regional E/I balance is to assess GABA and glutamate levels in the voxels of interest using MRS and thereby determine the directionality of the current polarity/parameters to optimize E/I. Similarly, tACS has been shown to have particularly long-lasting effects on cortical excitability and cognition when the stimulation frequency is tuned to the endogenous cortical firing frequency, as assessed by EEG (Neuling et al., 2013). This way, tES applications can be individually tailored. However, the high costs of neuroimaging may not always be feasible and more knowledge of the ideal balance required. Many of the current experiments exclude women due to the hormonal fluctuations and the influence on cortical excitation but if we want to eventually affect brain and behavior of the general population using tES, we must explore the relationship between the menstrual cycle and E/I further. The same applies to developing and aging populations. In the case of hormonal influences, blood measures of hormone levels may give indications of relative cortical excitability levels in women. However, more evidence is required to substantiate the evidence on the relationship between E/I and hormonal interactions.

Another solution, which might be a somewhat crude indicator, is individual variability in behavior. If E/I is related to brain oscillations and metabolic responses, which again are associated with behavioral response patterns, behavioral performance may distinguish at least extremely elevated or reduced levels of E/I. While behavioral performance does not capture the entire E/I variance or other factors that we mentioned here, it may still serve as a useful additional controlling factor for the variety of influential factors discussed here.

DISCUSSION

Evidence stemming from noninvasive brain stimulation studies suggests that there are separate subgroups of experimental subjects that differentially respond to stimulation. Specifically, up to half of them respond with reductions in excitability in response to the stimulation, whereas the other half responds, as expected, with increases in measures of excitability (Wassermann, 2002; Hamada et al., 2008; López Alonso et al., 2014). Such subgroups may have diminished many of the expected beneficial effects of tES in the past and identification of the type of responder before the application of tES would substantially help the outcome analysis and interpretation of tES effects. In order to achieve successful clinical intervention, this information is crucial for the user. We believe that the biological determinants of the subject response outcome depend on neurotransmitter balances, in particular glutamate and GABA, as their interaction defines the E/I balance in the area that is to be stimulated. The baseline in E/I balance might be differently skewed in each individual, such that some start off with higher relative excitation, whereas others have relatively low regional excitability. This will subsequently have differential effects on the capacity for the induction of plastic changes and therefore lead to different outcomes in experiments where each subject receives the same treatment. This would explain why in some cases up to half the sample responds to the enhanced excitability, whereas the same enhancement is disadvantageous in others (López Alonso et al., 2014). As Pavlov hypothesized more than 50 years ago, different personalities underlie different ratios between excitation and inhibition and therefore produce different behavioral outcomes (for a discussion, see Strelau, 1997). How these differences in cortical E/I balance arise is currently unknown, but it has been found that siblings show similar responses to brain stimulation, which suggests that there is either a heritable factor biasing the E/I balance, or that stimulation responses are similar in siblings due to some common morphological properties of their skulls and cortices (Wassermann, 2002).

For reasons of baseline neurotransmitter system activity, tES might lead to different results in different individuals. This can be due to the discussed factors and potential pre-existing vulnerabilities, as well as structural differences in cortical gray and white matter, skull and tissue thickness. The effects of tES can therefore be binary (effect vs. no effect), or they can show in varying degrees of the effect or even in negative effects. The outcome of the result does not always allow for inferences on the underlying mechanism, such that the uncertainty in current research interpretations is concerning. The degree of the response to tES may also vary with time of the day, the time point of menstrual cycle in women, environmental testing conditions, and general preexisting levels of neurotransmitter balances in the brain. These may further be influenced by medication or lifestyle preferences, such as smoking (as well as other methods of intoxication) or sleep patterns.

We would also like to note that our view implies that polarity-dependent effects of tES are not always straightforward and predictable. The common view that A-tDCS is generally excitatory and C-tDCS inhibitory has been challenged, as discussed here, and can be seen as a relatively crude average outcome. For example, the polarity-specific effect of tDCS depends on the organization, morphology and orientation of cortical neurons to the incoming current (Bikson et al., 2004; Kabakov et al., 2012; Rahman et al., 2013). Due to the curvature of an axon, there is always a combination between excitatory and slightly stronger inhibitory activity, such that the sum between these determines the net output (Kabakov et al., 2012).

For these reasons, it is possible that the biological processes underlying tES effects are even more complex than we suggest here. Despite the extensive research on inhibitory and excitatory effects of the current, the effects may not solely be explained by E/I. For instance, a subtle change in excitation and inhibition induced by weak current can alter network dynamics by simply changing the pattern of E/I. These changes are non-linear and the size of the effect depends on the current state of the network, affecting the rate and timing of neuronal firing (Reato et al., 2010). This means that even small simultaneous changes in the levels of excitation and inhibition can lead to a different outcome within the dynamics of the network.

Cellular tissue studies can provide more direct evidence for our idea in the future. However, investigating cellular E/I interactions in human higher-level cognition is currently not feasible. In order to fully understand the effects of tES on plasticity-behavior relationships, we have to understand the resulting formation of LTP and long-term depression (LTD) by the actions of NMDA and AMPA receptor activity (Huganir and Nicoll, 2013). Examining individual differences at the receptor level in humans is *in vivo* unfortunately is not feasible at the moment. It is also important to note that there is quite a leap from the interpretation of current effects at the receptor level in cell tissue and human behavioral studies. The bridge between molecular and human research consists of computational modeling of the current flow through different tissue configurations (for a comprehensive review see e.g., Bikson et al., 2012), which is a useful tool to understand current effects. In order to understand and predict the exact effects of tES (with its different types and parameters) we need to understand the cellular, broader cortical (e.g., regional interactions between brain areas) and behavioral effects of tES and how these are linked together. This link may be far simpler for lower-level skills, such as motor or perceptual brain functions, but more complex for higher-order cognitive abilities, including attention, working memory and arithmetic.

A potential problem with the majority of the evidence from tES research on cortical excitability is that it is all performed in the motor domain and may therefore not be generalizable to other behavioral and cognitive domains. For instance, the motor cortex may respond in fundamentally different patterns to other areas (e.g., in the prefrontal cortex). For example the observed reduction in inhibition associated with anodal tDCS and motor learning (Floyer-Lea et al., 2006; Stagg et al., 2009) stands in sharp contrast to the beneficial effect of cathodal inhibition on certain frontal cognitive functions (Weiss and Lavidor, 2012). In some domains cortical inhibition appears to be more beneficial than in others, especially considering cognitive functions involving attentional focus or the inhibition of irrelevant material, such as in the latter case. Therefore, one should be cautious about generalizing across domains.

MRS can be used to quantify concentrations of glutamate and GABA in different areas. As a measure of E/I balance, these quantifications are already used to distinguish healthy from psychiatric populations (e.g., Eichler and Meier, 2008; Yoon et al., 2010; Kubas et al., 2012). The addition of this neuroimaging technique or similarly EEG/MEG to measure oscillations, tES studies for the predetermination of E/I levels in potential subject pools would be very cost intensive. Nevertheless, we believe that this might clarify tES results and foster our understanding of both functional brain neurochemistry and tES methodology in the future.

CONCLUSION

Here we summarized the most well-known currently unpredictable factors influencing cortical excitability and plasticity and how the interaction of individual differences with the available multitude of stimulation parameters may influence the effects of noninvasive, plasticity-inducing electrical stimulation at the individual level. We conclude that the simple perception of tES polarity-specific neuronal modulation is an oversimplification of the complex effects and that the effects are currently far less predictable than assumed in the majority of the scientific community. We suggest that tES effects are moderated by pre-existing baseline E/I. Imbalances in E/I can be found in clinical or neuropsychiatric populations, during hormonal fluctuations (especially in women) and caused by interactions with the baseline neuronal activity, external influences, such as smoking or medication use, developmentally and age-related changes in E/I across the lifespan. Additional factors include individual differences in skull and cortical morphology, circadian influences that are currently not clarified, such as time of day or sleep deprivation, interactions with other neurotransmitter systems, and differential effects of tES due to unusual use of strategies in e.g., cognition. In addition, the current state of brain functioning and previous experiences can influence, or even flip polarity-dependent tDCS effects. For future research, it is of particular importance that scientists are aware of such variations and that they select their desired research populations with care in regard to potential unwanted noise in the data, and/or in some extreme cases the potential increase in seizure risk. These could be achieved by taking some of these factors into account, pre-assessing E/I levels or activation patterns using neuroimaging methods, in certain cases TMS, or at least behavioral patterns of performance.

ACKNOWLEDGMENTS

We would like to thank Michael Clayton for his comments. Beatrix Krause is supported by the Economic and Social Research Council (ESRC), the German Academic Exchange Service (DAAD), and the Studienstiftung des Deutschen Volkes. Roi Cohen Kadosh is a Wellcome Trust Career Development Fellow (0883781). Roi Cohen Kadosh filed a patent for an apparatus for improving and/or maintaining numerical ability.

REFERENCES

Alonzo, A., Brassil, J., Taylor, J. L., Martin, D., and Loo, C. K. (2012). Daily transcranial direct current stimulation (tDCS) leads to greater increases in cortical excitability than second daily transcranial direct current stimulation. *Brain Stimul.* 5, 208–213. doi: 10.1016/j.brs.2011.04.006

Antal, A., Terney, D., Poreisz, C., and Paulus, W. (2007). Towards unravelling task-related modulations of neuroplastic changes induced in the human motor cortex. *Eur. J. Neurosci.* 26, 2687–2691. doi: 10.1111/j.1460-9568.2007.05896.x

Batra, N. A., Seres-Mailo, J., Hanstock, C., Seres, P., Khudabux, J., Bellavance, F., et al. (2008). Proton magnetic resonance spectroscopy measurement of brain glutamate levels in premenstrual dysphoric disorder. *Biol. Psychiatry* 63, 1178–1184. doi: 10.1016/j.biopsych.2007.10.007

Batsikadze, G., Moliadze, V., Paulus, W., Kuo, M. F., and Nitsche, M. A. (2013). Partially non-linear stimulation intensity-dependent effects of direct current stimulation on motor cortex excitability in humans. *J. Physiol.* 591, 1987–2000. doi: 10.1113/jphysiol.2012.249730

Bavelier, D., Levi, D. M., Li, R. W., Dan, Y., and Hensch, T. K. (2010). Removing brakes on adult brain plasticity: from molecular to behavioral interventions. *J. Neurosci.* 30, 14964–14971. doi: 10.1523/jneurosci.4812-10.2010

Belousov, A. B. (2012). Novel model for the mechanisms of glutamate-dependent excitotoxicity: role of neuronal gap junctions. *Brain Res.* 1487, 123–130. doi: 10.1016/j.brainres.2012.05.063

Bikson, M., Inoue, M., Akiyama, H., Deans, J. K., Fox, J. E., Miyakawa, H., et al. (2004). Effects of uniform extracellular DC electric fields on excitability in rat hippocampal slices in vitro. *J. Physiol.* 557, 175–190. doi: 10.1113/jphysiol.2003.055772

Bikson, M., Rahman, A., and Datta, A. (2012). Computational models of transcranial direct current stimulation. *Clin. EEG Neurosci.* 43, 176–183. doi: 10.1177/1550059412445138

Bolognini, N., Fregni, F., Casati, C., Olgiati, E., and Vallar, G. (2010). Brain polarization of parietal cortex augments training-induced improvement of visual exploratory and attentional skills. *Brain Res.* 1349, 76–89. doi: 10.1016/j.brainres.2010.06.053

Brasil-Neto, J. P. (2012). Learning, memory and transcranial direct current stimulation. *Front. Psychiatry* 3:80. doi: 10.3389/fpsyt.2012.00080

Brem, A.-K., Fried, P. J., Horvath, J. C., Robertson, E. M., and Pascual-Leone, A. (2014). Is neuroenhancement by noninvasive brain stimulation a net zero-sum proposition? *Neuroimage* 85(Pt. 3), 1058–1068. doi: 10.1016/j.neuroimage.2013.07.038

Brignani, D., Ruzzoli, M., Mauri, P., and Miniussi, C. (2013). Is transcranial alternating current stimulation effective in modulating brain oscillations? *PLoS One* 8:e56589. doi: 10.1371/journal.pone.0056589

Brittain, J. S., Probert-Smith, P., Aziz, T. Z., and Brown, P. (2013). Tremor suppression by rhythmic transcranial current stimulation. *Curr. Biol.* 23, 436–440. doi: 10.1016/j.cub.2013.01.068

Cabeza, R. (2002). Hemispheric asymmetry reduction in older adults: the HAROLD model. *Psychol. Aging* 17, 85–100. doi: 10.1037//0882-7974.17.1.85

Caporale, N., and Dan, Y. (2008). Spike timing-dependent plasticity: a Hebbian learning rule. *Annu. Rev. Neurosci.* 31, 25–46. doi: 10.1146/annurev.neuro.31.060407.125639

Cohen Kadosh, R. (2013). Using transcranial electrical stimulation to enhance cognitive functions in the typical and atypical brain. *Transl. Neurosci.* 4, 20–33. doi: 10.2478/s13380-013-0104-7

Cohen Kadosh, R., Muggleton, N., Silvanto, J., and Walsh, V. (2010a). Double dissociation of format-dependent and number-specific neurons in human parietal cortex. *Cereb. Cortex* 20, 2166–2171. doi: 10.1093/cercor/bhp273

Cohen Kadosh, R., Soskic, S., Iuculano, T., Kanai, R., and Walsh, V. (2010b). Modulating neuronal activity produces specific and long-lasting changes in numerical competence. *Curr. Biol.* 20, 2016–2020. doi: 10.1016/j.cub.2010.10.007

Cramer, S. C., Nelles, G., Benson, R. R., Kaplan, J. D., Parker, R. A., Kwong, K. K., et al. (1997). A functional MRI study of subjects recovered from hemiparetic stroke. *Stroke* 28, 2518–2527. doi: 10.1161/01.str.28.12.2518

Cramer, S. C., Sur, M., Dobkin, B. H., O'brien, C., Sanger, T. D., Trojanowski, J. Q., et al. (2011). Harnessing neuroplasticity for clinical applications. *Brain* 134, 1591–1609. doi: 10.1093/brain/awr039

Datta, A., Truong, D., Minhas, P., Parra, L. C., and Bikson, M. (2012). Inter-individual variation during transcranial direct current stimulation and normalization of dose using MRI-derived computational models. *Front. Psychiatry* 3:91. doi: 10.3389/fpsyt.2012.00091

Dockery, C. A., Hueckel-Weng, R., Birbaumer, N., and Plewnia, C. (2009). Enhancement of planning ability by transcranial direct current stimulation. *J. Neurosci.* 29, 7271–7277. doi: 10.1523/jneurosci.0065-09.2009

Dorrn, A. L., Yuan, K., Barker, A. J., Schreiner, C. E., and Froemke, R. C. (2010). Developmental sensory experience balances cortical excitation and inhibition. *Nature* 465, 932–936. doi: 10.1038/nature09119

Edwards, D., Cortes, M., Datta, A., Minhas, P., Wassermann, E. M., and Bikson, M. (2013). Physiological and modeling evidence for focal transcranial electrical brain stimulation in humans: a basis for high-definition tDCS. *Neuroimage* 74, 266–275. doi: 10.1016/j.neuroimage.2013.01.042

Eichler, S. A., and Meier, J. C. (2008). E-I balance and human diseases - from molecules to networking. *Front. Mol. Neurosci.* 1:2. doi: 10.3389/neuro.02.002.2008

Epperson, C. N., Haga, K., Mason, G. F., Sellers, E., Gueorguieva, R., Zhang, W., et al. (2002). Cortical gamma-aminobutyric acid levels across the menstrual cycle in healthy women and those with premenstrual dysphoric disorder: a proton magnetic resonance spectroscopy study. *Arch. Gen. Psychiatry* 59, 851–858. doi: 10.1001/archpsyc.59.9.851

Epperson, C. N., O'malley, S., Czarkowski, K. A., Gueorguieva, R., Jatlow, P., Sanacora, G., et al. (2005). Sex, GABA and nicotine: the impact of smoking on cortical GABA levels across the menstrual cycle as measured with proton magnetic resonance spectroscopy. *Biol. Psychiatry* 57, 44–48. doi: 10.1016/j.biopsych.2004.09.021

Faden, A. I., Demediuk, P., Panter, S. S., and Vink, R. (1989). The role of excitatory amino acids and NMDA receptors in traumatic brain injury. *Science* 244, 798–800. doi: 10.1126/science.2567056

Falkenberg, L. E., Westerhausen, R., Specht, K., and Hugdahl, K. (2012). Resting-state glutamate level in the anterior cingulate predicts blood-oxygen level-dependent response to cognitive control. *Proc. Natl. Acad. Sci. U S A* 109, 5069–5073. doi: 10.1073/pnas.1115628109

Feurra, M., Pasqualetti, P., Bianco, G., Santarnecchi, E., Rossi, A., and Rossi, S. (2013). State-dependent effects of transcranial oscillatory currents on the motor system: what you think matters. *J. Neurosci.* 33, 17483–17489. doi: 10.1523/jneurosci.1414-13.2013

Finocchi, C., and Ferrari, M. (2011). Female reproductive steroids and neuronal excitability. *Neurol. Sci.* 32(Suppl. 1), S31–S35. doi: 10.1007/s10072-011-0532-5

Floyer-Lea, A., Wylezinska, M., Kincses, T., and Matthews, P. M. (2006). Rapid modulation of GABA concentration in human sensorimotor cortex during motor learning. *J. Neurophysiol.* 95, 1639–1644. doi: 10.1152/jn.00346.2005

Fujiyama, H., Hinder, M. R., Schmidt, M. W., Tandonnet, C., Garry, M. I., and Summers, J. J. (2012). Age-related differences in corticomotor excitability and inhibitory processes during a visuomotor RT task. *J. Cogn. Neurosci.* 24, 1253–1263. doi: 10.1162/jocn_a_00201

Gao, F., Edden, R. A., Li, M., Puts, N. A., Wang, G., Liu, C., et al. (2013). Edited magnetic resonance spectroscopy detects an age-related decline in brain GABA levels. *Neuroimage* 78, 75–82. doi: 10.1016/j.neuroimage.2013.04.012

Ge, S., and Dani, J. A. (2005). Nicotinic acetylcholine receptors at glutamate synapses facilitate long-term depression or potentiation. *J. Neurosci.* 25, 6084–6091. doi: 10.1523/jneurosci.0542-05.2005

Goto, N., Yoshimura, R., Moriya, J., Kakeda, S., Ueda, N., Ikenouchi-Sugita, A., et al. (2009). Reduction of brain gamma-aminobutyric acid (GABA) concentrations in early-stage schizophrenia patients: 3T Proton MRS study. *Schizophr. Res.* 112, 192–193. doi: 10.1016/j.schres.2009.04.026

Guleyupoglu, B., Schestatsky, P., Edwards, D., Fregni, F., and Bikson, M. (2013). Classification of methods in transcranial Electrical Stimulation (tES) and evolving strategy from historical approaches to contemporary innovations. *J. Neurosci. Methods* 219, 297–311. doi: 10.1016/j.jneumeth.2013.07.016

Hamada, M., Murase, N., Hasan, A., Balaratnam, M., and Rothwell, J. C. (2013). The role of interneuron networks in driving human motor cortical plasticity. *Cereb. Cortex* 23, 1593–1605. doi: 10.1093/cercor/bhs147

Hamada, M., Ugawa, Y., and Tsuji, S. (2008). High-frequency rTMS over the supplementary motor area for treatment of Parkinson's disease. *Mov. Disord.* 23, 1524–1531. doi: 10.1002/mds.22168

Harada, M., Kubo, H., Nose, A., Nishitani, H., and Matsuda, T. (2011). Measurement of variation in the human cerebral GABA level by in vivo MEGA-editing proton MR spectroscopy using a clinical 3 T instrument and its dependence on brain region and the female menstrual cycle. *Hum. Brain Mapp.* 32, 828–833. doi: 10.1002/hbm.21086

Hensch, T. K., and Bilimoria, P. M. (2012). Re-opening windows: manipulating critical periods for brain development. *Cerebrum* 2012:11.

Hensch, T. K., Fagiolini, M., Mataga, N., Stryker, M. P., Baekkeskov, S., and Kash, S. F. (1998). Local GABA circuit control of experience-dependent plasticity in developing visual cortex. *Science* 282, 1504–1508. doi: 10.1126/science.282.5393.1504

Hess, G., and Donoghue, J. P. (1994). Long-term potentiation of horizontal connections provides a mechanism to reorganize cortical motor maps. *J. Neurophysiol.* 71, 2543–2547.

Hess, G., and Donoghue, J. P. (1996). Long-term potentiation and long-term depression of horizontal connections in rat motor cortex. *Acta Neurobiol. Exp. (Wars)* 56, 397–405.

Huang, Y., Su, Y., Rorden, C., Dmochowski, J., Datta, A., and Parra, L. C. (2012). An automated method for high-definition transcranial direct current stimulation modeling. *Conf. Proc. IEEE Eng. Med. Biol. Soc.* 2012, 5376–5379. doi: 10.1109/EMBC.2012.6347209

Huber, R., Maki, H., Rosanova, M., Casarotto, S., Canali, P., Casali, A. G., et al. (2013). Human cortical excitability increases with time awake. *Cereb. Cortex* 23, 332–338. doi: 10.1093/cercor/bhs014

Huganir, R. L., and Nicoll, R. A. (2013). AMPARs and synaptic plasticity: the last 25 years. *Neuron* 80, 704–717. doi: 10.1016/j.neuron.2013.10.025

Iuculano, T., and Cohen Kadosh, R. (2013). The mental cost of cognitive enhancement. *J. Neurosci.* 33, 4482–4486. doi: 10.1523/jneurosci.4927-12.2013

Jackson, J. D., Balota, D. A., Duchek, J. M., and Head, D. (2012). White matter integrity and reaction time intraindividual variability in healthy aging and early-stage Alzheimer disease. *Neuropsychologia* 50, 357–366. doi: 10.1016/j.neuropsychologia.2011.11.024

Johnston, M. V. (2009). Plasticity in the developing brain: implications for rehabilitation. *Dev. Disabil. Res. Rev.* 15, 94–101. doi: 10.1002/ddrr.64

Kabakov, A. Y., Muller, P. A., Pascual-Leone, A., Jensen, F. E., and Rotenberg, A. (2012). Contribution of axonal orientation to pathway-dependent modulation of excitatory transmission by direct current stimulation in isolated rat hippocampus. *J. Neurophysiol.* 107, 1881–1889. doi: 10.1152/jn.00715.2011

Kanai, R., Chaieb, L., Antal, A., Walsh, V., and Paulus, W. (2008). Frequency-dependent electrical stimulation of the visual cortex. *Curr. Biol.* 18, 1839–1843. doi: 10.1016/j.cub.2008.10.027

Keeser, D., Meindl, T., Bor, J., Palm, U., Pogarell, O., Mulert, C., et al. (2011). Prefrontal transcranial direct current stimulation changes connectivity of resting-state networks during fMRI. *J. Neurosci.* 31, 15284–15293. doi: 10.1523/jneurosci.0542-11.2011

Knudsen, E. I. (2004). Sensitive periods in the development of the brain and behavior. *J. Cogn. Neurosci.* 16, 1412–1425. doi: 10.1162/0898929042304796

Krause, B., and Cohen Kadosh, R. (2013). Can transcranial electrical stimulation improve learning difficulties in atypical brain development? A future possibility for cognitive training. *Dev. Cogn. Neurosci.* 6, 176–194. doi: 10.1016/j.dcn.2013.04.001

Krause, B., Marquez-Ruiz, J., and Cohen Kadosh, R. (2013). The effect of transcranial direct current stimulation: a role for cortical excitation/inhibition balance? *Front. Hum. Neurosci.* 7:602. doi: 10.3389/fnhum.2013.00602

Kubas, B., Kulak, W., Sobaniec, W., Tarasow, E., Lebkowska, U., and Walecki, J. (2012). Metabolite alterations in autistic children: a 1H MR spectroscopy study. *Adv. Med. Sci.* 57, 152–156. doi: 10.2478/v10039-012-0014-x

Lang, N., Rothkegel, H., Reiber, H., Hasan, A., Sueske, E., Tergau, F., et al. (2011). Circadian modulation of GABA-mediated cortical inhibition. *Cereb. Cortex* 21, 2299–2306. doi: 10.1093/cercor/bhr003

Lang, N., Siebner, H. R., Ernst, D., Nitsche, M. A., Paulus, W., Lemon, R. N., et al. (2004). Preconditioning with transcranial direct current stimulation sensitizes the motor cortex to rapid-rate transcranial magnetic stimulation and controls the direction of after-effects. *Biol. Psychiatry* 56, 634–639. doi: 10.1016/j.biopsych.2004.07.017

Lasarge, C. L., Banuelos, C., Mayse, J. D., and Bizon, J. L. (2009). Blockade of GABA(B) receptors completely reverses age-related learning impairment. *Neuroscience* 164, 941–947. doi: 10.1016/j.neuroscience.2009.08.055

López Alonso, V., Cheeran, B., Río-Rodríguez, D., and Fernandez-Del-Olmo, M. (2014). Inter-individual variability in response to non-invasive brain stimulation paradigms. *Brain Stimul.* (in press).

McConnell, G. C., So, R. Q., Hilliard, J. D., Lopomo, P., and Grill, W. M. (2012). Effective deep brain stimulation suppresses low-frequency network oscillations in the basal ganglia by regularizing neural firing patterns. *J. Neurosci.* 32, 15657–15668. doi: 10.1523/jneurosci.2824-12.2012

Mcdonnell, M. N., Orekhov, Y., and Ziemann, U. (2007). Suppression of LTP-like plasticity in human motor cortex by the GABAB receptor agonist baclofen. *Exp. Brain Res.* 180, 181–186. doi: 10.1007/s00221-006-0849-0

Mcentee, W. J., and Crook, T. H. (1993). Glutamate: its role in learning, memory and the aging brain. *Psychopharmacology (Berl)* 111, 391–401. doi: 10.1007/bf02253527

Mekle, R., Mlynarik, V., Gambarota, G., Hergt, M., Krueger, G., and Gruetter, R. (2009). MR spectroscopy of the human brain with enhanced signal intensity at ultrashort echo times on a clinical platform at 3T and 7T. *Magn. Reson. Med.* 61, 1279–1285. doi: 10.1002/mrm.21961

Miniussi, C., Cappa, S. F., Cohen, L. G., Floel, A., Fregni, F., Nitsche, M. A., et al. (2008). Efficacy of repetitive transcranial magnetic stimulation/transcranial direct current stimulation in cognitive neurorehabilitation. *Brain Stimul.* 1, 326–336. doi: 10.1016/j.brs.2008.07.002

Moliadze, V., Antal, A., and Paulus, W. (2010). Electrode-distance dependent after-effects of transcranial direct and random noise stimulation with extracephalic reference electrodes. *Clin. Neurophysiol.* 121, 2165–2171. doi: 10.1016/j.clinph.2010.04.033

Moliadze, V., Atalay, D., Antal, A., and Paulus, W. (2012). Close to threshold transcranial electrical stimulation preferentially activates inhibitory networks before switching to excitation with higher intensities. *Brain Stimul.* 5, 505–511. doi: 10.1016/j.brs.2011.11.004

Murphy, K. M., Beston, B. R., Boley, P. M., and Jones, D. G. (2005). Development of human visual cortex: a balance between excitatory and inhibitory plasticity mechanisms. *Dev. Psychobiol.* 46, 209–221. doi: 10.1002/dev.20053

Muthukumaraswamy, S. D., Edden, R. A., Jones, D. K., Swettenham, J. B., and Singh, K. D. (2009). Resting GABA concentration predicts peak gamma frequency and fMRI amplitude in response to visual stimulation in humans. *Proc. Natl. Acad. Sci. U S A* 106, 8356–8361. doi: 10.1073/pnas.0900728106

Muthukumaraswamy, S. D., Evans, C. J., Edden, R. A., Wise, R. G., and Singh, K. D. (2012). Individual variability in the shape and amplitude of the BOLD-HRF correlates with endogenous GABAergic inhibition. *Hum. Brain Mapp.* 33, 455–465. doi: 10.1002/hbm.21223

Neuling, T., Rach, S., and Herrmann, C. S. (2013). Orchestrating neuronal networks: sustained after-effects of transcranial alternating current stimulation depend upon brain states. *Front. Hum. Neurosci.* 7:161. doi: 10.3389/fnhum.2013.00161

Neuling, T., Wagner, S., Wolters, C. H., Zaehle, T., and Herrmann, C. S. (2012). Finite-element model predicts current density distribution for clinical applications of tDCS and tACS. *Front. Psychiatry* 3:83. doi: 10.3389/fpsyt.2012.00083

Nitsche, M. A., Kuo, M. F., Karrasch, R., Wachter, B., Liebetanz, D., and Paulus, W. (2009). Serotonin affects transcranial direct current-induced neuroplasticity in humans. *Biol. Psychiatry* 66, 503–508. doi: 10.1016/j.biopsych.2009.03.022

Nitsche, M. A., Nitsche, M. S., Klein, C. C., Tergau, F., Rothwell, J. C., and Paulus, W. (2003). Level of action of cathodal DC polarisation induced inhibition of the human motor cortex. *Clin. Neurophysiol.* 114, 600–604. doi: 10.1016/s1388-2457(02)00412-1

Nitsche, M. A., and Paulus, W. (2001). Sustained excitability elevations induced by transcranial DC motor cortex stimulation in humans. *Neurology* 57, 1899–1901. doi: 10.1212/wnl.57.10.1899

Park, C. H., Chang, W. H., Park, J. Y., Shin, Y. I., Kim, S. T., and Kim, Y. H. (2013). Transcranial direct current stimulation increases resting state interhemispheric connectivity. *Neurosci. Lett.* 539, 7–10. doi: 10.1016/j.neulet.2013.01.047

Peterchev, A. V., Wagner, T. A., Miranda, P. C., Nitsche, M. A., Paulus, W., Lisanby, S. H., et al. (2012). Fundamentals of transcranial electric and magnetic stimulation dose: definition, selection and reporting practices. *Brain Stimul.* 5, 435–453. doi: 10.1016/j.brs.2011.10.001

Pinto, J. G., Hornby, K. R., Jones, D. G., and Murphy, K. M. (2010). Developmental changes in GABAergic mechanisms in human visual cortex across the lifespan. *Front. Cell. Neurosci.* 4:16. doi: 10.3389/fncel.2010.00016

Rahman, A., Reato, D., Arlotti, M., Gasca, F., Datta, A., Parra, L. C., et al. (2013). Cellular effects of acute direct current stimulation: somatic and synaptic terminal effects. *J. Physiol.* 591, 2563–2578. doi: 10.1113/jphysiol.2012.247171

Raz, N., Lindenberger, U., Rodrigue, K. M., Kennedy, K. M., Head, D., Williamson, A., et al. (2005). Regional brain changes in aging healthy adults: general trends, individual differences and modifiers. *Cereb. Cortex* 15, 1676–1689. doi: 10.1093/cercor/bhi044

Reato, D., Rahman, A., Bikson, M., and Parra, L. C. (2010). Low-intensity electrical stimulation affects network dynamics by modulating population rate and spike timing. *J. Neurosci.* 30, 15067–15079. doi: 10.1523/jneurosci.2059-10.2010

Reis, J., Schambra, H. M., Cohen, L. G., Buch, E. R., Fritsch, B., Zarahn, E., et al. (2009). Noninvasive cortical stimulation enhances motor skill acquisition over multiple days through an effect on consolidation. *Proc. Natl. Acad. Sci. U S A* 106, 1590–1595. doi: 10.1073/pnas.0805413106

Rivera, S. M., Reiss, A. L., Eckert, M. A., and Menon, V. (2005). Developmental changes in mental arithmetic: evidence for increased functional specialization in the left inferior parietal cortex. *Cereb. Cortex* 15, 1779–1790. doi: 10.1093/cercor/bhi055

Rojas, D. C., Singel, D., Steinmetz, S., Hepburn, S., and Brown, M. S. (2013). Decreased left perisylvian GABA concentration in children with autism and unaffected siblings. *Neuroimage* 86, 28–34. doi: 10.1016/j.neuroimage.2013.01.045

Romei, V., Rihs, T., Brodbeck, V., and Thut, G. (2008). Resting electroencephalogram alpha-power over posterior sites indexes baseline visual cortex excitability. *Neuroreport* 19, 203–208. doi: 10.1097/wnr.0b013e3282f454c4

Ross, L. A., Mccoy, D., Wolk, D. A., Coslett, H. B., and Olson, I. R. (2010). Improved proper name recall by electrical stimulation of the anterior temporal lobes. *Neuropsychologia* 48, 3671–3674. doi: 10.1016/j.neuropsychologia.2010.07.024

Ross, L. A., Mccoy, D., Wolk, D. A., Coslett, H. B., and Olson, I. R. (2011). Improved proper name recall in aging after electrical stimulation of the anterior temporal lobes. *Front. Aging Neurosci.* 3:16. doi: 10.3389/fnagi.2011.00016

Siebner, H. R., Lang, N., Rizzo, V., Nitsche, M. A., Paulus, W., Lemon, R. N., et al. (2004). Preconditioning of low-frequency repetitive transcranial magnetic stimulation with transcranial direct current stimulation: evidence for homeostatic plasticity in the human motor cortex. *J. Neurosci.* 24, 3379–3385. doi: 10.1523/jneurosci.5316-03.2004

Silvanto, J., Muggleton, N. G., Cowey, A., and Walsh, V. (2007). Neural adaptation reveals state-dependent effects of transcranial magnetic stimulation. *Eur. J. Neurosci.* 25, 1874–1881. doi: 10.1111/j.1460-9568.2007.05440.x

Silvanto, J., Muggleton, N., and Walsh, V. (2008). State-dependency in brain stimulation studies of perception and cognition. *Trends Cogn. Sci.* 12, 447–454. doi: 10.1016/j.tics.2008.09.004

Smith, M. J., Adams, L. F., Schmidt, P. J., Rubinow, D. R., and Wassermann, E. M. (2002). Effects of ovarian hormones on human cortical excitability. *Ann. Neurol.* 51, 599–603. doi: 10.1002/ana.10180

Smith, M. J., Keel, J. C., Greenberg, B. D., Adams, L. F., Schmidt, P. J., Rubinow, D. A., et al. (1999). Menstrual cycle effects on cortical excitability. *Neurology* 53, 2069–2072. doi: 10.1212/wnl.53.9.2069

Smith, A. E., Ridding, M. C., Higgins, R. D., Wittert, G. A., and Pitcher, J. B. (2009). Age-related changes in short-latency motor cortex inhibition. *Exp. Brain Res.* 198, 489–500. doi: 10.1007/s00221-009-1945-8

Snowball, A., Tachtsidis, I., Popescu, T., Thompson, J., Delazer, M., Zamarian, L., et al. (2013). Long-term enhancement of brain function and cognition using cognitive training and brain stimulation. *Curr. Biol.* 23, 987–992. doi: 10.1016/j.cub.2013.04.045

Stagg, C. J., Bachtiar, V., and Johansen-Berg, H. (2011). The role of GABA in human motor learning. *Curr. Biol.* 21, 480–484. doi: 10.1016/j.cub.2011.01.069

Stagg, C. J., Best, J. G., Stephenson, M. C., O'shea, J., Wylezinska, M., Kincses, Z. T., et al. (2009). Polarity-sensitive modulation of cortical neurotransmitters by transcranial stimulation. *J. Neurosci.* 29, 5202–5206. doi: 10.1523/jneurosci.4432-08.2009

Strelau, J. (1997). The contribution of pavlov's typology of CNS properties to personality research. *Eur. Psychol.* 2, 125–138. doi: 10.1027/1016-9040.2.2.125

Tecchio, F., Cancelli, A., Cottone, C., Tomasevic, L., Devigus, B., Zito, G., et al. (2013). Regional personalized electrodes to select transcranial current stimulation target. *Front. Hum. Neurosci.* 7:131. doi: 10.3389/fnhum.2013.00131

Teo, F., Hoy, K. E., Daskalakis, Z. J., and Fitzgerald, P. B. (2011). Investigating the role of current strength in tDCS modulation of working memory performance in healthy controls. *Front. Psychiatry* 2:45. doi: 10.3389/fpsyt.2011.00045

Terney, D., Chaieb, L., Moliadze, V., Antal, A., and Paulus, W. (2008). Increasing human brain excitability by transcranial high-frequency random noise stimulation. *J. Neurosci.* 28, 14147–14155. doi: 10.1523/JNEUROSCI.4248-08.2008

Trepel, C., and Racine, R. J. (2000). GABAergic modulation of neocortical long-term potentiation in the freely moving rat. *Synapse* 35, 120–128. doi: 10.1002/(sici)1098-2396(200002)35:2<120::aid-syn4>3.0.co;2-6

Truong, D. Q., Magerowski, G., Blackburn, G. L., Bikson, M., and Alonso-Alonso, M. (2013). Computational modeling of transcranial direct current stimulation (tDCS) in obesity: impact of head fat and dose guidelines. *Neuroimage Clin.* 2, 759–766. doi: 10.1016/j.nicl.2013.05.011

Turrigiano, G. G., and Nelson, S. B. (2000). Hebb and homeostasis in neuronal plasticity. *Curr. Opin. Neurobiol.* 10, 358–364. doi: 10.1016/s0959-4388(00)00091-x

Turrigiano, G. G., and Nelson, S. B. (2004). Homeostatic plasticity in the developing nervous system. *Nat. Rev. Neurosci.* 5, 97–107. doi: 10.1038/nrn1327

Wassermann, E. M. (2002). Variation in the response to transcranial magnetic brain stimulation in the general population. *Clin. Neurophysiol.* 113, 1165–1171. doi: 10.1016/s1388-2457(02)00144-x

Weiss, M., and Lavidor, M. (2012). When less is more: evidence for a facilitative cathodal tDCS effect in attentional abilities. *J. Cogn. Neurosci.* 24, 1826–1833. doi: 10.1162/jocn_a_00248

Wenk, G. L., Walker, L. C., Price, D. L., and Cork, L. C. (1991). Loss of NMDA, but not GABA-A, binding in the brains of aged rats and monkeys. *Neurobiol. Aging* 12, 93–98. doi: 10.1016/0197-4580(91)90047-n

Yoon, J. H., Maddock, R. J., Rokem, A., Silver, M. A., Minzenberg, M. J., Ragland, J. D., et al. (2010). GABA concentration is reduced in visual cortex in schizophrenia and correlates with orientation-specific surround suppression. *J. Neurosci.* 30, 3777–3781. doi: 10.1523/JNEUROSCI.6158-09.2010

Zaghi, S., Acar, M., Hultgren, B., Boggio, P. S., and Fregni, F. (2010). Noninvasive brain stimulation with low-intensity electrical currents: putative mechanisms of action for direct and alternating current stimulation. *Neuroscientist* 16, 285–307. doi: 10.1177/1073858409336227

Zheng, X., Alsop, D. C., and Schlaug, G. (2011). Effects of transcranial direct current stimulation (tDCS) on human regional cerebral blood flow. *Neuroimage* 58, 26–33. doi: 10.1016/j.neuroimage.2011.06.018

Zimmerman, M., and Hummel, F. (in press). "Brain stimulation and its role in neurological diseases," in *The Stimulated Brain*, ed K. Cohen Kadosh (Amsterdam: Elsevier).

2

Extraction and restoration of hippocampal spatial memories with non-linear dynamical modeling

Dong Song[1]*, Madhuri Harway[1], Vasilis Z. Marmarelis[1], Robert E. Hampson[2], Sam A. Deadwyler[2] and Theodore W. Berger[1]

[1] *Department of Biomedical Engineering, University of Southern California, Los Angeles, CA, USA*
[2] *Department of Physiology and Pharmacology, School of Medicine, Wake Forest University, Winston-Salem, NC, USA*

Edited by:
Mikhail Lebedev, Duke University, USA

Reviewed by:
Mikhail Lebedev, Duke University, USA
Yoshio Sakurai, Kyoto University, Japan
Yu Liu, The University of Tennessee Health Science Center, USA

Correspondence:
Dong Song, Department of Biomedical Engineering, University of Southern California, 403 Hedco Neuroscience Building, Los Angeles, CA 90089, USA
e-mail: dsong@usc.edu

To build a cognitive prosthesis that can replace the memory function of the hippocampus, it is essential to model the input-output function of the damaged hippocampal region, so the prosthetic device can stimulate the downstream hippocampal region, e.g., CA1, with the output signal, e.g., CA1 spike trains, predicted from the ongoing input signal, e.g., CA3 spike trains, and the identified input-output function, e.g., CA3-CA1 model. In order for the downstream region to form appropriate long-term memories based on the restored output signal, furthermore, the output signal should contain sufficient information about the memories that the animal has formed. In this study, we verify this premise by applying regression and classification modelings of the spatio-temporal patterns of spike trains to the hippocampal CA3 and CA1 data recorded from rats performing a memory-dependent delayed non-match-to-sample (DNMS) task. The regression model is essentially the multiple-input, multiple-output (MIMO) non-linear dynamical model of spike train transformation. It predicts the output spike trains based on the input spike trains and thus restores the output signal. In addition, the classification model interprets the signal by relating the spatio-temporal patterns to the memory events. We have found that: (1) both hippocampal CA3 and CA1 spike trains contain sufficient information for predicting the locations of the sample responses (i.e., left and right memories) during the DNMS task; and more importantly (2) the CA1 spike trains predicted from the CA3 spike trains by the MIMO model also are sufficient for predicting the locations on a single-trial basis. These results show quantitatively that, with a moderate number of unitary recordings from the hippocampus, the MIMO non-linear dynamical model is able to extract and restore spatial memory information for the formation of long-term memories and thus can serve as the computational basis of the hippocampal memory prosthesis.

Keywords: hippocampus, spatio-temporal pattern, spike, classification, regression, memory

INTRODUCTION

Cortical prosthesis is an emerging technology seeking to restore cognitive functions lost in diseases or injuries (Berger et al., 2005, 2010, 2011, 2012). It is achieved by bi-directional, closed-loop communications between the prosthetic device and the brain regions. This is distinct from sensory or motor prostheses, where one side of the communication is an external entity such as the sensory input (Loeb, 1990; Humayun et al., 1999) or the motor output (Mauritz and Peckham, 1987; Taylor et al., 2002; Nicolelis, 2003; Shenoy et al., 2003; Wolpaw and McFarland, 2004; Hochberg et al., 2006). Therefore, a cortical prosthesis must deal exclusively with the internal brain signals, in which sensory or motor information is embedded, by re-encoding the upstream (input) brain signals into the downstream (output) signals (**Figure 1A**).

For the past decade, we have been working on developing a hippocampal-cortical prosthesis for restoring the memory functions. Hippocampus is a brain region responsible for the creation of new long-term episodic memories (Milner, 1970; Squire and Zola-Morgan, 1991; Eichenbaum, 1999). Damage to the hippocampal areas can result in a permanent loss of such cognitive functions. In a normal hippocampus, short-term memories are encoded in the spatio-temporal patterns of spikes (i.e., spike trains) as the input from the entorhinal cortex. Memory information is then processed by the hippocampal feed-forward tri-synaptic pathway, which consists of dentate gyrus, CA3, and CA1 regions, and eventually transformed into the output spike trains to the subiculum, that is appropriate for the formation of long-term memories (**Figure 1B**). Although the exact nature of such a transformation or the underlying mechanisms is still largely unclear, it must be the neural signal (i.e., spike trains) flow from entorhinal cortex to dentate gyrus, to CA3, to CA1, and to subiculum, that enables the re-encoding of short-term memories into long-term memories. Maintaining the normal signal flow with a prosthetic device that bypasses a damaged or diseased hippocampal region provides a feasible way of restoring the lost long-term memory functions (**Figure 1A**).

For example, in our first-generation hippocampal memory prosthesis applications, we (a) record input spike trains from the

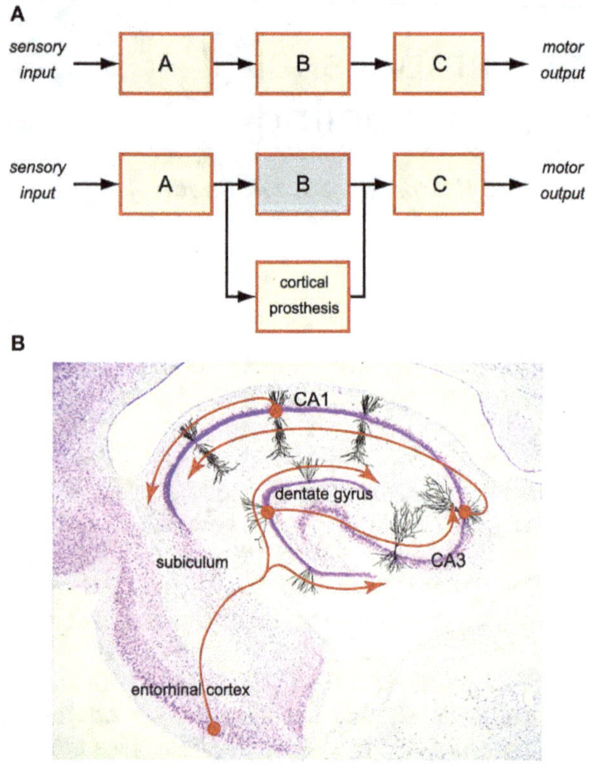

FIGURE 1 | Cortical prosthesis restores cognitive functions by bypassing the damaged brain region to maintain the brain signal flow. **(A)** Schematic diagram of a cortical prosthesis. **(B)** Intrinsic tri-synaptic pathway of the hippocampus.

CA3 region, (b) process them with a multi-input, multi-output (MIMO) non-linear dynamical model to predict the desired CA1 output spike trains, and (c) electrically stimulate the CA1 region with the predicted CA1 output patterns. Previous results have shown that, (a) the MIMO model can accurately predict the output spike trains in real time based on the ongoing input spike trains (Song et al., 2007, 2009a, 2013), and (b) the electrical stimulation can restore or even enhance the memory functions performed by the hippocampal CA3-CA1 system (Berger et al., 2011, 2012; Hampson et al., 2012a,b).

However, despite the success of demonstrating such a prosthesis, how the external behavioral events (i.e., memory events) are encoded in the two hippocampal regions and, more importantly, re-encoded by the prosthesis has not been clearly revealed, precisely due to the internal nature of the cortical prosthesis. In this study, we propose a new framework of modeling and representing the re-encoding process performed by a brain region at the *memory representation level*, as opposed to the *signal level* in our previous studies. In addition to ask the question, "What should the output signal be?" We further ask the question, "What do the signals mean?" Specifically, we combine our previously developed MIMO signal model (Song et al., 2007, 2009a, 2013), which predicts the output signal based on the input signal, with an additional memory decoding model that relates the input and/or output signals to the behaviors (memories) of the animal (**Figure 2**). The MIMO signal model is essentially a time-series regression model non-linear dynamically mapping the multiple output (CA1) signals to the multiple input (CA3) signals. On the other hand, the memory decoding model is a multi-input, signal-output (MISO) classification model identifying to which of a set of memory categories the spatio-temporal patterns of the input and/or output signals belong. The former model quantifies the input-output signal transformation, while the latter model decodes the memory by predicting the behavior.

The paper is organized as the follows. In section Materials and Methods, we formally formulate the modeling problem and provide the mathematical expressions. In section Results, we apply the methods to the modeling of the hippocampus during a memory-dependent task in rodents.

MATERIALS AND METHODS

BEHAVIORAL TASK AND ELECTROPHYSIOLOGICAL PROCEDURES

All animal procedures are reviewed and approved by the Institutional Animal Care and Use Committee of Wake Forest University, in accordance with US Department of Agriculture, International Association for the Assessment and Accreditation of Laboratory Animal Care and National Institutes of Health guidelines. Two male Long-Evans rats are trained to criterion on a two-lever, spatial delayed-non-match-to-sample (DNMS) task with random delay intervals (Deadwyler et al., 1996; Hampson et al., 1999). Animals perform the task by pressing (sample response) a single lever presented in one of the two positions in the sample phase (left or right). This event is called the "sample response." The lever is then retracted and the delay phase initiates; for the duration of the delay phase, the animal is required to nose-poke into a lighted device on the opposite wall. When the delay is ended, nose-poke light is extinguished, both levers are extended, and the animal is required to press the lever *opposite* to the sample lever. This event is called the "non-match response." If the correct lever is pressed, the animal is rewarded (**Figure 3**, top). A session includes approximately 100 successful DNMS tasks that each consists of two of the four behavioral events, i.e., right sample (RS) and left non-match (LN), or left sample (LS) and right non-match (RN).

Spike trains are obtained with multi-site recordings from different septo-temporal regions of the hippocampus of rats performing the DNMS task (**Figure 3**, bottom). For each hemisphere of the brain, a microwire multi-electrodes array (MEA) is surgically implanted into the hippocampus, with 8 electrodes in the CA3 (input) region and 8 electrodes in the CA1 (output) region. Spike trains are pre-screened based on mean firing rate and peri-event histogram. Perievent (−2 to +2 s) spike trains of the four behavioral events are extracted from each trial and then concatenated to form the datasets (**Figure 3**, bottom). The spike train data are discretized with a 2 ms bin size.

MIMO SIGNAL MODEL OF INPUT-OUTPUT SPIKE TRAIN TRANSFORMATION

The MIMO signal model of input-output spike train transformation takes the form of the sparse generalized Laguerre-Volterra model (SGLVM) we previously developed (Song et al., 2009a,b,

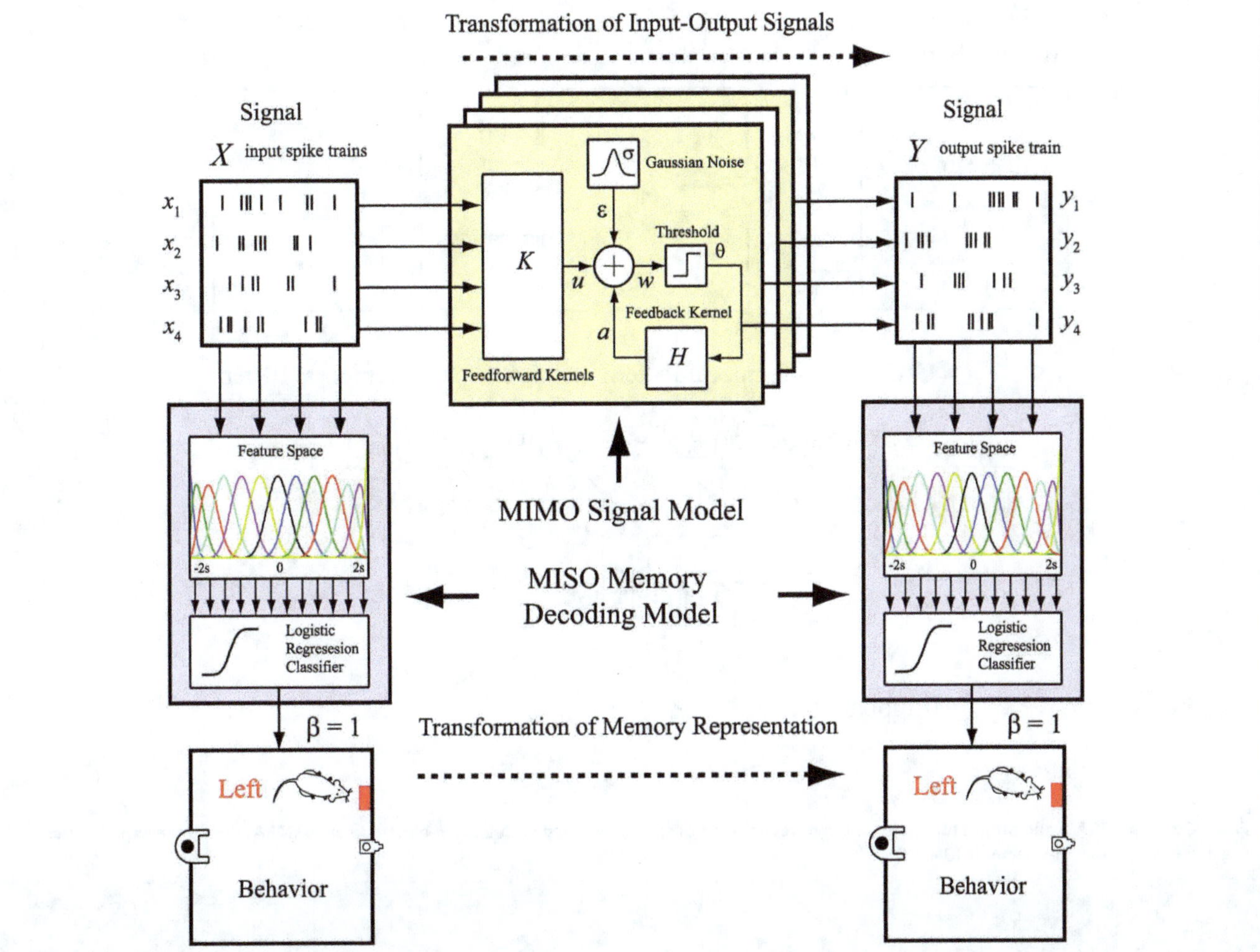

FIGURE 2 | MIMO signal model and MISO memory decoding model. The MIMO signal model predicts the output spatio-temporal patterns of spikes based on the ongoing input spatio-temporal patterns of spikes. The MISO memory decoding model predicts the memory (behavioral) events based on the input or output spatio-temporal patterns of spikes.

2013). In this approach, a MIMO model is a concatenation of a series of MISO models (not to be confused with the MISO classification model), that each can be considered a spiking neuron model (Song et al., 2006, 2007) (**Figure 2**). In this study, each MISO model consists of (a) MISO second-order Volterra kernels k transforming the input spike trains x to the synaptic potential u, (b) a Gaussian noise term ε capturing the stochastic properties of spike generation, (c) a threshold θ for generating output spikes y, (e) an adder generating the pre-threshold membrane potential w, and (d) a single-input, single-output first-order Volterra kernel h transforming the preceding output spikes to the spike-triggered feedback after-potential a. The model can be mathematical expressed as:

$$w = u(k, x) + a(h, y) + \varepsilon(\sigma) \tag{1}$$

$$y = \begin{cases} 0 \text{ when } w < \theta \\ 1 \text{ when } w \geq \theta \end{cases} \tag{2}$$

$$u(t) = k_0 + \sum_{n=1}^{N} \sum_{\tau=0}^{M_k} k_1^{(n)}(\tau) x_n(t-\tau) + \sum_{n=1}^{N} \sum_{\tau_1=0}^{M_k} \sum_{\tau_2=0}^{M_k} k_{2s}^{(n)}(\tau_1, \tau_2) x_n(t-\tau_1) x_n(t-\tau_2) \tag{3}$$

$$a(t) = \sum_{\tau=1}^{M_h} h(\tau) y(t-\tau) \tag{4}$$

The zeroth-order kernel, k_0, is the value of u when the input is absent. First-order kernels $k_1^{(n)}$ describe the first-order linear relation between the nth input x_n and u, as functions of the time intervals τ between the present time and the past time. Second-order self kernels $k_{2s}^{(n)}$ describe the second-order nonlinear interaction between pairs of spikes in the nth input x_n as they affect u. N is the number of inputs. M_k and M_h denote the memory lengths of the feedforward process and feedback process,

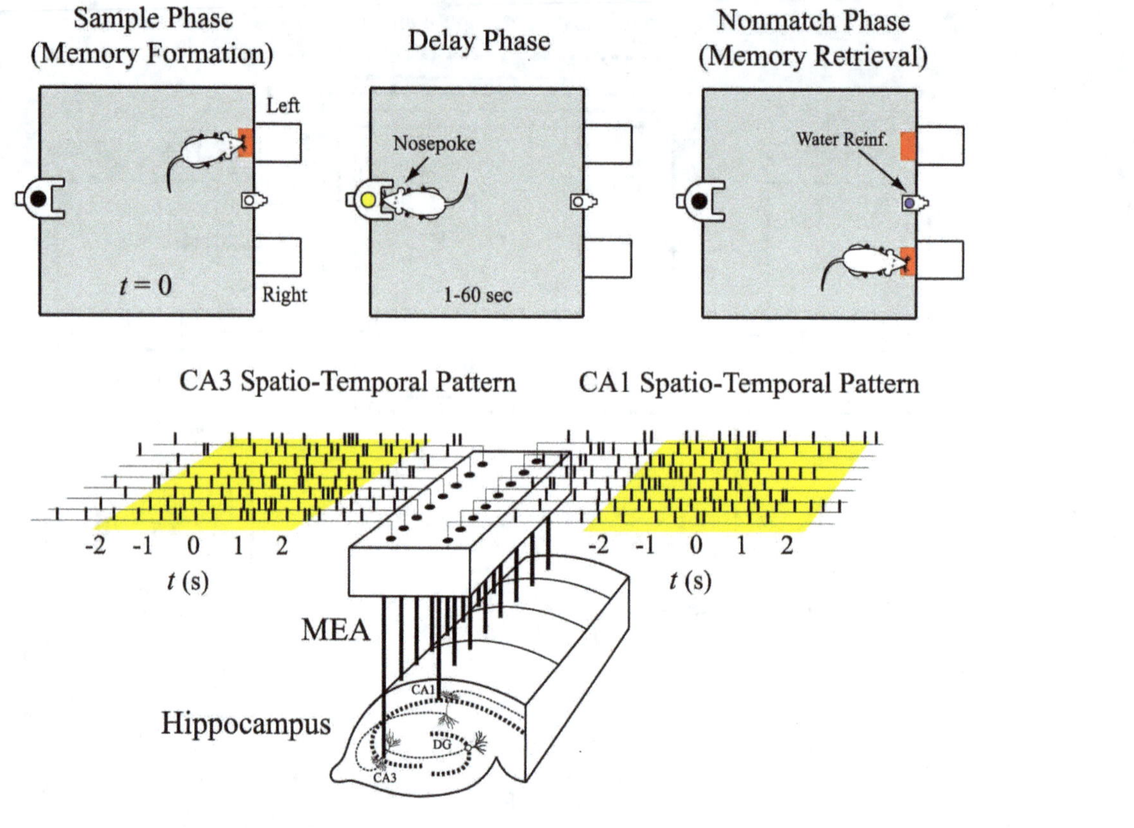

FIGURE 3 | Input (CA3) and output (CA1) spatio-temporal patterns of spikes recorded with a multi-electrode array (MEA) during the sample phase of the delayed-non-match-to-sample (DNMS) task.

respectively. They are chosen to be 2 s in this study. Second-order cross kernels and higher-order (e.g., third-order) kernels are not included in this study.

To facilitate model estimation and avoid overfitting, the Volterra kernels are expanded with Laguerre basis functions b as in Song et al. (2009c,d):

$$u(t) = c_0 + \sum_{n=1}^{N}\sum_{j=1}^{J} c_1^{(n)}(j)v_j^{(n)}(t) + \sum_{n=1}^{N}\sum_{j_1=1}^{J}\sum_{j_2=1}^{j_1} c_{2s}^{(n)}(j_1,j_2)v_{j_1}^{(n)}(t)v_{j_2}^{(n)}(t) \tag{5}$$

$$a(t) = \sum_{j=1}^{L} c_h(j)v_j^{(h)}(t) \tag{6}$$

where $v_j^{(n)}(t) = \sum_{\tau=0}^{M_k} b_j(\tau)x_n(t-\tau)$, $v_j^{(h)}(t) = \sum_{\tau=1}^{M_h} b_j(\tau)$ $y(t-\tau)$; $c_1^{(n)}$, $c_{2s}^{(n)}$, and c_h are the sought Laguerre expansion coefficients of $k_1^{(n)}$, $k_{2s}^{(n)}$, and h, respectively (c_0 is equal to k_0); J is the number of basis functions.

To achieve model sparsity, the coefficients are estimated with a composite penalized likelihood estimation method, i.e., group LASSO (Song et al., 2013). In maximum likelihood estimation (MLE), model coefficients are estimated by minimizing the negative log likelihood function $-l(c)$. In group LASSO, the composite penalized criterion is written as

$$\begin{aligned} S(c) &= -l(c) + \lambda\left(\sum_{n=1}^{N} \|c_1^{(n)}(j)\|_2^1 + \sum_{n=1}^{N} \|c_{2s}^{(n)}(j_1,j_2)\|_2^1\right) \\ &= -l(c) + \lambda\left(\sum_{n=1}^{N}\left(\sum_{j=1}^{J} c_1^{(n)}(j)^2\right)^{\frac{1}{2}} + \sum_{n=1}^{N}\left(\sum_{j_1=1}^{J}\sum_{j_2=1}^{j_1} c^{(n)}(j_1,j_2)^2\right)^{\frac{1}{2}}\right) \end{aligned} \tag{7}$$

where $\lambda \geq 0$ is a tuning parameter that controls the relative importance of the likelihood and the penalty term. When λ takes on a larger value, the estimation yields sparser result of the coefficients. λ is optimized with a two-fold cross-validation method.

MISO MEMORY DECODING MODEL OF SPATIO-TEMPORAL PATTERN OF SPIKES

The MISO memory decoding model of spike spatio-temporal patterns takes the form of the sparse generalized B-spline linear classification model (Song et al., 2013). In this approach, the feature space is defined as a set of B-spline basis functions for each neuron (input and/or output neurons depending on the application). The classifier is essentially the logistic regression (**Figure 2**).

B-splines are piecewise polynomials with smooth transitions between the adjacent pieces at a set of interior *knot* points. A polynomial spline of degree $d \geq 0$ on $[0, M]$ with $m > 0$ interior knot points and the knot sequence $\eta_0 = 0 < \eta_1 < \ldots < \eta_m < \eta_{m+1} = M$ is a function that is a polynomial of degree d between each pair of adjacent knots, and has d-1 continuous derivatives for $d = 1$. B-spline basis functions of degree d can be defined in a recursive fashion as

$$B_{j,d}(\tau) = \frac{\tau - \eta_j}{\eta_{j+d-1} - \eta_j} B_{j,d-1}(\tau) + \frac{\eta_{j+d} - \tau}{\eta_{j+d} - \eta_{j+1}} B_{j+1,d-1}(\tau) \quad (8)$$

where

$$B_{j,0}(\tau) = \begin{cases} 1 & \text{if } \eta_j < \tau < \eta_{j+1} \\ 0 & \text{otherwise} \end{cases} \quad (9)$$

For a given sequence of m knots and a fixed degree d, the total number of B-spline basis functions is $J = m + d + 1$.

Spatio-temporal patterns of spikes are projected to the B-spline feature space via inner product to yield the feature vectors as

$$z^{(n)}(j) = \sum_{\tau=0}^{M} B_j(\tau) x_n(\tau) \quad (10)$$

where M is the time widow for inner product. It is chosen to be from -2 to $+2$ s of the sample events (**Figure 3**, bottom). x_n is the nth neuron of the total N neurons included in analysis. Different from in the regression model, x can be CA3 and/or CA1 neurons depending on the context. $z^{(n)}(j)$ denotes the feature value of the nth neuron using the jth B-spline function. Therefore, z is a 1-by-JN vector. J is optimized in the range of 5–100 based on the out-of-sample prediction accuracy. In most of the cases, $J = 20$ is found to be optimal.

Since there are two possible behavioral outcomes, i.e., left or right position, the model output can be represented as a binary variable β. The classification model assumed by logistic regression is

$$P(\beta = 1|x) = \left[1 + \exp\left\{ -w_0 - \sum_{n=1}^{N} \sum_{j=1}^{J} w^{(n)}(j) z^{(n)}(j) \right\} \right]^{-1} \quad (11)$$

$$P(\beta = 0|x) = 1 - P(\beta = 1|x) \quad (12)$$

where w are the sought model coefficients; 1 and 0 represent left and right positions, respectively.

The linear classification rule is simply

$$\beta = \begin{cases} 1 & \text{if } \left\{ -w_0 - \sum_{n=1}^{N} \sum_{j=1}^{J} w^{(n)}(j) z^{(n)}(j) \right\} < 0 \\ 0 & \text{otherwise} \end{cases} \quad (13)$$

Compared with the MIMO regression model, the MISO classification model may suffer even more serious overfitting problem due to the high dimensional input (typically with hundreds of features) and the relatively small number of data points (typically 100 trials in this study). Therefore, $L1$ regularization (Lasso) is applied to achieve model sparsity and avoid overfitting as

$$S(c) = -l(c) + \lambda \left(\sum_{n=1}^{N} \sum_{j=1}^{J} ||w^{(n)}(j)||_2^1 \right) \quad (14)$$

Where $-l(c)$ and $\lambda = 0$ are the negative log likelihood function and the tuning parameter of the classification model, respectively. In this study, λ is optimized with a four-fold cross-validation method. By minimizing S, sparse weight matrix w are estimated and further used to reconstruct the classification feature matrix F with the B-spline basis functions as

$$F^{(n)}(\tau) = \sum_{j=1}^{J} B_j(\tau) w^{(n)}(j) \quad (15)$$

F can be directly used in the logistic regression along with the spatio-temporal pattern x as

$$P(\beta = 1|x) = \left[1 + \exp\left\{ -w_0 - \sum_{n=1}^{N} \sum_{t=1}^{M} F^{(n)}(\tau) x^{(n)}(t) \right\} \right]^{-1} \quad (16)$$

RESULTS

HIPPOCAMPAL CA3 AND CA1 ACTIVITIES CONTAINS SUFFICIENT INFORMATION FOR DECODING SPATIAL MEMORIES DURING THE DNMS TASK

First, we apply the MISO memory decoding model to the CA3 spike trains recorded during the sample phase of the DNMS tasks. For each sample event (left or right), we take the perievent spikes 2 s before and after the event with a 2 ms bin size. The spatio-temporal patterns of spikes are then N-by-2000 matrices, where N is the number of neurons. A session typically consists of 80–100 trials with roughly half being left sample trials and half being right sample trials. The spatio-temporal patterns are labeled with 1 for the left trials and 0 for the right trials. **Figure 4** (case #1) and **Figure 5** (case #2) show the spatio-temporal patterns from two animals with 26 and 43 CA3 neurons, respectively. For each position, four representative patterns and the overall patterns are shown. The overall patterns are obtained by smoothing the spike trains with B-spline functions and then summing across all trials for the specific position. It is evident that the two positions show different spatio-temporal patterns and the differences exist in specific time ranges of specific neurons (**Figures 4, 5**). The task

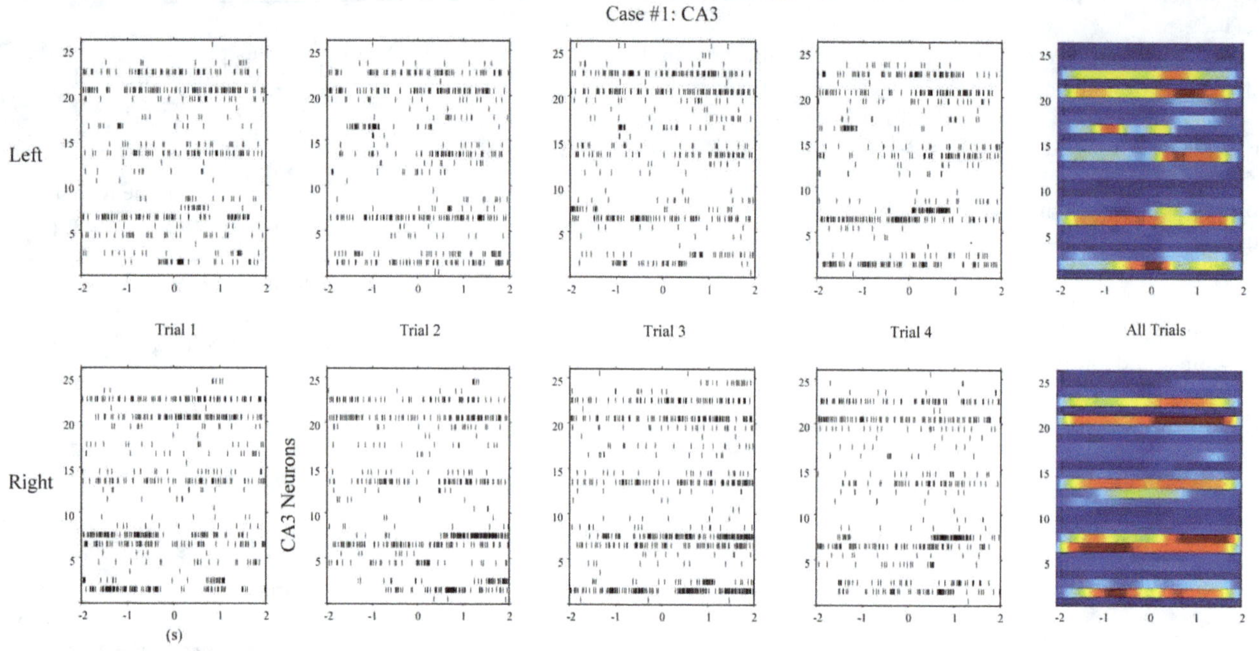

FIGURE 4 | Spatio-temporal patterns of spikes in the hippocampal CA3 (input) region during left and right sample events of the DNMS (case #1).

of the MISO memory decoding model is to identify these sparsely distributed differences from single trials of the spatio-temporal pattern and then predict the positions of the animal. Results show that the MISO memory decoding model can achieve a 100% out-of-sample prediction accuracy using the CA3 spatio-temporal patterns in both cases (**Figure 8**, top row).

Using the same method, we build MISO memory decoding models for the CA1 spike trains. **Figure 6** (case #1) and **Figure 7** (case #2) show the spatio-temporal patterns of CA1 during left and right trials (row 1 and 3) from the same two animals. There are 19 and 17 CA1 neurons recorded from these two animals, respectively. Similar to CA3, CA1 also show different spatio-temporal patterns during left and right trials. The prediction accuracy is 100% in one case and 91.3% in the other (**Figure 8**, middle row).

HIPPOCAMPAL CA1 ACTIVITIES CAN BE ACCURATELY PREDICTED BY THE MIMO SIGNAL MODEL BASED ON THE HIPPOCAMPAL CA3 ACTIVITIES

In the second step, we build MIMO signal models for the transformations from the CA3 spatio-temporal patterns to the CA1 spatio-temporal patterns. To build such a model, we concatenate CA3 perievent spike trains across all trials to form the input data and the corresponding CA1 spike trains to form the output data, and then apply our MIMO modeling method. The resulting SGLVM non-linear dynamically predicts the CA1 spikes based on the ongoing and past (within the memory window) CA3 spikes (Song et al., 2007, 2009a; Song and Berger, 2010). Results show that in both cases (**Figures 6**, **7**, row 2 and 4), the MIMO signal model can accurately predict the CA1 spatio-temporal patterns at both the single trial level (**Figures 6**, **7**, column 1–4) and the overall level (**Figures 6**, **7**, column 5). Importantly, a single set of the model coefficients are used for both the left and right trials. In other words, the estimated MIMO signal models are memory-invariant and can be used to predict the output signals without explicitly knowing what the events are (Song et al., 2011).

HIPPOCAMPAL CA1 ACTIVITIES PREDICTED BY THE MIMO SIGNAL MODEL CAN BE USED TO ACCURATELY DECODE THE SPATIAL MEMORY

Lastly, we build MISO memory decoding models for the CA1 spatio-temporal patterns predicted by the MIMO signal model, as opposed to the actual CA1 spatio-temporal patterns. Results show that the MISO memory decoding models can accurately predict the spatial memory based on the predicted CA1 patterns (**Figure 8**, bottom). The prediction accuracies are 91% and 87.5 for the two cases, respectively. Importantly, the MISO memory decoding model coefficients remain the same for the actual CA1 patterns and the predicted CA1 patterns. This indicates that the MIMO signal model has successfully transmitted the spatial information from CA3 to CA1 in the same form as it is encoded in the actual CA1 patterns. The MIMO signal model has not only *restored the signal*, but also *re-encoded the memory representations*.

SPATIAL INFORMATION IS SPARSELY DISTRIBUTED IN THE HIPPOCAMPAL CA1 AND CA3 SPATIO-TEMPORAL PATTERNS OF SPIKES

In order to gain more insights into how hippocampal CA3 and CA1 spike trains encode spatial information, we calculate Equation (15) and plot the classification weight matrices. These matrices have the same dimensions as their corresponding spatio-temporal patterns. In order to perform classification, we can simply calculate the dot products of the weight matrices and

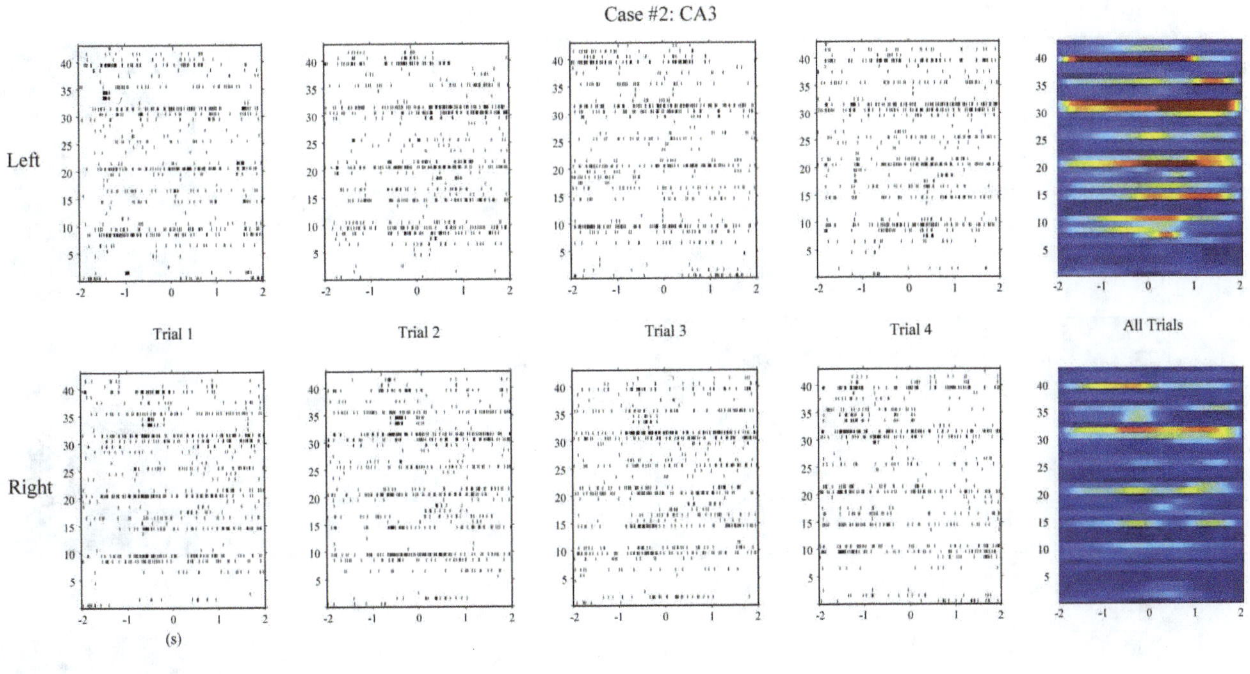

FIGURE 5 | Hippocampal CA3 spatio-temporal patterns from a different animal (case #2).

the corresponding spatio-temporal patterns (strictly speaking, the dot products of vectorized matrices), add the bias (i.e., w_0), and then use Equation (16) to predict the probability of the animal having left or right memories. **Figure 9** show results of CA3 and CA1 from the two animals. The CA1 weight matrices are for both the actual and MIMO predicted CA1 spatio-temporal patterns. In both cases, non-zero values (warm and cold colors represent positive and negative values, respectively) are sparsely distributed in the weight matrices. These results indicate that the spatial information exists in a redundant fashion in multiple ranges of the perievent intervals of multiple neurons. The MIMO signal model and the MISO memory decoding model jointly describe the re-encoding of the memory representations from CA3 to CA1.

DISCUSSIONS

Brain regions process and transmit information with spatio-temporal patterns of spikes. In order to build a cortical prosthesis to bypass a damaged brain region, it is necessary to restore the output signals of the damaged region and send it to the downstream region, so the information flow is maintained. We have shown intensively that non-linear dynamical MIMO models can predict accurately the output spatio-temporal patterns based on the ongoing input spatio-temporal patterns, and electrical stimulations of the output region following the predicted patterns can effectively restore and even enhance the memory function (Berger et al., 2011, 2012; Hampson et al., 2012a,b, 2013). The unique contribution of this paper is to combine the MIMO models with a new set of MISO memory decoding models so that the input and output signals can be related to the memory (behavioral) events and thus explain why it is possible for the downstream hippocampal region to correctly decode the MIMO model generated signals.

In our previous publications on the MIMO signal model (Song et al., 2006, 2007, 2009a,b, 2011, 2013; Song and Berger, 2010), the model goodness-of-fit are validated with a Kolmogorov-Smirnov (KS) test based on the time-rescaling theorem (Brown et al., 2002; Haslinger et al., 2010). This KS test is a powerful tool that allows the firing probability intensity function predicted by the MIMO model to be directly validated with the actual output spike train, and the model goodness-of-fit to be quantified statistically with confidence bounds. However, the KS test does not necessarily indicate whether the model goodness-of-fit is sufficient for decoding the behavior or restoring the cognitive function since it is developed only for quantifying the accuracy of the predicted point-process output signal. The typically used 95 or 99% confidence bounds will not guarantee a successful MIMO model for building the prosthesis. For example, a perfectly predicted output signal may contain no information about a specific memory of interest; on the other hand, a less accurately predicted output signal may still contain some or even sufficient information about the memory. The MISO memory decoding model described here directly quantifies the relations between output signals and memories, and provides a more functionally relevant measure to the model performance that is complementary to the KS test.

In hippocampal prosthesis applications, MISO memory decoding models are estimated with input-output data during the sample phase (−2 to 2 s). The reason is that, in the DNMS task, animals form the spatial memory (i.e., left or right level position) during the sample phase, retain the memory during the delay phase, and recall the memory during the non-match phase. Previous results have shown that MIMO model-based

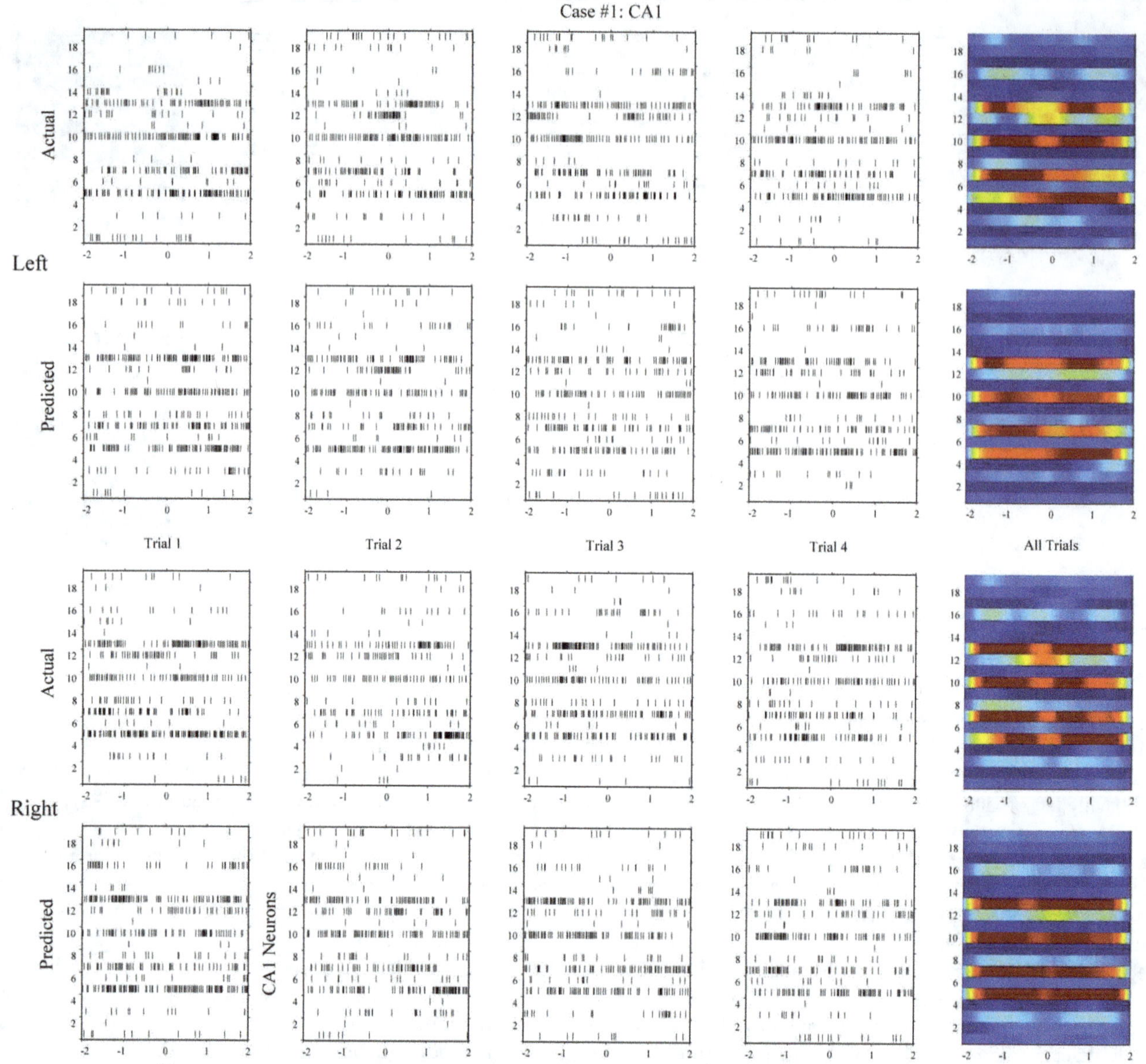

FIGURE 6 | Spatio-temporal patterns of spikes in the hippocampal CA1 (output) region during left and right events of the DNMS. For each position, the top row shows the actual CA1 spatio-temporal patterns; the bottom row shows the CA1 spatio-temporal patterns predicted by the MIMO model based on the ongoing CA3 spiking activities (case #1).

electrical stimulation restores and enhances the spatial memory during sample phases but not non-match phases (Berger et al., 2011, 2012; Hampson et al., 2012a), despite that the MIMO signal model is able to predict accurately the output signal during both sample and non-match phases (Song et al., 2011).

Hippocampus is a mainly feedforward network consisting of a large number of neurons. There are approximately 1 million, 330 thousand, and 420 thousand principal neurons in the rodent dentate gyrus, CA3, and CA1 regions, respectively (Amaral et al., 1990). However, despite the small number (tens to a hundred) of recorded neurons allowed by the current MEA technology, our hippocampal prosthesis has shown impressive success in both rodents and non-human primates during the spatial memory tasks. The main reason is that, at least during the DNMS task or the delayed match-to-sample (DMS) task, spatial memories (e.g., locations of the levels) are encoded in a highly redundant and distributed fashion in a large portion of the hippocampal neurons. As shown in this study, sampling a small number of neurons from the whole population still allows accurate extraction of spatial information.

The DNMS task is a highly restricted experimental paradigm that involves only two positions. Under normal conditions, however, the animal needs to form much more complex memories to maintain its normal life (Eichenbaum, 1999). A practical

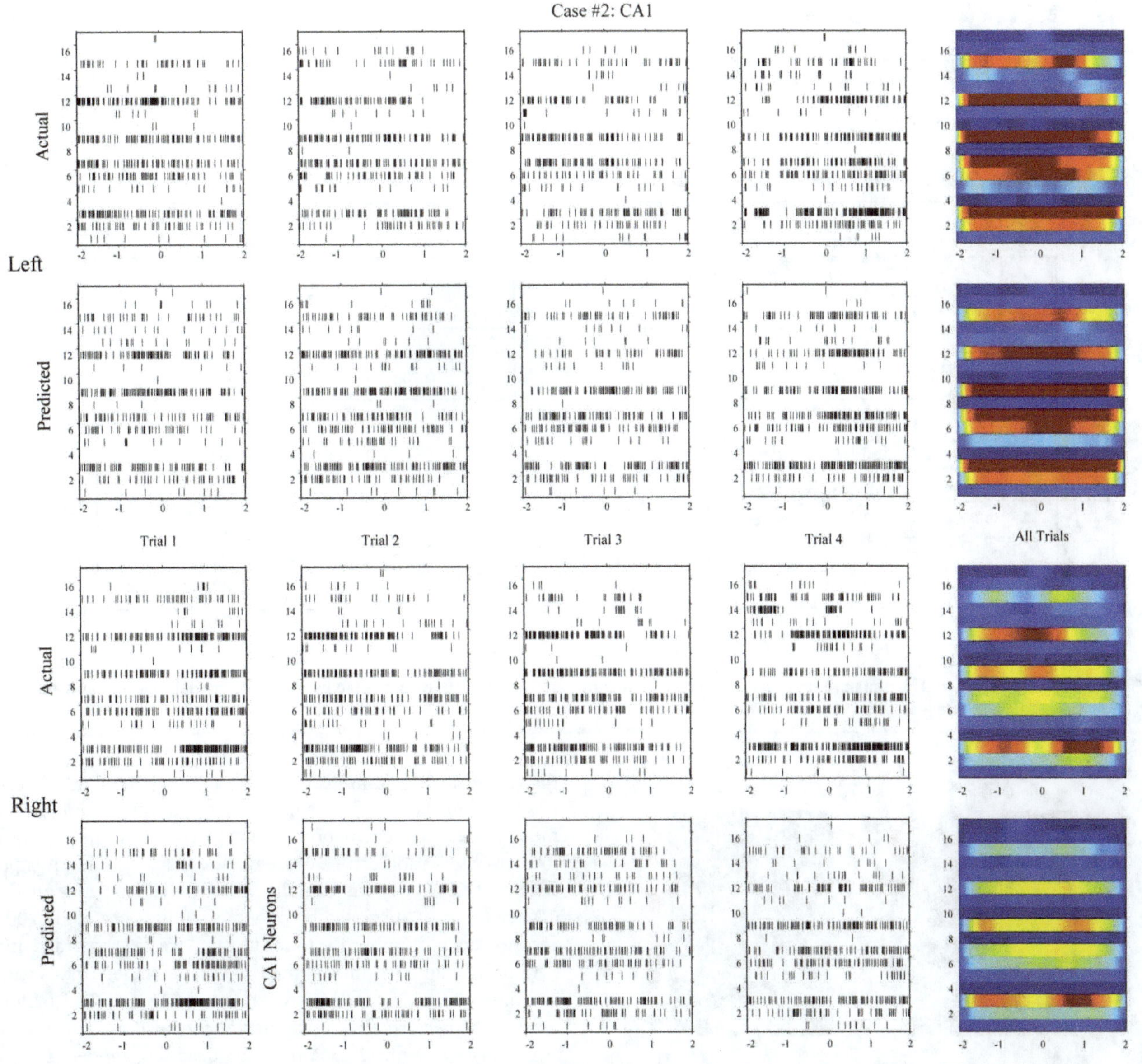

FIGURE 7 | Hippocampal CA1 spatio-temporal patterns (actual and MIMO model predicted) from a different animal (case #2).

hippocampal prosthesis should be able to extract and restore a large number of memories with the MIMO signal model and MISO memory decoding model. This will likely require (1) recording a larger number of hippocampal neurons to obtain more information necessary for decoding the episodic memories, (2) stimulating with more electrodes for generating richer output patterns to the downstream hippocampal region, and (3) developing more powerful MIMO signal model and MISO memory decoding model to more accurately restore the output signal and decode the memories. For example, the current MISO memory decoding model has binary (left or right) output; in order to decode more memories, it needs to be extended to handle multiple-category output. A natural solution is to use multinomial logistic regression (McCullagh and Nelder, 1989), instead of the standard binary-output logistic regression used in this study. Besides, other forms of discriminative models, e.g., support vector machine, or generative models, e.g., naive Bayes classifier, may be considered for their specific advantages. In addition, to collect input-output data for building multiple-memory models, new experimental paradigms involving multiple forms of behavioral events and sensory modalities need to be utilized (Hampson et al., 2012b). Nonetheless, the study described in the paper for the first time combines the regression model with the classification model to illustrate how memory-related information is encoded and re-encoded in the hippocampus, and has made a critical step toward building a hippocampal memory prosthesis.

Interestingly, in both cases in this study, the MISO memory decoding model shows higher prediction accuracy in the CA3

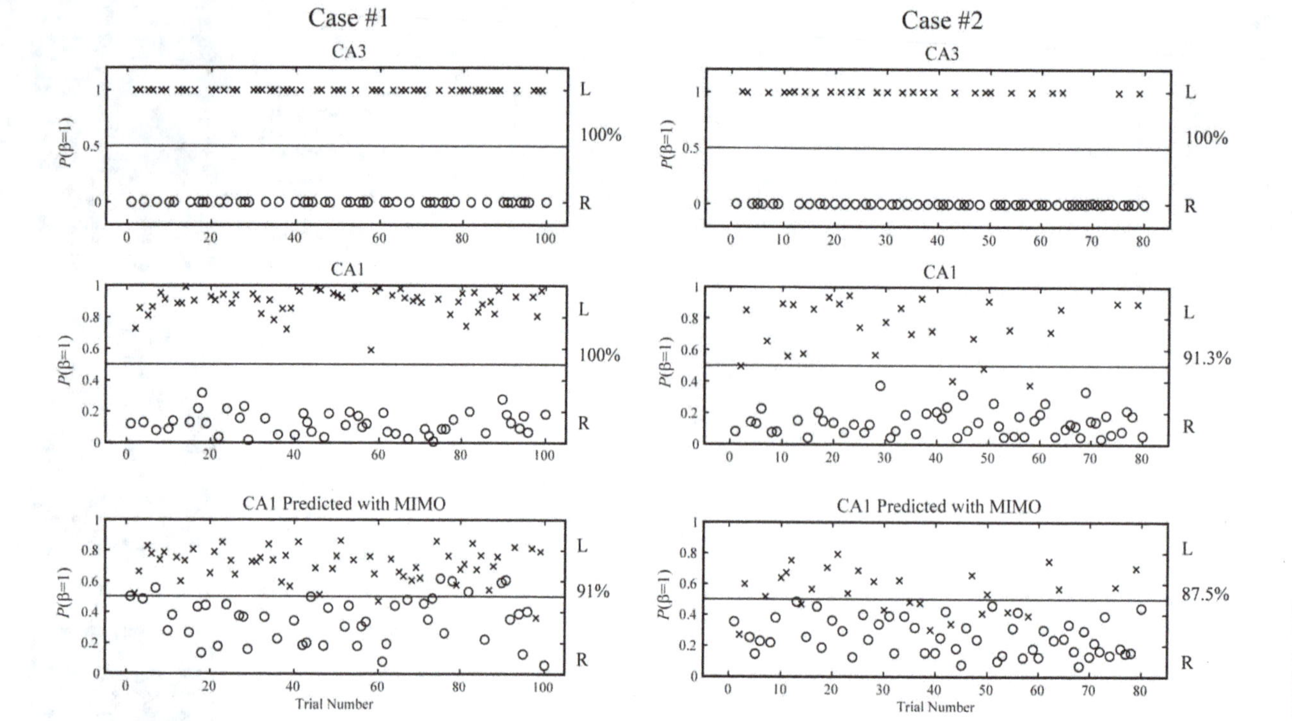

FIGURE 8 | Predicting spatial memory events based on inputs (CA3), outputs (CA1), or outputs predicted by the MIMO models (case #1 and #2). The horizontal lines in the middle represent the decision boundaries ($P = 0.5$).

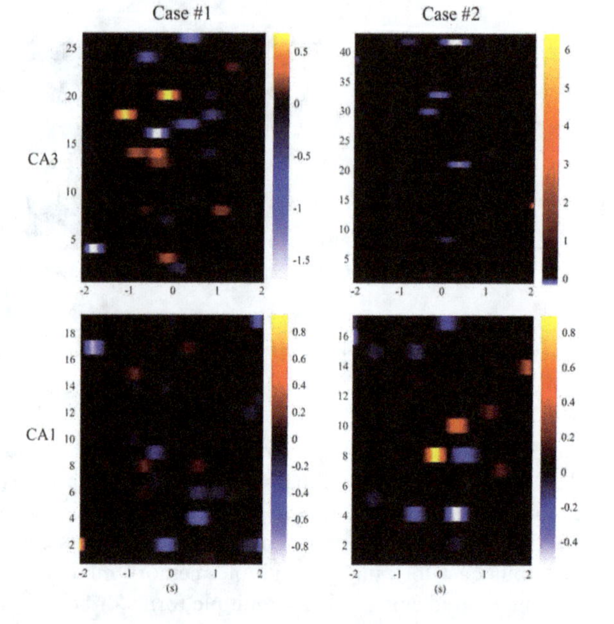

FIGURE 9 | Sparse classification feature matrices of the MISO memory decoding models (case #1 and #2). Black color represents zero-valued weights.

than in the actual CA1, and higher accuracy in the actual CA1 than in the predicted CA1. The latter is unsurprising since the predicted CA1 patterns are calculated with the MIMO signal model using the actual CA1 patterns as target signals, although the real-time calculation is driven by the ongoing CA3 patterns. It is thus unlikely for the predicted CA1 patterns to contain more memory-related information than the actual CA1 patterns. The former observation can be caused by two factors. First, it is possible that CA3 neurons contain more spatial information than CA1 neurons as suggested by previous studies (Lee et al., 2004). Second, it could simply due to the fact that we have recorded more CA3 units than CA1 units in the two cases included in this study. A more systematic, comparative study of CA3 and CA1 patterns needs to be performed to draw further conclusions.

In this study, the MISO memory decoding model takes the form of a B-spline, logistic regression model. The B-spline basis functions are utilized to reduce the model dimensionality and introduce a continuous metric for the similarities between spike trains. The optimal number of basis functions provides an estimate to the relevant temporal resolution of the spike trains. The logistic regression maps the spatio-temporal features to the probability of having a certain behavioral outcome. Despite the rather general model structure and the high prediction accuracy, however, this study does not necessarily suggest that the downstream hippocampal region decodes the CA1 spatio-temporal patterns in the same way. Instead, the main biological implications of this study are: first, the CA1 spatio-temporal patterns can be accurately predicted from the CA3 spatio-temporal patterns using a non-linear dynamical MIMO signal model; second, both CA3 and CA1 patterns contains sufficient information for decoding the memory events; third, the MIMO-model predicted CA1 patterns also contain sufficient information of the memory, and it must be this fact that makes the successful implementation of the hippocampal memory prostheses possible.

ACKNOWLEDGMENTS

This work was supported by the Defense Advanced Research Projects Agency (DARPA) through the Restorative Encoding Memory Integration Neural Device (REMIND) Program.

REFERENCES

Amaral, D. G., Ishizuka, N., and Claiborne, B. (1990). "Neurons, numbers and the hippocampal network," in *Progress in Brian Research,* Vol 83, eds J. Storm-Mathisen, J. Zimmer, and O. P. Ottersen (Amsterdam: Elsevier), 1–11.

Berger, T. W., Ahuja, A., Courellis, S. H., Deadwyler, S. A., Erinjippurath, G., Gerhardt, G. A., et al. (2005). Restoring lost cognitive function. *IEEE Eng. Med. Biol. Mag.* 24, 30–44. doi: 10.1109/MEMB.2005.1511498

Berger, T. W., Hampson, R. E., Song, D., Goonawardena, A., Marmarelis, V. Z., and Deadwyler, S. A. (2011). A cortical neural prosthesis for restoring and enhancing memory. *J. Neural Eng.* 8, 046017. doi: 10.1088/1741-2560/8/4/046017

Berger, T. W., Song, D., Chan, R. H. M., and Marmarelis, V. Z. (2010). The neurobiological basis of cognition: identification by multi-input, multioutput nonlinear dynamic modeling. *Proc. IEEE* 98, 356–374. doi: 10.1109/JPROC.2009.2038804

Berger, T. W., Song, D., Chan, R. H. M., Marmarelis,V. Z., LaCoss, J., Wills, J., et al. (2012). A hippocampal cognitive prosthesis: multi-input, multi-output nonlinear modeling and VLSI implementation. *IEEE Trans. Neural Syst. Rehabil. Eng.* 20, 198–211. doi: 10.1109/TNSRE.2012.2189133

Brown, E. N., Barbieri, R., Ventura, V., Kass, R. E., and Frank, L. M. (2002). The time-rescaling theorem and its application to neural spike train data analysis. *Neural Comput.* 14, 325–346. doi: 10.1162/08997660252741149

Deadwyler, S. A., Bunn, T., and Hampson, R. E. (1996). Hippocampal ensemble activity during spatial delayed-nonmatch-to-sample performance in rats. *J. Neurosci.* 16, 354–372.

Eichenbaum, H. (1999). The hippocampus and mechanisms of declarative memory. *Behav. Brain Res.* 103, 123–133. doi: 10.1016/S0166-4328(99)00044-3

Hampson, R. E., Gerhardt, G. A., Marmarelis, V. Z., Song, D., Opris, I., Santos, L., et al. (2012b). Facilitation and restoration of cognitive function in primate prefrontal cortex by a neuroprosthesis that utilizes minicolumn-specific neural firing. *J. Neural Eng.* 9, 056012. doi: 10.1088/1741-2560/9/5/056012

Hampson, R. E., Simeral, J. D., and Deadwyler, S. A. (1999). Distribution of spatial and nonspatial information in dorsal hippocampus. *Nature* 402, 610–614. doi: 10.1038/45154

Hampson, R. E., Song, D., Chan, R. H. M., Sweatt, A. J., Fuqua, J., Gerhardt, G. A., et al. (2012a). A nonlinear model for cortical prosthetics: memory facilitation by hippocampal ensemble stimulation. *IEEE Trans. Neural Syst. Rehabil. Eng.* 20, 184–197. doi: 10.1109/TNSRE.2012.2189163

Hampson, R. E., Song, D., Opris, I., Santos, L., Shin, D., Gerhardt, G. A., et al. (2013). Facilitation of memory encoding in primate hippocampus by a neuroprosthesis that promotes task specific neural firing. *J. Neural Eng.* 10, 066013. doi: 10.1088/1741-2560/10/6/066013

Haslinger, R., Pipa, G., and Brown, E. (2010). Discrete time rescaling theorem: determining goodness of fit for discrete time statistical models of neural spiking. *Neural Comput.* 22, 2477–2506. doi: 10.1162/NECO_a_00015

Hochberg, L. R., Serruya, M. D., Friehs, G. M., Mukand, J. A., Saleh, M., Caplan, A. H., et al. (2006). Neuronal ensemble control of prosthetic devices by a human with tetraplegia. *Nature* 442, 164–171. doi: 10.1038/nature04970

Humayun, M. S., de Juan, E., Weiland, J. D., Dagnelie, G., Katona, S., Greenberg, R., et al. (1999). Pattern electrical stimulation of the human retina. *Vision Res.* 39, 2569–2576. doi: 10.1016/S0042-6989(99)00052-8

Lee, I., Yoganarasimha, D., Rao, G., and Knierim, J. J. (2004). Comparison of population coherence of place cells in hippocampal subfields CA1 and CA3. *Nature* 430, 456–459. doi: 10.1038/nature02739

Loeb, G. E. (1990). Cochlear Prosthetics. *Annu. Rev. Neurosci.* 13, 357–371. doi: 10.1146/annurev.ne.13.030190.002041

Mauritz, K. H., and Peckham, H. P. (1987). Restoration of grasping functions in quadriplegic patients by Functional Electrical Stimulation (FES). *Int. J. Rehabil. Res.* 10, 57–61. doi: 10.1097/00004356-198712005-00010

McCullagh, P., and Nelder, J. A. (1989). *Generalized Linear Models.* Boca Raton, FL: Chapman & Hall/CRC. doi: 10.1007/978-1-4899-3242-6

Milner, B. (1970). "Memory and the medial temporal regions of the brain," in *Biology of Memory* eds K. H. Pribram and D. E. Broadbent (New York, NY: Academic Press), 29–50.

Nicolelis, M. A. L. (2003). Brain-machine interfaces to restore motor function and probe neural circuits. *Nat. Rev. Neurosci.* 4, 417–422. doi: 10.1038/nrn1105

Shenoy, K. V., Meeker, D., Cao, S. Y., Kureshi, S. A., Pesaran, B., Buneo, C. A., et al. (2003). Neural prosthetic control signals from plan activity. *Neuroreport* 14, 591–596. doi: 10.1097/00001756-200303240-00013

Song, D., and Berger, T. W. (2010). "Identification of nonlinear dynamics in neural population activity," in *Statistical Signal Processing for Neuroscience and Neurotechnology* ed K. G. Oweiss (Amsterdam: Elsevier), 103–128. doi: 10.1016/B978-0-12-375027-3.00004-1

Song, D., Chan, R. H., Marmarelis, V. Z., Hampson, R. E., Deadwyler, S. A., and Berger, T. W. (2007). Nonlinear dynamic modeling of spike train transformations for hippocampal-cortical prostheses. *IEEE Trans. Biomed. Eng.* 54, 1053–1066. doi: 10.1109/TBME.2007.891948

Song, D., Chan, R. H. M., Marmarelis, V. Z., Hampson, R. E., Deadwyler, S. A., and Berger, T. W. (2006). Physiologically plausible stochastic nonlinear kernel models of spike train to spike train transformation. *Conf. Proc. IEEE Eng. Med. Biol. Soc.* 1, 6129–6132. doi: 10.1109/IEMBS.2006.259253

Song, D., Chan, R. H. M., Marmarelis, V. Z., Hampson, R. E., Deadwyler, S. A., and Berger, T. W. (2009a). Nonlinear modeling of neural population dynamics for hippocampal prostheses. *Neural Netw.* 22, 1340–1351. doi: 10.1016/j.neunet.2009.05.004

Song, D., Chan, R. H. M., Marmarelis, V. Z., Hampson, R. E., Deadwyler, S. A., and Berger, T. W. (2009b). Sparse generalized Laguerre-Volterra model of neural population dynamics. *Conf. Proc. IEEE Eng. Med. Biol. Soc.* 2009, 4555–4558. doi: 10.1109/IEMBS.2009.5332719

Song, D., Chan, R. H. M., Marmarelis, V. Z., Hampson, R. E., Deadwyler, S. A., and Berger, T. W. (2011). Estimation and statistical validation of event-invariant nonlinear dynamic models of hippocampal CA3-CA1 population activities. *Conf. Proc. IEEE Eng. Med. Biol. Soc.* 2011, 3330–3333. doi: 10.1109/IEMBS.2011.6090903

Song, D., Marmarelis, V. Z., and Berger, T. W. (2009d). Parametric and non-parametric modeling of short-term synaptic plasticity. Part II: experimental study. *J. Comput. Neurosci.* 26, 21–37. doi: 10.1007/s10827-008-0098-2

Song, D., Wang, H., Tu, C. Y., Marmarelis, V. Z., Hampson, R. E., Deadwyler, S. A., et al. (2013). Identification of sparse neural functional connectivity using penalized likelihood estimation and basis functions. *J. Comput. Neurosci.* 35, 335–357. doi: 10.1007/s10827-013-0455-7

Song, D., Wang, Z., Marmarelis, V. Z., and Berger, T. W. (2009c). Parametric and non-parametric modeling of short-term synaptic plasticity. Part I: computational study. *J. Comput. Neurosci.* 26, 1–19. doi: 10.1007/s10827-008-0097-3

Squire, L. R., and Zola-Morgan, S. (1991). The medial temporal lobe memory system. *Science* 253, 1380–1386. doi: 10.1126/science.1896849

Taylor, D. M., Tillery, S. I. H., and Schwartz, A. B. (2002). Direct cortical control of 3D neuroprosthetic devices. *Science* 296, 1829–1832. doi: 10.1126/science.1070291

Wolpaw, J. R., and McFarland, D. J. (2004). Control of a two-dimensional movement signal by a noninvasive brain-computer interface in humans. *Proc. Natl. Acad. Sci. U.S.A.* 101, 17849–17854. doi: 10.1073/pnas.0403504101

3

What will this do to me and my brain? Ethical issues in brain-to-brain interfacing

Elisabeth Hildt*

Center for the Study of Ethics in the Professions, Illinois Institute of Technology, Chicago, IL, USA

Edited by:
Mikhail Lebedev, Duke University, USA

Reviewed by:
Markus Christen, University of Zurich, Switzerland
Hannah Maslen, University of Oxford, UK
Jens Clausen, University of Tuebingen, Germany

****Correspondence:***
Elisabeth Hildt, Center for the Study of Ethics in the Professions, Illinois Institute of Technology, 3241 S Federal Street, Chicago, 60616 IL, USA
e-mail: ehildt@iit.edu

Recent brain-to-brain interfacing studies provide proof of principle for the feasibility of various forms of direct information transfer between two brains, and may lead to the development of new approaches involving memory, emotions, or senses. What makes brain-to-brain interfaces unique is the transfer of information representing specific messages directly from one brain to another, without involving any activity of the peripheral nervous system or senses. The article discusses ethical issues that arise in neural interfacing. The focus is on the implications that brain-to-brain interfaces may have on the individual at the recipient side.

Keywords: ethics, brain-to-brain interfaces, research ethics, cross species experiments, agency, personal identity

INTRODUCTION

For several years now, brain-computer interfaces (BCIs) in which brain signals are used to navigate a computer, a prostheses or a technical device, have been developed in various experimental contexts (Wolpaw and Wolpaw, 2012; Grübler and Hildt, 2014). Researchers have recently taken the next step and run experiments based on connections between two brains. These so-called brain-to-brain interfaces (abbreviation: BBIs or BTBIs) involve not only a BCI component deriving information from a brain and sending it to a computer, but also a computer-brain interface (CBI) component delivering information to another brain. What results is technology-mediated brain-to-brain communication (B2B communication), i.e., direct communication between two brains that does not involve any activity of the peripheral nervous system. In what follows, ethical issues that arise in neural interfacing will be discussed after a short introduction to recent BBI experiments. In this, the focus will be on the implications BBIs may have on the individual at the CBI side of the BBI, i.e., on the recipient.

RECENT EXPERIMENTS

In their experiments involving a non-invasive BBI, Yoo et al. (2013) established functional links between the brain of a human volunteer and the brain of a rat. The human participant initiated an intention for intervention that was then transferred to an anesthetized rat's brain. This intention stimulated the motor area responsible for tail movement and led to involuntary tail movement. Technically, the experiment combined a BCI relying on EEG-based steady-state visual evoked potential and a CBI using transcranial focused ultrasound (FUS). FUS-based non-invasive neuromodulation of the rat brain was triggered by a computer when the human participant voluntarily started a thought process representing the intention to stimulate the rat brain. The intention was initiated by the participant looking at a strobe light flickering on a computer screen. In case of high synchronization, the FUS was triggered to transcranially modulate the anesthetized rat brain's motor cortex. Thus, the human subject was able to initiate (and thus control) the rat's tail movement via the BBI mediated "on–off" trigger.

In a similar experiment, Pais-Vieira et al. (2013) used a BBI to transfer behaviorally meaningful sensorimotor information from the brain of one rat (the "encoder" rat) to the brain of another rat (the "decoder" rat). In the study, while the encoder rat accomplished a sensorimotor task requiring the selection from two stimuli, cortical activity was recorded and transferred directly to the decoder rat's corresponding cortical areas via intracortical microstimulation. The sensorimotor information transferred via the BBI guided the decoder rat to learn similar behavioral choices, i.e., based solely on the neural patterns originating from the encoder rat. Furthermore, when the decoder animal's task performance was fed back to the encoder animal, continuous BBI operation influenced the encoder rat's neural activity and behavior. Overall, the BBI provided a "direct channel for behavioral information exchange" between two interconnected brains that allowed real-time sharing of sensorimotor information (Pais-Vieira et al., 2013, p. 6). The authors go on to state that these results "indicate that animal brain dyads or even brain networks could allow animal groups to synchronize their behaviors following neuronal-based cues." (Pais-Vieira et al., 2013, p. 6).

A related study not based on BBIs but involving a similar donor/recipient design, was done by Deadwyler et al. (2013). Via a mathematical model they derived information encoding patterns from the hippocampus of "donor" rats well trained in a specified paradigm and delivered the information via electrical stimulation to "recipient" rats that had never before been exposed to the specific character of this task. The transfer of the model-derived hippocampal firing pattern from the trained donor animals to naïve recipient animals via stimulation facilitated the recipient animals' task performance. As there was a time delay in between the encoding phase of the task and the behavioral response in the recipient animal, the study shows the transfer of a memory code, quite in contrast to the BBI-based study by Pais-Vieira et al. (2013) which relies on the immediate induction of a motor response.

Recently, Grau et al. (2014) provided the first example of conscious transmission of information between humans via a non-invasive BBI based on a BCI using motor imagery-controlled electroencephalography and a CBI that used transcranial magnetic stimulation (TMS) to induce the conscious perception of phosphenes, i.e., the experience of seeing light. The receiver subjects on the CBI side of the BBI were able to decipher the transmitted phosphene sequences carrying encrypted messages that coded for words such as hola" or "ciao."

Furthermore, there are speculations concerning possible future bidirectional BBI applications. For example, Yoo et al. (2013, p. 7) assume that "if both BCI and CBI are implemented between two awake human subjects, the information flow could be made bidirectional and communicative between apperceptive identities/individuals."

Possible future applications beyond the laboratory that have been envisioned include the use of BBIs in the military or in other professional contexts where they may allow for silent commands or may serve to synchronize behavior of a larger group of individuals. Further, applications may be seen in computer gaming, in enhancing human sensory capacities or in providing support to individuals with severe motor impairments (cf. Trimper et al., 2014).

NEED FOR ETHICAL REFLECTION

The recent studies provide proof of principle for the feasibility of various forms of direct information transfer between two brains, and may lead to the development of new approaches involving memory, emotions or senses. In view of these seminal publications on BBIs allowing information transfer between animals, between humans, and between animals and humans, there is a clear need for thorough ethical reflection.

BBIs combine the recording of brain signals on the side of the sender and brain stimulation on the side of the recipient. Each of these strategies raises a broad spectrum of ethical issues that are currently being discussed in contexts such as brain-computer interfaces, deep brain stimulation, or intrasurgical brain stimulation (Freudenstein et al., 2005; Grübler and Hildt, 2014; Unterrainer and Oduncu, 2015). What makes BBIs unique, however, is the transfer of information representing specific messages directly from one brain to another, without involving any activity of the peripheral nervous system or senses. On the side of the recipient, BBIs involve a form of information input not seen so far. Furthermore, whereas the specific "meaning" of the transferred signal is clearly defined by the technical system, the behavioral implications may be far from clear.

As BBI technology currently is in the very first stages of basic research, the ethical aspects raised in this contribution are speculative to a considerable degree. Nevertheless, it is important to reflect on these issues right now. The results will be of relevance to the design of possible future BBI studies involving human subjects and will give an idea of the broader implications and possible future uses of the BBI technology.

SOME GENERAL ASPECTS

But what exactly are the ethical issues possibly arising in brain-to-brain interfaces?

First of all, as in any kind of research involving human subjects, health-related safety issues have to be taken into consideration. In invasive systems that require surgery, there are risks concerning brain lesions. Furthermore, both in invasive and in non-invasive systems, some more indirect effects may arise: the recurring activation of specified pathways or brain regions both on the BCI part and the CBI part may influence brain functioning in various aspects.

In BBI use issues regarding agency, responsibility and liability undoubtedly will play a role (O'Brolchain and Gordijn, 2014; Vlek et al., 2014). Whereas traditional legal regulations concerning responsibility and liability in technology use may be applicable to BCIs, as suggested by several authors (Tamburrini, 2009; Clausen, 2011; Grübler, 2011), the fact that in BBIs two persons are involved complicates things considerably. The concept of "shared control" (Tamburrini, 2009), stating that in BCI use the user and the technical system together share control in achieving the output signal, undoubtedly applies to BBIs as well. Unlike in BCIs, however, there is not one person involved, but two, both of them not fully aware of their exact respective role in the system (cf. Vlek et al., 2014). Any ascription of responsibility for the outcome of any activity involving BBI functioning will be complicated by the BBI characteristic that the encoder may have initiated or significantly influenced a behavior or some sort of activity the decoder is performing (Trimper et al., 2014). Who is responsible for the consequences of activities in which BBIs are involved? The sender, i.e., the person involved in the BCI part? The recipient? The experimenter? The technical device? It may be speculated whether a concept of "hybrid agencies" (Suchman, 2007) involving several human actors might be applicable to BBIs.

Being part of a brain–brain dyad or a multi-brain system may also have complex repercussions on a person's concept of self, and raises questions concerning self-perception, individuality and body ownership (Hildt, 2011). For example, as an encoder, what is it like to be aware of another person exerting some behavior initiated or influenced by oneself? Will it be possible to clearly separate one's concept of self and the other?

Furthermore, complex problems with regard to privacy may arise, especially when the BCI component uses signals the sender is not aware of or signals the sender cannot control (Tamburrini, 2009; Trimper et al., 2014). Thus, it will be crucial to clearly define and explicitly state what kind of information will be transferred and to provide the sender with adequate measures to control the information transfer process. The same holds for the recipient in order to avoid the unconsented intrusion of information.

IMPLICATIONS FOR THE RECIPIENT

Imagine a BBI that transmits information that serves to mechanically make the decoder slightly move his left forefinger, in a method similar to the experiments run by Yoo et al. (2013) where BBI activity resulted in an anesthetized rat moving its tail. The recipient probably realizes that something is going on (his finger is moving in an automatic manner) and—being aware of the BBI and its usual function—will deduce that some information is being transferred. Thus, he probably will not ascribe authorship to himself for this movement. However, the situation will be different if the recipient is able to actively control the outcome of the information transfer, i.e., to actively control whether or not a certain movement finally occurs. For example, a person may be able to suppress the movement in question, or the BBI may solely confer a signal that serves as a stimulus for further action.

Now imagine a more flexible BBI in which various different patterns are enacted that elicit different types of reactions in the recipient. In case of five to ten different movement patterns conveyed via the BBI, would the recipient still be sure whether it is himself or the BBI that is initiating or controlling the movements? I have doubts. This uncertainty may lead him to erroneously ascribe authorship to himself for these movements (cf. Wegner, 2002; Vlek et al., 2014).

The same holds true, with even more complex implications, in cases where a BBI was able to elicit different types of emotions or memories. In a hypothetical situation where a BBI transmits a memory code that makes the recipient recall seeing a blue ball, the recipient may be clearly aware of the fact that his recurrent recalling of a blue ball may result from a BBI whose sole function is to elicit this urge. With a higher number of different stimulation patterns available, this connection will vanish so that it will be increasingly difficult for the recipient to know whether it is he or the BBI who induces a certain movement, emotion or memory. Furthermore, the transfer of emotions will considerably influence the recipient's overall well-being.

For example, in a scenario of memory transfer in humans, similar to the experiment in rats carried out by Deadwyler et al. (2013), the recipient would end up having two types of memories: his own genuine memories and the quasi-memories[1] transferred via the BBI technology. However, he would not be able to distinguish between his own genuine memories and the quasi-memories. As for quasi-memories, the same problems arise for quasi-olfactory experiences or for quasi-emotions elicited in the context of BBI use. The recipient would no longer know for certain which of his memories, sensory experiences or emotions are genuine and which are his quasi-memories, quasi-sensations or quasi-emotions resulting from BBI information transfer. In view of this, the recipient's sense of identity would be highly questioned [cf. the philosophical debate run by Shoemaker (1970), Williams (1976), Parfit (1984), and others].

In contrast, no direct identity issues arise in the conscious information transfer described by Grau et al. (2014). In their BBI experiment, the CBI elicits phosphenes in the recipient that code for specific words. The recipient is aware of the information transfer process which involves active deciphering.

NEURAL INTERFACING, NEURAL GRAFTING, AND CROSS SPECIES EXPERIMENTS

It is worthwhile to compare neural interfacing with the ethical issues raised by other biomedical approaches. In particular, neural tissue transplantation is of interest here since the strategies of neural interfacing and neural grafting both involve the possibility of additional content being transferred to a brain.

Neural tissue transplantation studies in Parkinson's disease patients were run mainly in the 1980s and 1990s. They aimed at replacing loss of dopaminergic neurons in the brains of Parkinson's disease patients by transplanting mesencephalic tissue from the developing brain of aborted human embryos and fetuses into the patient's brain (Barker et al., 2013).

In the context of these clinical grafting trials, guidelines were developed that addressed ethical issues in the retrieval and use of human embryonic and fetal material. Some of them, among other aspects, contain a paragraph that serves to exclude the possibility of "personality transfer" or any risk of transfer of individual characteristics from the brain tissue donor to the recipient (British Medical Association, 1988; Dickson, 1989; Boer, 1994). For example, the "NECTAR ethical guidelines for the retrieval and use of human embryonic or fetal donor tissue for experimental and clinical neurotransplantation and research" developed by the Network of European CNS Transplantation And Restoration (NECTAR), say in point 7: "Nervous tissue may be used for transplantation as suspended cell preparations or tissue fragments" (Boer, 1994, p. 3). Allowing only cell preparations or tissue fragments to be transplanted serves to avoid the transfer of any of the donor's individual characteristics to the graft recipient.

Even if for practical reasons a "personality transfer" or the transfer of individual characteristics is very unlikely to occur in brain tissue transplantations, the guidelines considered this concern by having a paragraph that explicitly rules out this possibility in clinical transplantation studies. BBIs, however, directly involve the very issue that these guidelines attempt to avoid in the case of clinical neural tissue transplantation: the transfer of individual characteristics from a donor to a recipient, such as for example in the transfer of a memory code. Whereas in neural grafting a material substrate, i.e., brain tissue, is transferred, in BBIs there is a direct transfer of information from one brain to another. What matters from an ethical point of view is the same in both approaches. The possibility of transfer of individual characteristics. This discrepancy points to a clear need for further reflection on the ethical issues involved in the transfer of information in BBIs involving humans.

Cross species neural interfacing experiments also raise tricky ethical issues (cf. Trimper et al., 2014). With regard to research involving animals containing human material (ACHM), some ethical reflection currently is going on. For example, the government-commissioned report "Animals Containing Human Material" from the UK Academy of Medical Sciences (2011) identifies a category (Category 2) of ethically sensitive research involving ACHM which should be approached with caution but

[1]The term "quasi-memory" has been coined by the American philosopher Sydney Shoemaker. He describes "quasi-memory knowledge" as "a kind of knowledge of past events such that someone's having this sort of knowledge of an event does involve there being a correspondence between his present cognitive state and a past cognitive and sensory state that was of the event, but such that this correspondence, although otherwise just like that which exists in memory, does not necessarily involve that past state's having been a state of the very same person who subsequently has the knowledge." (Shoemaker, 1970, p. 271).

could go ahead if approval by a specialist committee on a case-by-case basis is obtained (cf. Abbott, 2011). Among others, this category includes research that involves the modification of animal brains, other than non-human primates, "that may make the brain function potentially more 'human-like"' (Academy of Medical Sciences, 2011, p. 110).

The introduction of more "human-like" function into an animal brain via BBIs is not totally out of reach. A possible example is the BBI-induced transfer of the ability to distinguish between different words or commands (such as left, right, up, down) and to behave accordingly. Thus, some of the considerations of animals containing human material may apply to BBI technologies as well. Furthermore, in BBIs, information transfer may also emanate from an animal to a human being. For example, (Trimper et al., 2014, p. 2) speculate on possible future interspecies BBI uses such as enhancing human sensory systems or "aiding in search-and-rescue operations, linking our brains with those of the search-and-rescue animal. " In analogy to the point raised above with regard to animals containing human material (ACHM), there is a clear need for further reflection on the ethical issues involved in attempts to modify the brains of humans in ways that might result in some "animal-like" functions.

CONCLUSION

Current BBI research opens up fascinating new communication pathways but also raises considerable practical and ethical questions. One of the central questions is whether there actually is a need for direct brain-to-brain communication. At least at the moment, it seems doubtful whether there are broader applications for such a complex, rigid and expensive technology. Furthermore, in view of the complex ethical implications arising in the BBI recipient described above, the spectrum of possible ethically acceptable BBIs seems rather limited.

REFERENCES

Abbott, A. (2011). Regulations proposed for animal-human chimaeras. *Nature* 475, 438. doi: 10.1038/475438a

Academy of Medical Sciences. (2011). *Animals Containing Human Material.* Available online at: http://www.acmedsci.ac.uk/policy/policy-projects/animals-containing-human-material/

Barker, R. A., Barrett, J., Mason, S. L., and Björklund, A. (2013). Fetal dopaminergic transplantation trials and the future of neural grafting in Parkinson's disease. *Lancet Neurol.* 12, 84–91. doi: 10.1016/S1474-4422(12)70295-8

Boer, G. J., on behalf of the Network of European CNS Transplantation and Restoration (NECTAR). (1994). Ethical guidelines for the use of human embryonic or fetal tissue for experimental and clinical neurotransplantation and research. *J. Neurol.* 242, 1–13. doi: 10.1007/BF00920568

British Medical Association. (1988). BMA guidelines on the use of fetal tissue. *Lancet* 1, 1119.

Clausen, J. (2011). Conceptual and ethical issues with brain-hardware interfaces. *Curr. Opin. Psychiatry* 24, 495–501. doi: 10.1097/YCO.0b013e32834bb8ca

Deadwyler, S. A., Berger, T. W., Sweatt, A. J., Song, D., Chan, R. H., Opris, I., et al. (2013). Donor/recipient enhancement of memory in rat hippocampus. *Front. Syst. Neurosci.* 7:120. doi: 10.3389/fnsys.2013.00120

Dickson, J. (1989). Fetal tissue transplants win U.K. approval. *Science* 245, 464–465. doi: 10.1126/science.2756428

Freudenstein, D., Gharabaghi, A., and Tatagiba, M. (2005). "Erhalt der Funktion: Überwachung der Sprache bei Operationen am Gehirn," in *Neurowissenschaften und Menschenbild, Mentis,* eds E.-M. Engels, and E. Hildt (Paderborn: Mentis verlag), 35–55.

Grau, C., Ginhoux, R., Riera, A., Nguyen, T. L., Chauvat, H., Berg, M., et al. (2014). Conscious brain-to-brain communication in humans using non-invasive technologies. *PLoS ONE* 9:e105225. doi: 10.1371/journal.pone.0105225

Grübler, G. (2011). Beyond the responsibility gap. Discussion note on responsibility and liability in the use of brain-computer interfaces. *AI Soc.* 26, 377–382. doi: 10.1007/s00146-011-0321-y

Grübler, G., and Hildt, E. (eds.). (2014). *Brain-Computer Interfaces in their Ethical, Social and Cultural Contexts.* Dordrecht: Springer. doi: 10.1007/978-94-017-8996-7

Hildt, E. (2011). Brain-computer interaction and medical access to the brain: individual, social and ethical implications. *Stud. Ethics Law Technol.* 4. doi: 10.2202/1941-6008.1143. Available online at: http://www.degruyter.com/view/j/selt.2011.4.3/selt.2011.4.3.1143/selt.2011.4.3.1143.xml

O'Brolchain, F., and Gordijn, B. (2014). "Brain-computer interfaces and user responsibility," in Brain-Computer Interfaces in their Ethical, Social and Cultural Contexts, eds G. Grübler, and E. Hildt (Dordrecht: Springer), 163–182.

Pais-Vieira, M., Lebedev, M., Kunicki, C., Wank, J., and Nicolelis, M. A. L. (2013). A brain-to-brain interface for real-time sharing of sensorimotor information. *Sci. Rep.* 3, 1319. doi: 10.1038/srep01319

Parfit, D. (1984). *Reasons and Persons.* Oxford University Press: Oxford.

Shoemaker, S. (1970). Persons and their pasts. *Am. Philos. Q.* 7, 269–285.

Suchman, L. A. (2007). *Human-Machine Reconfigurations. Plans and Situated Actions,* 2nd *Edn.* Cambridge: Cambridge University Press.

Tamburrini, G. (2009). Brain to computer communication: ethical perspectives on interaction models. *Neuroethics* 2, 137–149. doi: 10.1007/s12152-009-9040-1

Trimper, J. B., Wolpe, P. R., and Rommelfanger, K. S. (2014). When "I" becomes "We": ethical implications of emerging brain-to-brain interfacing technologies. *Front. Neuroeng.* 7:4. doi: 10.3389/fneng.2014.00004

Unterrainer, M., and Oduncu, F. S. (2015). The ethics of deep brain stimulation (DBS). *Med. Health Care Philos.* doi: 10.1007/s11019-015-9622-0. [Epub ahead of print].

Vlek, R., van Acken, J.-P., Beursken, E., Roijendijk, L., and Haselager, P. (2014). "BCI and a user's judgment of agency," in *Brain-Computer Interfaces in their Ethical, Social and Cultural Contexts,* eds G. Grübler, and E. Hildt (Dordrecht: Springer), 193–202.

Wegner, D. M. (2002). *The Illusion of Conscious Will.* Cambridge, MA: MIT Press.

Williams, B. (1976). *Problems of the Self.* Cambridge: Cambridge University Press.

Wolpaw, J. R., and Wolpaw, E. W. (eds.). (2012). *Brain-Computer Interfaces. Principles and Practice.* Oxford: Oxford University Press. doi: 10.1093/acprof:oso/9780195388855.001.0001

Yoo, S.-S., Kim, H., Filandrianos, E., Taghados, S. J., and Park, S. (2013). Non-invasive brain-to-brain interface (BBI): establishing functional links between two brains. *PLoS ONE* 8:e60410. doi: 10.1371/journal.pone.0060410

4

Changes in cerebellar activity and inter-hemispheric coherence accompany improved reading performance following Quadrato Motor Training

Tal Dotan Ben-Soussan[1,2]*†, Keren Avirame[1,3†], Joseph Glicksohn[1,4], Abraham Goldstein[1,5], Yuval Harpaz[1] and Michal Ben-Shachar[1,6]

[1] *The Leslie and Susan Gonda (Goldschmied) Multidisciplinary Brain Research Center, Bar-Ilan University, Ramat-Gan, Israel*
[2] *Research Institute for Neuroscience, Education and Didactics, Cognitive Neurophysiology Laboratory, Patrizio Paoletti Foundation, Assisi, Italy*
[3] *Department of Neurology, Charité - Universitätsmedizin, Berlin, Germany*
[4] *Department of Criminology, Bar-Ilan University, Ramat-Gan, Israel*
[5] *Department of Psychology, Bar-Ilan University, Ramat-Gan, Israel*
[6] *Department of English, Linguistics Division, Bar-Ilan University, Israel*

Edited by:
Mikhail Lebedev, Duke University, USA

Reviewed by:
Froylán Gómez-lagunas, UNAM, Mexico
Panagiotis D. Bamidis, Aristotle University of Thessaloniki, Greece

****Correspondence:***
Tal Dotan Ben-Soussan, Research Institute for Neuroscience, Education and Didactics, Cognitive Neurophysiology Laboratory, Patrizio Paoletti Foundation, via Cristoforo Cecci 2, 06081 - Santa Maria degli Angeli, Assisi (PG), Italy
e-mail: research@fondazionepatriziopaoletti.org

† These authors have contributed equally to this work.

Dyslexia is a multifactorial reading deficit that involves multiple brain systems. Among other theories, it has been suggested that cerebellar dysfunction may be involved in dyslexia. This theory has been supported by findings from anatomical and functional imaging. A possible rationale for cerebellar involvement in dyslexia could lie in the cerebellum's role as an oscillator, producing synchronized activity within neuronal networks including sensorimotor networks critical for reading. If these findings are causally related to dyslexia, a training regimen that enhances cerebellar oscillatory activity should improve reading performance. We examined the cognitive and neural effects of Quadrato Motor Training (QMT), a structured sensorimotor training program that involves sequencing of motor responses based on verbal commands. Twenty-two adult Hebrew readers (12 dyslexics and 10 controls) were recruited for the study. Using Magnetoencephalography (MEG), we measured changes in alpha power and coherence following QMT in a within-subject design. Reading performance was assessed pre- and post-training using a comprehensive battery of behavioral tests. Our results demonstrate improved performance on a speeded reading task following one month of intensive QMT in both the dyslexic and control groups. Dyslexic participants, but not controls, showed significant increase in cerebellar oscillatory alpha power following training. In addition, across both time points, inter-hemispheric alpha coherence was higher in the dyslexic group compared to the control group. In conclusion, the current findings suggest that the combination of motor and language training embedded in QMT increases cerebellar oscillatory activity in dyslexics and improves reading performance. These results support the hypothesis that the cerebellum plays a role in skilled reading, and begin to unravel the underlying mechanisms that mediate cerebellar contribution in cognitive and neuronal augmentation.

Keywords: dyslexia, MEG, motor training, cerebellum, alpha power, coherence, reading

INTRODUCTION

Reading is a basic ability necessary in every-day life. Failure to acquire literacy early in the schooling years may have serious consequences for an individual's academic achievements, well-being and employment prospects. Dyslexia, which is characterized by difficulties with accurate and fluent word recognition, poor spelling and decoding abilities, is the most common learning disability, with a prevalence rate of about 10% in school-age children (Deffenbacher et al., 2004). Longitudinal studies further indicate that dyslexia is a chronic condition that persists into adulthood (Shaywitz et al., 2008).

Difficulties in learning to read are commonly thought to derive from impaired phonemic representations and phonological processing (Bradley and Bryant, 1983; Ramus, 2004). This phonological deficit has been associated with aberrant cortical responses and altered asymmetry of activity in frontal and temporal language- and reading-related areas (Ramus, 2004; Dufor et al., 2007; Gabrieli, 2009), as well as with structural and functional abnormalities of the cerebellum (Pernet et al., 2009b).

The involvement of the cerebellum in higher cognitive functions such as language was once a controversial issue (Leiner et al., 1993; Rao et al., 2001). However, much evidence has been gathered in recent years to support this view. Initially, studies in patients with cerebellar disease reported significant deficits in verbal fluency (Akshoomoff et al., 1992; Appollonio et al., 1993). Later, cerebellar involvement was found in other aspects of language, such as phonological and semantic processing (for reviews see Stoodley and Schmahmann, 2009; Stoodley and Stein, 2011). In addition, structural imaging demonstrated that lower cerebellar declive volumes are associated with impaired reading abilities, suggesting that the cerebellum may be a biomarker of dyslexia (Pernet et al., 2009b). In fact, the cerebellar and frontal differences between dyslexics and controls are the most consistent (for reviews see Pernet et al., 2009a,b). For example, Eckert et al. (2003) found that the volume of the right anterior lobe of the cerebellum significantly distinguished dyslexic from control participants, and was correlated with reading measured by a single-word reading task.

According to broader theories, dyslexia is not limited to phonological difficulties but encompasses a wide range of neurodevelopmental deficits that can be traced back to the sensorimotor systems (Stein, 2001; Galaburda et al., 2006). It follows that difficulties in phonological processing related to dyslexia are secondary to impairments in basic sensory and motor processing. Some posit an impairment at an early stage in which fast incoming sensory information is processed in the magnocellular system (Stein and Walsh, 1997), while others have suggested a fundamental deficit in the integration of rapidly successive transient signals (Tallal et al., 1996) or in the detection of regularities in sound sequences (Oganian and Ahissar, 2012). These approaches all put forward the premise that sensorimotor alterations might be the source of the core reading impairments observed in dyslexia.

Although the role of the motor system in dyslexia is still controversial, it is by no means a novel proposal that dyslexia involves a motor component. Already in the 1930's, Orton observed abnormal clumsiness in dyslexic children. He suggested that clumsy children could have difficulties in learning complex body movements as well as movements which are necessary for speech and writing (Orton, 1937). Studies of dyslexic participants have found impaired motor performance in a variety of tasks such as speed of tapping, heel-toe placement, rapid successive finger opposition, accuracy in copying, learning and execution of motor sequence (Nicolson et al., 2001; De Kleine and Verwey, 2009). This body of evidence supports the claims regarding the functional interactions between motor control systems, language and reading (for reviews see Hickok et al., 2011; Buckner, 2013).

The importance of cerebellar oscillatory function in neuroplasticity (Swinnen, 2002; De Zeeuw et al., 2011) and its role in motor acquisition, such as bimanual skills (e.g., Andres et al., 1999), have long been acknowledged in studies related to motor learning. Since impaired motor skills were often observed in dyslexics, some researchers attributed dyslexics' cognitive and motor deficiencies to abnormal development and functioning of the cerebellum (Nicolson et al., 1999, 2001). These findings lead to the claim that the role of the cerebellum is not limited to regulating the rate, force, rhythm, and accuracy of movements, but also the speed, capacity, consistency and appropriateness of cognitive processes (Schmahmann, 2004; Hölzel et al., 2011; Buckner, 2013).

Consequently, several training studies aimed to improve reading through integrated sensory stimulation, incorporating visuomotor and vestibular home-based exercise program lasting 6 months (Reynolds et al., 2003; Reynolds and Nicolson, 2007). In their study, the intervention group improved in a range of motor skills, such as cerebellar/vestibular and eye movement tests, as well as in the Dyslexia Screening Test, more than the control group. Although the authors could only speculate about the neural mechanisms underlying these motor and cognitive improvements, they pointed to the involvement of cerebellar function in mediating these behavioral changes. In order to improve reading and spelling in dyslexia, other studies investigated the effect of normalizing oscillatory activity on reading and spelling using neurofeedback (Breteler et al., 2010). Following 10 weeks of neurofeedback training, the intervention group showed improved spelling in contrast to the control group; however, no improvement was found in reading performance in either group. In addition, a significant increase in alpha coherence was found, which was interpreted as an indication that attentional processes account for the observed improvement in spelling, while no correlation was found between the two measures. So far, the link between training-induced changes in cerebellar alpha oscillatory activity and reading skills remained unexplored.

In the current study, we explore the possible potential interactions between sensorimotor and reading systems, and the role of the cerebellum as a mediator between them. In a preliminary attempt to understand the causal relationship between these constructs and their role in dyslexia, we examined how reading skills change as a result of a highly-structured form of sensorimotor training. We applied *Quadrato Motor Training* (QMT), a new sensorimotor whole-body training that involves following a structured set of simple oral instructions, by stepping to the instructed corner in a square. Recently, we demonstrated that one session of QMT can improve cognitive function, including creativity and spatial cognition, in comparison to two alternative training regimens that did not combine motor and cognitive aspects (Ben-Soussan et al., 2013, 2014). In the current study, the QMT is applied for a period of one month, in order to test its efficacy in inducing plasticity.

We have chosen magneto-encephalography (MEG) as the main tool for assessing changes in brain activity, due to its excellent resolution in the temporal domain, as well as its superiority to EEG in terms of effective spatial resolution (Kanda et al., 2000; Genow et al., 2004). In fact, it has been explicitly argued that MEG could be an excellent tool for evaluating the neural correlates of training-induced changes in dyslexia because of its ability to localize the sources of the alpha activation in parallel to the examination of long-distance alpha coherence (Salmelin, 2007). Further theoretical motivation for this choice is provided by the temporal sampling framework (TSF), which has been recently proposed to connect the observed sensorimotor deficits in dyslexia to temporal alterations in neuronal oscillations (Goswami, 2011). We therefore set out to examine the effects of QMT in a group of adult dyslexics and matched controls using MEG alpha power and coherence as electrophysiological dependent measures, as well as reading performance and verbal fluency as cognitive measures.

We hypothesized that dyslexics would show reduced alpha power, altered alpha coherence and lower reading skills at baseline in comparison to controls. We further hypothesized that QMT would increase cerebellar alpha power due to the important role of cerebellar alpha power in voluntary action (Tesche and Karhu, 2000; Ivry et al., 2002). Increased cerebellar alpha power would then serve to normalize alpha coherence (Basar et al., 1997; Andres et al., 1999; Silberstein et al., 2003; Silberstein, 2006; Güntekin and Basar, 2010) and improve reading (Goswami, 2011). We therefore tested whether a 4-week period of daily QMT would: (a) Enhance alpha power and normalize alpha coherence in dyslexic adults; (b) Enhance reading performance. Finally, we tested whether changes in alpha power and inter-hemispheric alpha coherence would correlate with behavioral changes in reading.

METHODS

PARTICIPANTS

Twenty-two native Hebrew speakers participated in the study: 12 dyslexic participants (5 females and 7 males; mean age = 30 (±6); years of education = 15 (±1)) and 10 controls (7 females and 3 males; mean age = 27 (±5); years of education = 14(±2)). We recruited volunteers who had been previously diagnosed as dyslexic by a clinical or educational psychologist and had a documented history of reading and spelling difficulties. We excluded participants who were further diagnosed with comorbid disorders, including Attention Deficit Hyperactivity Disorder (ADHD), Attention Deficit Disorder (ADD) and developmental coordination disorder (Ramus et al., 2003). All participants provided written informed consent to take part in the study.

PROCEDURE

The study included three phases: pre-training assessment, QMT training, and post-training assessment (See **Figure 1**). The pre-training session (Day 1) included the following components in this fixed order: (a) Cognitive testing (about 30 min, see Section Cognitive Tasks below); (b) MEG measurements (about 15 min, see Section MEG Data Acquisition below); and (c) QMT training (about 7 min, see Section Quadrato Motor Training below). Post-training assessment took place at the lab on Day 29, and included the cognitive and MEG components as on Day 1 in the same order using matched versions of the cognitive tasks (see Section Cognitive Tasks). Due to technical problems, one dyslexic participant did not complete the behavioral tasks; additionally,

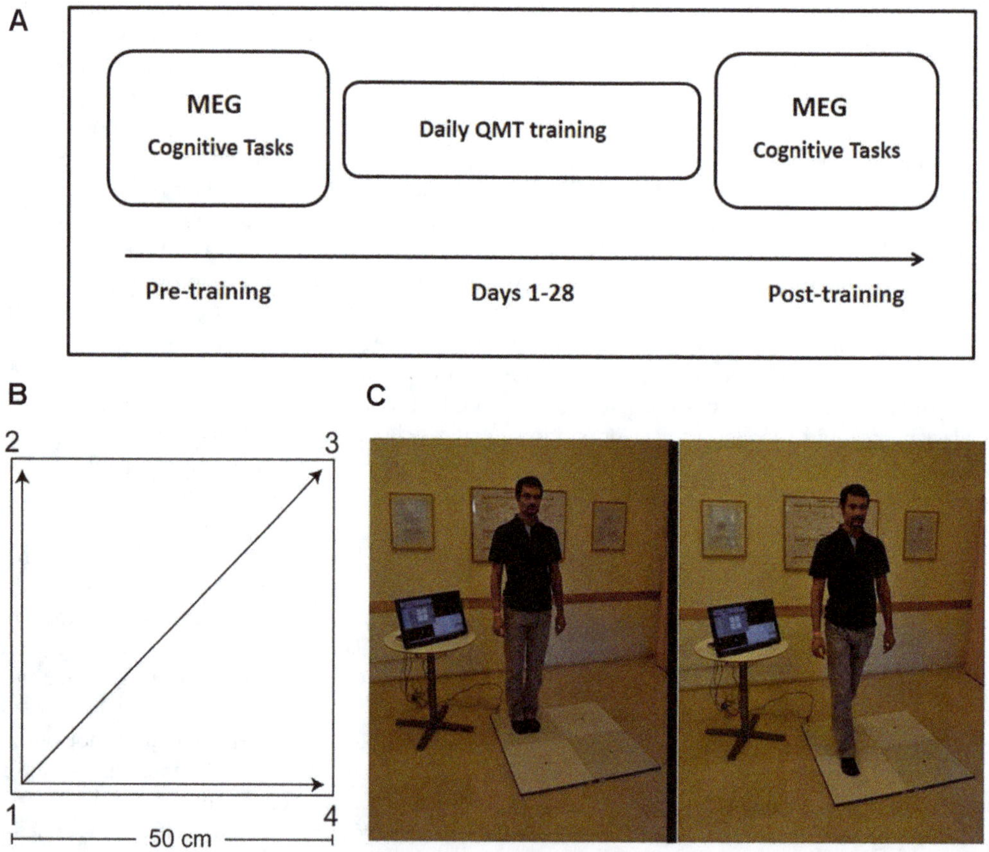

FIGURE 1 | Study design and Quadrato Motor Training. (A) Experimental protocol. MEG and behavioral measurements were conducted before and after 4 weeks of QMT training (see text for details). Two different versions of the cognitive tests were presented pre- and post-training in a counterbalanced order. **(B)** The spatial layout of the training space. **(C)** Practice setup. The trainee listens to recorded instructions and takes a step towards the target point. Figure adapted from Ben-Soussan et al. (2014). Quadrato Motor Training = QMT; Magnetoencephalography = MEG.

the behavioral data for the post-training verbal fluency tasks was incomplete for two dyslexic and one control participants. In those cases where participants failed to complete certain behavioral tests, their MEG measurements were still included in the analysis of the MEG data in order to increase statistical power given the small sample size.

QUADRATO MOTOR TRAINING

The participant stood in a quiet room at one corner of a 0.5 m × 0.5 m square and made movements in response to verbal instructions given by an audio tape recording. Participants were instructed to keep the eyes focused straight ahead and their hands loose at the side of the body. They were also told to immediately continue with the next instruction and not to stop due to mistakes. At each corner, there are three possible directions to move. The training thus consists of 12 possible movements (**Figure 1**). The daily training consisted of a sequence of 69 commands, lasting 7 min. Two variables that were addressed in other studies of motor learning are limb velocity and the decision regarding the responding limb (Criscimagna-Hemminger et al., 2002; Donchin et al., 2003). In order to control these parameters, we used a movement-sequence paced at a rate of an average of 0.5 Hz (similar to a slow walking rate), and we instructed the participants to begin all movements with the leg closest to the center of the square. Starting on day 2, daily QMT sessions were conducted by the participants at home. Home training lasted 27 consecutive days (from Day 2 to Day 28), and lasted 7 min each day.

COGNITIVE TASKS

The cognitive tasks were performed before the MEG measurement, and lasted for about 30 min. The order of tasks was fixed, starting with the reading test, category-based fluency and then letter-based fluency task. Each task had two different versions, and each of these versions was assigned to the pre- or post-training session in a counterbalanced manner across subjects.

Reading test

This test examines single-word reading speed and accuracy. A list of forty five written Hebrew words of increasing difficulty was presented and participants were asked to accurately read as many words as possible from the list in 1 min. The level of difficulty of the words was controlled in terms of word length and number of syllables. In order to minimize learning effects from the pre-test to the post-test, two non-overlapping word lists were created. Each list was presented either before or after training, in a counterbalanced manner. The two lists of 45 words were sampled from a database of rated Hebrew words (Levy-Drori and Henik, 2006), and were matched item-by-item for concreteness, availability of context, familiarity, number of letters and number of syllables. Since several participants from the control group finished the list of words in less than 1 min, the final score represents the number of words which were read correctly in the first 30 s.

Category-based fluency task

Participants were asked to say in 1 min as many words as possible belonging to a given semantic category. Two semantic categories were used alternately: (a) Animals; (b) Fruits and vegetables. One category was presented in the pre-training session (Day 1) and the other in the post-training session (Day 29), and the order of the categories was counterbalanced across subjects. Fruits and vegetables were treated as one category in order to avoid the ambiguity between botanical definitions and common usage (as in "avocado"). These categories were chosen because they have comparable norms, and in order to avoid test-retest influence by repeating the same category (Kavé, 2005).

Letter-based fluency task

Participants were asked to say in one minute as many words as possible that start with a given letter. We used two Hebrew letters: Bet (/b/) and Gimel (/g/). One letter served for pre-training and the other for post-training, and the order of the categories was counterbalanced across subjects. These letters were chosen because they have comparable norms, and in order to avoid test-retest influence by repeating the same letter (Kavé, 2005).

MEG DATA ACQUISITION

Power and coherence measures were collected using the MEG at the beginning and at the end of the month, after performing the cognitive tasks. MEG recordings were conducted with a whole-head 248-channel magnetometer array (4-D Neuroimaging, Magnes 3600 WH) in a magnetically shielded room. During the Rest condition, the participants were asked to refrain from moving and from falling asleep. In addition, the participants were asked to keep their eyes closed, in order to reduce ocular artifacts in the measured signals and to facilitate the localization of potential generator regions of the alpha resting–state oscillations (Goldman et al., 2002). Data acquisition took 15 min. We also collected MEG data using two active tasks which will be reported elsewhere. Before acquiring the data, the head-shape of each subject was digitized. Reference coils located approximately 30 cm above the head oriented by the x, y and z axes were used to record environmental noise. Three accelerometers, one for each axis, attached to the MEG gantry were used to record building vibrations in order to remove artifacts caused by them. The data were digitized at a sampling rate of 1017.25 Hz, and a 0.1 to 400 Hz band-pass filter was used online. The 50 Hz line power fluctuations were recorded directly from the power-line in order to remove the artifact on the MEG sensors.

PREPROCESSING MEG DATA

Power line, heartbeat, and vibration artifacts were removed automatically (Tal and Abeles, 2013). The data were then divided into 1 s epochs. Muscle artifact was estimated by examining the absolute value of all the MEG channels for every epoch, after applying a 20 Hz high-pass filter. For each epoch, the mean absolute value was computed. These values were then converted to z-scores, and epochs with z-scores greater than 3 standard deviations were rejected. Eye blinks were not considered as possible artifact for the alpha power processing, because the participants had their eyes closed and did not blink. Some eye movement artifact was still present in the data, but this was in a lower frequency range and was negligible in the alpha frequency range. Two of the 248 channels were noisy (one of the channels registered a constant zero value and the other exceeded 1 nanotesla); these channels were therefore excluded from all sensor and source level analysis. For left-right coherence computation, their homolog channels were omitted as well.

SOURCE LOCALIZATION

Source localization was applied for the alpha (7–13 Hz) frequency band. Synthetic Aperture Magnetometry (SAM) beamforming (Robinson and Vrba, 1999) was used with multiple spheres forward solution based on the digitized headshape. The neural activity was estimated for a grid of points covering the volume of the brain with 5 mm intervals. The power of activity was calculated for every grid point and for every epoch. Since raw beamforming results are biased toward deep sources it was necessary to normalize the images in order to keep the noise level equal throughout the whole volume of the brain. For this purpose, a pseudo-*z* score was calculated by averaging the power of every location, across epochs, divided by its noise estimate. The noise estimate was determined by the weights (the spatial filter). Deep sources generally have weights with higher values and are therefore noisier. Dividing the power of activity by the square of the weight norm can compensate for this bias (see Equation 3 in Sekihara et al., 2004). The absolute value of the weights of a particular location serves as a noise estimate. The resulting images represent the increase of alpha compared to noise, without being biased to deep sources. The pseudo-*z* value for each location was visualized as the color of voxels in the resulting functional images. The images were transformed to Talairach space by fitting a template MRI to the individual headshapes using SPM8 (Friston et al., 2007) and FieldTrip (Open Source Software for Advanced Analysis of MEG, Oostenveld et al., 2011) packages used with Matlab® R2010b. In order to control for multiple comparisons, a simulation was applied using an Analysis of Functional NeuroImages (AFNI) function (AlphaSim) which determines the probability to get significant clusters of different sizes at random. According to the simulation, at current parameters (given the template brain and spatial resolution used), clusters of voxels with a *p*-value smaller than 0.05 and exceeding one cubic cm (8 voxels) do not count as random noise. We decided to be even more conservative and to take only clusters containing more than 20 voxels at a threshold of $p < 0.005$ (Bunge et al., 2001).

COHERENCE

The coherence between left and right sensors was computed using FieldTrip. The data were first baseline-corrected by subtracting the mean of every epoch from the MEG traces. Eighteen channels located along the midline of the helmet were omitted from the coherence analysis, because these channels are likely to present with high coherence based on proximity, since spatially close sensors are likely to pick up very similar activities (Lehnertz et al., 2014).

Fourier transform was then computed using a spectral smoothing box of 1 Hz (meaning that the 10 Hz bin includes 9 to 11 Hz oscillations). The frequencies per time window were computed using a DPSS bell-shaped window. The resulting complex spectrum was used to assess coherence between each channel and its homolog. The coherence value of the 18 channels located along the mid-line of the helmet was set to one, representing perfect coherence between each channel and itself (the vertical red line in **Figure 4**). The coherence was projected onto a two-dimensional map of the sensor array, using the same left-right coherence value for the left as well as the right sensor, thus creating symmetrical maps of coherence. After the creation of the maps, channels *close* to the midline were excluded from the statistical analysis (in addition to the midline channels). This step was necessary because channels near the midline had high coherence values which did not represent cortical coherence, but simply the fact that the activity of one brain region was measured by two nearby channels. The channel pairs chosen were at least 11 cm apart in order to avoid "false coherence" resulting from close channels that pick up the same source and covered the lateral area of increased coherence (greater than 0.3; **Figure 4**). This procedure resulted in 59 channel pairs for which left-right coherence was statistically evaluated. Usually when studying inter-hemispheric differences, coherence is computed for one artifact-free channel for each region (e.g., from frontal, central, parietal, and temporal regions) and is computed for channels located in the corresponding regions of the two hemispheres (Osipova et al., 2003; Kikuchi et al., 2011). In fact, the number of chosen pairs is conventionally determined by *apriori* assumptions and therefore restricted to particular regions of interest. However, due to the exploratory nature of the current study, it was important to expand the search across multiple sensors.

STATISTICAL ANALYSIS

Mixed design ANOVA was used to test the effects of QMT on performance in the reading and verbal fluency tasks, with Training (pre-training, post-training) as a within-subject factor and Group (dyslexic, control) as a between-subjects factor. Statistical parametric maps were produced from MEG data using the AFNI package (Cox, 2012). Mixed design ANOVA was used to test the effects of QMT on alpha activity, i.e., alpha power and alpha coherence. Pearson correlation was used to test the association between behavioral and neuronal changes. The correlation threshold was $p < 0.05$. *Post hoc* comparisons were conducted using *t*-tests.

RESULTS

COGNITIVE RESULTS

Reading task

Performance on the speeded reading task was entered into a 2 (Group) by 2 (Training) ANOVA. First, a significant main effect for Group [$F_{(1,19)} = 7.80$, $p < 0.05$] was observed, indicating that, across both time points, the number of words correctly read by the controls ($M = 38.5$, SD = 6.3) was higher than the number of words correctly read by the dyslexic participants ($M = 27.6$, SD = 10.7). Secondly, the analysis yielded a main effect for Training [$F_{(1,19)} = 6.89$, $p < 0.05$], showing that QMT improved single-word reading performance across both groups (see **Figure 2**). Finally, the interaction between Training and Group was not significant ($p > 0.9$).

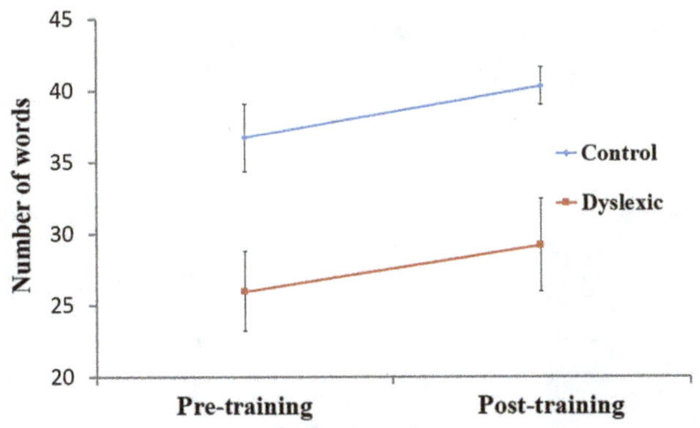

FIGURE 2 | Reading performance pre- and post-training. Number of words read correctly (mean ± SEM) in 30 s, pre- and post-training in the dyslexic (red) and control (blue) groups.

Table 1 | Mean scores of letter-based and category-based fluency tasks as a function group and training.

	Letter				Category			
	Pre Mean	SD	Post Mean	SD	Pre Mean	SD	Post Mean	SD
Dyslexic	8.7	2.4	9.0	1.9	23.9	5.2	24.9	4.3
Control	10.9	3.1	10.4	2.1	23.8	5.1	25.6	4.0

Verbal fluency

We conducted two separate analyses for the category-based and letter-based fluency tasks using a 2 (Group) by 2 (Training) ANOVA. No significant main effects or interactions were found, for either the category-based or the letter-based fluency task. The mean scores (i.e., number of words generated in 1 min) of the control participants for the category-based or letter-based fluency were similar to the norms (Kavé, 2005).

Based on previous studies demonstrating significant differences in phonological fluency between dyslexic and controls (Rack et al., 1992; Reid et al., 2007), we conducted a planned comparison between the groups for letter-based fluency, separately for pre- and post-QMT. While a marginally significant difference in phonological fluency was found pre-training between the dyslexic and control groups [$t_{(19)} = 2.08$, $p = 0.051$], no such difference was found following the training. In addition, no differences were found between the groups in semantic fluency, neither before nor after training. See **Table 1**.

MEG RESULTS

Between-group differences in cerebellar alpha power

We first examined the effect of QMT on alpha power using a mixed design ANOVA, with Training as a within-subject factor and Group (Dyslexia, Control) as a between-subjects factor, for each voxel. The ANOVA revealed a significant Group × Training interaction in a cluster in the right cerebellum. The center of mass of this cluster was located in the right culmen (Talairach coordinates (in mm): 12, −37, −22; $F_{(1,20)} = 13.3$, $p < 0.0025$; See **Figure 3A**). Before training, cerebellar alpha power was significantly lower in the dyslexic group compared to the control group ($t_{(20)} = 3.88$, $p = 0.001$). Following 4 weeks of daily QMT, cerebellar alpha power significantly increased in the dyslexic group ($t_{(11)} = 3.08$, $p = 0.01$) in contrast to the control group which showed no significant change following training (see **Figure 3B**).

The ANOVA also revealed a significant Group × Training interaction for three frontal clusters, located in the right superior frontal gyrus (SFG) (Talairach coordinates in (mm): 23, 53, 17) [$F_{(1,20)} = 16.08$, $p < 0.001$], supplementary motor area (SMA) (Talairach coordinates in (mm): 13, 18, 42) [$F_{(1,20)} = 22.41$, $p < 0.001$] and the left middle frontal gyrus (Talairach coordinates in (mm): −27, 8, 57) [$F_{(1,20)} = 16.01$, $p < 0.001$]. While there were no significant differences between the groups in these areas prior to training, the control group showed a significant decrease in alpha power in the left medial frontal gyrus (MFG) ($t_{(9)} = 4.54$, $p < 0.005$), right SFG ($t_{(9)} = 3.73$, $p < 0.005$) and SMA ($t_{(9)} = 3.69$, $p < 0.005$) following 4 weeks of daily QMT. On the other hand, the opposite pattern was observed in the dyslexic group in which alpha power increased in the right SFG ($t_{(11)} = 2.66$, $p < 0.05$).

Coherence

Inter-hemispheric alpha coherence was tested using a mixed design 2-way ANOVA for each of the 59 channels, with Training as within-subject factor and Group as between-subjects factor. Across both time points, inter-hemispheric alpha coherence was significantly higher in the dyslexic group compared to the control group for five channel pairs ($F_{(1,21)} > 8.35$, $p < 0.01$, uncorrected; See **Figure 4**). No main effect for Training or interaction was found.

Neuro-cognitive correlations

In order to study the possible associations between change in alpha activity and change in reading performance, we calculated Pearson correlations between behavioral and neuronal change within each group. This analysis was motivated by previous studies relating reading, cerebellar activity and alpha coherence (Nicolson et al., 2001; Weiss and Mueller, 2003; Arns et al., 2007). Change in speeded reading was calculated as the difference between the number of words read correctly in 30 s before and after training. Change in cerebellar alpha power was calculated as the difference between pre- and post- training cerebellar alpha power of the cluster which was found to have the significant Group × Training interaction. Change in inter-hemispheric alpha coherence was calculated as the difference between pre- and post-training values of the bilateral temporal alpha coherence. No significant correlation was found between change in cerebellar alpha power and change in reading in the two groups. Yet, as can be seen in **Figure 5**, change in temporal alpha coherence was positively correlated with the change in reading score ($r = 0.58$, $p < 0.05$, $n = 11$; uncorrected) in the dyslexic group but not in the control group. Using the Fisher r-to-z transformation, we calculated the z value to assess the significance of the difference between two correlation coefficients. The results indicated a significant difference between the two correlation values ($z = 1.87$, $p < 0.05$).

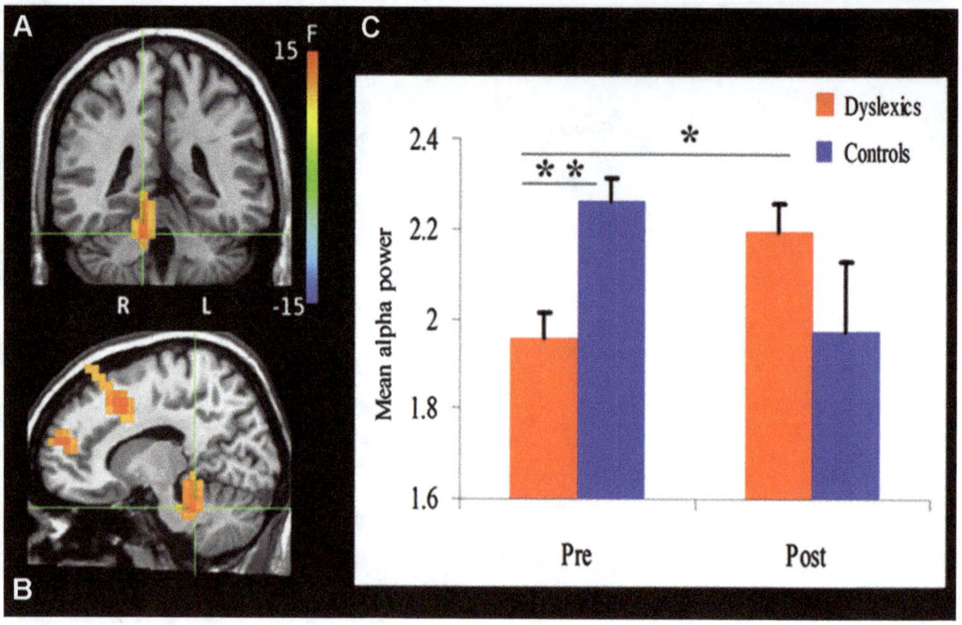

FIGURE 3 | Changes in alpha power. (A) and **(B)** demonstrate the significant clusters resulting from the Group (dyslexics, controls) by Training (pre-training, post-training) interaction. Voxels are colored by the *F* statistics, overlaid on coronal **(A)** and sagittal **(B)** views. The statistical map is thresholded at $p <$ 0.0025 in addition to a cluster size threshold of 20 voxels. The focus point (green cross) is positioned in the right culmen (Talairach coordinate: 12, −37, −22). **(C)** The bar graph shows alpha power as a function of Group and Training (mean + SEM). * $p = 0.01$; ** $p = 0.001$.

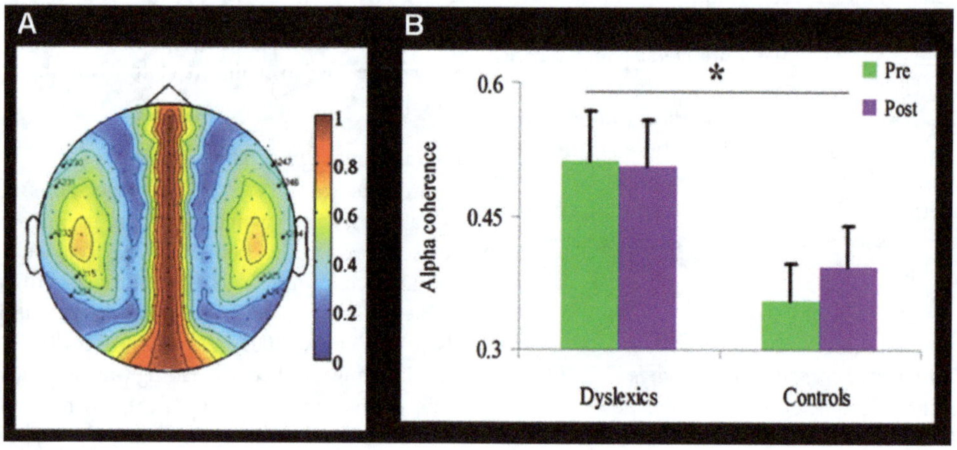

FIGURE 4 | Alpha coherence in the dyslexic and control groups. **(A)** Group differences in inter-hemispheric alpha coherence. The coherence was higher over temporal channels in the dyslexic group compared with the control group (* $p < 0.01$, uncorrected). **(B)** Temporal alpha coherence as a function of Group and Training (mean + SEM), demonstrating significant group differences between the dyslexic and control groups (* $p < 0.01$, uncorrected), as well as a null effect of the training in the dyslexic group and a trend toward an increase in alpha coherence in the control group.

DISCUSSION

Our results contribute two novel findings with regards to the cerebellar involvement in dyslexia: First, we show that cerebellar alpha activity prior to training is lower in dyslexics compared to controls. Second, a 4-week training program enhanced cerebellar alpha activity in dyslexics, but not in controls. Two other important findings are reported here for the first time: First, QMT over a period of 4 weeks improves reading speed in adults, and second, the improvement in reading performance is associated with increase in temporal alpha coherence in the dyslexic group. Below, we discuss these results in the context of different approaches to dyslexia and examine the possible role of the cerebellum in this neurodevelopmental disorder.

QMT ENHANCES PERFORMANCE IN A SPEEDED READING TASK

This study was inspired by the controversial body of research that examines the connection between reading and the sensorimotor

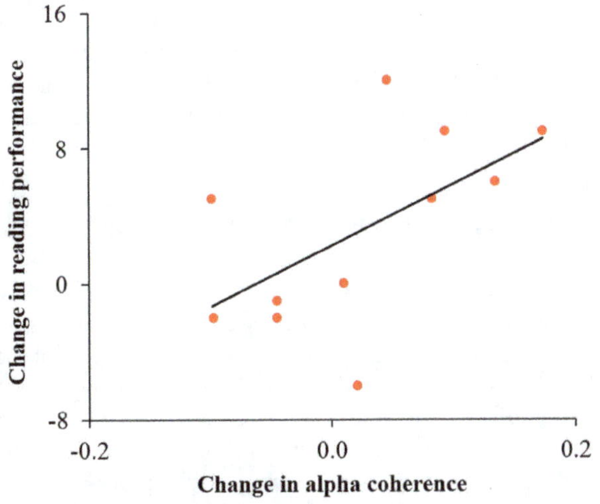

FIGURE 5 | Correlation between change in temporal alpha coherence and change in reading performance in the dyslexic group. Change in alpha coherence, calculated by the subtraction of pre- from post-training, was positively correlated with the change in number of words read correctly in 30 s ($r = 0.58$, $p < 0.05$).

systems (e.g., Flöel et al., 2003; Pulvermüller, 2005), in the context of novel discoveries about the benefit of daily sensorimotor practice for cognition (Ben-Soussan et al., 2013). We found improved reading skills in both groups as a result of 4-week QMT. Commonly, experimental studies attempt to enhance reading abilities and phonological functions by providing a training program for the target skill. Here we show that sensorimotor training might be beneficial for improving reading skills even though the practice relies on faculties that are not directly related to reading. Indeed, the QMT is based on a series of motor responses to verbal commands, which involve functions such as spatial cognition and response inhibition (Ben-Soussan et al., 2014). QMT-related improvement in the speeded reading task was found using different stimulus lists at each time point (pre- and post-training) and is thus considered to result from QMT and not from test-retest effects. This finding is also in agreement with previous results showing cognitive improvement in non-dyslexics adults even following short term QMT (Ben-Soussan et al., 2013, 2014).

In addition to group differences in reading score measured at baseline, a trend of a lower score in the phonological fluency task was observed pre-training in dyslexics compared to controls. This trend was not observed following 4 weeks of daily QMT, suggesting that QMT helped in normalizing the performance on this task. Again, the use of different categories at each time point (pre- and post-training) provided support to the interpretation that it is probably the QMT that normalized performance and not the repetition of the task. In addition, no differences were found between the groups in semantic fluency, neither before nor after training. This supports the view that dyslexia is more related to phonological than to semantic impairment (Leggio et al., 2000).

QMT ENHANCES CEREBELLAR ALPHA POWER IN DYSLEXIC ADULTS

In line with our hypothesis, cerebellar alpha power was significantly lower in the dyslexic group prior to training in comparison to the control group (see **Figure 3C**). Importantly, following 4 weeks of daily QMT, we found that cerebellar alpha significantly increased in the dyslexic group in the right culmen, a region which has been previously reported to be related to language processing (Luke et al., 2002; Pernet et al., 2009a,b; Rudner et al., 2013). This finding may reflect the role of the cerebellum as a general timing mechanism for both sensorimotor and cognitive processes (Ivry, 1997; Tesche and Karhu, 2000; Ivry et al., 2002; Tesche et al., 2007), such as the acquisition of sensorimotor skills and response readiness (Martin et al., 2006). It might also be linked to the critical involvement of the cerebellum in the coordination of smooth movements, maintenance of balance and posture, visually guided movements and motor learning (for review see Manto et al., 2012), which are inherent components of the QMT.

In addition to cerebellar changes, we found differences between dyslexics and controls in frontal alpha activity following 4 weeks of daily QMT. While alpha power in the left MFG and SMA significantly decreased in the control group, the dyslexic group showed increased alpha power in right SFG. These regions have been previously reported to be related to movement and language processing (Binder et al., 1997; Eckert et al., 2003; Neumann et al., 2004). Contrary to the dyslexics, the control group showed a trend towards a reduction in cerebellar alpha power; however, there was a notable increase of the control group's dispersion around the mean, which might account for the lack of statistical significance of this effect. In line with previous findings on motor practice, it is possible that the reduction of frontal and cerebellar activity indicates that practice became simpler as control of movement and coordination improve (Lacourse et al., 2004).

Previous work based on one session of training reported decreased frontal alpha activity in healthy young subjects (Ben-Soussan et al., 2013). This decreased frontal activity was mostly observed following simple motor training, indicating that changes in these regions might be related to motor learning as well as action observation and intention understanding (Exner et al., 2002; Dapretto et al., 2005). These results are compatible with Goldberg et al. (2006) who reported a complete segregation between self-related and sensorimotor activity in relevant cortical regions using functional neuroimaging. Their results showed that frontal regions were functionally inactive during sensorimotor tasks and active during self-engaged tasks. It is therefore possible that reduced activity of frontal regions at rest in controls signifies automaticity of sensorimotor components as a result of the repetition of the same sequence of QMT for 4 weeks.

ALPHA COHERENCE IN DYSLEXIC ADULTS COMPARED TO CONTROLS

Alpha coherence is important for cognitive and sensory processing (Weiss and Mueller, 2003; Ben-Soussan et al., 2013). Previously, EEG studies revealed increased coherence in dyslexic children, especially between temporal areas during rest (Shiota et al., 2000; Arns et al., 2007). Contrary to prior results showing increased inter-hemispheric alpha coherence following a single session of QMT (Ben-Soussan et al., 2013), in the current study neither group showed a significant increase in alpha coherence following one month of daily QMT. It should be noted that the previous results were obtained using EEG and not MEG. In fact, calculating connectivity from sensor level recordings is not straightforward, as these recordings are highly dependent on the effects of field spread. In other words, coherence measured by MEG reflects fewer sources because the spatial scale of the MEG sensors is smaller resulting in inflated estimates. Moreover, EEG and MEG are different in their sensitivity to radial and tangential dipoles (Srinivasan et al., 2007). This points to the necessity to integrate different methods in the study of training-induced plasticity.

Importantly, in the current study coherence analysis confirmed increased inter-hemispheric alpha coherence in the dyslexic group compared to the control group across time points. The increased inter-hemispheric coherence, especially between the temporal areas, may reflect the connection between left and right superior temporal sulci, which are considered to be necessary for phonological processing (Hickok and Poeppel, 2004). These findings converge with independent data from diffusion imaging showing that children with lower phonological and reading skills have higher anisotropy in temporal-callosal fiber tracts (Ben-Shachar et al., 2007; Dougherty et al., 2007).

Consequently, we propose that the increased coherence found in the dyslexic group may reflect a compensation mechanism (Roberts and Kraft, 1989; Arns et al., 2007). This suggestion further accords with the view that both left and right posterior superior temporal cortices are required for phonological processing (Hickok and Poeppel, 2007). Indeed, earlier models of dyslexia promoted the premise that complex cognitive functions, such as the translation of graphic symbols into a phonemic code, depend on component processes from both cerebral hemispheres, and that at least some subtypes of dyslexia may be due to abnormal inter-hemispheric communication (Gazzaniga, 1973; Gladstone and Best, 1985; Wolff et al., 1990). The association between change in coherence and reading performance revealed a significant positive correlation only in the dyslexic group, suggesting that the underlying mechanisms of improved reading observed in this study are connected with increased inter-hemispheric communication in the alpha range. Due to the low power of the correlation analysis ($N = 11$) and the non-significant effect of training on alpha coherence, this finding should be treated as suggestive, and should be tested in future larger MEG studies of developmental dyslexia. Nonetheless, the positive correlation reveals that participants who showed higher improvement of speeded reading also demonstrated increased bilateral temporal alpha coherence, in addition to the general increase in coherence observed in dyslexia. Some researchers aimed at normalizing brain activity (and consequently ameliorating behavioral and cognitive deficits) in various developmental disorders by suppressing hyper-connectivity (Pineda et al., 2012). Similarly, in stroke rehabilitation, applying brain stimulation to inhibit inappropriate activity of non-specialized areas has been argued to offer an effective avenue of treatment (Naeser et al., 2005). However, ameliorating cognitive deficits in developmental disorders may not necessarily be achieved through suppressing abnormal connectivity, because the observed hyper-connectivity does not necessarily reflect a dysfunction (Arns et al., 2007). Indeed, findings from neurofeedback training show that, contrary to the expected effects, 6 months of training induced an increase in alpha coherence, which might be related to improved attention (Breteler et al., 2010).

TOWARDS A NEW APPROACH TO UNDERSTANDING AND TREATING DYSLEXIA

Existing methods of treating dyslexia usually rely on phonetic and reading materials which aim at dealing directly with the linguistic impairments. Nevertheless, dyslexia, as well as other developmental disorders, should not be interpreted as being impairments in a single cognitive process (Castles and Coltheart, 1993; Pernet et al., 2009a). These cognitive impairments should rather be regarded as the endpoint of an abnormal developmental process, reflecting the interactions of multiple potentially deficient processes as well as compensatory processes (Thomas and Karmiloff-Smith, 2002). The current study attempted to investigate dyslexia-related differences in specific regions, in inter-hemispheric coherence, and in response to intervention. In this way, the differences between groups in the training-induced electrophysiological effects may provide further insight into the deficient and compensatory processes that characterize dyslexia.

In line with our results, we suggest that both the deficient cerebellar alpha power and possibly compensatory alpha coherence may be connected to the cerebellum's role as a generator of alpha activity, and that sensorimotor training may lead to cerebellar plasticity which could eventually rebalance the system. In this respect, altered cerebellar oscillatory activity may be the source of the deficit in dyslexia since it could be viewed as a neural system that mediates cortical communication (Andres et al., 1999; Silberstein et al., 2003). Our preliminary findings also disclose that sensorimotor training can be a practical intervention in dyslexia because of its potential to facilitate cerebellar oscillatory activity. Exploring how neuronal oscillation and cerebellar function change as a result of training may have valuable implications for educational neuroscience.

LIMITATIONS

The current study is a preliminary attempt to examine empirically the question of system modulation, which is required for improving reading in dyslexia. The main limitations of the current study are the small sample size and the use of only one training paradigm. The choice of QMT was made based on previous studies in which it was demonstrated that cognitive changes, namely increased creativity and improved spatial cognition, are QMT specific, and are not observed in two control groups (Ben-Soussan et al., 2013, 2014). In the future, a study on a larger sample that includes several training regimes may extend the current results. In future research, it would be important to include a passive control group; in particular, a dyslexic passive control group would ensure that any test-retest effects that were controlled for with normal-readers and with the two different versions of the tasks are not different in participants with dyslexia.

So far, EEG studies have generally avoided studying cerebellar function because of the complex folding of the cerebellar cortex. As for MEG, signals can be obtained from the cerebellum especially within the alpha range (Ivry, 2000; Park et al., 2011). However, source localization makes it difficult to distinguish between signals arising in the cerebellar cortex and deep nuclei. Thus, our results should be interpreted keeping these limitations in mind. Regarding the coherence analysis, the statistical significance was not corrected for 59 comparisons and should be therefore evaluated with caution. However, since no previous study has shown similar left-right coherence effects it was impossible for us to focus on channels of interest and reduce the number of multiple comparisons. The results we report here can therefore be considered as exploratory, and should be confirmed in future studies. We expect that future studies will utilize independent imaging methods in order to examine the role of the cerebellum in reading and dyslexia, and the impact of QMT on cerebellar activity and connectivity.

CONCLUSIONS

The current MEG study is in line with previous studies suggesting that dyslexia may be related to cerebellar dysfunction. Four weeks of daily QMT enhances reading performance and cerebellar alpha oscillations in dyslexic participants. In addition, improved reading performance in dyslexics correlates with inter-hemispheric temporal alpha coherence. Our results suggest that cerebellar impairment in dyslexia can be modulated by sensorimotor training. Most importantly, the investigation of training-induced effects on reading performance provides a unique opportunity to gain insight into the relation between behavioral and neuronal changes. A better understanding of the functional coordination between cortical regions and the cerebellum would be necessary to pinpoint some of the underlying sources of dyslexia and to create training paradigms for clinical purposes. The current study provides an important step in bringing together different approaches to study the sources and treatment of dyslexia and the scientific value of sensorimotor training.

ACKNOWLEDGMENTS

We would like to thank the participants who let us examine their minds and brains. This study was supported by the Italy-Israel R&D Cooperation Program (Number 44186) awarded to Joseph Glicksohn and Tal Dotan Ben-Soussan and by the Israeli Center of Research Excellence (I-CORE) in Cognition (I-CORE Program 51/11).

REFERENCES

Akshoomoff, N. A., Courchesne, E., Press, G. A., and Iragui, V. (1992). Contribution of the cerebellum to neuropsychological functioning: evidence from a case of cerebellar degenerative disorder. *Neuropsychologia* 30, 315–328. doi: 10.1016/0028-3932(92)90105-u

Andres, F. G., Mima, T., Schulman, A. E., Dichgans, J., Hallett, M., and Gerloff, C. (1999). Functional coupling of human cortical sensorimotor areas during bimanual skill acquisition. *Brain* 122, 855–870. doi: 10.1093/brain/122.5.855

Appollonio, I. M., Grafman, J., Schwartz, V., Massaquoi, S., and Hallett, M. (1993). Memory in patients with cerebellar degeneration. *Neurology* 43, 1536–1536. doi: 10.1212/wnl.43.8.1536

Arns, M., Peters, S., Breteler, R., and Verhoeven, L. (2007). Different brain activation patterns in dyslexic children: evidence from EEG power and coherence patterns for the double-deficit theory of dyslexia. *J. Integr. Neurosci.* 6, 175–190. doi: 10.1142/s0219635207001404

Basar, E., Schurmann, M., Basar-Eroglu, C., and Karakas, S. (1997). Alpha oscillations in brain functioning: an integrative theory. *Int. J. Psychophysiol.* 26, 5–29. doi: 10.1016/s0167-8760(97)00753-8

Ben-Shachar, M., Dougherty, R. F., and Wandell, B. A. (2007). White matter pathways in reading. *Curr. Opin. Neurobiol.* 17, 258–270. doi: 10.1016/j.conb.2007.03.006

Ben-Soussan, T. D., Berkovich-Ohana, A., Glicksohn, J., and Goldstein, A. (2014). A suspended act: increased reflectivity and gender-dependent electrophysiological change following Quadrato Motor Training. *Front. Psychol.* 5:55. doi: 10.3389/fpsyg.2014.00055

Ben-Soussan, T. D., Glicksohn, J., Goldstein, A., Berkovich-Ohana, A., and Donchin, O. (2013). Into the square and out of the box: the effects of Quadrato Motor Training on creativity and alpha Coherence. *PLoS One* 8:e55023. doi: 10.1371/journal.pone.0055023

Binder, J. R., Frost, J. A., Hammeke, T. A., Cox, R. W., Rao, S. M., and Prieto, T. (1997). Human brain language areas identified by functional magnetic resonance imaging. *J. Neurosci.* 17, 353–362.

Bradley, L., and Bryant, P. E. (1983). Categorizing sounds and learning to read: a causal connection. *Nature* 301, 419–421. doi: 10.1038/301419a0

Breteler, M. H., Arns, M., Peters, S., Giepmans, I., and Verhoeven, L. (2010). Improvements in spelling after QEEG-based neurofeedback in dyslexia: a randomized controlled treatment study. *Appl. Psychophysiol. Biofeedback* 35, 5–11. doi: 10.1007/s10484-009-9105-2

Buckner, R. L. (2013). The cerebellum and cognitive function: 25 years of insight from anatomy and neuroimaging. *Neuron* 80, 807–815. doi: 10.1016/j.neuron.2013.10.044

Bunge, S. A., Ochsner, K. N., Desmond, J. E., Glover, G. H., and Gabrieli, J. D. (2001). Prefrontal regions involved in keeping information in and out of mind. *Brain* 124, 2074–2086. doi: 10.1093/brain/124.10.2074

Castles, A., and Coltheart, M. (1993). Varieties of developmental dyslexia. *Cognition* 47, 149–180. doi: 10.1016/0010-0277(93)90003-e

Cox, R. W. (2012). AFNI: what a long strange trip it's been. *Neuroimage* 62, 743–747. doi: 10.1016/j.neuroimage.2011.08.056

Criscimagna-Hemminger, S. E., Donchin, O., Gazzaniga, M. S., and Shadmehr, R. (2002). Learning dynamics of reaching movements generalizes from dominant to non-dominant arm. *J. Neurophysiol.* 89, 168–176. doi: 10.1152/jn.00622.2002

Dapretto, M., Davies, M. S., Pfeifer, J. H., Scott, A. A., Sigman, M., Bookheimer, S. Y., et al. (2005). Understanding emotions in others: mirror neuron dysfunction in children with autism spectrum disorders. *Nat. Neurosci.* 9, 28–30. doi: 10.1038/nn1611

De Kleine, E., and Verwey, W. B. (2009). Motor learning and chunking in dyslexia. *J. Mot. Behav.* 41, 331–338. doi: 10.3200/jmbr.41.4.331-338

De Zeeuw, C. I., Hoebeek, F. E., Bosman, L. W., Schonewille, M., Witter, L., and Koekkoek, S. K. (2011). Spatiotemporal firing patterns in the cerebellum. *Nat. Rev. Neurosci.* 12, 327–344. doi: 10.1038/nrn3011

Deffenbacher, K. E., Kenyon, J. B., Hoover, D. M., Olson, R. K., Pennington, B. F., DeFries, J. C., et al. (2004). Refinement of the 6p21. 3 quantitative trait locus influencing dyslexia: linkage and association analyses. *Hum. Genet.* 115, 128–138. doi: 10.1007/s00439-004-1126-6

Donchin, O., Francis, J. T., and Shadmehr, R. (2003). Quantifying generalization from trial-by-trial behavior of adaptive systems that learn with basis functions: theory and experiments in human motor control. *J. Neurosci.* 23, 9032–9045.

Dougherty, R. F., Ben-Shachar, M., Deutsch, G. K., Hernandez, A., Fox, G. R., and Wandell, B. A. (2007). Temporal-callosal pathway diffusivity predicts phonological skills in children. *Proc. Natl. Acad. Sci. U S A* 104, 8556–8561. doi: 10.1073/pnas.0608961104

Dufor, O., Serniclaes, W., Sprenger-Charolles, L., and Démonet, J. F. (2007). Top-down processes during auditory phoneme categorization in dyslexia: a PET study. *Neuroimage* 34, 1692–1707. doi: 10.1016/j.neuroimage.2006.10.034

Eckert, M. A., Leonard, C. M., Richards, T. L., Aylward, E. H., Thomson, J., and Berninger, V. W. (2003). Anatomical correlates of dyslexia: frontal and cerebellar findings. *Brain* 126, 482–494. doi: 10.1093/brain/awg026

Exner, C., Koschack, J., and Irle, E. (2002). The differential role of premotor frontal cortex and basal ganglia in motor sequence learning: evidence from focal basal ganglia lesions. *Learn. Mem.* 9, 376–386. doi: 10.1101/lm.48402

Flöel, A., Ellger, T., Breitenstein, C., and Knecht, S. (2003). Language perception activates the hand motor cortex: implications for motor theories of speech perception. *Eur. J. Neurosci.* 18, 704–708. doi: 10.1046/j.1460-9568.2003.02774.x

Friston, K. J., Ashburner, J. T., Kiebel, S. J., Nichols, T. E., and Penny, W. D. (2007). *Statistical Parametric Mapping: The Analysis of Functional Brain Images.* London: Academic Press.

Gabrieli, J. D. (2009). Dyslexia: a new synergy between education and cognitive neuroscience. *Science* 325, 280–283. doi: 10.1126/science.1171999

Galaburda, A. M., LoTurco, J., Ramus, F., Fitch, R. H., and Rosen, G. D. (2006). From genes to behavior in developmental dyslexia. *Nat. Neurosci.* 9, 1213–1217. doi: 10.1038/nn1772

Gazzaniga, M. S. (1973). Brain theory and minimal brain dysfunction. *Ann. N Y Acad. Sci.* 205, 89–92. doi: 10.1111/j.1749-6632.1973.tb43166.x

Genow, A., Hummel, C., Scheler, G., Hopfengärtner, R., Kaltenhäuser, M., Buchfelder, M., et al. (2004). Epilepsy surgery, resection volume and MSI localization in lesional frontal lobe epilepsy. *Neuroimage* 21, 444–449. doi: 10.1016/j.neuroimage.2003.08.029

Gladstone, M., and Best, C. T. (1985). "Developmental dyslexia: the potential role of interhemispheric collaboration in reading acquisition," in *Hemispheric Function Collaboration in the Child*, ed C. T. Best (San Francisco: Academic Press), 87–118.

Goldberg, I. I., Harel, M., and Malach, R. (2006). When the brain loses its self: prefrontal inactivation during sensorimotor processing. *Neuron* 50, 329–339. doi: 10.1016/j.neuron.2006.03.015

Goldman, R. I., Stern, J. M., Engel, J. Jr., and Cohen, M. S. (2002). Simultaneous EEG and fMRI of the alpha rhythm. *Neuroreport* 13, 2487–2492. doi: 10.1097/00001756-200212200-00022

Goswami, U. (2011). A temporal sampling framework for developmental dyslexia. *Trends Cogn. Sci.* 15, 3–10. doi: 10.1016/j.tics.2010.10.001

Güntekin, B., and Basar, E. (2010). A new interpretation of P300 responses upon analysis of coherences. *Cogn. Neurodynm.* 4, 107–118. doi: 10.1007/s11571-010-9106-0

Hickok, G., and Poeppel, D. (2004). Dorsal and ventral streams: a framework for understanding aspects of the functional anatomy of language. *Cognition* 92, 67–99. doi: 10.1016/j.cognition.2003.10.011

Hickok, G., and Poeppel, D. (2007). The cortical organization of speech processing. *Nat. Rev. Neurosci.* 8, 393–402. doi: 10.1038/nrn2113

Hickok, G., Houde, J., and Rong, F. (2011). Sensorimotor integration in speech processing: computational basis and neural organization. *Neuron* 69, 407–422. doi: 10.1016/j.neuron.2011.01.019

Hölzel, B. K., Carmody, J., Vangel, M., Congleton, C., Yerramsetti, S. M., Gard, T., et al. (2011). Mindfulness practice leads to increases in regional brain gray matter density. *Psychiatry Res.* 191, 36–43. doi: 10.1016/j.pscychresns.2010.08.006

Ivry, R. (1997). Cerebellar timing systems. *Int. Rev. Neurobiol.* 41, 555–573. doi: 10.1016/s0074-7742(08)60370-0

Ivry, R. (2000). Exploring the role of the cerebellum in sensory anticipation and timing: commentary on Tesche and Karhu. *Hum. Brain Mapp.* 9, 115–118. doi: 10.1002/(sici)1097-0193(200003)9:3<115::aid-hbm1>3.3.co;2-x

Ivry, R. B., Spencer, R. M., Zelaznik, H. N., and Diedrichsen, J. (2002). The cerebellum and event timing. *Ann. N Y Acad. Sci.* 978, 302–317. doi: 10.1111/j.1749-6632.2002.tb07576.x

Kanda, M., Nagamine, T., Ikeda, A., Ohara, S., Kunieda, T., Fujiwara, N., et al. (2000). Primary somatosensory cortex is actively involved in pain processing in human. *Brain Res.* 853, 282–289. doi: 10.1016/s0006-8993(99)02274-x

Kavé, G. (2005). Phonemic fluency, semantic fluency and difference scores: normative data for adult Hebrew speakers. *J. Clin. Exp. Neuropsychol.* 27, 690–699. doi: 10.1080/13803390490918499

Kikuchi, M., Shitamichi, K., Yoshimura, Y., Ueno, S., Remijn, G. B., Hirosawa, T., et al. (2011). Lateralized theta wave connectivity and language performance in 2-to 5-year-old children. *J. Neurosci.* 31, 14984–14988. doi: 10.1523/jneurosci.2785-11.2011

Lacourse, M. G., Turner, J. A., Randolph-Orr, E., Schandler, S. L., and Cohen, M. J. (2004). Cerebral and cerebellar sensorimotor plasticity following motor imagery-based mental practice of a sequential movement. *J. Rehabil. Res. Dev.* 41, 505–524. doi: 10.1682/jrrd.2004.04.0505

Leggio, M. G., Silveri, M. C., Petrosini, L., and Molinari, M. (2000). Phonological grouping is specifically affected in cerebellar patients: a verbal fluency study. *J. Neurol. Neurosurg. Psychiatry* 69, 102–106. doi: 10.1136/jnnp.69.1.102

Lehnertz, K., Ansmann, G., Bialonski, S., Dickten, H., Geier, C., and Porz, S. (2014). Evolving networks in the human epileptic brain. *Physica D* 267, 7–15. doi: 10.1016/j.physd.2013.06.009

Leiner, H. C., Leiner, A. L., and Dow, R. S. (1993). Cognitive and language functions of the human cerebellum. *Trends Neurosci.* 16, 444–447. doi: 10.1016/0166-2236(93)90072-t

Levy-Drori, S., and Henik, A. (2006). Concreteness and context availability in lexical decision tasks. *Am. J. Psychol.* 119, 45–65. doi: 10.2307/20445318

Luke, K. K., Liu, H. L., Wai, Y. Y., Wan, Y. L., and Tan, L. H. (2002). Functional anatomy of syntactic and semantic processing in language comprehension. *Hum. Brain Mapp.* 16, 133–145. doi: 10.1002/hbm.10029

Manto, M., Bower, J. M., Conforto, A. B., Delgado-García, J. M., da Guarda, S. N. F., Gerwig, M., et al. (2012). Consensus paper: roles of the cerebellum in motor control—the diversity of ideas on cerebellar involvement in movement. *Cerebellum* 11, 457–487. doi: 10.1007/s12311-011-0331-9

Martin, T., Houck, J. M., Bish, J. P., Kičić, D., Woodruff, C. C., Moses, S. N., et al. (2006). MEG reveals different contributions of somatomotor cortex and cerebellum to simple reaction time after temporally structured cues. *Hum. Brain Mapp.* 27, 552–561. doi: 10.1002/hbm.20200

Naeser, M. A., Martin, P. I., Nicholas, M., Baker, E. H., Seekins, H., Kobayashi, M., et al. (2005). Improved picture naming in chronic aphasia after TMS to part of right Broca's area: an open-protocol study. *Brain Lang.* 93, 95–105. doi: 10.1016/j.bandl.2004.08.004

Neumann, K., Euler, H. A., Gudenberg, A. W. V., Giraud, A. L., Lanfermann, H., Gall, V., et al. (2004). The nature and treatment of stuttering as revealed by fMRI: a within-and between-group comparison. *J. Fluency Disord.* 28, 381–410. doi: 10.1016/j.jfludis.2003.07.003

Nicolson, R. I., Fawcett, A. J., and Dean, P. (2001). Developmental dyslexia: the cerebellar deficit hypothesis. *Trends Neurosci.* 24, 508–511. doi: 10.1016/s0166-2236(00)01896-8

Nicolson, R. I., Fawcett, A. J., Berry, E. L., Jenkins, I. H., Dean, P., and Brooks, D. J. (1999). Association of abnormal cerebellar activation with motor learning difficulties in dyslexic adults. *Lancet* 353, 1662–1667. doi: 10.1016/s0140-6736(98)09165-x

Oganian, Y., and Ahissar, M. (2012). Poor anchoring limits dyslexics' perceptual, memory and reading skills. *Neuropsychologia* 50, 1895–1905. doi: 10.1016/j.neuropsychologia.2012.04.014

Oostenveld, R., Fries, P., Maris, E., and Schoffelen, J. M. (2011). FieldTrip: open source software for advanced analysis of MEG, EEG and invasive electrophysiological data. *Comput. Intell. Neurosci.* 2011:156869. doi: 10.1155/2011/156869

Orton, S. T. (1937). *Reading, Writing and Speech Problems in Children.* New York: Norton.

Osipova, D., Ahveninen, J., Kaakkola, S., Jääskeläinen, I. P., Huttunen, J., and Pekkonen, E. (2003). Effects of scopolamine on MEG spectral power and coherence in elderly subjects. *Clin. Neurophysiol.* 114, 1902–1907. doi: 10.1016/s1388-2457(03)00165-2

Park, H., Kang, E., Kang, H., Kim, J. S., Jensen, O., Chung, C. K., et al. (2011). Cross-frequency power correlations reveal the right superior temporal gyrus as a hub region during working memory maintenance. *Brain Connect.* 1, 460–472. doi: 10.1089/brain.2011.0046

Pernet, C., Andersson, J., Paulesu, E., and Demonet, J. F. (2009a). When all hypotheses are right: a multifocal account of dyslexia. *Hum. Brain Mapp.* 30, 2278–2292. doi: 10.1002/hbm.20670

Pernet, C., Poline, J., Demonet, J., and Rousselet, G. (2009b). Brain classification reveals the right cerebellum as the best biomarker of dyslexia. *BMC Neurosci.* 10:67. doi: 10.1186/1471-2202-10-67

Pineda, J. A., Juavinett, A., and Datko, M. (2012). Self-regulation of brain oscillations as a treatment for aberrant brain connections in children with autism. *Med. Hypotheses* 79, 790–798. doi: 10.1016/j.mehy.2012.08.031

Pulvermüller, F. (2005). Brain mechanisms linking language and action. *Nat. Rev. Neurosci.* 6, 576–582. doi: 10.1038/nrn1706

Rack, J. P., Snowling, M. J., and Olson, R. K. (1992). The nonword reading deficit in developmental dyslexia: a review. *Read. Res. Q.* 27, 29–53.

Ramus, F. (2004). Neurobiology of dyslexia: a reinterpretation of the data. *Trends Neurosci.* 27, 720–726. doi: 10.1016/j.tins.2004.10.004

Ramus, F., Pidgeon, E., and Frith, U. (2003). The relationship between motor control and phonology in dyslexic children. *J. Child Psychol. Psychiatry* 44, 712–722. doi: 10.1111/1469-7610.00157

Rao, S. M., Mayer, A. R., and Harrington, D. L. (2001). The evolution of brain activation during temporal processing. *Nat. Neurosci.* 4, 317–323. doi: 10.1038/85191

Reid, A. A., Szczerbinski, M., Iskierka-Kasperek, E., and Hansen, P. (2007). Cognitive profiles of adult developmental dyslexics: theoretical implications. *Dyslexia* 13, 1–24. doi: 10.1002/dys.321

Reynolds, D., and Nicolson, R. I. (2007). Follow-up of an exercise-based treatment for children with reading difficulties. *Dyslexia* 13, 78–96. doi: 10.1002/dys.331

Reynolds, D., Nicolson, R. I., and Hambly, H. (2003). Evaluation of an exercise-based treatment for children with reading difficulties. *Dyslexia* 9, 48–71. doi: 10.1002/dys.235

Roberts, T. A., and Kraft, R. H. (1989). Developmental differences in the relationship between reading comprehension and hemispheric alpha patterns: an EEG study. *J. Educ. Psychol.* 81, 322–328. doi: 10.1037/0022-0663.81.3.322

Robinson, S. E., and Vrba, J. (1999). "Functional neuroimaging by synthetic aperture magnetometry (SAM)," in *Recent Advances in Biomagnetism*, eds T. Yoshimoto, M. Kotani, S. Kuriki, H. Karibe and N. Nakasato (Sendai: Tohuku University Press), 302–305.

Rudner, M., Karlsson, T., Gunnarsson, J., and Rönnberg, J. (2013). Levels of processing and language modality specificity in working memory. *Neuropsychologia* 51, 656–666. doi: 10.1016/j.neuropsychologia.2012.12.011

Salmelin, R. (2007). Clinical neurophysiology of language: the MEG approach. *Clin. Neurophysiol.* 118, 237–254. doi: 10.1016/j.clinph.2006.07.316

Schmahmann, J. D. (2004). Disorders of the cerebellum: ataxia, dysmetria of thought and the cerebellar cognitive affective syndrome. *J. Neuropsychiatry Clin. Neurosci.* 16, 367–378. doi: 10.1176/appi.neuropsych.16.3.367

Sekihara, K., Nagarajan, S. S., Poeppel, D., and Marantz, A. (2004). Asymptotic SNR of scalar and vector minimum-variance beamformers for neuromagnetic source reconstruction. *IEEE Trans. Biomed. Eng.* 51, 1726–1734. doi: 10.1109/tbme.2004.827926

Shaywitz, S. E., Morris, R., and Shaywitz, B. A. (2008). The education of dyslexic children from childhood to young adulthood. *Annu. Rev. Psychol.* 59, 451–475. doi: 10.1146/annurev.psych.59.103006.093633

Shiota, M., Koeda, T., and Takeshita, K. (2000). Cognitive and neurophysiological evaluation of Japanese dyslexia. *Brain Dev.* 22, 421–426. doi: 10.1016/s0387-7604(00)00167-4

Silberstein, R. B. (2006). Dynamic sculpting of brain functional connectivity and mental rotation aptitude. *Prog. Brain Res.* 159, 63–76. doi: 10.1016/s0079-6123(06)59005-3

Silberstein, R. B., Danieli, F., and Nunez, P. L. (2003). Fronto-parietal evoked potential synchronization is increased during mental rotation. *Neuroreport* 14, 67–71. doi: 10.1097/00001756-200301200-00013

Srinivasan, R., Winter, W. R., Ding, J., and Nunez, P. L. (2007). EEG and MEG coherence: measures of functional connectivity at distinct spatial scales of neocortical dynamics. *J. Neurosci. Methods* 166, 41–52. doi: 10.1016/j.jneumeth.2007.06.026

Stein, J. (2001). The magnocellular theory of developmental dyslexia. *Dyslexia* 7, 12–36. doi: 10.1002/dys.186

Stein, J., and Walsh, V. (1997). To see but not to read; the magnocellular theory of dyslexia. *Trends Neurosci.* 20, 147–152. doi: 10.1016/s0166-2236(96)01005-3

Stoodley, C. J., and Schmahmann, J. D. (2009). Functional topography in the human cerebellum: a meta-analysis of neuroimaging studies. *Neuroimage* 44, 489–501. doi: 10.1016/j.neuroimage.2008.08.039

Stoodley, C. J., and Stein, J. F. (2011). The cerebellum and dyslexia. *Cortex* 47, 101–116. doi: 10.1016/j.cortex.2009.10.005

Swinnen, S. P. (2002). Intermanual coordination: from behavioural principles to neural-network interactions. *Nat. Rev. Neurosci.* 3, 348–359. doi: 10.1038/nrn807

Tal, I., and Abeles, M. (2013). Cleaning MEG artifacts by external cues. *J. Neurosci. Methods* 217, 31–38. doi: 10.1016/j.jneumeth.2013.04.002

Tallal, P., Miller, S. L., Bedi, G., Byma, G., Wang, X., Nagarajan, S. S., et al. (1996). Language comprehension in language-learning impaired children improved with acoustically modified speech. *Science* 271, 81–84. doi: 10.1126/science.271.5245.81

Tesche, C. D., Moses, S. N., Houck, J. M., Martin, T., Hanlon, F. M., Jackson, E., et al. (2007). Dynamics of frontal and cerebellar activation during aversive conditioning: an MEG study. *Int. Congr. Ser.* 1300, 437–440. doi: 10.1016/j.ics.2007.02.057

Tesche, C. D., and Karhu, J. J. (2000). Anticipatory cerebellar responses during somatosensory omission in man. *Hum. Brain Mapp.* 9, 119–142. doi: 10.1002/(sici)1097-0193(200003)9:3<119::aid-hbm2>3.3.co;2-i

Thomas, M., and Karmiloff-Smith, A. (2002). Are developmental disorders like cases of adult brain damage? Implications from connectionist modelling. *Behav. Brain Sci.* 25, 727–750. doi: 10.1017/s0140525x02000134

Weiss, S., and Mueller, H. M. (2003). The contribution of EEG coherence to the investigation of language. *Brain Lang.* 85, 325–343. doi: 10.1016/s0093-934x(03)00067-1

Wolff, P. H., Michel, G. F., Ovrut, M., and Drake, C. (1990). Rate and timing precision of motor coordination in developmental dyslexia. *Dev. Psychol.* 26, 349–359. doi: 10.1037/0012-1649.26.3.349

5

What limits the performance of current invasive brain machine interfaces?

Gytis Baranauskas *

Neurophysiology Laboratory, Neuroscience Institute, Lithuanian University of Health Sciences, Kaunas, Lithuania

Edited by:
Mikhail Lebedev, Duke University, USA

Reviewed by:
Mikhail Lebedev, Duke University, USA
Imran Khan Niazi, Aalborg University, Denmark
Philip Kennedy, Neural Signals Inc., USA

***Correspondence:**
Gytis Baranauskas, Neurophysiology Laboratory, Neuroscience Institute, Lithuanian University of Health Sciences, Eiveniu g. 4, LT-50009 Kaunas, Lithuania
e-mail: gytis11@yahoo.com

The concept of a brain-machine interface (BMI) or a computer-brain interface is simple: BMI creates a communication pathway for a direct control by brain of an external device. In reality BMIs are very complex devices and only recently the increase in computing power of microprocessors enabled a boom in BMI research that continues almost unabated to this date, the high point being the insertion of electrode arrays into the brains of 5 human patients in a clinical trial run by Cyberkinetics with few other clinical tests still in progress. Meanwhile several EEG-based BMI devices (non-invasive BMIs) were launched commercially. Modern electronics and dry electrode technology made possible to drive the cost of some of these devices below few hundred dollars. However, the initial excitement of the direct control by brain waves of a computer or other equipment is dampened by large efforts required for learning, high error rates and slow response speed. All these problems are directly related to low information transfer rates typical for such EEG-based BMIs. In invasive BMIs employing multiple electrodes inserted into the brain one may expect much higher information transfer rates than in EEG-based BMIs because, in theory, each electrode provides an independent information channel. However, although invasive BMIs require more expensive equipment and have ethical problems related to the need to insert electrodes in the live brain, such financial and ethical costs are often not offset by a dramatic improvement in the information transfer rate. Thus the main topic of this review is why in invasive BMIs an apparently much larger information content obtained with multiple extracellular electrodes does not translate into much higher rates of information transfer? This paper explores possible answers to this question by concluding that more research on what movement parameters are encoded by neurons in motor cortex is needed before we can enjoy the next generation BMIs.

Keywords: brain machine interface, brain computer interface, extracellular recordings, information, throughput, multichannel recordings

Although the idea of a direct control of devices by human mind can be tracked down to the first experiments relating brain signals to behavior (Humphrey et al., 1970; Kennedy et al., 1992; Kennedy and Bakay, 1998; Wolpaw et al., 2002; Mussa-Ivaldi and Miller, 2003), only the advent of more powerful computer technologies in the last few decades enabled routine testing of these ideas in the environment of a scientific laboratory and, in some cases, in real life (Chapin et al., 1999; Taylor et al., 2002; Carmena et al., 2003; Velliste et al., 2008). This lead to the use of term "brain machine interface" (BMI) for such devices and in the last 15 years the number of papers published per year in the field of BMI increased exponentially (**Figure 1**). During this period it has been demonstrated that not only rats (Chapin et al., 1999) and monkeys (Wessberg et al., 2000) but also humans can control both a computer cursor and a prosthetic arm by their brain activity (Kennedy et al., 2000; Wolpaw and McFarland, 2004; Hochberg et al., 2006, 2012; Kim et al., 2008). Although already in late '90s Kennedy and his colleagues employed a single electrode in human patients to conditionally control activity of single units (Kennedy and Bakay, 1998) and then a computer cursor Kennedy et al., 2000), usually only experiments with multiple electrodes are considered to be relevant to BMIs of today and the tests with a robotic lever in rats are viewed as the birth of the modern BMI concept (Chapin et al., 1999; Lebedev and Nicolelis, 2006). Thus for electrode arrays it is possible to claim that in less than a decade the idea of BMI made a jump from the animal research to the tests in humans (Hochberg et al., 2006), a spectacular achievement.

However, did we achieve a qualitative improvement in invasive BMIs? This paper tries to answer this question by applying a single measure- information transfer rate. Although it may be viewed as a rather narrow-minded approach to evaluate the progress in a large field of science and technology by applying a single measure, the author believes that such a unified approach can be very useful in determining the strategy for future development of research and technology. This view is shared by a number of researchers as attested by a recent focused review on the topic (Tehovnik et al., 2013), a few reviews on EEG-based non-invasive BMIs (Wolpaw et al., 2000, 2002; Haselager, 2013), some papers on invasive BMIs (Gilja et al., 2012) and the position taken by the Defense Advanced Research Project Agency (DARPA), which funded many outstanding labs in the field of invasive BMI during

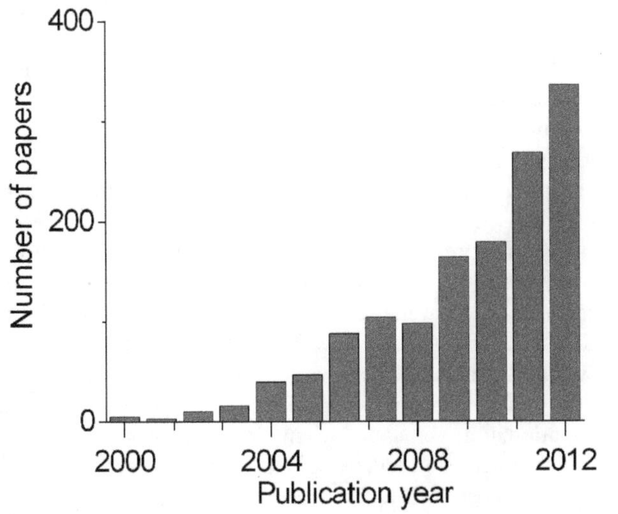

FIGURE 1 | The number of papers published each year with terms "Brain Machine Interface," PubMed search data.

the last few decades (Judy, 2012). The agency states that higher information transfer rates and increased durability/stability of BMI devices are the primary goals for this field of research (Judy, 2012). The information transfer rate is directly related to the ability to control a device (Tonet et al., 2008; Haselager, 2013; also see below) and may not be easily applied to some recently proposed new applications of BMIs such as restoration of neuronal function (Grosse-Wentrup et al., 2011). Nevertheless, device control remains the mainstream of BMI research and in these applications the information transfer rates can be used as the main quantitative measure to evaluate the overall system performance (Tonet et al., 2008; Haselager, 2013; Tehovnik et al., 2013).

Originally the mathematical information theory was developed to help optimize the communication line capacity (Shannon, 1948); these lines were mainly used for telegraph at that time, however, the theory is sufficiently general to be applied to any communication line, including the one used for a device control in BMI and the theory provides a quantitative measure, information content, that is independent of how BMI functions.

Even though to quantify BMI performance we employ just a single measure, the information transfer rate, we are still facing a daunting task to estimate information content in behavioral tasks that are used for BMI capability demonstration. The mathematical information theory determines what it takes to reproduce "at one point either exactly or approximately a message selected at another point" in space and time (Shannon, 1948). Shannon talks about a message selected from a set of messages and it is not important what is actually written in the message, the only thing that matters is how many such messages can be chosen, the number of possible selections. In a center-out reaching behavioral task, which is frequently used for BMI demonstrations (Taylor et al., 2002; Wolpaw and McFarland, 2004; Mulliken et al., 2008) and in which typically a subject has to choose several targets on the screen by moving a cursor from a central location, one message can correspond to one target. If during all runs 8 different targets were presented, we have 8 different messages. The information content is measured as a logarithm of number of choices to base of 2; for 8 messages with an equal probability to be presented the information content will be $\log_2(8) = 3$. By taking into account the error rates and the time needed to accomplish the task one can obtain the information transfer rate values (Tonet et al., 2008; Tehovnik et al., 2013). However, this approach has caveats and such a simple information content estimate is insufficient when we evaluate BMI performance. In this task the target relative size affects the subject performance and the larger target size will lead to higher information transfer rate even though no actual change in BMI performance will be present. The question of such task difficulty has been investigated in a number of papers on human-computer interactions (Fitts, 1954; MacKenzie and Buxton, 1992) and the Fitts' law is probably the best for evaluation of information content in such tasks. For other types of tasks, such as reaching and grasping (Carmena et al., 2003), the parameters determining task difficulty can be only guessed and there is a need of experimental data that information content of such tasks is evaluated. As long as no such experimental data exist, we are limited to these BMI studies that employ center-out reaching task. Luckily, this behavioral task is, probably, the most frequently used behavioral task in invasive BMI research from early on and even by limiting analysis to the center-out reaching task a trend in invasive BMI performance can be detected and few conclusions made.

In this review the author will try to show that the fundamental issues of biology but not computer power or electronic circuit capabilities are the limiting factors in achieving higher information transfer rates in invasive BMIs of today. More specifically, the author believes that, to increase invasive BMI performance, a more profound understanding about what neurons encode in motor areas of our brain is necessary and, actually, such BMIs can be a testing ground for new ideas on what kind of information is present in neuronal signals.

The paper is organized as follows. First, differences between invasive and non-invasive BMIs will be explained in brief. Second, the relationship between the information transfer rates and practical applications is discussed; examples from both invasive and non-invasive BMI will be presented. Third, technological factors that affect information rates in invasive BMIs will be evaluated. Finally, two examples of high information transfer rates in invasive BMIs will be analyzed and the strategies to improve information transfer rates will be suggested.

Today the term BMI can be applied to very different devices, from head caps with electrodes for electro-encephalogram (EEG) recording, in which EEG signal is transformed to commands for letter selection on a computer screen (Wolpaw et al., 2002; Krusienski et al., 2008) to implanted electrode arrays in monkey or, less frequently, rat and human brains, enabling a robotic arm control (Hochberg et al., 2006; Nicolelis and Lebedev, 2009). Since there are vast technological differences between a head-cap with electrodes for EEG and an array of wires inserted into the brain to record single neurons or field potentials of neuronal assemblies, usually all BMIs are broadly divided into two groups (Wolpaw et al., 2002; Tonet et al., 2008):

(1) Non-invasive BMIs, mainly EEG-based, although there are also systems that use muscle signals (EMG), gaze direction (Surakka et al., 2004; Oskoei and Hu, 2007; Tuisku et al., 2012) and other signals that do not require a surgical intervention.
(2) Invasive BMIs, these systems require a surgical intervention for electrode insertion and include not only electrode arrays inserted into the cortex but also electrodes implanted into the body for peripheral nerve activity detection (Navarro et al., 2005) or any other type of BMI that require extensive surgical procedure, for instance, cochlear implants (Moller, 2006).

These two classes of BMIs can be separated not only on the basis of technological differences but also on the basis of ethical problems associated with surgery in invasive BMIs. Invasive BMIs always require at least some surgery, which could be painful and, possibly, risky and there is always a question if such risks are offset by the benefits of BMI. In addition, invasive BMIs are usually much more expensive than non-invasive ones. Therefore, the expectation bar for invasive BMIs is higher than for non-invasive BMIs.

In spite of differences, all BMIs can be defined as devices that process information detected in the brain activity; the extracted information is used to determine the subject's intent and to control a computer cursor or a prosthesis. Thus, from information theory point of view the key characteristic of such a device is the amount of information transferred per unit of time, or channel capacity if we use Shannon's terms (Shannon, 1948) or throughput as it is called in many recent papers (Tonet et al., 2008; Gilja et al., 2012). An attempt to take a unified approach in the BMI research dates back to at least the first international meeting on non-invasive BMIs (Wolpaw et al., 2000). However, the use of information transfer rates became more common in the field of invasive BMIs only recently (Simeral et al., 2011; Gilja et al., 2012; Flint et al., 2013). Thus it is not an accident that the mentioned above DARPA initiative aimed to advance significantly the development of the upper-limb prosthesis technology places the information transfer rates at the center of its stated goals. The main reason for such an emphasis on information transfer rates is that in the design of neuroprosthesis this rate determines the functionality of a device (Tonet et al., 2008; Haselager, 2013). To understand that, we can take a wheelchair controlled by BMI as an example. One of the most important features of a wheelchair is the ability to stop it in case of emergency. The information transfer rate can be directly translated into the time required for such a command, because the command has 1 bit of information. Since typical EEG-based BMIs have information transfer rates of 0.25–0.5 bits/s (Wolpaw et al., 2002; Allison et al., 2012), for a EEG-based BMI it will take at least 2–4 s to stop a wheelchair. This is hardly acceptable because even at a very moderate speed of 0.5–1 m/s the wheelchair will move 1–2 m before it will stop. Although for non-emergency cases one can anticipate when to stop but if something unexpected happens there is no time for preparation, thus at least two-fold faster information transfer rates are needed for efficient stopping of a wheelchair in case of emergency.

More complex behaviors such as an arm movement correspond to much higher information transfer rates. To give an example, Paul Fitts in his famous paper (Fitts, 1954) estimated that in a simple tapping task human subject routinely achieve ~10 bit/s information transfer rates. It is likely that the control of a robotic arm with many degrees of freedom will require even higher information transfer rates. Human speech can be used as another example of a typical information rate routinely achieved by our brains. In a slow human speech ~100 words are produced each minute, or 1–2 words per second. If we use word recognition perplexity to estimate information content of each word (Brown et al., 1992), then each English word contains ~7.5 bits of information on average, corresponding to 7–15 bit/s of information transfer rates in a slow human speech. These examples show that fluent interactions with human beings require information transfer rates of $\geq\sim$10 bit/s and, keeping in mind that information unit, a bit, is defined in a logarithmic scale, this information transfer rate is several orders of magnitude higher than achieved by most BMIs today, usually <3 bit/s (see below). It may be argued that some human patients could benefit even from such low information transfer rates (Wolpaw et al., 2002) but an example with a wheelchair shows that even for such patients increasing these rates is critical for at least some functions.

Lower information transfer rates mean less fun as it has been discovered by companies making EEG-based devices for entertainment. A number of devices are already on the market such as several toys made by Neurosky, Mindball made by Interactive Productline and few others. Although Neurosky claims that several of its toys had "a phenomenal success," all these devices, according to their users, share one thing in common- they are difficult to control. More specifically, not only it takes time to learn to use them but also the achieved control is unreliable. Some users even claimed that actually no control was achieved by such devices, in many cases brain signals are of low quality because of the presence of artifacts (Fatourechi et al., 2007). Thus in spite of relatively low prices of some of these devices, the lowest being approximately 100$, the user experience is still somehow limited in spite of attractiveness of the idea to directly control a device by thought.

From the point view of information theory, unreliable control is equivalent to low information transfer rates. Today EEG-based BMIs are limited to information transfer rates of <0.5 bit/s (Klobassa et al., 2009; Townsend et al., 2010). To put this number in perspective, we can take as a benchmark information transfer rates achieved by human subjects in a simple motor task of tapping (Fitts, 1954) and in speech recognition employing cochlear implants, the first BMIs used in large numbers (Mussa-Ivaldi and Miller, 2003). The gap between the EEG-based BMI information transfer rate of 0.5 bit/s and the 10 bit/s rate achieved in both cochlear implants used for human speech recognition (Dunn et al., 2010), and the tapping task is frightening. Since the bit scale is logarithmic, a difference of 10 bits in information content corresponds to 1000 times higher information content. It is true that cochlear implants, so far the only invasive BMIs in wide use, started slowly in 50 and 60 s. The first users of cochlear implants were able to have only some comprehension of sounds but not speech, corresponding to very low information transfer rates, probably of the order of few bits per second (Moller, 2006). However, the ability to recognize human speech was, almost certainly, a key to their widespread use and today >40,000 (by some estimates >20,000) of these devices have been implanted (Rauschecker and Shannon, 2002).

These considerations should suffice to convince the reader that, at least to some degree, progress in the development of BMIs can be evaluated by looking at how much information transfer rates were improved over the years of research. In non-invasive BMIs there is a consensus that current limit is ~0.5 bit/s and it is largely unchanged in the last 10–15 years (Wolpaw et al., 2002; Krusienski et al., 2008; Townsend et al., 2010). This notion is less obvious for invasive BMIs. One problem in this field is that only recently the need for a uniform measure of information content has been more widely recognized and employed in the result description (Li et al., 2009; Simeral et al., 2011; Gilja et al., 2012; Flint et al., 2013). Although to calculate the information content of a behavioral task the information theory allows the use of almost any movement parameter such as the target number or the target coordinate (Tonet et al., 2008; Tehovnik et al., 2013), to have a meaningful comparison of BMI performance in different tasks, the comparison that permits to decide which algorithm, parameter choice or configuration of BMI is better, we need to take into account the difficulty of task. The concept of difficulty can be easily explained in a center-out reaching task (Taylor et al., 2002; Hochberg et al., 2006), in which a subject has to reach from the monitor center a target located some distance from the initial position. Although it is possible to take the logarithm of the number of targets as the information content of such a task, intuitively it seems obvious that larger targets are easier to reach. Fitts' studies for one-dimensional tasks of this type confirmed that target size but not number of targets determines how long it takes to reach the target (Fitts, 1954). He introduced an index of difficulty, defined as

$$I_d = -log_2 \frac{W_s}{2A} \ bits/response,$$

where W_s is the target size ("tolerance range" in the original paper) and A is the average amplitude of movements, corresponding to the average distance to the target. Importantly, Fitts showed that for this measure of difficulty the limit of human performance was always the same, 10 bits/s, independent of target size, distance to the target etc. Thus, if this index of difficulty is used as the information content of the task, then differences in center-out task performance should indicate differences in the BMI performance but not the task difficulty. Although attempts were made to extend this method to 2D and 3D tasks (MacKenzie and Buxton, 1992), there is no consensus what difficulty measure should be used in such cases. Recently an alternative approach has been suggested, SNR, a logarithm of the ratio of the actual value variance to the mean squared error of the predicted values (Li et al., 2009). It is reminiscent of the index of difficulty, where target size is substituted by the mean square of the predicted values and the average amplitude of movements by the actual value variance. However, first it has to be demonstrated experimentally that SNR evaluates correctly the difficulty of a behavioral task. SNR is only one possible measure to evaluate BMI performance in motor tasks, one can invent many other measures and the question is what these measures tell us. If exactly the same task is performed by different BMIs, it is straightforward to compare the performance of these BMIs. However, if tasks differ even in a single parameter, be it target presentation time or movement speed, it is much more difficult to compare the performance of these BMIs. We need a measure that represents BMI performance in a task-independent manner, something what Fitts demonstrated for human performance in several different tasks: his difficulty measure returned similar performance values (<20% change) for movement distances covering more than one order of magnitude (Fitts, 1954). If SNR is an objective measure of BMI performance it should produce the same or similar value for all tasks performed by the same BMI; to verify this statement we need experimental data.

For a symmetrical center-out reaching task the above Fitts' formula can be easily applied because distance to all targets is the same. Therefore in this review the analysis of BMI performance is limited to a single behavioral task, the center-out reaching task. Luckily, a sufficiently large number of studies employed this task over the span of more than one decade and the results from probably the best laboratories in the field of BMI can be included (**Figure 2**). The results presented in **Figure 2** show little or no improvement in the information transfer rates over ~10 years of research except for two data points, marked in red and black (**Figure 2**). These two outliers will be discussed below. If we neglect the outliers, the obvious question is why so much effort resulted in not much improvement in probably the main parameter determining the performance of invasive BMIs? A number of brilliant people were involved in this type of research and there must be a serious reason why we see little progress toward improvement in this key parameter. The next few paragraphs will be devoted to an attempt to answer this question. First the issues of technology will be very briefly explained, with a focus on the question if the current state of computer power, electrode technology impedes to achieve higher information transfer rates. Then an answer to the main question of this paper, how to improve the performance of invasive BMIs, will be sought.

In invasive devices typically >20 of electrodes are used to pick up extracellularly brain signals (Schwartz et al., 2006, 2001). Usually, these brain signals are the so-called "single units," representing action potentials of one or few neurons (Harris et al., 2000). When more than one single-unit is present in the trace from one electrode, spike sorting procedure is employed for their separation (Lewicki, 1998). In some cases local field potentials and multi-unit signals are also used for BMIs, these signals represent large populations of neurons (Andersen et al., 2004; Buzsáki et al., 2012; Aggarwal et al., 2013). How much information can be present in such recordings and how does the recording technology limit this amount of information?

It is much debated how much information a single action potential encodes. In visual system information rates up to ~1 bit/spike and >10 bit/s have been reported (Buracas et al., 1998). If all recorded single neurons were independent with no correlation between their action potential firing times, 10 neurons would correspond to 10 independent information channels and suffice to achieve information transfer rates of >100 bit/s (10 × 10). This rate is many orders of magnitude higher than typical rates of 1–2 bit/s achieved in invasive BMIs (**Figure 2**). In visual system

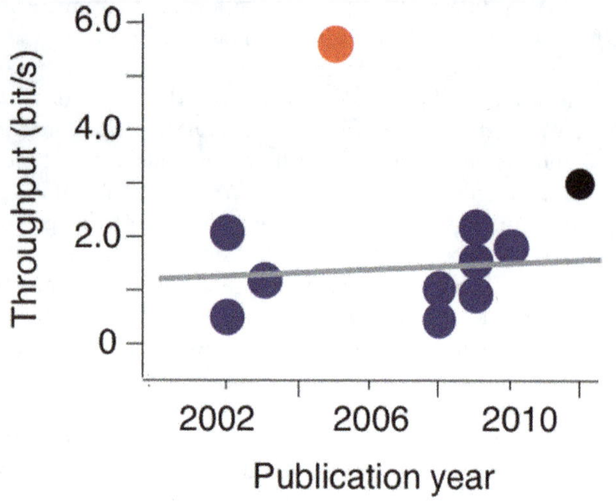

FIGURE 2 | Information transfer rates or throughput estimated for center-out reaching task (blue and black circles) and for "GO" cue task (red circle) in BMI papers. Most data were taken from supplemental material of Gilja et al. (2012) while the "GO" cue data are for Santhanam et al. (2006) study. The line represents a linear fit for all blue data points; there was no significant increase in information transfer rates in this time period.

neurons seem to be rather independent in information coding (Ecker et al., 2010), suggesting that potentially the information transfer rates that can be achieved with tens of recorded neurons in invasive BMIs is huge, well above the required 10 bits/s for fluent interaction with humans (see above) and magnitudes of order higher than currently achieved rates. One explanation for low information transfer rates achieved in current invasive BMIs could be that in motor systems only relatively few neurons encode large amounts of information and correlation between neurons is sufficiently high to reduce the amount of information encoded by the whole neuronal population (Carmena et al., 2003; Lebedev et al., 2008; Ecker et al., 2010). This inference is supported by the fact that for BMI control the pooled single unit information content is not much higher than the one found in the local field potential and multiunit signals, which are presumably the averages of large neuronal populations and individual differences of neurons are canceled out (Buzsáki et al., 2012; Aggarwal et al., 2013). In fact one of the best BMI performances in the terms of information transfer rates was achieved with no spike sorting, i.e., no neuron separation at each single electrode was used (Gilja et al., 2012).

One may argue that, since spike sorting procedure requires relatively high signal-to-noise ratio (Lewicki, 1998), low signal-to-noise ratio obtained with electrode arrays may result in poorly-separated single units, containing action potentials from more than one neuron, and the real independence of single neurons will be masked by such a contaminated single neuron signal (Ecker et al., 2010). However, in electrode arrays each recording site is sufficiently distant (>150 μm) from the other recording sites to ensure that no action potentials from the same neuron will be recorded by two recordings sites (Henze et al., 2000). Nevertheless, in electrode arrays correlation has been observed even for single units from different recording sites, corresponding to distinct, non-overlapping neuronal signals, thus it is unlikely that signal quality can account for relatively strong correlation between single units in motor system (Nicolelis and Lebedev, 2009; Ifft et al., 2013). These correlations between single units changed during learning to perform motor tasks, a clear indication that they are genuine and related to the motor control (Ifft et al., 2013). Finally, one of the best BMI performances in the terms of information transfer rates was achieved with no spike sorting, indicating that recorded single unit signal quality was not a limiting factor (Gilja et al., 2012). Thus it can be concluded that it is unlikely that insufficient quality of the electrode signal or amplification and filtration of the electrode signal limits the performance of current BMIs.

Another limitation of current technology is the number of simultaneously supported channels, usually it is the number of electrodes employed and the number of signal channels amplified and processed. The largest current systems can support up to 256 independent channels (Blackrock Microsystems, Salt Lake City, USA) while the largest electrode arrays may contain up to 96 electrodes. In one of the first papers on invasive BMIs it has been claimed that an almost unlimited accuracy of limb movement predictions could be achieved by increasing the number of recorded neurons (Wessberg et al., 2000). It was estimated that 400–500 of simultaneously recorded neurons would permit to achieve 90% accuracy. However, as the number of electrodes and simultaneously recorded neurons increased, the obtained data suggest no dramatic improvement beyond the first 40–100 neurons (Carmena et al., 2003; supplementary material in Gilja et al., 2012). Recently, based on a more extensive dataset, a logarithmic dependence of BMI performance (measured as SNR, see above) on the number of recorded neurons has been proposed (Lebedev and Nicolelis, 2011). It can be shown that essentially it is the same relationship suggested previously (Wessberg et al., 2000). It is asserted that with >10,000 of neurons the BMI performance would be on par with native hand (Lebedev and Nicolelis, 2011). Obviously the final proof of this claim will be an experiment with >10,000 recorded neurons. For now, several cautionary remarks can be made. The log/log scale is deceiving when a relatively narrow range of values is used, less than two orders of magnitude for recorded neuron numbers (from 2–3 to <200) and less than one order for SNR (from 0 to ~8 in $10^*\log_{10}$ scale, corresponding to 1–6.3, Figure 2 in Lebedev and Nicolelis, 2011); we still need to see if the same relationship holds for additional >2 orders for neuronal numbers and ~2 orders for SNR. Second, the graph is based on data tracking monkey walking, it is a stereotyped repetitive movement and it is not clear if the same relationship will hold for voluntary movements. One more note on the neuronal numbers regards neuron selection process in planar electrode arrays that are employed in most invasive BMIs of today. Since in such an array all electrodes are permanently fixed to the same platform it is impossible to adjust the penetration depth individually resulting in suboptimal location of electrode tips. It has been claimed that this is a serious issue that may compromise dramatically the BMI performance (Mulliken et al., 2008). In this paper it is shown that a better selection of <10 neurons in BMI with a flexible array with movable electrodes permits to achieve the same or even better performance than in a BMI with a rigid array and 10 times more recorded single units (~80). Nevertheless, the achieved performance is not better than reported previously; and probably it is safe to say that at least for the foreseeable future we will not achieve significantly higher information transfer rates by employing much larger arrays if no other changes are introduced.

The final note in support of the statement that currently technology is not a limiting factor in achieving higher information transfer rates in invasive BMIs is the absence of a clear increase in the information transfer rates in the last 10 years although the computer technology and electronics improved significantly, there were also advances in the electrode technology.

Clearly, this analysis on how the recording technology limits the amount of information present in the traces of extracellular electrodes is very brief. Nevertheless, it should be sufficient to state that electrode design, signal amplification and filtration, spike detection and sorting is unlikely to limit the information content present in these traces and there is a hope that the information content could be increased if the number of electrodes is increased >10 times. Then we have to accept the fact that in invasive BMI papers the recorded neurons probably encode only the reported amount of information about the predicted movement parameters. This conclusion is based in part on the fact that, for a given pair of parameters, let's say the neuronal spike rate and the cursor coordinate x, the information theory provides a precise formula to calculate the mutual information which is directly related to the maximal ability to estimate the value of one parameter when we know the value of the second parameter; in our example it would be the ability of the neuronal spike rate to predict the cursor coordinate x (Nelken and Chechik, 2007). Most algorithms that are used for movement control such as Kalman filters are known to efficiently utilize available information and it is unlikely that these algorithms dramatically limit the performance of BMIs. An example of an algorithm that does improve BMI performance nearly two-fold provided here below (Gilja et al., 2012) is largely based on a change of the movement parameters that are used for prediction but not the filters itself, the filters in the study were essentially a modified version of Kalman filter used by others also. We should remember that the information content is always calculated for a certain set of parameters that we want to predict and the information theory does not provide a recipe which parameters we should choose. It is possible in the same neuronal data set to find larger information quantity encoded by neurons if another movement parameter is chosen. To give an example, motor neurons may encode both the velocity and the position of a hand and but more velocity information is usually found in these neurons (Kim et al., 2011; Simeral et al., 2011). Thus, it is crucial to determine behavioral task or movement parameters for which the information quantity encoded by neurons is the highest. Essentially it is equivalent to asking what information the recorded neurons encode.

The presence of significant correlation between the measured parameter and the recorded neuronal activity does not mean that the recorded neuronal population is involved in determination of that parameter; correlation alone does not prove the presence of a causal link (Cramer, 2003; MacKinnon et al., 2007; Guilford and Fruchter, 1973). Actually in one of the papers considered to be a forerunner of the BMI concept (Fetz and Finocchio, 1971; Mussa-Ivaldi and Miller, 2003) the authors were asking very similar question: if we see a correlation between neuronal activity and muscle activity and movements, do these neurons participate in the generation of these movements? Since it was possible to force some neurons to be active when no muscle activity was present, even though just minutes before their activity correlated with the muscle activity, the answer was that correlation alone is not sufficient for such a claim.

BMIs may offer a new way to explore this issue. Intuitively it seems that the most efficient BMI will employ for the device control those parameters that are associated with the highest information content in the recorded neurons; this notion is confirmed by the information theory (Nelken and Chechik, 2007). Below two examples will be discussed to demonstrate how an unorthodox choice of parameters used for prediction enabled a dramatic increase in the information transfer rates in BMI.

One such an example has been reported by Shenoy group for the standard center-out reaching task (Gilja et al., 2012). Although in this case, similarly to the previous BMIs employing the center-out reaching task, the population of recorded neurons predicted the continuous movement parameters such as cursor position and velocity, there was a change in the coordinate system. Instead of trying to predict the cursor velocity with the respect to the observer, in other words instead of using a coordinate system fixed to the observer, it was assumed that the monkey always aims to the target, thus the coordinate axis was rotating toward the target as the cursor moved on. Although this modification was used only to predict cursor movements during algorithm training with brain control, the key fact is that such a modification of training introduced a coordinate system transformation for the velocity estimates. This modification alone significantly improved the information transfer rate in this task by <1 bit/s (less than two-fold). Although a relatively modest improvement, it was sufficient to achieve the best performance in this type of task (black circle in **Figure 2**) and to bring the target reach time to the range similar of the native hand (Gilja et al., 2012). A possible critique of this particular paper can be that apparently no limb fixation was used. In a number of studies it has been shown that there is a decrease in BMI performance following limb fixation (reviewed in Tehovnik et al., 2013). Nevertheless, it should be noted that Gilja and his colleagues demonstrated an improvement in BMI performance that resulted following the introduction of the new algorithm while all other conditions including hand fixation remained unchanged. Hence, the modification of coordinate system for algorithm training was sufficient to improve BMI performance by almost two fold. In addition, the same algorithm was used in an ALS patient with very limited hand movements and the achieved information transfer rate was well above the reported rates for similar patients (Henderson et al., 2013).

In invasive BMIs based on electrode arrays implanted in monkeys, the maximal reported information transfer rate was obtained in a 2006 study performed by the same Shenoy group (red circle in **Figure 2**, Santhanam et al., 2006). In contrast to all previous and most subsequent invasive BMI embodiments in monkeys, in this BMI the recorded neuronal population did not predict a parameter related to the continuous movement of a cursor such as velocity or coordinates, instead the recorded neuronal population was used to directly predict which target was chosen by the monkey. In the task employed in the study a monkey had to choose a limited number of targets following the "GO" cue and the algorithm predicted which target was chosen, no attempt to identify the movement trajectory was made. This change alone permitted to increase the information transfer rate from typical 0.8–1.5 bit/s to >6 bit/s. Such a >4 bit/s increase corresponds to more than one order increase in the information content. Although care was taken to have no eye movements during the period used to predict which target was chosen, it is clear that the signal used in this study is related to vision- the monkey had first to see the location of the target and then in one way or another this target location in the visual field of the monkey was reflected in the activity of neurons in the pre-motor area of the cortex.

This approach is somehow similar to the one taken in one of the most efficient forms of non-invasive BMIs in the terms of information transfer rates- row-column flickering based spellers (Wolpaw et al., 2002; Krusienski et al., 2008). In these spellers a subject watches a matrix of letters and symbols on a computer screen and each column or row increases in intensity for a brief period of time, 60–100 ms. Following 3–15 repetitions an accuracy >90% can be achieved. In non-invasive BMIs such an approach can routinely achieve information transfer rates of 0.25–0.5 bit/s, only two times less than it is achieved in standard center-out reaching tasks of invasive BMIs (**Figure 2**). Similarly to (Santhanam et al., 2006); most spellers use a vision related signal, either steady state evoked potentials (SSVEPs, reviewed in Vialatte et al., 2010) or P300, which in case of the EEG-based spellers is likely to be related to gaze (Brunner et al., 2010) and is clearly triggered by a visual signal. In spite of this similarity in the origins of the control signal, assuming that the "GO" cue task in Santhanam et al. (2006) and the speller tasks are similar, the invasive BMI is a clear winner with information transfer rates higher by >5 bit/s. This difference (>6 bit/s and 0.5 bit/s) correspond to a >~40 fold increase in the information transfer rates and only 3–4 bit/s shy of the rates typical for cochlear implants, ~10 bit/s. Thus, although the signal used by Santhanam and his colleagues is somehow similar to the non-invasive, EEG-based BMI signals P300 and SSVEP (Wolpaw et al., 2002), there is a dramatic difference in information transfer rates between invasive and non-invasive BMIs. May be we are not that far from electrode-array based invasive BMIs suitable for clinical applications?

The last example of an efficient invasive BMI presented here (Santhanam et al., 2006) suggests that the type of information encoded by the recorded neuronal signals in the cortical premotor areas is actually very different from what we usually think it is. This cortical area was used by many invasive BMIs although primary motor cortex may better predict upper limb movements (Wessberg et al., 2000; Carmena et al., 2003). It is difficult to compare information content in reaching and grasping tasks because we need to know the statistics of movements with and without BMI control, correlation coefficients alone cannot be directly translated into information content and, as explained above, the new suggested measure SNR (Li et al., 2009; Fitzsimmons et al., 2009) has not been validated experimentally. Although intuitively it may seem that, because of the 3-dimensionality and many degrees of freedom involved, 3D tasks correspond to large information transfer rates, Fitts' and subsequent studies on information content of human reaching movements suggest that a simple ratio of the target size (determined by the variability of the hand movement at the end point) to the distance to the target defines the information content of these movements (Fitts, 1954; MacKenzie and Buxton, 1992). Thus even for 3D tasks the information transfer rates may be similar to the ones present in 1D and 2D tasks, the data on which are shown in **Figure 2**.

If in the 3D-tasks the achieved information transfer rates are similar to the 2D-tasks, few bits per second, then may be these pre-motor neurons encode something that is not directly related to the movement trajectory? At least one study suggests that the answer is yes. It is clear that in Santhanam et al. (2006), study the pre-motor cortex neuronal signal that predicted targets was related to vision even though eyes were fixed during the period used for prediction; this choice of signal permitted to achieve the information transfer rates higher by >3–4 bit/s or by one order of magnitude compared to BMIs predicting movement. If such high information transfer rates can be achieved for a vision-related signal, maybe there is something fundamental that we are missing from the motor signal in primary and pre-motor areas? The "GO" cue permitted synchronization of all neuronal responses and a very brief time window of 250 ms could be used for decoding (Santhanam et al., 2006), something that is impossible to apply for a continuous movement decoding. It has been shown that the first few hundreds of milliseconds contain most information about the movement in the center-out reaching task (Taylor et al., 2003), indicating that after these first moments something is changed. The results of Gilja et al. (2012), suggest that the trick could be the changing coordinate system, in other words neurons encode in a coordinate system that is not fixed with respect to the subject's body/torso but moves together with the hand approaching the target.

It should be noted that, at least in theory, there is an entirely different method to achieve high information transfer rates, at least when we deal with very few neurons. It is the so-called conditional modulation that was used in 70 s (Fetz and Finocchio, 1971; Schmidt et al., 1978). It has been shown that rates up to >1 bit/s can be achieved with a single neuron (in an 8-target task the average time to target was 1.35 s, 97.5% correct, p. 359 in Schmidt et al., 1978). Similar approach was used by Kennedy and his colleagues when a single electrode was implanted in a human patient though much lower information transfer rates were achieved (<0.5 bit/s, Kennedy and Bakay, 1998). In a direct test of this idea in BMI the information transfer rates of 0.2–0.5 bit/s were achieved (Moritz and Fetz, 2011). A further modification of this approach is to directly stimulate muscles by a signal generated by such modulated neuronal activity (Moritz et al., 2008). The main question for this method is, can several neurons or groups of neurons be simultaneously modulated in independent fashion? It is known that monkeys are capable to voluntary modify the firing rates of neighboring neurons in opposite direction (Fetz and Baker, 1973); however it has yet to be shown if the same principle can be applied in BMI with at least 5–10 neurons.

Nevertheless, potentially, such a method could offer very high information transfer rates even with a limited number of channels offered by current recording technologies.

As a final note, it should be added that there are new directions in BMI research that are difficult to evaluate from the point of view of information transfer rates. One such an example can be the recent demonstration that electrical stimulation of sensory areas may provide a sensation of a surface texture (O'Doherty et al., 2011). The difficulty of the task was low- the target size was almost the same as the distance between the targets and the estimated Fitts' difficulty of the task is <1.5 bit. For the achieved travel times between targets >1 s, the estimated information transfer rate was <1.5 bit/s, no improvement over typical rates in the center-out reaching task. However, this analysis misses the fact that in some case, due to brain stimulation, a monkey was able to determine if the target touched by the monkey was correct in less than <0.35 s. Even though it is only a yes or no decision and errors were present, the estimated information transfer rate is >2.5 bit/s. In addition one has to take into account that stimulation was performed in packets at 10 Hz, thus in reality the information transfer rates of >3 bit/s could be present. Furthermore, the texture sensation may be extremely valid for human patients to improve their comfort level with new BMI devices that would make this new technology more acceptable for the patients. The information transfer rates alone cannot be used to evaluate the performance of BMI also in an entirely new trend in BMI research- neuronal restoration (Grosse-Wentrup et al., 2011). Nevertheless, for device control information transfer rates offer a universal measure of BMI performance and may prove to be very useful in better understanding of our brain function.

In summary, the provided examples suggest that we still don't have sufficient understanding about what is encoded in premotor and motor areas of the cortex in order to achieve high rates of information transfer in invasive BMIs. Probably more effort should be devoted to understanding what kind of information is represented in recorded neuronal populations while technology issues seem to be secondary, at least for now. Research on invasive BMIs provides an unparalleled opportunity to test hypothesis on how movements are encoded in the brain. It seems that neurons in cortical pre-motor areas process a significant component of vision- or/and intention-related information that can be used to better predict movements; probably future BMIs should take into account this type of information. It is known that visual feedback is important for accurate hand movements (Saunders and Knill, 2003); in all invasive BMIs subjects can see the position of a cursor or a device. However, during decoding of neuronal signals vision-related or intention-related information is almost never used for invasive BMI control; probably, because it seems to contradict the idea of BMI, namely to predict movements from neuronal activity without other additional information. Since by far the best result in the center-out or similar tasks was achieved in an invasive BMI that does use intention- or/and vision- related information, maybe it is an indication that our brains never tries to predict limb coordinates alone but always combines different types of information and these different types of information are processed by neurons in cortical pre-motor areas and used to reach the desired target. There is nothing new in this idea (Hoshi and Tanji, 2004) and it should be no surprise that the use of intention or vision-related information permitted to Santhanam et al. to achieved maximal rate of 6 bit/s in invasive BMI, not much worse than it is achieved in natural movements, ~10 bit/s, thus assuring us that one day we will have prosthetic arms, controlled by brain almost as efficiently as we can control our own hands.

ACKNOWLEDGMENTS

This work was funded by the European Social Fund under the Global Grant measure.

REFERENCES

Aggarwal, V., Mollazadeh, M., Davidson, A. G., Schieber, M. H., and Thakor, N. V. (2013). State-based decoding of hand and finger kinematics using neuronal ensemble and LFP activity during dexterous reach-to-grasp movements. *J. Neurophysiol.* 109, 3067–3081. doi: 10.1152/jn.01038.2011

Allison, B. Z., Dunne, S., Leeb, R., Millan, J. D. R., and Nijholt, A. (2012). *Towards Practical Brain-computer Interfaces.* Heidelberg; New York, NY; Dordrecht, London: Springer.

Andersen, R. A., Musallam, S., and Pesaran, B. (2004). Selecting the signals for a brain-machine interface. *Curr. Opin. Neurobiol.* 14, 720–726. doi: 10.1016/j.conb.2004.10.005

Brown, P. F., Pietra, V. J. D., Mercer, R. L., Pietra, S. A. D., and Lai, J. C. (1992). An estimate of an upper bound for the entropy of english. *Comput. Linguist.* 18, 31–40.

Brunner, P., Joshi, S., Briskin, S., Wolpaw, J. R., Bischof, H., and Schalk, G. (2010). Does the "P300" speller depends on eye gaze? *J. Neural. Eng.* 7, 056013. doi: 10.1088/1741-2560/7/5/056013

Buracas, G. T., Zador, A. M., DeWeese, M. R., and Albright, T. D. (1998). Efficient discrimination of temporal patterns by motion-sensitive neurons in primate visual cortex. *Neuron* 20, 959–969. doi: 10.1016/S0896-6273(00)80477-8

Buzsáki, G., Anastassiou, C. A., and Koch, C. (2012). The origin of extracellular fields and currents–EEG, ECoG, LFP and spikes. *Nat. Rev. Neurosci.* 13, 407–420. doi: 10.1038/nrn3241

Carmena, J. M., Lebedev, M. A., Crist, R. E., O'Doherty, J. E., Santucci, D. M., Dimitrov, D. F., et al. (2003). Learning to control a brain-machine interface for reaching and grasping by primates. *PLoS Biol.* 1:E42. doi: 10.1371/journal.pbio.0000042

Chapin, J. K., Moxon, K. A., Markowitz, R. S., and Nicolelis, M. A. (1999). Real-time control of a robot arm using simultaneously recorded neurons in the motor cortex. *Nat. Neurosci.* 2, 664–670. doi: 10.1038/10223

Cramer, D. (2003). A cautionary tale of two statistics: partial correlation and standardized partial regression. *J. Psychol.* 137, 507–511. doi: 10.1080/00223980309600632

Dunn, C. C., Noble, W., Tyler, R. S., Kordus, M., Gantz, B. J., and Ji, H. (2010). Bilateral and unilateral cochlear implant users compared on speech perception in noise. *Ear Hear.* 31, 296–298. doi: 10.1097/AUD.0b013e3181c12383

Ecker, A. S., Berens, P., Keliris, G. A., Bethge, M., Logothetis, N. K., and Tolias, A. S. (2010). Decorrelated neuronal firing in cortical microcircuits. *Science* 327, 584–587. doi: 10.1126/science.1179867

Fatourechi, M., Bashashati, A., Ward, R. K., and Birch, G. E. (2007). EMG and EOG artifacts in brain computer interface systems: a survey. *J. Clin. Neurophysiol.* 118, 480–494. doi: 10.1016/j.clinph.2006.10.019

Fetz, E. E., and Baker, M. A. (1973). Operantly conditioned patterns on precentral unit activity and correlated responses in adjacent cells and contralateral muscles. *J. Neurophysiol.* 36, 179–204.

Fetz, E. E., and Finocchio, D. V. (1971). Operant conditioning of specific patterns of neural and muscular activity. *Science* 174, 431–435. doi: 10.1126/science.174.4007.431

Fitts, P. M. (1954). The information capacity of the human motor system in controlling the amplitude of movement. *J. Exp. Psychol.* 47, 381–391. doi: 10.1037/h0055392

Fitzsimmons, N. A., Lebedev, M. A., Peikon, I. D., and Nicolelis, M. A. (2009). Extracting kinematic parameters for monkey bipedal walking from cortical neuronal ensemble activity (2009). *Front. Integr. Neurosci.* 3:3. doi: 10.3389/neuro.07.003.2009

Flint, R. D., Wright, Z. A., Scheid, M. R., and Slutzky, M. W. (2013). Long term, stable brain machine interface performance using local field potentials and multiunit spikes. *J. Neural Eng.* 10, 056005. doi: 10.1088/1741-2560/10/5/056005

Gilja, V., Nuyujukian, P., Chestek, C. A., Cunningham, J. P., Yu, B. M., Fan, J. M., et al. (2012). A high-performance neural prosthesis enabled by control algorithm design. *Nat. Neurosci.* 15, 1752–1757. doi: 10.1038/nn.3265

Grosse-Wentrup, M., Mattia, D., and Oweiss, K. (2011). Using brain-computer interfaces to induce neural plasticity and restore function. *J. Neural Eng.* 8:025004. doi: 10.1088/1741-2560/8/2/025004

Guilford, J. P., and Fruchter, B. (1973). *Fundamental Statistics in Psychology and Education*. 5th Edn. New York, NY: McGraw-Hill Book Co.

Harris, K. D., Henze, D. A., Csicsvari, J., Hirase, H., and Buzsáki, G. (2000). Accuracy of tetrode spike separation as determined by simultaneous intracellular and extracellular measurements. *J. Neurophysiol.* 84, 401–414.

Haselager, P. (2013). Did I do that? Brain–computer interfacing and the sense of agency. *Minds Mach.* 23, 405–418. doi: 10.1007/s11023-012-9298-7

Henderson, J. M., Giljam V., Pandarinath, C., Blabe, C., Hochberg, L. R., and Shenoy, K. V. (2013). High performance computer cursor control using neuronal ensemble recordings from the motor cortex of a person with ALS. *Neurosurgery* 60, 184. doi: 10.1227/01.neu.0000432784.58847.74

Henze, D. A., Borhegyi, Z., Csicsvari, J., Mamiya, A., Harris, K. D., and Buzsáki, G. (2000). Intracellular features predicted by extracellular recordings in the hippocampus *in vivo*. *J. Neurophysiol.* 84, 390–400.

Hochberg, L. R., Bacher, D., Jarosiewicz, B., Masse, N. Y., Simeral, J. D., Vogel, J., et al. (2012). Reach and grasp by people with tetraplegia using a neurally controlled robotic arm. *Nature* 485, 372–375. doi: 10.1038/nature11076

Hochberg, L. R., Serruya, M. D., Friehs, G. M., Mukand, J. A., Saleh, M., Caplan, A. H., et al. (2006). Neuronal ensemble control of prosthetic devices by a human with tetraplegia. *Nature* 442, 164–171. doi: 10.1038/nature04970

Hoshi, E., and Tanji, J. (2004). Functional specialization in dorsal and ventral premotor areas. *Prog. Brain Res.* 143, 507–511. doi: 10.1016/S0079-6123(03)43047-1

Humphrey, D. R., Schmidt, E. M., and Thompson, W. D. (1970). Predicting measures of motor performance from multiple cortical spike trains. *Science* 170, 758–762. doi: 10.1126/science.170.3959.758

Ifft, P. J., Shokur, S., Lebedev, M. A., and Nicolelis, M. A. (2013). A brain-machine interface enables bimanual arm movements in monkeys. *Sci. Transl. Med.* 5, 210ra154. doi: 10.1126/scitranslmed.3006159

Judy, J. W. (2012). Neural interfaces for upper-limb prosthesis control: opportunities to improve long-term reliability. *IEEE Pulse* 3, 57–60. doi: 10.1109/MPUL.2011.2181026

Kennedy, P. R., and Bakay, R. A. (1998). Restoration of neural output from a paralyzed patient by a direct brain connection. *Neuroreport* 9, 1707–1711. doi: 10.1097/00001756-199806010-00007

Kennedy, P. R., Bakay, R. A., Moore, M. M., and Adams, K. (2000). Direct control of a computer from the human central nervous system. *IEEE Trans. Rehabil. Eng.* 8, 198–202. doi: 10.1109/86.847815

Kennedy, P. R., Bakay, R. A., and Sharpe, S. M. (1992). Behavioral correlates of action potentials recorded chronically inside the Cone Electrode. *Neuroreport* 3, 605–608. doi: 10.1097/00001756-199207000-00015

Kim, S.-P., Simeral, J. D., Hochberg, L. R., Donoghue, J. P., and Black, M. J. (2008). Neural control of computer cursor velocity by decoding motor cortical spiking activity in humans with tetraplegia. *J. Neural Eng.* 5, 455–476. doi: 10.1088/1741-2560/5/4/010

Kim, S.-P., Simeral, J. D., Hochberg, L. R., Donoghue, J. P., Friehs, G. M., and Black, M. J. (2011). Point-and-click cursor control with an intracortical neural interface system by humans with tetraplegia. *IEEE Trans. Neural Syst. Rehabil. Eng.* 19, 193–203. doi: 10.1109/TNSRE.2011.2107750

Klobassa, D. S., Vaughan, T. M., Brunner, P., Schwartz, N. E., Wolpaw, J. R., Neuper, C., et al. (2009). Toward a high-throughput auditory P300-based brain-computer interface. *Clin. Neurophysiol.* 120, 1252–1261. doi: 10.1016/j.clinph.2009.04.019

Krusienski, D. J., Sellers, E. W., McFarland, D. J., Vaughan, T. M., and Wolpaw, J. R. (2008). Toward enhanced P300 speller performance. *J. Neurosci. Methods* 167, 15–21. doi: 10.1016/j.jneumeth.2007.07.017

Lebedev, M. A., and Nicolelis, M. A. L. (2006). Brain-machine interfaces: past, present and future. *Trends Neurosci.* 29, 536–546. doi: 10.1016/j.tins.2006.07.004

Lebedev, M. A., and Nicolelis, M. A. L. (2011). Toward a whole-body neuroprosthetic. *Prog. Brain Res.* 194, 47–60. doi: 10.1016/B978-0-444-53815-4.00018-2

Lebedev, M. A., O'Doherty, J. E., and Nicolelis, M. A. (2008). Decoding of temporal intervals from cortical ensemble activity. *J. Neurophysiol.* 99, 166–186. doi: 10.1152/jn.00734.2007

Lewicki, M. S. (1998). A review of methods for spike sorting: the detection and classification of neural action potentials. *Netw. Bristol Engl.* 9, R53–R78. doi: 10.1088/0954-898X/9/4/001

Li, Z., O'Doherty, J. E., Hanson, T. L., Lebedev, M. A., Henriquez, C. S., and Nicolelis, M. A. L. (2009). Unscented Kalman filter for brain-machine interfaces. *PLoS ONE* 4:e6423. doi: 10.1371/journal.pone.0006243

MacKenzie, I. S., and Buxton, W. (1992). "Extending Fitts Law to two-dimensional tasks," in *Proceedings of the SIGCHI Conference on Human Factors in Computing Systems, series CHI '92*, (New York, NY: ACM), 219–226. doi: 10.1145/142750.142794

MacKinnon, D. P., Fairchild, A. J., and Fritz, M. S. (2007). Mediation analysis. *Annu. Rev. Psychol.* 58, 593–614. doi: 10.1146/annurev.psych.58.110405.085542

Moller, A. R. (2006). "History of cochlear impalnts and auditory brainstem implants," in *Cohlear and Brainstem Implants. Adv. Otorhinolaryngology.* (Basel: Karger), 1–10.

Moritz, C. T., and Fetz, E. E. (2011). Volitional control of single cortical neurons in a brain machine interface. *J. Neural. Eng.* 8, 025017. doi: 10.1088/1741-2560/8/2/025017

Moritz, C. T., Perlmutter, S. I., and Fetz, E. E. (2008). Direct control of paralyzed muscles by cortical neurons. *Nature* 456, 639–643. doi: 10.1038/nature07418

Mulliken, G. H., Musallam, S., and Andersen, R. A. (2008). Decoding trajectories from posterior parietal cortex ensembles. *J. Neurosci.* 28, 12913–12926. doi: 10.1523/JNEUROSCI.1463-08.2008

Mussa-Ivaldi, F. A., and Miller, L. E. (2003). Brain-machine interfaces: computational demands and clinical needs meet basic neuroscience. *Trends Neurosci.* 26, 329–334. doi: 10.1016/S0166-2236(03)00121-8

Navarro, X., Krueger, T. B., Lago, N., Micera, S., Stieglitz, T., and Dario, P. (2005). A critical review of interfaces with the peripheral nervous system for the control of neuroprostheses and hybrid bionic systems. *J. Peripher. Nerv. Syst.* 10, 229–258. doi: 10.1111/j.1085-9489.2005.10303.x

Nelken, I., and Chechik, G. (2007). Information theory in auditory research. *Hear. Res.* 229, 94–105. doi: 10.1016/j.heares.2007.01.012

Nicolelis, M. A. L., and Lebedev, M. A. (2009). Principles of neural ensemble physiology underlying the operation of brain-machine interfaces. *Nat. Rev. Neurosci.* 10, 530–540. doi: 10.1038/nrn2653

O'Doherty, J. E., Lebedev, M. A., Ifft, P. J., Zhuang, K. Z., Shokur, S., Bleuler, H. et al. (2011). Active tactile exploration using a brain-machine-brain interface. *Nature* 479, 228–231. doi: 10.1038/nature10489

Oskoei, M. A., and Hu, H. (2007). Myoelectric control systems- a survey. *Biomed. Signal Process. Control* 2, 275–294. doi: 10.1016/j.bspc.2007.07.009

Rauschecker, J. P., and Shannon, R. V. (2002). Sending sound to the brain. *Science* 295, 1025–1029. doi: 10.1126/science.1067796

Santhanam, G., Ryu, S. I., Yu, B. M., Afshar, A., and Shenoy, K. V. (2006). A high-performance brain-computer interface. *Nature* 442, 195–198. doi: 10.1038/nature04968

Saunders, J. A., and Knill, D. C. (2003). Humans use continuous visual feedback from the hand to control fast reaching movements. *Exp. Brain Res.* 152, 341–352. doi: 10.1007/s00221-003-1525-2

Schmidt, E. M., McIntosh, J. S., Durelli, L., and Bak, M. J. (1978). Fine control of operantly conditioned firing patterns of cortical neurons. *Exp. Neurol.* 61, 349–369. doi: 10.1016/0014-4886(78)90252-2

Schwartz, A. B., Cui, X. T., Weber, D. J., and Moran, D. W. (2006). Brain-controlled interfaces: movement restoration with neural prosthetics. *Neuron* 52, 205–220. doi: 10.1016/j.neuron.2006.09.019

Schwartz, A. B., Taylor, D. M., and Tillery, S. I. (2001). Extraction algorithms for cortical control of arm prosthetics. *Curr. Opin. Neurobiol.* 11, 701–707. doi: 10.1016/S0959-4388(01)00272-0

Shannon, C. E. (1948). Mathematical theory of communication. *Bell Syst. Tech. J.* 27, 379–423, 623–656. doi: 10.1002/j.1538-7305.1948.tb00917.x

Simeral, J. D., Kim, S.-P., Black, M. J., Donoghue, J. P., and Hochberg, L. R. (2011). Neural control of cursor trajectory and click by a human with tetraplegia 1000 days after implant of an intracortical microelectrode array. *J. Neural Eng.* 8, 025027. doi: 10.1088/1741-2560/8/2/025027

Surakka, V., Illi, M., and Isokoski, P. (2004). Gazing and frowning as a new human-computer interaction technique. *ACM Trans. Appl. Percept.* 1, 40–56. doi: 10.1145/1008722.1008726

Taylor, D. M., Tillery, S. I. H., and Schwartz, A. B. (2002). Direct cortical control of 3D neuroprosthetic devices. *Science* 296, 1829–1832. doi: 10.1126/science.1070291

Taylor, D. M., Tillery, S. I. H., and Schwartz, A. B. (2003). Information conveyed through brain-control: cursor versus robot. *IEEE Trans. Neural. Syst. Rehab. Eng.* 11, 195–199. doi: 10.1109/TNSRE.2003.814451

Tehovnik, E. J., Woods, L. C., and Slocum, W. M. (2013). Transfer of information by BMI. *Neuroscience* 255, 134–146. doi: 10.1016/j.neuroscience.2013.10.003

Tonet, O., Marinelli, M., Citi, L., Rossini, P. M., Rossini, L., Megali, G., et al. (2008). Defining brain-machine interface applications by matching interface performance with device requirements. *J. Neurosci. Methods* 167, 91–104. doi: 10.1016/j.jneumeth.2007.03.015

Townsend, G., LaPallo, B. K., Boulay, C. B., Krusienski, D. J., Frye, G. E., Hauser, C. K., et al. (2010). A novel P300-based brain-computer interface stimulus presentation paradigm: moving beyond rows and columns. *Clin. Neurophysiol.* 121, 1109–1120. doi: 10.1016/j.clinph.2010.01.030

Tuisku, O., Surakka, V., Vanhala, T., Rantanen, V., and Lekkala, J. (2012). Wireless Face Interface: using voluntary gaze direction and facial muscle activations for human–computer interaction. *Interact. Comput.* 24, 1–9. doi: 10.1016/j.intcom.2011.10.002

Velliste, M., Perel, S., Spalding, M. C., Whitford, A. S., and Schwartz, A. B. (2008). Cortical control of a prosthetic arm for self-feeding. *Nature* 453, 1098–1101. doi: 10.1038/nature06996

Vialatte, F.-B., Maurice, M., Dauwels, J., and Cichocki, A. (2010). Steady state visually evoked potentials: focus on essential paradigms and future perspectives. *Prog. Neurobiol.* 90, 418–438. doi: 10.1016/j.neurobio.2009.11.005

Wessberg, J., Stambaugh, C. R., Kralik, J. D., Beck, P. D., Laubach, M., Chapin, J. K., et al. (2000). Real-time prediction of hand trajectory by ensembles of cortical neurons in primates. *Nature* 408, 361–365. doi: 10.1038/35042582

Wolpaw, J. R., Birbaumer, N., Heetderks, W. J., McFarland, D. J., Peckham, P. H., Schalk, G., et al. (2000). Brain-computer interface technology: a review of the first international meeting. *IEEE Trans. Rehabil. Eng.* 8, 164–173.

Wolpaw, J. R., Birbaumer, N., McFarland, D. J., Pfurtscheller, G., and Vaughan, T. M. (2002). Brain-computer interfaces for communication and control. *Clin. Neurophysiol.* 113, 767–791. doi: 10.1016/S1388-2457(02)00057-3

Wolpaw, J. R., and McFarland, D. J. (2004). Control of a two-dimensional movement signal by a noninvasive brain-computer interface in humans. *Proc. Natl. Acad. Sci. U.S.A.* 101, 17849–17854. doi: 10.1073/pnas.0403504101

6

Boosting visual cortex function and plasticity with acetylcholine to enhance visual perception

Jun Il Kang*[1,2], *Frédéric Huppé-Gourgues*[1] and *Elvire Vaucher*[1]

[1] *École d'optométrie, Université de Montréal, Montréal, QC, Canada*
[2] *Département de Neuroscience, Université de Montréal, Montréal, QC, Canada*

Edited by:
Mikhail Lebedev, Duke University, USA

Reviewed by:
Michael A. Silver, University of California at Berkeley, USA
Pietro Pietrini, University of Pisa Medical School, Italy

****Correspondence:***
Elvire Vaucher, École d'optométrie, Université de Montréal, CP 6128 succursale centre-ville, Montréal QC H3C 3J7, Canada
e-mail: elvire.vaucher@umontreal.ca

The cholinergic system is a potent neuromodulatory system that plays critical roles in cortical plasticity, attention and learning. In this review, we propose that the cellular effects of acetylcholine (ACh) in the primary visual cortex during the processing of visual inputs might induce perceptual learning; i.e., long-term changes in visual perception. Specifically, the pairing of cholinergic activation with visual stimulation increases the signal-to-noise ratio, cue detection ability and long-term facilitation in the primary visual cortex. This cholinergic enhancement would increase the strength of thalamocortical afferents to facilitate the treatment of a novel stimulus while decreasing the cortico-cortical signaling to reduce recurrent or top-down modulation. This balance would be mediated by different cholinergic receptor subtypes that are located on both glutamatergic and GABAergic neurons of the different cortical layers. The mechanisms of cholinergic enhancement are closely linked to attentional processes, long-term potentiation (LTP) and modulation of the excitatory/inhibitory balance. Recently, it was found that boosting the cholinergic system during visual training robustly enhances sensory perception in a long-term manner. Our hypothesis is that repetitive pairing of cholinergic and sensory stimulation over a long period of time induces long-term changes in the processing of trained stimuli that might improve perceptual ability. Various non-invasive approaches to the activation of the cholinergic neurons have strong potential to improve visual perception.

Keywords: attention, cholinergic system, cognitive enhancement, cortical plasticity, nicotinic receptors, muscarinic receptors, perceptual learning, visual cortex

INTRODUCTION

Boosting the brain's functioning during rehabilitation paradigms might help individuals with cognitive or sensory deficits to better recover their abilities. In this review, we will examine how the cholinergic system might help in this regard by specifically focusing on visual function. Recent knowledge about the cellular and functional organization of the primary visual cortex (V1) is particularly interesting for the deciphering of the neurobiological mechanisms of perceptual learning and its modulation by the cholinergic system. V1 is the first cortical step of the integration of complex visual stimuli and is decisive in the selection of specific stimuli from the visual field. This process further orients processing in higher cognitive cortical areas involved in elaboration of fine visual conscious perception. Thus, cholinergic modulation of visual processing in V1 would have strong effects on the fine-tuning of perception and the acquisition of memory traces.

Perceptual learning is the long-term improvement of the ability to detect or discriminate specific sensory stimuli without interfering with or diminishing other skills that results from training over a sustained period of time (Fahle and Poggio, 2002; Fahle, 2009; Roelfsema et al., 2010). In vision, improvements in the discrimination of specific attributes of a stimulus, such as its orientation (Ramachandran and Braddick, 1973; Fiorentini and Berardi, 1980; Mayer, 1983), contrast (Hua et al., 2010) or vernier acuity (McKee and Westheimer, 1978), have been demonstrated using such paradigms. Increases in visual capacity should go together with increases in the numbers of neurons that encode the trained stimulus in the V1 and the expansions of the cortical maps that represent the stimulus (Kilgard and Merzenich, 1998). The signal-to-noise ratio is usually increased. The connectivity between neurons and efficiency of the neuronal transmission, i.e., the strength of the input they transmit as well as the short processing time, should also be increased. Changes in dendritic spines number, morphology and synaptic plasticity (i.e., long-lasting modifications of the strength of the post-synaptic electrical signal) have also been demonstrated during perceptual learning (Gilbert and Li, 2012). However, it should be assumed that the neurons involved in perceptual learning increase the amount of information that they carry while preserving their primary selective response properties (Gilbert et al., 2001). Perceptual learning is also facilitated either by attention (Ahissar and Hochstein, 1993) or reinforcement by reward expectation (Seitz et al., 2009); both of these process enhance neuronal transmission efficiency.

Perceptual learning or increased cortical processing of specific stimuli is generally achieved with repetitive training. It has been recently suggested that it can also be boosted by neuromodulation and extrinsic control of the cerebral neuromodulatory systems by electrical or pharmacological means. The cholinergic system, which uses acetylcholine (ACh) as a neurotransmitter, is particularly relevant because it widely innervates V1 and alters the efficiency of neurons. The injection of ACh or its analogs into V1 has been shown to increase neuronal responses and trigger synaptic plasticity (Gu, 2003) and cortical plasticity (Bear and Singer, 1986). More specifically, the administration of ACh during visual processing increases thalamocortical input while reducing intracortical recurrence (Gil et al., 1997; Disney et al., 2007; Soma et al., 2013a) and thus enhances specific stimulus processing and output. This diversity of the actions of ACh is due to the ubiquitous localization of both ionotropic nicotinic receptors (nAChRs) and metabotropic muscarinic receptors (mAChRs) in V1 (Levey et al., 1991; Disney et al., 2006; Amar et al., 2010), which are involved in the facilitation of cortical activity and synchronized cortical activity. In addition to the direct and acute effects of ACh, an increasing number of studies have recently shown that repetitive cholinergic activation of the visual cortex has also the ability to enhance visual perception. The repetitive pairing of ACh release with exposure to a visual stimulus improves several visual capacities, such as contrast sensitivity (Mayer, 1983; Hua et al., 2010), motion detection (Rokem and Silver, 2010), working memory (Furey et al., 2000; Bentley et al., 2004), texture discrimination (Beer et al., 2013) and visual acuity (Kang et al., 2014) in both humans and animals. Many animal studies have also demonstrated the involvement of the cholinergic system in perceptual learning in different sensory modalities, including olfaction (Wilson et al., 2004) and audition (Bakin and Weinberger, 1996). These improvements suggest that paired visual and cholinergic stimulation induces perceptual learning possibly via synaptic and cortical modifications linked to attention mechanisms (Herrero et al., 2008) or reward expectation (Chubykin et al., 2013) and cortical plasticity. The repetition of such pairings would result in a more efficient processing and increased automaticity of visual stimuli. This could be related to reduced strength of connectivity between attention regions and V1 (Ricciardi et al., 2013) and a role of ACh in perceptual inference and repetition suppression (Moran et al., 2013).

Our research hypothesis proposes that cholinergic effects in V1 contribute to perceptual learning and can thus be used to voluntarily develop one's brain capacity and aid the restoration of visual function. In the present review, we will discuss how ACh might improve perceptual capacities, particularly during repetitive stimulation paired with visual stimulation, which are related to its roles in the long-term enhancement of cortical responsiveness and cortical plasticity (**Figure 1**). Specifically, we will first discuss the diverse effects of ACh on V1 neuron function and connectivity and relate these effects to the background theory of the cholinergic modulation of neural mechanisms and brain function. To assess these neuronal mechanisms, we will primarily discuss studies that have been performed in rodents and non-human primates (for more information about cholinergic effects on human cognition, see Drevets et al., 2008; Bentley et al., 2011).

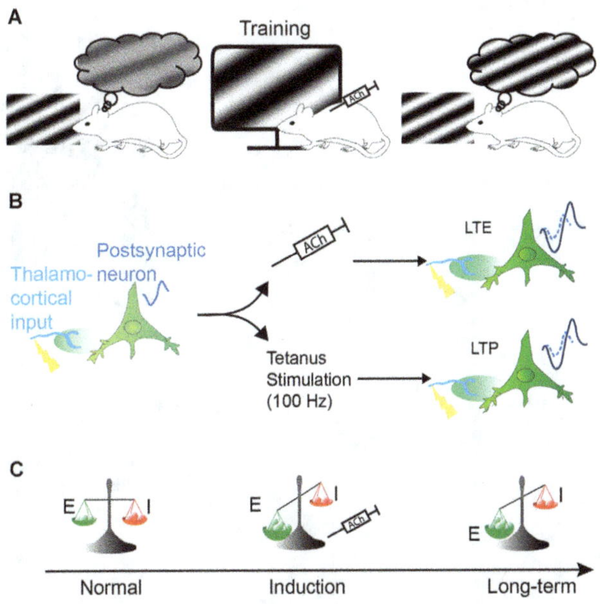

FIGURE 1 | Hypothesis of the effect of the cholinergic system on visual perception. Increase of perceptual capacity (perceptual learning) can be obtained by naturally or artificially activating the cholinergic system during sensory training. This perceptual learning might be achieved by long-term facilitation of cortical responses and/or change of the excitatory/inhibitory balance. **(A)** Representation of the improvement of visual perception in the rat by pairing the presentation of a specific sinusoidal grating coupled to cholinergic system activation (represented by injection of acetylcholine, ACh). **(B)** Long-term enhancement (LTE) of the cortical responses by ACh (upper path) share common features with classical long-term potentiation (LTP, lower path): visual stimulation of presynaptic input evokes small responses (represented by a resulting small visual evoked potential (VEP) signal waveform) in post-synaptic neurons. If paired to cholinergic activation, the presynaptic stimulation induces a long-term enhancement of neuronal responses (upper path, represented by an increased VEP signal waveform). This mechanism is similar to LTP where theta-burst stimulation (100 Hz) in lateral geniculate nucleus (LGN) induces an increase of postsynaptic potentiation in the cortex (lower path). VEP signals are imaginary waveform to compare neuronal response magnitude, as recorded in our previous experiments. **(C)** Cortical plasticity induced by ACh could also result from a change in excitatory and inhibitory balance by changing the strength of the excitatory synapse over inhibitory synapses, resulting in long-term modification of cortical responses.

ORGANIZATION OF THE CHOLINERGIC SYSTEM IN V1

Cholinergic fibers are distributed throughout the cortical layers of V1 (Lysakowski et al., 1989; Avendaño et al., 1996; Mechawar et al., 2000), which suggests that ACh might affect every step of visual processing (**Figure 2A**).

LOCAL EFFECT OF THE CHOLINERGIC FIBERS

The cholinergic system influences the local network by diffuse transmission rather than by synaptic transmission (Descarries et al., 1997; Yamasaki et al., 2010). This property is related to the fact that ACh is released from the varicosities that are distributed along the cholinergic axons and that these varicosities show only rare synaptic organizations at the ultrastructural level (Umbriaco et al., 1994; Vaucher and Hamel, 1995; Mechawar et al., 2000).

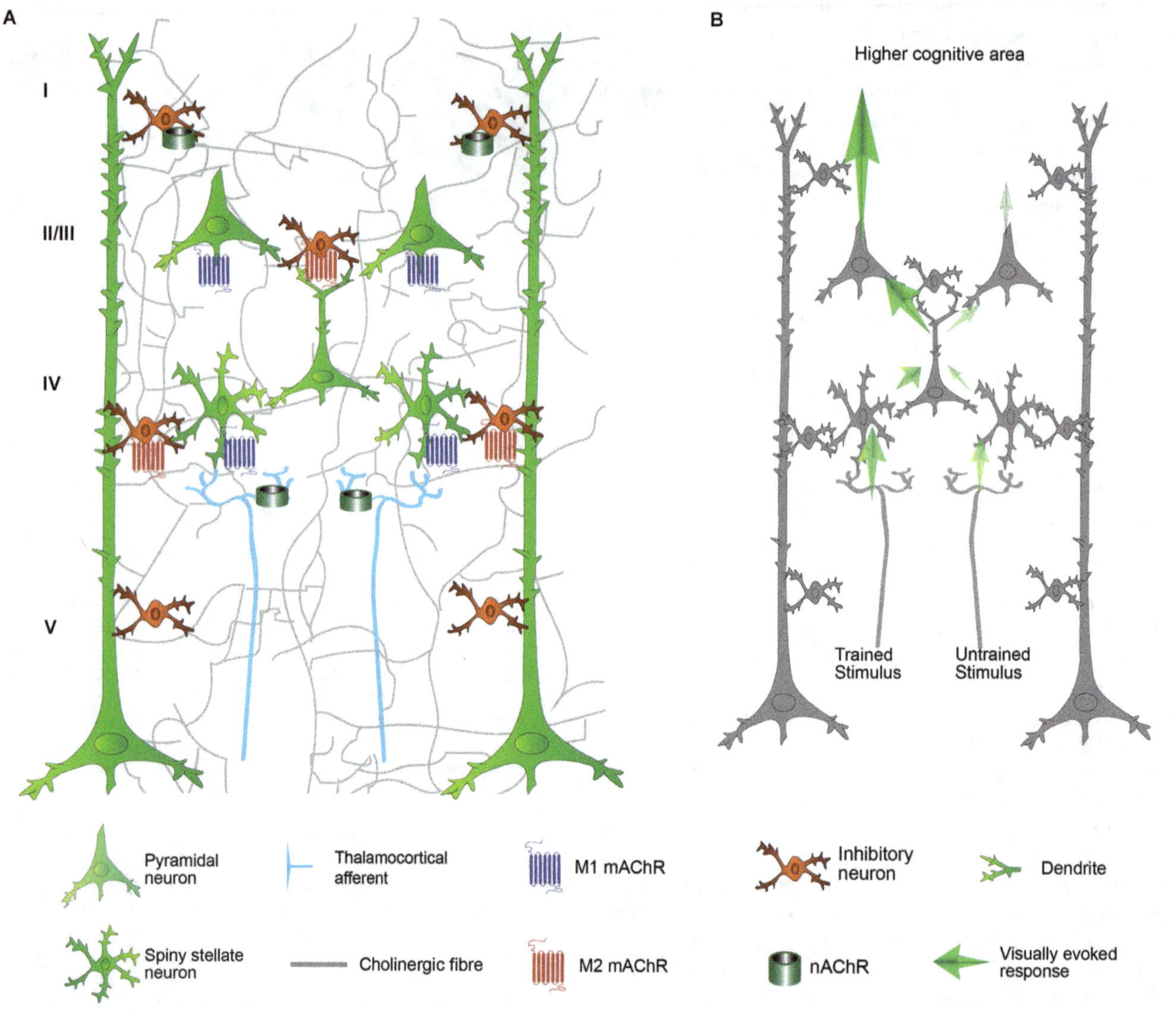

FIGURE 2 | Schematic representation of the primary visual cortex (V1) and its cholinergic modulation on cortical processing. (A) Thalamocortical afferent (light blue fibers) from LGN conveying stimulus information reach spiny stellate neuron in the layer IV. The input is transferred to the layer II/III, then layer V and to higher visual area. The cholinergic activation modulates the visual processing in virtually all the levels of V1 connectivity by nicotinic (green cylinder) and muscarinic (seven transmembrane domains molecules) receptors. **(B)** Cortical processing after VS/HDB training. The cortical processing for the trained stimulus is significantly enhanced after VS/HDB training but un-trained stimulus processing is not affected. Note that the input from the thalamus is similar but the feedforward propagation is increased. Excitatory influences are shown in blue arrows. The strength of the response enhancement is represented by the contrast of the arrow. Layer VI and horizontal connections are omitted for clarity.

However, the modulation of the cortex by ACh is not widespread and is primarily selective and adapted to the local microfunction due to the differential distribution of varicosities along the cholinergic axons (Zhang et al., 2011) and the differential distribution of the cholinergic receptor subtypes on different neuronal targets. Moreover, ACh release might be triggered by local neuronal activity to induce locally restricted rather than generalized action of the cholinergic system (Laplante et al., 2005). The variety of the cholinergic receptors and their distributions convey subtype-specific functions (Thiele, 2013; Groleau et al., 2014). In V1, AChRs exhibit differential subtype densities across the cortical layers (I-VI) on both excitatory (Gulledge et al., 2009; Thiele, 2013) and inhibitory neurons (Hashimoto et al., 1994). The distinct actions of cholinergic receptors can be related to differences in the conductances of the ionotropic receptor nAChRs for Na^+, K^+ ($\alpha_4\beta_2$) and Ca^{2+} (α_7) (Rang, 2003) and in the intracellular pathways of the different subtypes of the G-protein coupled mAChRs. Amongst the five mAChR subtypes identified, the M1, M3 and M5 mAChRs are coupled with Gq/11 proteins, which activate phospholipase C and lead to increases in intracellular Ca^{2+} and the M2 and M4 mAChRs are bound with Gi protein that inhibits adenylyl cyclase, which leads to a decrease in cAMP, the inhibition of voltage-gated Ca^{2+} channels and an increased K^+ efflux (Caulfield and Birdsall, 1998; Wess, 2003). In addition,

M1 promotes the opening of NMDARs and induces LTP in the hippocampus (Buchanan et al., 2010; Giessel and Sabatini, 2010).

CHOLINERGIC FIBERS ACTIVATION IN V1

Stimulation of the cholinergic system in V1 can be achieved via the administration of ACh analogs (e.g., carbachol), cholinergic receptor agonists (e.g., nicotine and selective mAChR drugs) or cholinesterase inhibitors or through electrical or optogenetic stimulation of the cholinergic neurons that project to V1. The cholinergic neurons that project to V1 are located in the basal forebrain (BF), particularly the ventral pallidum, substantia innominata and the horizontal limb of the diagonal band of Broca (HDB; Gaykema et al., 1990; Laplante et al., 2005). Although the nucleus basalis magnocellularis is the main cholinergic nucleus of the BF which innervates the cortical mantle, it projects only weakly to V1 (Luiten et al., 1987; Vaucher and Hamel, 1995); nevertheless, some studies report that the stimulation of this nucleus might induce functional changes in the visual cortex (Goard and Dan, 2009; Pinto et al., 2013). Moreover, although there are GABAergic neurons in the BF, many studies have confirmed that the effects of BF stimulation are identical to those of intracerebral injections of ACh agonists and are primarily mediated by the cholinergic fibers (Dauphin et al., 1991; Ma and Suga, 2005; Dringenberg et al., 2007; Kocharyan et al., 2008; Kang and Vaucher, 2009). There are also intrinsic cholinergic neurons that represent only 10–15% of the total cortical innervation (Eckenstein et al., 1988; Chédotal et al., 1994), and the involvement of these neurons in cortical processing remains unclear.

ACETYLCHOLINE MODULATES THE FLOW OF VISUAL INFORMATION IN V1

The efficiencies of the cortical inputs and outputs are altered by the different cholinergic receptors in both the glutamatergic and GABAergic systems according to the cortical layer, neuron and receptor subtype reached by ACh (**Figure 2**). V1 integrates visual information via different pathways that include the following: the feedforward thalamocortical pathways, V1 intracortical connectivities, and the feedback influence from higher cortical areas (**Figure 3**). The visual information arriving to layer IV of V1 from the lateral geniculate nucleus (LGN) is considered to be the dominant thalamocortical visual pathway. In contrast, the intracortical pathway might arise from neighboring neurons, local recurrent axons or more broadly from horizontal networks. The cholinergic system induces facilitation, suppression or does not affect the visual cells. Direct local effects of ACh might be opposed to the indirect effects of ACh due to neuronal interactions across layers. The general picture of the cholinergic influence on V1 is that the response to a stimulus is increased by cholinergic modulation in the thalamocortical pathway while the intracortical influence is suppressed. The cholinergic influence described in the following paragraph represents the acute effects in V1 that can participate in attention and trigger perceptual learning. The effects of the cholinergic system on long-range corticocortical relationships are also of interest but are beyond the scope of this review.

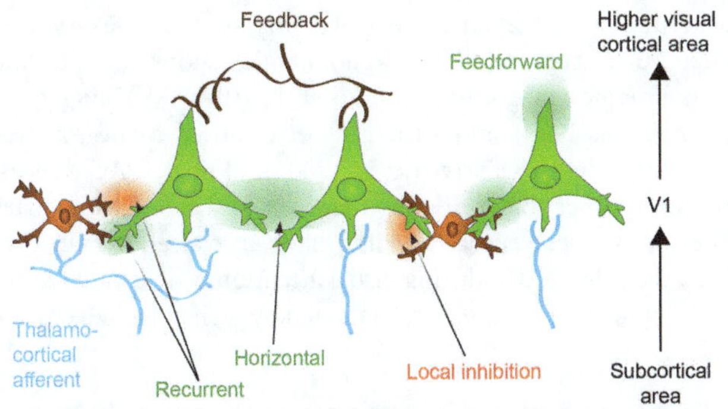

FIGURE 3 | Neuronal connectivity within the primary visual cortex (V1). Neurons from V1 receive thalamocortical (in blue) and corticocortical inputs originating from upper cortical areas (feedback control, in brown). The thalamocortical information is integrated within V1 and further transmitted to upper cortical areas (feedforward transmission). The activation of neurons might enhance activation or inhibition of neighboring neuron by the horizontal connections or through the local inhibitory interneurons. Recurrent connections auto-regulates neuronal activity (see text for more details). Excitatory effect is expressed as green color and inhibitory effect as red.

CHOLINERGIC MODULATION OF THALAMOCORTICAL INPUTS

Cortical responses to sensory stimuli transmitted by the LGN are amplified during learning and experience-dependent plasticity to emphasize relevant information (Sarter et al., 2005; Wang et al., 2013). These thalamic afferents are of prime relevance because they define the receptive fields and other properties of V1 neurons. Complex information is extracted according to its properties (e.g., orientation) via projections to different columns (in primates) or specific cells (in rodents). Cholinergic activation in this layer induces a general increase in responsiveness regardless of the features of the visual stimuli (e.g., orientation; Disney et al., 2012), which allows the cortex to respond reliably to weak stimulation (Disney et al., 2007). ACh increases the thalamocortical input through presynaptic nAChRs on the thalamocortical fibers (Gil et al., 1997; Disney et al., 2007; **Figures 2A, 4**). The M1 mAChR also amplifies the spiny stellate cell/pyramidal cell response through a postsynaptic intracellular pathway (Gu, 2003), but inhibition through the M4 mAChR has also been observed on spiny neurons in the somatosensory cortex (Eggermann and Feldmeyer, 2009). Interestingly, the cholinergic facilitation of thalamocortical inputs in sensory cortex slices is ACh-concentration dependent. High doses of ACh enhance the thalamocortical afferents both *in vitro* and in computational models (Hasselmo, 2006; Deco and Thiele, 2011). Together, these results indicate that, under conditions of high levels of ACh release, the enhancement of the thalamocortical inputs in layer IV facilitates the transmission of sensory information and induces experience-dependent plasticity (e.g., learning).

CHOLINERGIC MODULATION OF INTRACORTICAL INTERACTIONS

In addition to the enhancement of thalamocortical inputs, ACh might modulate intracortical connectivity either by suppressing lateral inhibition (Kimura and Baughman, 1997; Metherate et al., 2005; Metherate, 2011) or suppressing the spread of the excitation of thalamic inputs (Kimura et al., 1999; Silver et al., 2008). The presynaptic mAChRs that are located on the glutamatergic fibers induce a suppression of the intracortical neurons (Gil et al., 1997), although the inhibition of GABAergic terminals induces a disinhibition of the pyramidal cells (Ji and Dani, 2000; Christophe et al., 2002; Seeger et al., 2004; Salgado et al., 2007). Intracortical connectivity modulates the response intensity and the output of V1 neurons (**Figure 3**). The lateral connections also synchronize the firing of similar neuronal populations (Gilbert and Wiesel, 1989; Lien and Scanziani, 2013), which allows for lateral correlation between neurons with similar orientation preferences during typical perceptual learning tasks (e.g., the Vernier acuity test) (Ramalingam et al., 2013). The differential action of ACh on lateral connections might simultaneously enhance specific modules of the same orientation (lateral correlation) while depressing adjacent irrelevant modules (McGuire et al., 1991; Stettler et al., 2002). A recent study using optogenetics showed that inhibition of the intracortical excitatory neurons leads to a receptive field reduction (Li et al., 2013), and this finding is consistent with the effect of ACh release in V1 (Roberts et al., 2005; Zinke et al., 2006) and the increases in the population receptive fields of M1/M3 mAChR knock-out mice (Groleau et al., 2014). Furthermore, an ACh esterase inhibitor reduces surround suppression in a perceptual study in humans (Kosovicheva et al., 2012), which could be indicative of a weakening of lateral connections. Hasselmo (2006) proposed that high ACh levels suppress the magnitude of feedback excitation, whereas low ACh levels result in weaker afferent input to the cortex. Similarly, Deco and Thiele (2011) also proposed that high ACh levels decrease the intracortical interactions and that low ACh increase these interactions. The hypothesis of these authors was confirmed in an *in vitro* study that showed that the enhancement of the recurrent cortical activity in low-dose ACh conditions was independent of the thalamocortical input (Wester and Contreras, 2013). Together, these results suggest that during intense ACh release, the intracortical connections are inhibited, which relieves the sensory cortices from recurrent connections. However, in low concentration of ACh situations, the lateral connections might amplify the thalamocortical activity amongst similarly tuned neurons.

These effects have primarily been recorded within layer II/III; however, in layers I, V and VI, which are primarily involved in feedback mechanisms, ACh might also influence feedforward processing by interacting with neurons in layers IV and II/III (De Pasquale and Sherman, 2012). Layer I neurons are densely innervated by the cholinergic projections (Vaucher and Hamel, 1995; Mechawar et al., 2000). It has been shown that inhibitory actions mediated by AChRs can suppress layer II/III (Zinke et al., 2006; Alitto and Dan, 2012; Soma et al., 2013b) and layer V pyramidal neuron activity (Lucas-Meunier et al., 2009; Amar et al., 2010) and can also inhibit the cortical GABAergic network and thus result in the disinhibition of the majority of the cortical layers (Christophe et al., 2002). It has been observed that local ACh application primarily suppresses the activity of layer VI neurons (Disney et al., 2012), which can alter the activation of all of the layers of V1 in a linear manner via the intracortical pathway (Olsen et al., 2012) and alter the activation of the thalamocortical fibers (Cudeiro and Sillito, 2006; Sillito et al., 2006). Cholinergic action might thus disinhibit the activities of other layers by suppressing layer VI. Topical injections of ACh into layer V produce the predominant effect of facilitation of the regular and fast-spiking cells (Soma et al., 2013b), although local ACh activation seems to decrease excitatory drive through presynaptic M1 mAChRs (Kimura and Baughman, 1997) and to increase inhibitory drive through M3 mAChRs (Amar et al., 2010). Similarly, an increase in the activation of GABAergic neurons activation in layer V has been observed following repetitive BF/visual pairing (Kang et al., 2014). Layer V pyramidal neurons send dense projections to the superior colliculus and diverse thalamic nuclei that are involved in focused attention.

Finally, ACh can promote the co-activation of different cortical areas and layers which might be an efficient method for the selection of visual information via a summation of the temporally coincident presynaptic spikes (Fries et al., 2007). It has been shown that visually driven gamma power is differentially distributed across the layers of V1 (Xing et al., 2012) and that gamma oscillations can be induced by cholinergic stimulation (Rodriguez et al., 2004; Bhattacharyya et al., 2013).

In conclusion, BF stimulation that facilitates the release of ACh in multiple layers of V1 might act in diverse manners and results in the enhancement of visual stimulus-driven responses. The pre-amplified responses of layer IV are filtered out by GABAergic neurons of layer II/III to transfer task-relevant information to higher visual cortical areas. The activated synaptic connections can be modulated by layers V and VI or by the feedback mechanism of layer I. Differential responses across layers might be integrated by the synchronization of their activities in the gamma-band to facilitate visual processes.

CELLULAR EFFECTS OF ACETYLCHOLINE IN V1-RELATED ATTENTION

Most of these cellular mechanisms contribute to attentional mechanisms in V1. Attention increases the cortical response to stimuli (i.e., the signal) while lowering interference from the background (i.e., the noise). Several animal studies have described deficits of attention following cholinergic lesions or injections of cholinergic antagonists (Voytko et al., 1994; McGaughy and Sarter, 1998, 1999) and ACh has been shown to be involved in attention in V1 (Herrero et al., 2008). However, ACh release promotes rather than initiates attention. Because ACh-mediated attention and perceptual learning have crucial effects on each other, the role of ACh during visual attention is delineated in the following section to better understand how ACh enhances cortical functioning.

CHOLINERGIC INVOLVEMENT IN BOTTOM-UP AND TOP-DOWN ATTENTION

ACh has been suggested to control the balance between bottom-up and top-down processing through attentional mechanisms (Yu and Dayan, 2002, 2005; Sarter et al., 2005). This influence is mediated by pre-synaptic thalamocortical nAChRs (Gil et al., 1997; Disney et al., 2007). Attention that is prompted by the properties of a stimulus, i.e., the saliency of the stimulus relative to the background, is said to be bottom-up attention, whereas attention that is prompted by the voluntary direction of focus toward a specific stimulus is defined as top-down attention. Although it can be difficult to separate bottom-up and top-down attentional control (Ansorge et al., 2010; Egeth et al., 2010; Eimer and Kiss, 2010; Theeuwes, 2010), some studies have shown that cholinergic activity influences bottom-up attention. The effect of ACh on bottom-up attention might occur not only in V1 but also in early processing areas such as the thalamus. For example, the direct injection of 192-IgG saporin into the BF causes a complete loss of cholinergic projections to the neocortex but causes restricted fiber lesions when injected into V1. The injection of 192-IgG saporin into the BF but not V1 affects performance in the sustained attention task (McGaughy and Sarter, 1998, 1999). In addition, compared to controls and ex-smokers, human smokers have been shown to exhibit increased subcortical activity during an attentional task (Nestor et al., 2011). These data indicate that attentional dysfunction following cholinergic lesions might be due to the disruption of detection processes that are independent of V1. However, there is no direct evidence of cholinergic enhancement effect in bottom-up attention in human studies (Rokem et al., 2010). In contrast, there is a growing body of evidence showing that ACh is involved in top-down attention. Direct effects of ACh on attention in the visual cortex have been measured (Herrero et al., 2008; Bauer et al., 2012). Specifically, Herrero et al. provided direct evidence that ACh in V1 enhances the cortical response to an attentional demand (Herrero et al., 2008). It has also been shown that lesions to the cholinergic system impair attention performance and increase neuronal activity in the PFC upon the presentation of distractors (which trigger top-down attention) (Gill et al., 2000). Taken together, these results indicate that ACh can facilitate task-relevant learning in V1 by promoting attentional states in both top-down and bottom-up manners.

CHOLINERGIC MODULATION OF RESPONSE GAIN

Response gain modulation by ACh has frequently been observed (Disney et al., 2007; Aggelopoulos et al., 2011; Bhattacharyya et al., 2013; Soma et al., 2013a) and follows the gain control model at least in terms of the contrast-response function. Increasing thalamocortical pathway input in a context-independent manner while context-dependent intracortical suppression occurs might facilitate the transmission of information related to novel stimuli. In V1, context-dependent (i.e., increases in the maximal response) and independent (i.e., increases in the baseline response) gain control due to cholinergic effects have both been observed (80% and 20%, respectively) without any laminar bias (Soma et al., 2013b). These findings could be related to the optimization of the gain of supragranular pyramidal cells controlled by ACh which could result in the detection of novel stimuli and hence perceptual learning (Moran et al., 2013). Interestingly, gain modulation was proposed as function that underlies of attentional control (Keitel et al., 2013) and network connectivity (Haider and McCormick, 2009). The high gain that results from the amplification of the responses of excited neurons is similar to attention processes (Servan-Schreiber et al., 1990; Eldar et al., 2013) and hence facilitates learning. Taken together, these results suggest that ACh might assist in visual perceptual learning via modulation of cortical responses through gain control in both stimulus-dependent and -independent manners.

CELLULAR EFFECTS OF ACETYLCHOLINE IN V1 IN RELATION TO CORTICAL PLASTICITY

Learning and perceptual learning are sustained by cortical plasticity which triggers anatomical reorganization of the cortical connectivity. The cholinergic system plays also a key role in cortical plasticity. For example, the blockade of cholinergic activation via cholinergic antagonists or cholinergic fiber lesions results in robust impairment of learning in rats (Conner et al., 2003; Dotigny et al., 2008) and ocular dominance plasticity in kittens (Bear and Singer, 1986). In acute preparations, cholinergic pairing is also involved in plasticity as observed in the cat auditory cortex; the application of ACh during acoustic processing alters the receptive fields of single neurons in a tone-specific manner (Metherate and Weinberger, 1990). The pairing of cholinergic and auditory stimulation also leads to the reorganization of the cortical map (Kilgard and Merzenich, 1998); i.e., an enlargement of the representation of the specifically trained frequency. Cholinergic pairing with sensory stimulation also induces long-lasting effects on cortical responsiveness observed in both the visual cortex (Dringenberg et al., 2007; Kang et al., 2014) and the somatosensory cortex (Verdier and Dykes, 2001). Cortical plasticity is essential for the occurrence of perceptual learning (for review see Fahle, 2009), although not systematic, cholinergic-sensory paired activation would thus facilitate the induction of perceptual learning in the sensory cortices (Reed et al., 2011).

CHOLINERGIC MODULATION OF LONG-TERM CORTICAL RESPONSIVENESS

At the neuronal level, ACh has been shown to contribute to cortical plasticity through both the acute and long-term modulation of synaptic responses (Sato et al., 1987; Soma et al., 2012). The impairment of learning by cholinergic antagonists is similar to the effect of blocking cortical plasticity mechanisms and LTP with NMDA receptor (NMDAR) antagonists (Morris et al., 1986; Artola and Singer, 1987; Cooke and Bear, 2010). In most situations, LTP in the visual cortex induced by high theta-burst stimulation (100 Hz) (Heynen and Bear, 2001; Dringenberg et al., 2007) has been found to be NMDAR-dependent. Interestingly, cholinergic system-induced cortical plasticity has also been found to be NMDAR-dependent (Verdier and Dykes, 2001; Dringenberg et al., 2007; Kang and Vaucher, 2009) but independent of theta-burst stimulation (Kirkwood et al., 1999; **Figure 1B**). Previous studies in hippocampal slices have shown that NMDAR opening during LTP induction is facilitated by mAChR activation (Buchanan et al., 2010) and administration of ACh to pyramidal neurons (Shinoe et al., 2005). Additionally, NMDAR-dependent long-term facilitation of synaptic responses is associated with ACh release in V1, and LTP is impaired in the visual cortices of mAChR knock-out mice (Origlia et al., 2006).

CHOLINERGIC MODULATION OF THE EXCITATION-INHIBITION BALANCE

Another contribution of the cholinergic system to cortical plasticity mechanisms in V1 is the alteration of the excitatory and inhibitory (E-I) balance (**Figure 1C**). The excitatory and inhibitory synaptic inputs tend to equilibrate during maturation to optimally tune the neurons according to sensory experiences

(Hensch et al., 1998; Sun et al., 2010) during the critical period; i.e., the post-natal time window during which mammals visual cortices are highly plastic that terminates with the maturation of the neurons. It has been proposed that disrupting the E-I balance can re-open the critical period after maturation (Hensch, 2004). Neuromodulation can also disrupt the E-I balance and contribute to cortical plasticity. Recent studies have also demonstrated numerous examples of cortical plasticity that are modified by the inhibitory system (Hensch, 2005). The onset of the critical period is accelerated by GABAA inhibitory receptor activation (Fagiolini and Hensch, 2000; Iwai et al., 2003). Conversely, it is also possible to re-induce plasticity after the critical period by reducing the inhibitory drive via the injection of GABAA receptor antagonists (Harauzov et al., 2010). As the inhibitory system is strongly modulated by the cholinergic system through the protein Lynx1 (Takesian and Hensch, 2013), which acts as a brake on nAChR-dependent plasticity (Morishita et al., 2010), by nAChRs (Christophe et al., 2002; Arroyo et al., 2012), or by mAChRs (Salgado et al., 2007), cholinergic activation might modulate the E-I balance and facilitate cortical plasticity in adults that would promote perceptual learning. An interaction between the cholinergic and GABAergic systems has been shown to occur following BF stimulation that increases the activation of Parvalbumin-positive (PV+) neurons through mAChRs (Dotigny et al., 2008; Alitto and Dan, 2012). Interestingly, Alitto and Dan used an optogenetic method to show that the nAChRs on vasoactive intestinal peptide-positive (VIP+) neurons and layer I neurons can inhibit excitatory and PV+ neurons (Christophe et al., 2002).

The cholinergic modulation of V1 thus promotes cortical plasticity through LTP-like long-term enhancement of synaptic responses to subsequent presentations of a visual stimulus and through control of the excitatory-inhibitory balance that regulate the strength of cortical output and internal connectivity. The cortical plasticity induced by cholinergic stimulation could transfer the acute cholinergic effect into long-term scale to produce visual precision.

REPETITIVE CHOLINERGIC STIMULATION TRIGGERS PERCEPTUAL LEARNING

In summary, acute effects of cholinergic activation might amplify the thalamocortical response that promotes the transmission of sensory inputs. Intensive release of ACh might also inhibit intracortical interactions and relieve the internal brake on processing in the sensory cortices. Simultaneously, neurons with similar tuning characteristics (e.g., orientation) are co-activated via lateral connections to enhance the transfer of visual information. This cholinergic alternation might contribute to gain control modulation in both stimulus-dependent or and -independent manners and prioritize the processing of selected visual stimuli; this process might be linked to attention and is the first step of perceptual learning. The cholinergic activation also induces the NMDAR-dependent LTP-like long-term enhancement (i.e., cortical plasticity) and relief of the brakes on plasticity by altering the E-I balance. The repetitive coupling of visual and cholinergic stimulation results in reinforcement of all of these acute mechanisms and generate gamma-band synchronization. This would result in the consolidation of the synaptic strengths of new and existing neuronal connections, facilitation of the processing of certain thalamocortical inputs while suppressing others. It has been shown that increases in the cortical responses by expanding the number of neurons to a stimulation (via increases in the strength of the connections) would improve perceptual capacity (Anton-Erxleben and Carrasco, 2013). The repetitive cholinergic-visual stimulation would also increase the efficiency and automaticity of these selected pathways. These processes contribute to perceptual learning.

REPETITIVE CHOLINERGIC STIMULATION PROMOTES LONG-TERM POTENTIATION

As mentioned above, ACh can induce NMDAR-dependent long-term modifications of postsynaptic glutamatergic neurons which are related to memory formation. The opening of the NMDAR launches a second messenger cascade and guides the expression of synaptic glutamate receptors (Regehr and Tank, 1990; Zhong et al., 2006) but also activates autoregulated kinases that confer a persistent improved response of the neuron to the stimulus. Immunohistochemistry for the c-Fos, which is an immediate early gene and also a transcription factor for synaptogenesis genes, has revealed that c-Fos is increased in layer II/III pyramidal neurons following a repetitive BF/visual stimulation (Kang et al., 2014), which may be indicative of the formation of new synapses and LTP mechanisms. Repetitive pairing of the cholinergic and visual stimulation also induces morphological reorganization, i.e., increase in the numbers of cholinergic varicosities in the proximity of the neurons that are sensitive to the orientation of the stimulus (Zhang et al., 2011). This increased number of cholinergic inputs, along with postsynaptic mechanisms, would increase and consolidate the response of the activated neurons to ameliorate its long-term efficiency. Thus repetitive cholinergic stimulation might enhance the encoding of the memory and morphological modifications.

REPETITIVE CHOLINERGIC STIMULATION PROMOTES STIMULUS SELECTION AND AMPLIFICATION

We suggest that selection of decisive inputs is controlled by the cholinergic system and contributes to the specific enhancement of a particular stimulus in perceptual learning. Modulation of the orientation selectivity of the neurons provides a great example of the possible improvement of perceptual sensitivity. Training of the rat to a preferred or a non-preferred orientation might increase the cortical response for this orientation (Cooke and Bear, 2010; **Figure 4**). These mechanisms are facilitated by repetitive cholinergic activation, which improve orientation discrimination of human or rats (Rokem and Silver, 2010; Kang et al., 2014). Repetitive cholinergic stimulation coupled with a certain orientation stimulus might favor the discrimination of this stimulus by two different cellular mechanisms (**Figure 4**). First, ACh can harmonize the activation of the whole dendritic tree of layer II/III neurons to preserve their orientation selectivity and confer responsiveness to new orientation—the dendrites of the layer II/III neurons receive inputs randomly over all of their branches, some of which are selective for the neurons'

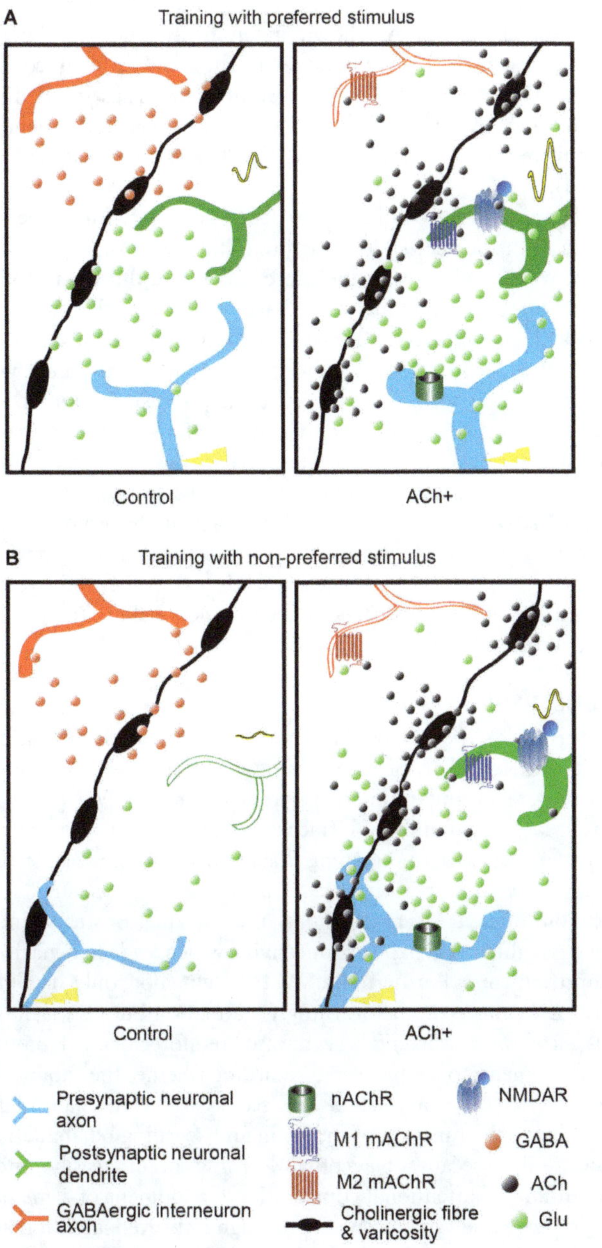

FIGURE 4 | Summary of the effect of acetylcholine on neuronal transmission of the visual inputs. The varicose cholinergic fiber (black fiber with swellings) can act on excitatory input (blue axon), neighboring GABAergic inhibitory input (red axon) and on V1 neurons (green dendrite). Excitatory/inhibitory influences are represented by red and green dots, respectively. Cholinergic activation (ACh+, right panel) is represented by black dots. The cortical response to the stimulus is represented by a VEP signal waveform which changes are elicited by increased numbers of neurons responding to the trained stimulus or increased neurons efficiency. **(A)** Response of the V1 neuron after a training with preferred stimulus coupled to cholinergic activation (right panel, ACh+) or without (left panel, control). The cortical response to this stimulus is increased (high VEP signal waveform in right panel compared to small VEP signal waveform in left panel). In presence of cholinergic activation the inhibitory influence is reduced by M2 muscarinic receptors (mAChRs), the postsynaptic excitatory influence is increased by M1 mAChRs located on the postsynaptic neuron *(Continued)*

FIGURE 4 | Continued
and nAChRs located on the thalamocortical fiber and a long-term effect is triggered by NMDA receptor activation, compared to normal condition (control, left panel). In a normal visual process (control) local or recurrent inhibition via GABAergic interneuron (in red) blocks the development to a long-term modification. **(B)** Response of the V1 neuron after a training with non-preferred stimulus coupled to cholinergic activation (right panel, ACh+) or without (left panel, control). The neuronal response to this stimulus is increased (small VEP signal waveform in right panel compared to flat VEP signal waveform in left panel). In normal condition (control, left panel), non-preferred orientation stimulus does not evoke activation in postsynaptic neurons in V1. Weak thalamocortical innervation is suppressed by GABAergic inhibition and hence fails to transmit to postsynaptic neuron. Acetylcholine can amplify the weak presynaptic input (ACh+) by nicotinic receptors and activates postsynaptic neuron through M1 muscarinic receptor. GABAergic inhibition is suppressed by M2 muscarinic receptor and NMDA receptor opening occurs leading to long-term modification.

un-preferred orientations (Jia et al., 2010). Second, the cholinergic system can enhance orientation discrimination through its interaction with the GABAergic system which assists in the sharpening (Isaacson and Scanziani, 2011) of the convergent input in the layer II/III neurons (Nassi and Callaway, 2009) but also filters out task-relevant information during perceptual learning (Roberts and Thiele, 2008). PV+ and somatostatin-positive (SOM+) GABAergic neurons are particularly involved in orientation tuning in V1 (Atallah et al., 2012; Wilson et al., 2012). It has been shown that the specific activation of PV+ neurons in V1 improves orientation discrimination abilities in awake rats during perceptual learning (Lee et al., 2012) and repetitive coupling of ACh to visual stimulation activates the V1 GABAergic neurons (Dotigny et al., 2008; Kang et al., 2014).

Thus repetitive cholinergic pairing to sensory training enhances the cortical response to trained feature of the sensory stimulus that increases the influence of the feedforward afferent.

REPETITIVE CHOLINERGIC STIMULATION PROMOTES PERCEPTUAL LEARNING RELATED TO ATTENTION, REWARD EXPECTATION AND CONNECTIVITY

Repetitive cholinergic stimulation first promotes attentional mechanisms that are necessary to perceptual learning (Ahissar and Hochstein, 1993; Schoups et al., 2001; Li et al., 2004; Mukai et al., 2007). These attentional processes might be also related to synchronization in the gamma band (30–90 Hz) (Fries et al., 2008) induced by repetitive cholinergic stimulation which has been proposed to facilitate the transfer of the visual information to higher visual areas. ACh can also promote task-irrelevant perceptual learning that occurs in the absence of conscious effort (Skrandies and Fahle, 1994; Watanabe et al., 2002; Gutnisky et al., 2009). Compared to task-relevant learning, which utilizes focused attention as reinforcement, studies of task-irrelevant learning have suggested that reward serves as the reinforcement signal (Seitz et al., 2009; Chubykin et al., 2013). During task-irrelevant learning, the response to a feature on which attention was not directed can also be enhanced (Watanabe et al., 2001; Giordano et al., 2009; Gutnisky et al., 2009). Interestingly, rewards can affect the visual response in V1 (Shuler and Bear, 2006), and the cholinergic system can influence reward timing expectancy (Chubykin et al., 2013). To reconcile studies showing a role of attention in perceptual learning or not, Roelfsema proposed that the attentional feedback signal related to the cholinergic system that enhances the plasticity of task-relevant features in the visual cortex also causes the inhibition of task-irrelevant features so that their plasticity is switched off (Roelfsema et al., 2010).

To a cognitive point of view, by modulating synaptic transmission in V1 and modifying the cortical dynamics, ACh can also participates in the perceptual inference to increase the strength of the representation of trained stimuli and reduce the sensory noise (Yu and Dayan, 2002) and induce sensory precision (Moran et al., 2013). It might suppress the top-down sources in the balance between top-down and bottom-up information integration in V1 (Yu and Dayan, 2005). This is in agreement with a recent study demonstrating that the cholinergic enhancement reduces the connectivity strength between cortical regions involved in attention and V1 (Ricciardi et al., 2013) and reduce the activity in frontoparietal regions (Furey et al., 2008). This suggests an increased neural efficiency in the processing of the trained stimulus that leads to an improved perceptual task performance (Ricciardi et al., 2013) linked to an automation of the cortical processing and a reduction of the attentional load required to process the trained stimulus (Furey, 2011).

Together, the findings from recent work using different techniques suggests that cholinergic pairing induces perceptual learning via different mechanisms that include the following: (1) the use of the layer II/III GABAergic system to filter the pre-amplified response from layer IV; (2) NMDAR-dependent modification at the postsynaptic level to induce long-term augmentations of individual neurons, and an increase in the numbers of cholinergic varicosities to facilitate ACh release; and (3) changes in the efficiency of the connectivity between cortical areas and bottom-up and top-down control.

CLINICAL PERSPECTIVES OF CHOLINERGIC MODULATION OF BRAIN'S FUNCTION

Similar with experimental data, some clinical studies have demonstrated that enhancing cholinergic system improves perception (Furey et al., 2000; Bentley et al., 2004; Wilson et al., 2004; Rokem and Silver, 2010; Beer et al., 2013; Ricciardi et al., 2013). Clinically, a method to enhance cholinergic function might involve the use of ACh esterase inhibitors, such as physostigmine, galantamine, rivastigmine or donepezil. Nicotine is also a well-known molecule that enhances cognitive function. These drugs are currently used to the treatment of Alzheimer's disease or diverse dementia. Orally administered nicotine or smoking improve attentional performance (Nestor et al., 2011; Newhouse et al., 2011), learning (Riekkinen and Riekkinen, 1997; Olausson et al., 2004), attention (Thiel et al., 2005; Nestor et al., 2011) and memory consolidation (Beer et al., 2013) through the activation of nAChRs. Increases in ACh action due to the administration of acetylcholinesterase inhibitors or direct mAChRs agonists alleviate cognitive deficits in Alzheimer's disease (Cummings, 2003), Parkinson's disease (Fagerström et al., 1994; Holmes et al., 2011) and schizophrenia patients (Shekhar et al., 2008). An $\alpha 7$ nAChR agonist is also used as a cognitive enhancer in patients with schizophrenia (Freedman, 2013) and Alzheimer's disease (Hilt et al., 2009). As shown in an fMRI study, cholinergic action potentiates communication efficiency between cortical areas (Wylie et al., 2012). The use of these drugs in cholinergically healthy subjects might also be beneficial for enhancing cognitive function (Buchanan et al., 2008; Demeter and Sarter, 2013).

Some pharmacological approaches have been developed to increase the perceptual learning in healthy humans. Performance improvements following the use of donepezil during a motion direction discrimination task have confirmed that systemic blockade of ACh esterase can induce perceptual learning (Rokem and Silver, 2010, 2013). Cholinergic amplifications paired with sensory stimulations might also be a promising approach to accelerating visual recovery following lesions to the retina or the optical nerve. If the neuronal mechanisms that occur during perceptual learning and after retinal lesions are similar (Gilbert and Li, 2012) (i.e., they both involve changes in the responsiveness of cortical neurons to inputs from outside the neurons' preferred receptive fields (Darian-Smith and Gilbert, 1994)), then ACh might also aid to boost structural and functional plasticity of the visual cortex to recover from losses of retinal input.

CONCLUSION

In this review, we proposed that the neuromodulator ACh, which is known for its involvement in attention and learning, might participate in and promote perceptual learning. We proposed that, via the inhibition of intracortical feedback, ACh can render V1 more sensitive to incoming thalamocortical information and enhance sensory performance. During visual processing, ACh acts on different layers to amplify the encoding of weak stimuli by strengthening synaptic connectivity, which leads to behavioral improvements. Furthermore, ACh might not only facilitate task-relevant perceptual learning via attention but also facilitate task-irrelevant learning via reward reinforcement. However, much remains to be uncovered regarding whether the cholinergic system has the potential to be used as a key mechanism for improving the function of the brain and speeding rehabilitation. Specifically, because perceptual learning occurs easily under conditions of attentional control, the development of a method to improve one's brain capacity through improved attention and cholinergic stimulation is very attractive.

ACKNOWLEDGMENTS

Authors acknowledge the financial support of the Canadian Institutes of Health Research (CIHR, MOP-111003), the Natural Sciences and Engineering Research council of Canada (NSERC, 238835–2011), the FRQS Vision Research Network and the Ecole d'optométrie, Université de Montréal. Authors are thankful to Micheline P. Gloin for help with the artwork.

REFERENCES

Aggelopoulos, N. C., Liebe, S., Logothetis, N. K., and Rainer, G. (2011). Cholinergic control of visual categorization in macaques. *Front. Behav. Neurosci.* 5:73. doi: 10.3389/fnbeh.2011.00073

Ahissar, M., and Hochstein, S. (1993). Attentional control of early perceptual learning. *Proc. Natl. Acad. Sci. U S A* 90, 5718–5722. doi: 10.1073/pnas.90.12.5718

Alitto, H. J., and Dan, Y. (2012). Cell-type-specific modulation of neocortical activity by basal forebrain input. *Front. Syst. Neurosci.* 6:79. doi: 10.3389/fnsys.2012.00079

Amar, M., Lucas-Meunier, E., Baux, G., and Fossier, P. (2010). Blockade of different muscarinic receptor subtypes changes the equilibrium between excitation and inhibition in rat visual cortex. *Neuroscience* 169, 1610–1620. doi: 10.1016/j.neuroscience.2010.06.019

Ansorge, U., Horstmann, G., and Scharlau, I. (2010). Top-down contingent attentional capture during feed-forward visual processing. *Acta Psychol. (Amst)* 135, 123–126. doi: 10.1016/j.actpsy.2010.05.008

Anton-Erxleben, K., and Carrasco, M. (2013). Attentional enhancement of spatial resolution: linking behavioural and neurophysiological evidence. *Nat. Rev. Neurosci.* 14, 188–200. doi: 10.1038/nrn3443

Arroyo, S., Bennett, C., Aziz, D., Brown, S. P., and Hestrin, S. (2012). Prolonged disynaptic inhibition in the cortex mediated by slow, non-α7 nicotinic excitation of a specific subset of cortical interneurons. *J. Neurosci.* 32, 3859–3864. doi: 10.1523/JNEUROSCI.0115-12.2012

Artola, A., and Singer, W. (1987). Long-term potentiation and NMDA receptors in rat visual cortex. *Nature* 330, 649–652. doi: 10.1038/330649a0

Atallah, B. V., Bruns, W., Carandini, M., and Scanziani, M. (2012). Parvalbumin-expressing interneurons linearly transform cortical responses to visual stimuli. *Neuron* 73, 159–170. doi: 10.1016/j.neuron.2011.12.013

Avendaño, C., Umbriaco, D., Dykes, R. W., and Descarries, L. (1996). Acetylcholine innervation of sensory and motor neocortical areas in adult cat: a choline acetyltransferase immunohistochemical study. *J. Chem. Neuroanat.* 11, 113–130. doi: 10.1016/0891-0618(96)00132-9

Bakin, J. S., and Weinberger, N. M. (1996). Induction of a physiological memory in the cerebral cortex by stimulation of the nucleus basalis. *Proc. Natl. Acad. Sci. U S A* 93, 11219–11224. doi: 10.1073/pnas.93.20.11219

Bauer, M., Kluge, C., Bach, D., Bradbury, D., Heinze, H. J., Dolan, R. J., et al. (2012). Cholinergic enhancement of visual attention and neural oscillations in the human brain. *Curr. Biol.* 22, 397–402. doi: 10.1016/j.cub.2012.01.022

Bear, M. F., and Singer, W. (1986). Modulation of visual cortical plasticity by acetylcholine and noradrenaline. *Nature* 320, 172–176. doi: 10.1038/320172a0

Beer, A. L., Vartak, D., and Greenlee, M. W. (2013). Nicotine facilitates memory consolidation in perceptual learning. *Neuropharmacology* 64, 443–451. doi: 10.1016/j.neuropharm.2012.06.019

Bentley, P., Driver, J., and Dolan, R. J. (2011). Cholinergic modulation of cognition: insights from human pharmacological functional neuroimaging. *Prog. Neurobiol.* 94, 360–388. doi: 10.1016/j.pneurobio.2011.06.002

Bentley, P., Husain, M., and Dolan, R. J. (2004). Effects of cholinergic enhancement on visual stimulation, spatial attention and spatial working memory. *Neuron* 41, 969–982. doi: 10.1016/s0896-6273(04)00145-x

Bhattacharyya, A., Veit, J., Kretz, R., Bondar, I., and Rainer, G. (2013). Basal forebrain activation controls contrast sensitivity in primary visual cortex. *BMC Neurosci.* 14:55. doi: 10.1186/1471-2202-14-55

Buchanan, R. W., Conley, R. R., Dickinson, D., Ball, M. P., Feldman, S., Gold, J. M., et al. (2008). Galantamine for the treatment of cognitive impairments in people with schizophrenia. *Am. J. Psychiatry* 165, 82–89. doi: 10.1176/appi.ajp.2007.07050724

Buchanan, K. A., Petrovic, M. M., Chamberlain, S. E., Marrion, N. V., and Mellor, J. R. (2010). Facilitation of long-term potentiation by muscarinic M(1) receptors is mediated by inhibition of SK channels. *Neuron* 68, 948–963. doi: 10.1016/j.neuron.2010.11.018

Caulfield, M. P., and Birdsall, N. J. (1998). International union of pharmacology. XVII. Classification of muscarinic acetylcholine receptors. *Pharmacol. Rev.* 50, 279–290.

Chédotal, A., Cozzari, C., Faure, M. P., Hartman, B. K., and Hamel, E. (1994). Distinct choline acetyltransferase (ChAT) and vasoactive intestinal polypeptide (VIP) bipolar neurons project to local blood vessels in the rat cerebral cortex. *Brain Res.* 646, 181–193. doi: 10.1016/0006-8993(94)90076-0

Christophe, E., Roebuck, A., Staiger, J. F., Lavery, D. J., Charpak, S., and Audinat, E. (2002). Two types of nicotinic receptors mediate an excitation of neocortical layer I interneurons. *J. Neurophysiol.* 88, 1318–1327. doi: 10.1152/jn.00199.2002

Chubykin, A. A., Roach, E. B., Bear, M. F., and Shuler, M. G. (2013). A cholinergic mechanism for reward timing within primary visual cortex. *Neuron* 77, 723–735. doi: 10.1016/j.neuron.2012.12.039

Conner, J. M., Culberson, A., Packowski, C., Chiba, A. A., and Tuszynski, M. H. (2003). Lesions of the basal forebrain cholinergic system impair task acquisition and abolish cortical plasticity associated with motor skill learning. *Neuron* 38, 819–829. doi: 10.1016/s0896-6273(03)00288-5

Cooke, S. F., and Bear, M. F. (2010). Visual experience induces long-term potentiation in the primary visual cortex. *J. Neurosci.* 30, 16304–16313. doi: 10.1523/JNEUROSCI.4333-10.2010

Cudeiro, J., and Sillito, A. M. (2006). Looking back: corticothalamic feedback and early visual processing. *Trends Neurosci.* 29, 298–306. doi: 10.1016/j.tins.2006.05.002

Cummings, J. L. (2003). Use of cholinesterase inhibitors in clinical practice: evidence-based recommendations. *Am. J. Geriatr. Psychiatry* 11, 131–145. doi: 10.1097/00019442-200303000-00004

Darian-Smith, C., and Gilbert, C. D. (1994). Axonal sprouting accompanies functional reorganization in adult cat striate cortex. *Nature* 368, 737–740. doi: 10.1038/368737a0

Dauphin, F., Lacombe, P., Sercombe, R., Hamel, E., and Seylaz, J. (1991). Hypercapnia and stimulation of the substantia innominata increase rat frontal cortical blood flow by different cholinergic mechanisms. *Brain Res.* 553, 75–83. doi: 10.1016/0006-8993(91)90232-k

Deco, G., and Thiele, A. (2011). Cholinergic control of cortical network interactions enables feedback-mediated attentional modulation. *Eur. J. Neurosci.* 34, 146–157. doi: 10.1111/j.1460-9568.2011.07749.x

Demeter, E., and Sarter, M. (2013). Leveraging the cortical cholinergic system to enhance attention. *Neuropharmacology* 64, 294–304. doi: 10.1016/j.neuropharm.2012.06.060

De Pasquale, R., and Sherman, S. M. (2012). Modulatory effects of metabotropic glutamate receptors on local cortical circuits. *J. Neurosci.* 32, 7364–7372. doi: 10.1523/JNEUROSCI.0090-12.2012

Descarries, L., Gisiger, V., and Steriade, M. (1997). Diffuse transmission by acetylcholine in the CNS. *Prog. Neurobiol.* 53, 603–625. doi: 10.1016/s0301-0082(97)00050-6

Disney, A. A., Aoki, C., and Hawken, M. J. (2007). Gain modulation by nicotine in macaque v1. *Neuron* 56, 701–713. doi: 10.1016/j.neuron.2007.09.034

Disney, A. A., Aoki, C., and Hawken, M. J. (2012). Cholinergic suppression of visual responses in primate V1 is mediated by GABAergic inhibition. *J. Neurophysiol.* 108, 1907–1923. doi: 10.1152/jn.00188.2012

Disney, A. A., Domakonda, K. V., and Aoki, C. (2006). Differential expression of muscarinic acetylcholine receptors across excitatory and inhibitory cells in visual cortical areas V1 and V2 of the macaque monkey. *J. Comp. Neurol.* 499, 49–63. doi: 10.1002/cne.21096

Dotigny, F., Ben Amor, A. Y., Burke, M., and Vaucher, E. (2008). Neuromodulatory role of acetylcholine in visually-induced cortical activation: behavioral and neuroanatomical correlates. *Neuroscience* 154, 1607–1618. doi: 10.1016/j.neuroscience.2008.04.030

Drevets, W. C., Price, J. L., and Furey, M. L. (2008). Brain structural and functional abnormalities in mood disorders: implications for neurocircuitry models of depression. *Brain Struct. Funct.* 213, 93–118. doi: 10.1007/s00429-008-0189-x

Dringenberg, H. C., Hamze, B., Wilson, A., Speechley, W., and Kuo, M. C. (2007). Heterosynaptic facilitation of in vivo thalamocortical long-term potentiation in the adult rat visual cortex by acetylcholine. *Cereb. Cortex* 17, 839–848. doi: 10.1093/cercor/bhk038

Eckenstein, F. P., Baughman, R. W., and Quinn, J. (1988). An anatomical study of cholinergic innervation in rat cerebral cortex. *Neuroscience* 25, 457–474. doi: 10.1016/0306-4522(88)90251-5

Egeth, H. E., Leonard, C. J., and Leber, A. B. (2010). Why salience is not enough: reflections on top-down selection in vision. *Acta Psychol. (Amst)* 135, 130–132; discussion 133–139. doi: 10.1016/j.actpsy.2010.05.012

Eggermann, E., and Feldmeyer, D. (2009). Cholinergic filtering in the recurrent excitatory microcircuit of cortical layer 4. *Proc. Natl. Acad. Sci. U S A* 106, 11753–11758. doi: 10.1073/pnas.0810062106

Eimer, M., and Kiss, M. (2010). The top-down control of visual selection and how it is linked to the N2pc component. *Acta Psychol. (Amst)* 135, 100–102. doi: 10.1016/j.actpsy.2010.04.010

Eldar, E., Cohen, J. D., and Niv, Y. (2013). The effects of neural gain on attention and learning. *Nat. Neurosci.* 16, 1146–1153. doi: 10.1038/nn.3428

Fagerström, K. O., Pomerleau, O., Giordani, B., and Stelson, F. (1994). Nicotine may relieve symptoms of Parkinson's disease. *Psychopharmacology (Berl)* 116, 117–119. doi: 10.1007/bf02244882

Fagiolini, M., and Hensch, T. K. (2000). Inhibitory threshold for critical-period activation in primary visual cortex. *Nature* 404, 183–186. doi: 10.1038/35004582

Fahle, M. (2009). Perceptual learning and sensomotor flexibility: cortical plasticity under attentional control? *Philos. Trans. R. Soc. Lond. B Biol. Sci.* 364, 313–319. doi: 10.1098/rstb.2008.0267

Fahle, M., and Poggio, T. (2002). *Perceptual Learning.* Cambridge, Mass.: MIT Press.

Fiorentini, A., and Berardi, N. (1980). Perceptual learning specific for orientation and spatial frequency. *Nature* 287, 43–44. doi: 10.1038/287043a0

Freedman, R. (2013). α7-Nicotinic acetylcholine receptor agonists for cognitive enhancement in schizophrenia. *Annu. Rev. Med.* 65, 245–261. doi: 10.1146/annurev-med-092112-142937

Fries, P., Nikolić, D., and Singer, W. (2007). The gamma cycle. *Trends Neurosci.* 30, 309–316. doi: 10.1016/j.tins.2007.05.005

Fries, P., Womelsdorf, T., Oostenveld, R., and Desimone, R. (2008). The effects of visual stimulation and selective visual attention on rhythmic neuronal synchronization in macaque area V4. *J. Neurosci.* 28, 4823–4835. doi: 10.1523/JNEUROSCI.4499-07.2008

Furey, M. L. (2011). The prominent role of stimulus processing: cholinergic function and dysfunction in cognition. *Curr. Opin. Neurol.* 24, 364–370. doi: 10.1097/WCO.0b013e328348bda5

Furey, M. L., Pietrini, P., and Haxby, J. V. (2000). Cholinergic enhancement and increased selectivity of perceptual processing during working memory. *Science* 290, 2315–2319. doi: 10.1126/science.290.5500.2315

Furey, M. L., Ricciardi, E., Schapiro, M. B., Rapoport, S. I., and Pietrini, P. (2008). Cholinergic enhancement eliminates modulation of neural activity by task difficulty in the prefrontal cortex during working memory. *J. Cogn. Neurosci.* 20, 1342–1353. doi: 10.1162/jocn.2008.20092

Gaykema, R. P., Luiten, P. G., Nyakas, C., and Traber, J. (1990). Cortical projection patterns of the medial septum-diagonal band complex. *J. Comp. Neurol.* 293, 103–124. doi: 10.1002/cne.902930109

Giessel, A. J., and Sabatini, B. L. (2010). M1 muscarinic receptors boost synaptic potentials and calcium influx in dendritic spines by inhibiting postsynaptic SK channels. *Neuron* 68, 936–947. doi: 10.1016/j.neuron.2010.09.004

Gil, Z., Connors, B. W., and Amitai, Y. (1997). Differential regulation of neocortical synapses by neuromodulators and activity. *Neuron* 19, 679–686. doi: 10.1016/s0896-6273(00)80380-3

Gilbert, C. D., and Li, W. (2012). Adult visual cortical plasticity. *Neuron* 75, 250–264. doi: 10.1016/j.neuron.2012.06.030

Gilbert, C. D., Sigman, M., and Crist, R. E. (2001). The neural basis of perceptual learning. *Neuron* 31, 681–697. doi: 10.1016/s0896-6273(01)00424-x

Gilbert, C. D., and Wiesel, T. N. (1989). Columnar specificity of intrinsic horizontal and corticocortical connections in cat visual cortex. *J. Neurosci.* 9, 2432–2442.

Gill, T. M., Sarter, M., and Givens, B. (2000). Sustained visual attention performance-associated prefrontal neuronal activity: evidence for cholinergic modulation. *J. Neurosci.* 20, 4745–4757.

Giordano, A. M., McElree, B., and Carrasco, M. (2009). On the automaticity and flexibility of covert attention: a speed-accuracy trade-off analysis. *J. Vis.* 9, 30.1–30.10. doi: 10.1167/9.3.30

Goard, M., and Dan, Y. (2009). Basal forebrain activation enhances cortical coding of natural scenes. *Nat. Neurosci.* 12, 1444–1449. doi: 10.1038/nn.2402

Groleau, M., Nguyen, H. N., Vanni, M., Huppé-Gourgues, F., Casanova, C., and Vaucher, E. (2014). Impaired functional organization in the visual cortex of muscarinic receptors knock-out mice. *Neuroimage* 98, 233–242. doi: 10.1016/j.neuroimage.2014.05.016

Gu, Q. (2003). Contribution of acetylcholine to visual cortex plasticity. *Neurobiol. Learn. Mem.* 80, 291–301. doi: 10.1016/s1074-7427(03)00073-x

Gulledge, A. T., Bucci, D. J., Zhang, S. S., Matsui, M., and Yeh, H. H. (2009). M1 receptors mediate cholinergic modulation of excitability in neocortical pyramidal neurons. *J. Neurosci.* 29, 9888–9902. doi: 10.1523/JNEUROSCI.1366-09.2009

Gutnisky, D. A., Hansen, B. J., Iliescu, B. F., and Dragoi, V. (2009). Attention alters visual plasticity during exposure-based learning. *Curr. Biol.* 19, 555–560. doi: 10.1016/j.cub.2009.01.063

Haider, B., and McCormick, D. A. (2009). Rapid neocortical dynamics: cellular and network mechanisms. *Neuron* 62, 171–189. doi: 10.1016/j.neuron.2009.04.008

Harauzov, A., Spolidoro, M., DiCristo, G., De Pasquale, R., Cancedda, L., Pizzorusso, T., et al. (2010). Reducing intracortical inhibition in the adult visual cortex promotes ocular dominance plasticity. *J. Neurosci.* 30, 361–371. doi: 10.1523/JNEUROSCI.2233-09.2010

Hashimoto, T., Shu, H., and Kuriyama, K. (1994). Muscarinic M1 receptor mediated inhibition of GABA release from rat cerebral cortex. *Neurochem. Int.* 24, 389–394. doi: 10.1016/0197-0186(94)90117-1

Hasselmo, M. E. (2006). The role of acetylcholine in learning and memory. *Curr. Opin. Neurobiol.* 16, 710–715. doi: 10.1016/j.conb.2006.09.002

Hensch, T. K. (2004). Critical period regulation. *Annu. Rev. Neurosci.* 27, 549–579. doi: 10.1146/annurev.neuro.27.070203.144327

Hensch, T. K. (2005). Critical period plasticity in local cortical circuits. *Nat. Rev. Neurosci.* 6, 877–888. doi: 10.1038/nrn1787

Hensch, T. K., Fagiolini, M., Mataga, N., Stryker, M. P., Baekkeskov, S., and Kash, S. F. (1998). Local GABA circuit control of experience-dependent plasticity in developing visual cortex. *Science* 282, 1504–1508. doi: 10.1126/science.282.5393.1504

Herrero, J. L., Roberts, M. J., Delicato, L. S., Gieselmann, M. A., Dayan, P., and Thiele, A. (2008). Acetylcholine contributes through muscarinic receptors to attentional modulation in V1. *Nature* 454, 1110–1114. doi: 10.1038/nature07141

Heynen, A. J., and Bear, M. F. (2001). Long-term potentiation of thalamocortical transmission in the adult visual cortex in vivo. *J. Neurosci.* 21, 9801–9813.

Hilt, D., Gawryl, M., and Koenig, G. (2009). Safety, tolerability and cognitive effects of a novel α7 nicotinic receptor agonist in Alzheimer's disease patients on stable donepezil or rivastigmine therapy. *Alzheimers Dement.* 5:e32. doi: 10.1016/j.jalz.2009.07.147

Holmes, A. D., Copland, D. A., Silburn, P. A., and Chenery, H. J. (2011). Acute nicotine enhances strategy-based semantic processing in Parkinson's disease. *Int. J. Neuropsychopharmacol.* 14, 877–885. doi: 10.1017/S1461145710001665

Hua, T., Bao, P., Huang, C. B., Wang, Z., Xu, J., Zhou, Y., et al. (2010). Perceptual learning improves contrast sensitivity of V1 neurons in cats. *Curr. Biol.* 20, 887–894. doi: 10.1016/j.cub.2010.03.066

Isaacson, J. S., and Scanziani, M. (2011). How inhibition shapes cortical activity. *Neuron* 72, 231–243. doi: 10.1016/j.neuron.2011.09.027

Iwai, Y., Fagiolini, M., Obata, K., and Hensch, T. K. (2003). Rapid critical period induction by tonic inhibition in visual cortex. *J. Neurosci.* 23, 6695–6702.

Ji, D., and Dani, J. A. (2000). Inhibition and disinhibition of pyramidal neurons by activation of nicotinic receptors on hippocampal interneurons. *J. Neurophysiol.* 83, 2682–2690.

Jia, H., Rochefort, N. L., Chen, X., and Konnerth, A. (2010). Dendritic organization of sensory input to cortical neurons in vivo. *Nature* 464, 1307–1312. doi: 10.1038/nature08947

Kang, J. I., Groleau, M., Dotigny, F., Giguère, H., and Vaucher, E. (2014). Visual training paired with electrical stimulation of the basal forebrain improves orientation-selective visual acuity in the rat. *Brain Struct. Funct.* 219, 1493–1507. doi: 10.1007/s00429-013-0582-y

Kang, J. I., and Vaucher, E. (2009). Cholinergic pairing with visual activation results in long-term enhancement of visual evoked potentials. *PLoS One* 4:e5995. doi: 10.1371/journal.pone.0005995

Keitel, C., Andersen, S. K., Quigley, C., and Müller, M. M. (2013). Independent effects of attentional gain control and competitive interactions on visual stimulus processing. *Cereb. Cortex* 23, 940–946. doi: 10.1093/cercor/bhs084

Kilgard, M. P., and Merzenich, M. M. (1998). Cortical map reorganization enabled by nucleus basalis activity. *Science* 279, 1714–1718. doi: 10.1126/science.279.5357.1714

Kimura, F., and Baughman, R. W. (1997). Distinct muscarinic receptor subtypes suppress excitatory and inhibitory synaptic responses in cortical neurons. *J. Neurophysiol.* 77, 709–716.

Kimura, F., Fukuda, M., and Tsumoto, T. (1999). Acetylcholine suppresses the spread of excitation in the visual cortex revealed by optical recording: possible differential effect depending on the source of input. *Eur. J. Neurosci.* 11, 3597–3609. doi: 10.1046/j.1460-9568.1999.00779.x

Kirkwood, A., Rozas, C., Kirkwood, J., Perez, F., and Bear, M. F. (1999). Modulation of long-term synaptic depression in visual cortex by acetylcholine and norepinephrine. *J. Neurosci.* 19, 1599–1609.

Kocharyan, A., Fernandes, P., Tong, X. K., Vaucher, E., and Hamel, E. (2008). Specific subtypes of cortical GABA interneurons contribute to the neurovascular coupling response to basal forebrain stimulation. *J. Cereb. Blood Flow Metab.* 28, 221–231. doi: 10.1038/sj.jcbfm.9600558

Kosovicheva, A. A., Sheremata, S. L., Rokem, A., Landau, A. N., and Silver, M. A. (2012). Cholinergic enhancement reduces orientation-specific surround suppression but not visual crowding. *Front. Behav. Neurosci.* 6:61. doi: 10.3389/fnbeh.2012.00061

Laplante, F., Morin, Y., Quirion, R., and Vaucher, E. (2005). Acetylcholine release is elicited in the visual cortex, but not in the prefrontal cortex, by patterned visual stimulation: a dual in vivo microdialysis study with functional correlates in the rat brain. *Neuroscience* 132, 501–510. doi: 10.1016/j.neuroscience.2004.11.059

Lee, S. H., Kwan, A. C., Zhang, S., Phoumthipphavong, V., Flannery, J. G., Masmanidis, S. C., et al. (2012). Activation of specific interneurons improves V1 feature selectivity and visual perception. *Nature* 488, 379–383. doi: 10.1038/nature11312

Levey, A. I., Kitt, C. A., Simonds, W. F., Price, D. L., and Brann, M. R. (1991). Identification and localization of muscarinic acetylcholine receptor proteins in brain with subtype-specific antibodies. *J. Neurosci.* 11, 3218–3226.

Li, Y. T., Ibrahim, L. A., Liu, B. H., Zhang, L. I., and Tao, H. W. (2013). Linear transformation of thalamocortical input by intracortical excitation. *Nat. Neurosci.* 16, 1324–1330. doi: 10.1038/nn.3494

Li, W., Piëch, V., and Gilbert, C. D. (2004). Perceptual learning and top-down influences in primary visual cortex. *Nat. Neurosci.* 7, 651–657. doi: 10.1038/nn1255

Lien, A. D., and Scanziani, M. (2013). Tuned thalamic excitation is amplified by visual cortical circuits. *Nat. Neurosci.* 16, 1315–1323. doi: 10.1038/nn.3488

Lucas-Meunier, E., Monier, C., Amar, M., Baux, G., Frégnac, Y., and Fossier, P. (2009). Involvement of nicotinic and muscarinic receptors in the endogenous cholinergic modulation of the balance between excitation and inhibition in the young rat visual cortex. *Cereb. Cortex* 19, 2411–2427. doi: 10.1093/cercor/bhn258

Luiten, P. G., Gaykema, R. P., Traber, J., and Spencer, D. G. Jr. (1987). Cortical projection patterns of magnocellular basal nucleus subdivisions as revealed by anterogradely transported phaseolus vulgaris leucoagglutinin. *Brain Res.* 413, 229–250. doi: 10.1016/0006-8993(87)91014-6

Lysakowski, A., Wainer, B. H., Bruce, G., and Hersh, L. B. (1989). An atlas of the regional and laminar distribution of choline acetyltransferase immunoreactivity in rat cerebral cortex. *Neuroscience* 28, 291–336. doi: 10.1016/0306-4522(89)90180-2

Ma, X., and Suga, N. (2005). Long-term cortical plasticity evoked by electric stimulation and acetylcholine applied to the auditory cortex. *Proc. Natl. Acad. Sci. U S A* 102, 9335–9340. doi: 10.1073/pnas.0503851102

Mayer, M. J. (1983). Practice improves adults' sensitivity to diagonals. *Vision Res.* 23, 547–550. doi: 10.1016/0042-6989(83)90130-x

McGaughy, J., and Sarter, M. (1998). Sustained attention performance in rats with intracortical infusions of 192 IgG-saporin-induced cortical cholinergic deafferentation: effects of physostigmine and FG 7142. *Behav. Neurosci.* 112, 1519–1525. doi: 10.1037//0735-7044.112.6.1519

McGaughy, J., and Sarter, M. (1999). Effects of ovariectomy, 192 IgG-saporin-induced cortical cholinergic deafferentation and administration of estradiol on sustained attention performance in rats. *Behav. Neurosci.* 113, 1216–1232. doi: 10.1037/0735-7044.113.6.1216

McGuire, B. A., Gilbert, C. D., Rivlin, P. K., and Wiesel, T. N. (1991). Targets of horizontal connections in macaque primary visual cortex. *J. Comp. Neurol.* 305, 370–392. doi: 10.1002/cne.903050303

McKee, S. P., and Westheimer, G. (1978). Improvement in vernier acuity with practice. *Percept. Psychophys.* 24, 258–262. doi: 10.3758/bf03206097

Mechawar, N., Cozzari, C., and Descarries, L. (2000). Cholinergic innervation in adult rat cerebral cortex: a quantitative immunocytochemical description. *J. Comp. Neurol.* 428, 305–318. doi: 10.1002/1096-9861(20001211)428:2<305::aid-cne9>3.0.co;2-y

Metherate, R. (2011). Functional connectivity and cholinergic modulation in auditory cortex. *Neurosci. Biobehav. Rev.* 35, 2058–2063. doi: 10.1016/j.neubiorev.2010.11.010

Metherate, R., Kaur, S., Kawai, H., Lazar, R., Liang, K., and Rose, H. J. (2005). Spectral integration in auditory cortex: mechanisms and modulation. *Hear. Res.* 206, 146–158. doi: 10.1016/j.heares.2005.01.014

Metherate, R., and Weinberger, N. M. (1990). Cholinergic modulation of responses to single tones produces tone-specific receptive field alterations in cat auditory cortex. *Synapse* 6, 133–145. doi: 10.1002/syn.890060204

Moran, R. J., Campo, P., Symmonds, M., Stephan, K. E., Dolan, R. J., and Friston, K. J. (2013). Free energy, precision and learning: the role of cholinergic neuromodulation. *J. Neurosci.* 33, 8227–8236. doi: 10.1523/jneurosci.4255-12.2013

Morishita, H., Miwa, J. M., Heintz, N., and Hensch, T. K. (2010). Lynx1, a cholinergic brake, limits plasticity in adult visual cortex. *Science* 330, 1238–1240. doi: 10.1126/science.1195320

Morris, R. G., Anderson, E., Lynch, G. S., and Baudry, M. (1986). Selective impairment of learning and blockade of long-term potentiation by an N-methyl-D-aspartate receptor antagonist, AP5. *Nature* 319, 774–776. doi: 10.1038/319774a0

Mukai, I., Kim, D., Fukunaga, M., Japee, S., Marrett, S., and Ungerleider, L. G. (2007). Activations in visual and attention-related areas predict and correlate with the degree of perceptual learning. *J. Neurosci.* 27, 11401–11411. doi: 10.1523/jneurosci.3002-07.2007

Nassi, J. J., and Callaway, E. M. (2009). Parallel processing strategies of the primate visual system. *Nat. Rev. Neurosci.* 10, 360–372. doi: 10.1038/nrn2619

Nestor, L., Mccabe, E., Jones, J., Clancy, L., and Garavan, H. (2011). Differences in "bottom-up" and "top-down" neural activity in current and former cigarette smokers: evidence for neural substrates which may promote nicotine abstinence through increased cognitive control. *Neuroimage* 56, 2258–2275. doi: 10.1016/j.neuroimage.2011.03.054

Newhouse, P. A., Potter, A. S., Dumas, J. A., and Thiel, C. M. (2011). Functional brain imaging of nicotinic effects on higher cognitive processes. *Biochem. Pharmacol.* 82, 943–951. doi: 10.1016/j.bcp.2011.06.008

Olausson, P., Jentsch, J. D., and Taylor, J. R. (2004). Nicotine enhances responding with conditioned reinforcement. *Psychopharmacology (Berl)* 171, 173–178. doi: 10.1007/s00213-003-1575-y

Olsen, S. R., Bortone, D. S., Adesnik, H., and Scanziani, M. (2012). Gain control by layer six in cortical circuits of vision. *Nature* 483, 47–52. doi: 10.1038/nature10835

Origlia, N., Kuczewski, N., Aztiria, E., Gautam, D., Wess, J., and Domenici, L. (2006). Muscarinic acetylcholine receptor knockout mice show distinct synaptic plasticity impairments in the visual cortex. *J. Physiol.* 577, 829–840. doi: 10.1113/jphysiol.2006.117119

Pinto, L., Goard, M. J., Estandian, D., Xu, M., Kwan, A. C., Lee, S. H., et al. (2013). Fast modulation of visual perception by basal forebrain cholinergic neurons. *Nat. Neurosci.* 16, 1857–1863. doi: 10.1038/nn.3552

Ramachandran, V. S., and Braddick, O. (1973). Orientation-specific learning in stereopsis. *Perception* 2, 371–376. doi: 10.1068/p020371

Ramalingam, N., McManus, J. N., Li, W., and Gilbert, C. D. (2013). Top-down modulation of lateral interactions in visual cortex. *J. Neurosci.* 33, 1773–1789. doi: 10.1523/jneurosci.3825-12.2013

Rang, H. P. (2003). *Pharmacology.* Edinburgh; Toronto: Churchill Livingstone.

Reed, A., Riley, J., Carraway, R., Carrasco, A., Perez, C., Jakkamsetti, V., et al. (2011). Cortical map plasticity improves learning but is not necessary for improved performance. *Neuron* 70, 121–131. doi: 10.1016/j.neuron.2011.02.038

Regehr, W. G., and Tank, D. W. (1990). Postsynaptic NMDA receptor-mediated calcium accumulation in hippocampal CA1 pyramidal cell dendrites. *Nature* 345, 807–810. doi: 10.1038/345807a0

Ricciardi, E., Handjaras, G., Bernardi, G., Pietrini, P., and Furey, M. L. (2013). Cholinergic enhancement reduces functional connectivity and BOLD variability in visual extrastriate cortex during selective attention. *Neuropharmacology* 64, 305–313. doi: 10.1016/j.neuropharm.2012.07.003

Riekkinen, M., and Riekkinen, P. Jr. (1997). Nicotine and D-cycloserine enhance acquisition of water maze spatial navigation in aged rats. *Neuroreport* 8, 699–703. doi: 10.1097/00001756-199702100-00024

Roberts, M. J., and Thiele, A. (2008). Spatial integration and its moderation by attention and acetylcholine. *Front. Biosci.* 13, 3742–3759. doi: 10.2741/2963

Roberts, M. J., Zinke, W., Guo, K., Robertson, R., Mcdonald, J. S., and Thiele, A. (2005). Acetylcholine dynamically controls spatial integration in marmoset primary visual cortex. *J. Neurophysiol.* 93, 2062–2072. doi: 10.1152/jn.00911.2004

Rodriguez, R., Kallenbach, U., Singer, W., and Munk, M. H. (2004). Short- and long-term effects of cholinergic modulation on gamma oscillations and response synchronization in the visual cortex. *J. Neurosci.* 24, 10369–10378. doi: 10.1523/jneurosci.1839-04.2004

Roelfsema, P. R., van Ooyen, A., and Watanabe, T. (2010). Perceptual learning rules based on reinforcers and attention. *Trends Cogn. Sci.* 14, 64–71. doi: 10.1016/j.tics.2009.11.005

Rokem, A., Landau, A. N., Garg, D., Prinzmetal, W., and Silver, M. A. (2010). Cholinergic enhancement increases the effects of voluntary attention but does not affect involuntary attention. *Neuropsychopharmacology* 35, 2538–2544. doi: 10.1038/npp.2010.118

Rokem, A., and Silver, M. A. (2010). Cholinergic enhancement augments magnitude and specificity of visual perceptual learning in healthy humans. *Curr. Biol.* 20, 1723–1728. doi: 10.1016/j.cub.2010.08.027

Rokem, A., and Silver, M. A. (2013). The benefits of cholinergic enhancement during perceptual learning are long-lasting. *Front. Comput. Neurosci.* 7:66. doi: 10.3389/fncom.2013.00066

Salgado, H., Bellay, T., Nichols, J. A., Bose, M., Martinolich, L., Perrotti, L., et al. (2007). Muscarinic M2 and M1 receptors reduce GABA release by Ca2+ channel modulation through activation of PI3K/Ca2+ -independent and PLC/Ca2+ -dependent PKC. *J. Neurophysiol.* 98, 952–965. doi: 10.1152/jn.00060.2007

Sarter, M., Hasselmo, M. E., Bruno, J. P., and Givens, B. (2005). Unraveling the attentional functions of cortical cholinergic inputs: interactions between signal-driven and cognitive modulation of signal detection. *Brain Res. Brain Res. Rev.* 48, 98–111. doi: 10.1016/j.brainresrev.2004.08.006

Sato, H., Hata, Y., Masui, H., and Tsumoto, T. (1987). A functional role of cholinergic innervation to neurons in the cat visual cortex. *J. Neurophysiol.* 58, 765–780.

Schoups, A., Vogels, R., Qian, N., and Orban, G. (2001). Practising orientation identification improves orientation coding in V1 neurons. *Nature* 412, 549–553. doi: 10.1038/35087601

Seeger, T., Fedorova, I., Zheng, F., Miyakawa, T., Koustova, E., Gomeza, J., et al. (2004). M2 muscarinic acetylcholine receptor knock-out mice show deficits in behavioral flexibility, working memory and hippocampal plasticity. *J. Neurosci.* 24, 10117–10127. doi: 10.1523/jneurosci.3581-04.2004

Seitz, A. R., Kim, D., and Watanabe, T. (2009). Rewards evoke learning of unconsciously processed visual stimuli in adult humans. *Neuron* 61, 700–707. doi: 10.1016/j.neuron.2009.01.016

Servan-Schreiber, D., Printz, H., and Cohen, J. D. (1990). A network model of catecholamine effects: gain, signal-to-noise ratio and behavior. *Science* 249, 892–895. doi: 10.1126/science.2392679

Shekhar, A., Potter, W. Z., Lightfoot, J., Lienemann, J., Dube, S., Mallinckrodt, C., et al. (2008). Selective muscarinic receptor agonist xanomeline as a novel treatment approach for schizophrenia. *Am. J. Psychiatry* 165, 1033–1039. doi: 10.1176/appi.ajp.2008.06091591

Shinoe, T., Matsui, M., Taketo, M. M., and Manabe, T. (2005). Modulation of synaptic plasticity by physiological activation of M1 muscarinic acetylcholine receptors in the mouse hippocampus. *J. Neurosci.* 25, 11194–11200. doi: 10.1523/jneurosci.2338-05.2005

Shuler, M. G., and Bear, M. F. (2006). Reward timing in the primary visual cortex. *Science* 311, 1606–1609. doi: 10.1126/science.1123513

Sillito, A. M., Cudeiro, J., and Jones, H. E. (2006). Always returning: feedback and sensory processing in visual cortex and thalamus. *Trends Neurosci.* 29, 307–316. doi: 10.1016/j.tins.2006.05.001

Silver, M. A., Shenhav, A., and D'esposito, M. (2008). Cholinergic enhancement reduces spatial spread of visual responses in human early visual cortex. *Neuron* 60, 904–914. doi: 10.1016/j.neuron.2008.09.038

Skrandies, W., and Fahle, M. (1994). Neurophysiological correlates of perceptual learning in the human brain. *Brain Topogr.* 7, 163–168. doi: 10.1007/bf01186774

Soma, S., Shimegi, S., Osaki, H., and Sato, H. (2012). Cholinergic modulation of response gain in the primary visual cortex of the macaque. *J. Neurophysiol.* 107, 283–291. doi: 10.1152/jn.00330.2011

Soma, S., Shimegi, S., Suematsu, N., and Sato, H. (2013a). Cholinergic modulation of response gain in the rat primary visual cortex. *Sci. Rep.* 3:1138. doi: 10.1038/srep01138

Soma, S., Shimegi, S., Suematsu, N., Tamura, H., and Sato, H. (2013b). Modulation-specific and laminar-dependent effects of acetylcholine on visual responses in the rat primary visual cortex. *PLoS One* 8:e68430. doi: 10.1371/journal.pone.0068430

Stettler, D. D., Das, A., Bennett, J., and Gilbert, C. D. (2002). Lateral connectivity and contextual interactions in macaque primary visual cortex. *Neuron* 36, 739–750. doi: 10.1016/s0896-6273(02)01029-2

Sun, Y. J., Wu, G. K., Liu, B. H., Li, P., Zhou, M., Xiao, Z., et al. (2010). Fine-tuning of pre-balanced excitation and inhibition during auditory cortical development. *Nature* 465, 927–931. doi: 10.1038/nature09079

Takesian, A. E., and Hensch, T. K. (2013). Balancing plasticity/stability across brain development. *Prog. Brain Res.* 207, 3–34. doi: 10.1016/b978-0-444-63327-9.00001-1

Theeuwes, J. (2010). Top-down and bottom-up control of visual selection. *Acta Psychol. (Amst)* 135, 77–99. doi: 10.1016/j.actpsy.2010.02.006

Thiel, C. M., Zilles, K., and Fink, G. R. (2005). Nicotine modulates reorienting of visuospatial attention and neural activity in human parietal cortex. *Neuropsychopharmacology* 30, 810–820. doi: 10.1038/sj.npp.1300633

Thiele, A. (2013). Muscarinic signaling in the brain. *Annu. Rev. Neurosci.* 36, 271–294. doi: 10.1146/annurev-neuro-062012-170433

Umbriaco, D., Watkins, K. C., Descarries, L., Cozzari, C., and Hartman, B. K. (1994). Ultrastructural and morphometric features of the acetylcholine innervation in adult rat parietal cortex: an electron microscopic study in serial sections. *J. Comp. Neurol.* 348, 351–373. doi: 10.1002/cne.903480304

Vaucher, E., and Hamel, E. (1995). Cholinergic basal forebrain neurons project to cortical microvessels in the rat: electron microscopic study with anterogradely transported phaseolus vulgaris leucoagglutinin and choline acetyltransferase immunocytochemistry. *J. Neurosci.* 15, 7427–7441.

Verdier, D., and Dykes, R. W. (2001). Long-term cholinergic enhancement of evoked potentials in rat hindlimb somatosensory cortex displays characteristics of long-term potentiation. *Exp. Brain Res.* 137, 71–82. doi: 10.1007/s002210000646

Voytko, M. L., Olton, D. S., Richardson, R. T., Gorman, L. K., Tobin, J. R., and Price, D. L. (1994). Basal forebrain lesions in monkeys disrupt attention but not learning and memory. *J. Neurosci.* 14, 167–186.

Wang, L., Kloc, M., Gu, Y., Ge, S., and Maffei, A. (2013). Layer-specific experience-dependent rewiring of thalamocortical circuits. *J. Neurosci.* 33, 4181–4191. doi: 10.1523/JNEUROSCI.4423-12.2013

Watanabe, T., Nanez, J. E. Sr., Koyama, S., Mukai, I., Liederman, J., and Sasaki, Y. (2002). Greater plasticity in lower-level than higher-level visual motion processing in a passive perceptual learning task. *Nat. Neurosci.* 5, 1003–1009. doi: 10.1038/nn915

Watanabe, T., Nanez, J. E., and Sasaki, Y. (2001). Perceptual learning without perception. *Nature* 413, 844–848. doi: 10.1038/35101601

Wess, J. (2003). Novel insights into muscarinic acetylcholine receptor function using gene targeting technology. *Trends Pharmacol. Sci.* 24, 414–420. doi: 10.1016/s0165-6147(03)00195-0

Wester, J. C., and Contreras, D. (2013). Differential modulation of spontaneous and evoked thalamocortical network activity by acetylcholine level in vitro. *J. Neurosci.* 33, 17951–17966. doi: 10.1523/jneurosci.1644-13.2013

Wilson, D. A., Fletcher, M. L., and Sullivan, R. M. (2004). Acetylcholine and olfactory perceptual learning. *Learn. Mem.* 11, 28–34. doi: 10.1101/lm.66404

Wilson, N. R., Runyan, C. A., Wang, F. L., and Sur, M. (2012). Division and subtraction by distinct cortical inhibitory networks in vivo. *Nature* 488, 343–348. doi: 10.1038/nature11347

Wylie, K. P., Rojas, D. C., Tanabe, J., Martin, L. F., and Tregellas, J. R. (2012). Nicotine increases brain functional network efficiency. *Neuroimage* 63, 73–80. doi: 10.1016/j.neuroimage.2012.06.079

Xing, D., Yeh, C. I., Burns, S., and Shapley, R. M. (2012). Laminar analysis of visually evoked activity in the primary visual cortex. *Proc. Natl. Acad. Sci. U S A* 109, 13871–13876. doi: 10.1073/pnas.1201478109

Yamasaki, M., Matsui, M., and Watanabe, M. (2010). Preferential localization of muscarinic M1 receptor on dendritic shaft and spine of cortical pyramidal cells and its anatomical evidence for volume transmission. *J. Neurosci.* 30, 4408–4418. doi: 10.1523/jneurosci.5719-09.2010

Yu, A. J., and Dayan, P. (2002). Acetylcholine in cortical inference. *Neural Netw.* 15, 719–730. doi: 10.1016/s0893-6080(02)00058-8

Yu, A. J., and Dayan, P. (2005). Uncertainty, neuromodulation and attention. *Neuron* 46, 681–692. doi: 10.1016/j.neuron.2005.04.026

Zhang, Z. W., Kang, J. I., and Vaucher, E. (2011). Axonal varicosity density as an index of local neuronal interactions. *PLoS One* 6:e22543. doi: 10.1371/journal.pone.0022543

7

Pharmacological cognitive enhancement—how neuroscientific research could advance ethical debate

Hannah Maslen[1]*, Nadira Faulmüller[2,3] and Julian Savulescu[4]

[1] Oxford Martin School, University of Oxford, Oxford, UK
[2] Department of Experimental Psychology, University of Oxford, Oxford, UK
[3] Department Values, Technology and Innovation, Delft University of Technology, Delft, Netherlands
[4] Oxford Uehiro Centre for Practical Ethics, University of Oxford, Oxford, UK

Edited by:
Mikhail Lebedev, Duke University, USA

Reviewed by:
Elisabeth Hildt, University of Mainz, Germany
Brendon Boot, Harvard University Medical School, USA
Patricia Anne O'Malley, Miami Valley Hospital Center of Nursing Excellence, USA

***Correspondence:**
Hannah Maslen, Oxford Martin School, University of Oxford, 34 Broad Street, Oxford, OX1 3BD, UK
e-mail: hannah.maslen@philosophy.ox.ac.uk

There are numerous ways people can improve their cognitive capacities: good nutrition and regular exercise can produce long-term improvements across many cognitive domains, whilst commonplace stimulants such as coffee temporarily boost levels of alertness and concentration. Effects like these have been well-documented in the medical literature and they raise few (if any) ethical issues. More recently, however, clinical research has shown that the off-label use of some pharmaceuticals can, under certain conditions, have modest cognition-improving effects. Substances such as methylphenidate and modafinil can improve capacities such as working memory and concentration in some healthy individuals. Unlike their more mundane predecessors, these methods of "cognitive enhancement" are thought to raise a multitude of ethical issues. This paper presents the six principal ethical issues raised in relation to pharmacological cognitive enhancers (PCEs)—issues such as whether: (1) the medical safety-profile of PCEs justifies restricting or permitting their elective or required use; (2) the enhanced mind can be an "authentic" mind; (3) individuals might be coerced into using PCEs; (4), there is a meaningful distinction to be made between the treatment vs. enhancement effect of the same PCE; (5) unequal access to PCEs would have implications for distributive justice; and (6) PCE use constitutes cheating in competitive contexts. In reviewing the six principal issues, the paper discusses how neuroscientific research might help advance the ethical debate. In particular, the paper presents new arguments about the contribution neuroscience could make to debates about justice, fairness, and cheating, ultimately concluding that neuroscientific research into "personalized enhancement" will be essential if policy is to be truly informed and ethical. We propose an "ethical agenda" for neuroscientific research into PCEs.

Keywords: cognitive enhancement, brain function augmentation, ethics, modafinil, ritalin, justice, cheating, personalized enhancement

INTRODUCTION

Recent research in neuroscience and pharmacology has demonstrated that various pharmaceuticals can have modest cognition-enhancing effects in healthy individuals (for reviews, see Repantis et al., 2010; Husain and Mehta, 2011). For example, some studies have shown that modafinil—originally developed for the treatment of narcolepsy—can improve various dimensions of cognitive function in sleep-deprived (Wesensten et al., 2005; Thomas and Kwong, 2006) and non-sleep-deprived healthy adults (Turner et al., 2003; Müller et al., 2004). Similarly, methylphenidate—originally developed for the treatment of Attention Deficit Hyperactivity Disorder (ADHD)—has been shown to improve spatial working memory and planning in healthy adults (Elliott et al., 1997; Mehta et al., 2000).

Unlike the more mundane methods for improving cognitive function—such as exercise and good nutrition (Dresler et al., 2012)—these pharmaceutical cognitive enhancers (PCEs) are thought to raise a host of ethical issues for individuals and society (Greely et al., 2008; Bostrom and Sandberg, 2009). At the individual level, concerns are raised about medical safety and side effects, the authenticity of the enhanced mind and the value of achievements facilitated by pharmaceutical intervention. At the societal level, ethical questions can be asked about whether the availability of PCEs would increase or undermine equality, and about whether individuals will be directly or indirectly coerced into using PCEs. Further normative questions emerge particularly in the healthcare setting: should we be drawing a sharp line between treatment and enhancement and should individuals be given access to PCEs through medical professionals?

In this paper, we outline the key issues at stake in the normative debate about pharmacological cognitive enhancement (PCE) and, for each issue, suggest the contribution that neuroscientific research could make. The greatest contribution will be made to the discussions surrounding the safety and efficacy of PCEs. Although the question of what harms are worth risking in the pursuit of certain benefits is to a large extent normative, the dearth of evidence about the effectiveness and safety of PCEs in real-world contexts renders the discussion mostly hypothetical at this point. More research on the risks of dependency is also urgently needed. Data of this kind will be crucial for discussions about regulation, and for debates about the permissibility of requiring or encouraging people to use PCEs.

In addition to the contribution neuroscience will make to understanding the risk-benefit profiles of PCEs, we suggest that a more nuanced understanding of the neural systems affected by different substances will enrich the debate about whether PCE use constitutes cheating. Also related to cheating, we further suggest that the neuroscientific evidence on the functional trade-offs precipitated by some PCE adds an important dimension to the debate about whether achievements facilitated by PCEs should be seen to be effortless and involve little sacrifice. Drawing together our conclusions, we propose an "ethical agenda" for future neuroscientific research on PCE. This agenda sets out what sort of research would help move the ethical debates forward, and why. Resolving these debates will be crucial for ensuring that society responds to the increasing use of PCE in the most responsible, fair and rational way. For a summary of our "ethical agenda" for neuroscientific research, see **Table 1**.

OVERVIEW OF PHARMACOLOGICAL COGNITIVE ENHANCEMENT

What it means to "enhance" is notoriously difficult to pin down. To enhance is essentially to improve or increase, but what this improvement must be relative to is not obvious. On the broadest definitions of enhancement, some capacity is enhanced if it is improved relative to its prior level of functioning such that it increases the individual's chances of leading a good life—enhancement thus occurs regardless of how well- or poorly-functioning the capacity originally was (Savulescu et al., 2011). On more restrictive definitions of enhancement, a capacity is enhanced if it is improved beyond a particular point—perhaps a species mean or agreed "normal" level of functioning (c.f. Sabin and Daniels, 1994). Others define enhancement as any improvement which goes beyond correcting pathology. For example: "A

Table 1 | Summary of ethical agenda for neuroscientific research.

Suggested type of study	Advancement in ethical debate
Longitudinal studies investigating the long-term safety profile of PCEs	This is perhaps the most pressing task for neuroscientists. The long-term, real-world safety profile of PCEs is of considerable import to potential users and to all debates about PCE ethics and policy. In relation to the latter concerns, longitudinal studies will advance ethical debates about: (1) whether PCEs should be placed on the open market for enhancement purposes (and with what restrictions), and (2) whether employees doing particular types of jobs can legitimately be required to take PCEs
Identification of pathology associated with mental or psychiatric disorders or limitations to enable classificatory separation of conditions which are diseases from those which constitute normal human variation	Will advance the ethical debate about whether the administration and effects of particular PCEs constitute treatment or enhancement, and how resources should be deployed accordingly
Identification of the effects of PCEs in targeted and specified populations of ethical significance, such as those who are worst off. In particular, further research into the baseline effect should be conducted	Will advance the debate about distributive justice and access to PCEs. If PCEs have differential effects on those who are already worst off, this will be highly relevant to their permissibility and just distribution
More precise distinction between the different cognitive effects of different PCEs	Will (1) be of central relevance to whether certain putative PCEs will be used for enhancement and, if so, in which contexts and (2) advance the debate on cheating in competitive contexts: some effects (e.g., creativity) might be considered more unfair than others (e.g., wakefulness) and enhancing motivation vs. enhancing effectiveness might be considered relevant to the value of any resulting achievements
Investigation of the functional trade-offs associated with different PCEs	Will (1) be of central relevance to whether certain putative PCEs will be used for enhancement and, if so, in which contexts and will (2) advance the debate about the nature of the sacrifice possibly required for achievements to have value. It will also (3) advance the debate about the practicality and legitimacy of requiring certain people to take PCEs
Pursuit of a "personalized enhancement" approach to bring us closer to understanding what effect any particular PCE will have in any particular person	Will be relevant to many (if not all) ethical debates and policy considerations including: (1) whether particular people could legitimately be required to take PCEs in certain contexts, (2) who should be given priority access to which PCEs, (3) whether unequal effects have ramifications for cheating. Only when we can predict the *personal* benefits and costs of enhancement can policy be truly informed and ethical

cognitively enhanced person [...] is not necessarily somebody with particularly high (let alone super-human) cognitive capacities. A cognitively enhanced person, rather, is somebody who has benefited from an intervention that improves the performance of some cognitive subsystem without correcting some specific, identifiable pathology or dysfunction of that subsystem" (Bostrom and Sandberg, 2009). In this paper, we adopt the broader understanding of cognitive enhancement. We do this in part because the substances currently available and likely to be available in the near future effect only modest improvements (Husain and Mehta, 2011), but also because we believe that any line intended to mark the point at which an improvement counts as enhancement necessarily involves a value judgement involving normative (ethical) considerations.

Most of the substances cited as putative PCEs were originally developed for clinical use, to treat conditions that are at least partly characterized by some observable cognitive defect. Here, again, it is sometimes difficult to decide what should count as a cognitive *defect*. However, in the case of defective or deficient capacities, decisions must be made about where to place the line to determine who should receive medical attention and resources. For example, two of the substances receiving the most attention from those interested in enhancement—methylphenidate and modafinil—were originally developed to treat the symptoms of ADHD and narcolepsy, respectively. More recently, however, these substances have been used off-label by healthy individuals to improve their memories, level of alertness, or powers of concentration (e.g., Maher, 2008). Other substances with some modest enhancing effects on cognition include donepezil, dopamine agonists (such as d-amphetamine, bromocriptine, and pergolide), guanfacine, atomoxetine, reboxetine, galantamine, rivastigmine, and memantine. Working pharmacologically in different ways, these substances have been shown to improve cognitive functions such as response inhibition, working memory, episodic memory, attention, vigilance, and incidental learning (see de Jongh et al., 2008; Lanni et al., 2008; Husain and Mehta, 2011). However, this limited evidence of effectiveness should be cautiously considered alongside studies producing null results and some evidence of task-specific impairments (see Hall and Lucke, 2010 and Advokat, 2010 for less optimistic reviews of the scientific literature on PCE).

The prospect of being able to enhance any of these cognitive functions probably would be attractive to many individuals. Whether the goal of such enhancement would be to perform better at work, to learn a skill or language quicker, to decrease the need for rest in leisure time, or even just to experience one's mind as "sharper," improving cognition would presumably come with many benefits. Data from various prevalence studies indicate that there are groups of individuals who use some of the substances listed above for purposes of studying, to combat jet-lag or even to facilitate completion of household chores (for a review of student uses, see Smith and Farah, 2011; see also Maher, 2008).

Whilst the neuroscientific literature is reporting some modest enhancement effects of these substances on the cognition of healthy individuals (c.f. Husain and Mehta, 2011), the ethical literature has been raising and responding to a variety of issues pertaining to their use (for overview see Greely et al., 2008; Bostrom and Sandberg, 2009). Some of these issues are practical, some socio-political and others relate to the individual user. The overarching goal is to ascertain how permissible and how moral PCE use is and how society and regulatory bodies should respond to it. Although the ethical debate is principally a normative enterprise, it cannot reach firm conclusions about how to proceed based purely on hypothetical reasoning and untutored speculation: it must be informed by neuroscientific research providing the empirical facts about PCEs. In what follows, we outline the key issues in the enhancement debate, emphasizing where we think neuroscientific research might have particular importance for the normative debate.

ETHICAL DEBATE AND THE RELEVANCE OF NEUROSCIENTIFIC RESEARCH

MEDICAL SAFETY AND EFFECTIVENESS

In many ethical discussions of cognitive enhancers the first issue to be raised (often to be set aside so that there can be any further discussion at all) is whether cognitive enhancers are *medically safe* to use. Since there are no longitudinal studies yet examining the long-term use of pharmaceuticals such as modafinil and methylphenidate, some authors argue that we currently do not know enough about the potential dangers and that the availability and use of PCEs should be avoided on this basis (e.g., Drabiak-Syed, 2011; Boot et al., 2012).

Despite the huge interest in PCE from philosophers and scientists, the evidence of their *effectiveness* is still inconclusive. Moreover, where there is evidence of enhancement effects, they often tend to be limited to improvements on specific tasks, are only seen at certain dosages and are not observed in all people (Ragan et al., 2013; Farah et al., 2014). Crucially, it must be remembered that the degree and nature of any cognitive improvements will be different for each PCE and so no sweeping claims should be made about the effectiveness of PCEs in general. In terms of both effectiveness and safety, it should also be noted that short term studies carried out in laboratory settings are not representative of long term use in real world contexts.

In his meta-analysis of randomized controlled trials of methyphendidate, Repantis et al. (2010) found a significant improvement in the long-term memory of healthy participants, particularly when there was a longer interval between the learning phase and recall. However, the meta-analysis revealed no significant improvements in attention, mood or executive functions. Similar findings emerged from Farah et al.'s (2014) review of more than fifty experiments on the effects of amphetamine and methylphenidate: they found convincing evidence of an enhancing effect of stimulants on learning under some circumstances, specifically when the retention interval between study and test was longer than an hour, but not at shorter intervals. They also concluded that the evidence for improvement of executive functions was much less clear. There is some evidence to suggest that the effects of methylphenidate on cognitive control are only significantly positive in participants whose performance on placebo was lowest (Smith and Farah, 2011).

In relation to the effectiveness of modafinil, Farah et al.'s (2014) recent review of single dose studies of modafinil concluded that there is clear evidence of enhanced executive function and memory for sleep-deprived individuals but, for rested adults, whilst there were some positive findings for specific tasks such as those requiring inhibitory control, there were also a large number of null results and the occasional finding of impairment. They refer to this pattern—of limited improvements on some specific tasks and impairment on others—as being "familiar" for PCEs.

There are also some reviews of the effectiveness of anti-dementia medications for cognitive enhancement. These include acetylcholinesterase inhibitors such as donepezil, rivastigmine, and galantamine. A review conducted by Repantis (2013) concluded that the few existing studies of effects in healthy participants provide no consistent evidence for a neuroenhancement effect. In the case of, donepezil there was some evidence to suggest improvements on retention of training on complex aviation tasks (Yesavage et al., 2002), improvements in verbal memory and episodic memory (Gron et al., 2005). However, other studies showed no or limited effects on memory and attention and two others showed transient impairment of episodic memory (Beglinger et al., 2004, 2005). The same pattern of results suggesting enhancement in some cases but no effect or even impairment in others can be seen for donepezil. Further, a review of the efficacy of these putative cognitive enhancers for patients with mild cognitive impairment concluded that they did not improve cognition or function among patients with low-level impairment (Tricco et al., 2013).

The *medical safety* of PCEs varies from substance to substance, and side effects relate not only to the direct pharmacological effects but also to broader psychological and physiological changes. The review conducted by Repantis (2013) concluded that in the majority of trials, the drugs were well tolerated. However, side effects were noted. In relation to methylphenidate, side effects included increased heart rate and some instances of increases in blood pressure. Headaches, anxiety, nervousness, dizziness, drowsiness, and insomnia were also typical complaints.

Repantis (2013) summarizes similar side effects for modafinil, where adverse reactions included headache, dizziness, gastrointestinal complaints (e.g., nausea, abdominal pain, dry mouth), increased diuresis, palpitations, nervousness, restlessness, and sleep disturbances and insomnia (especially in studies with non-sleep deprived individuals). In their recent review, Ragan et al. (2013) highlight the fact that modafinil was reviewed by the European Medicines Agency (2010), who concluded that it should not be prescribed for obstructive sleep apnea, shift-work sleep disorder, and idiopathic hypersomnia because of the risks of serious skin reaction, suicidality, depression, psychosis, and adverse cardiovascular events.

In relation to anti-dementia drugs, Repantis (2013) concluded that, in the majority of the trials in healthy adults, donepezil was well tolerated. However, some side effects were reported in some participants, including gastrointestinal complaints (e.g., nausea), headaches, dizziness, nightmares, and insomnia. The meta analysis of anti-dementia drugs for people with mild cognitive impairment (Tricco et al., 2013) revealed that patients taking these medications experienced significantly more nausea, diarrhea, vomiting, and headaches than patients taking placebo. The authors also suggest that patients taking these medications might be at greater cardiac risk, with one study finding a higher incidence of bradycardia among patients who received galantamine.

As Farah et al. (2014) emphasize, there is another type of risk that should not be ignored in a consideration of the safety of PCEs. Many pharmaceuticals, especially stimulants, present a risk of dependence. The authors cite a nationwide survey analyzed by Kroutil et al. (2006) which estimates that almost one in twenty nonmedical users of prescription stimulants meet the criteria for dependence or abuse (For further discussion of the potential for addiction in student populations see Outram, 2010 and White et al., 2006).

Finally, as Ragan et al. (2013) point out, there is no such thing as a completely safe drug, only a drug whose benefits outweigh its drawbacks. However, it is also worth emphasizing that, even if there are long-term risks associated with these substances, this does not (by itself) mean that they should automatically be prohibited. There are serious risks associated with many activities that the state permits because it is believed that individuals should decide for themselves whether these risks are worth taking. Dangerous sports and cosmetic surgery both come with risks, but the value some individuals attach to the respective sporting experiences and cosmetic effects justifies giving these individuals the choice to take risks in their pursuit.

This caveat notwithstanding, and taking into account potential costs to the healthcare system, greater knowledge about safety and efficacy will allow regulators to decide whether the decision about which risks are worth taking should be put in the hands of consumers (for a detailed discussion of the way risks and benefits should be assessed for cognitive enhancement devices, such as brain stimulators, see Maslen et al., 2014). The ethical debate about the level of risk consumers should be allowed to take is of great practical importance when it comes to making policy recommendations. In addition, the question of whether the harms of a certain PCE outweigh its benefits will be important to discussions about the permissibility of requiring individuals to use PCEs and about the possible need to protect individuals from pressure to take any of the substances under discussion.

Finally, the empirical project of identifying the different effects PCEs have across a different individuals (c.f. Husain and Mehta, 2011) is likely to feed into the normative debate about which effects (for which individuals) constitute a form of treatment and which effects (for which individuals) constitute enhancement. We discuss these and other ethical issues in what follows.

AUTHENTICITY AND NATURALNESS

There are a bundle of related ethical issues that are sometimes raised under the broad heading of *authenticity* (see Bublitz and Merkel, 2009; Juth, 2011). Some of these pertain to numerical personal identity—do individuals become categorically different persons when they transform themselves via enhancement? (DeGrazia, 2005)—some consider less drastically what it is for an individual to be to be more or less his or her "real" self (The President's Council on Bioethics, 2003), and other ethical concerns pertain to what it is to be, and function as, a human being (Kass, 2003).

The principal tenet underlying authenticity objections against the use of PCEs is that individuals are most themselves when they are in their "natural," unaltered state. If capacities and characteristics fundamental to one's identity are changed, then the individual is recast as an altered or inauthentic person (e.g., Elliott, 1999). This argument is premised on the idea that there is a "real," true self, and that this real self is to be preserved as much as possible. However, this assumption can be challenged: individuals often (and understandably) try to improve themselves in ways that allow them to more successfully achieve their goals. Being autonomous is to form goals for how one's life is to go, including what kind of person to be. On this model of authenticity as autonomy, whether PCE is authentic depends on whether it helps a person to achieve her autonomous goals. For example, an individual might teach him or herself motivational strategies to overcome his or her naturally lazy disposition; another individual might use techniques from cognitive behavior therapy to overcome his or her propensity for generalized anxiety (e.g., Butler et al., 2006) or shyness, or gregariousness, or bad temper, or gullibility. Such strategies may not render the individuals inauthentic, but rather assist them in removing barriers that otherwise prevent them from maximizing self-actualization. Correspondingly, if PCEs can, for example, help an individual to concentrate better so that he or she can achieve the goals he or she values, this acts in service of authenticity rather than undermines it. There is great human variation, and variation within individuals subject to many intrinsic and extrinsic factors (see Kahane and Savulescu, 2013). Even if the authentic self were defined, it seems likely that many factors interfere and PCEs may reduce the effect of such influences.

However, some deny that authenticity is reducible to autonomy. Such writers (e.g., Taylor, 1991) appeal to a "real self." But even on such an account, the real self may be complex and multifaceted. Often people have a range of qualities and they may use PCEs to bring out some of their qualities, while suppressing others. Thus, whether an enhanced self compromises the real self depends on what constitutes a person's real self and what the effect of the PCE is—both questions for cognitive science. If PCEs merely amplify, rather than add entirely new qualities, then they enable the self to evolve, rather than replacing one individual with a set of attributes with another with different attributes.

There is a related but different concern about *naturalness.* The idea that enhancements will take us too far from what it is to be human altogether is often accompanied by the idea that too much technological intervention will lead to an overmechanization of the mind. The activities in which we engage—and, more importantly, the ways in which we engage in them—are said to have a certain quality to them that makes them "human" activities (President's Council on Bioethics, 2003). In this vein, Kass (2003) argues that since individuals play no role in bringing about the effects of biomedical interventions, they cannot understand these effects "in human terms." His suggestion is that whereas the effects of studying or training are "intelligible" to us, the effects of direct interventions are not comprehensible and thus our use of them departs "from "genuine," unmediated, and (in principle) self-transparent human activity" (p. 23).

However, we argue that we make use of many directly-acting substances, in medicine and in leisure, that do not result in departure from "genuine" human activity. Just because their pharmacological mechanisms are not understood by the average person does not mean that they cannot be made sense of as part of a human narrative. Kass cites alcohol, caffeine and nicotine as not having the same unintelligible quality as direct biomedical interventions. He says this is because "we use these agents not as pure chemicals but in forms and social contexts that, arguably, give them a meaning different from what they would have were we to take them as pills" (p. 22). An obvious objection to Kass' resistance to PCEs would be to add PCEs to beverages, as caffeine currently is. It would then be "intelligible" in the same way that caffeine is said to be "intelligible." Moreover, if intelligibility can be conferred by social context then the social context of, for example, studying, or conducting research should equally make PCEs part of a comprehensible human enterprise. Perhaps his distinction between the forms alcohol, caffeine, and nicotine tend to take, and the form of a simple pill, is supposed to indicate that the former are enjoyed for themselves, rather than being instrumental to achieve some goal. However, studies have reported that some individuals take PCEs for recreational purposes (see Smith and Farah, 2011) and it is common knowledge that caffeine is regularly used exclusively for alertness and for performance enhancement. Even if it might be the case in lay people's current perceptions (cf. Faulmüller et al., 2013; Schelle et al., 2014), from a normative stance it cannot be that form and context make all the difference between the human intelligibility of an espresso and a caffeine pill and a PCE.

The core of such an "intelligibility" objection may be that PCEs and other new technologies work in ways entirely alien to the way the human mind normally works, adding a completely new way of being. For example, chips inserted into the human brain that allowed us to perceive other people's thoughts directly would be entirely new. Neuroscience can assist by unravelling the way the mind does work, and does not, and by enabling categorization of enhancers into those which harness natural processes, and those that introduce entirely new capacities. Most enhancers at present appear to harness existing neurobiological physiology, though exactly how many enhance performance remains to be determined.

The ethical debate about authenticity and naturalness is unlikely to be advanced solely by the findings of neuroscientific research. The disagreement is partly a normative one about what constitutes the "real" self and whether our "real" selves are the selves we are most prone to being or the selves that we aspire to develop in to—or whether it makes sense to speak of "real" selves at all. Qualitative research, such as that conducted by Singh (2005) or Bolt and Schermer (2009), will helpfully provide a clearer picture of the sorts of experiences individuals have when taking PCEs.

In summary, it is important to recognize that most PCEs, if not all, harness innate biological systems, for example, affecting release, reuptake or sensitivity to neurotransmitters that cause cognitive activity. They do not at present introduce radical "new ways of being" divorced from the ordinary human way—they really just provide "more of the same." Indeed, humans vary in the ways in which their cognitive systems function and in some cases, PCEs may bring those at the lower end of normal up to the level of function of those in the mid to upper range.

More importantly, we suggest that what matters more than whether the experiences are in some sense authentic is whether the individual wants and values the effects of the PCE and whether the individual is autonomous in his or her decision to use PCE. This, we suggest, is a legitimate concern and is addressed in the following section.

COERCION

If PCEs were to become more commonplace, then employers might start to require their employees to use PCEs. The Academy of Medical Sciences et al. (2012) suggested in a recent report that "[O]ccupations that require particular patterns of focus could benefit from enhancements that facilitate achieving such patterns. For example, surgeons may need to be able to concentrate for extended periods, whereas other jobs such as air traffic control can require very rapid reactions during periods of relative uniformity. As an extrapolation to this, it is possible that in these high-responsibility occupations enhancement could be seen as a moral obligation, or even demanded by the public." (p. 38, for a discussion see also Maslen et al., in press). The US Airforce has already approved the use of modafinil by its pilots (Caldwell and Caldwell, 2005) and some medical practitioners are beginning to wonder whether enhancement might be required of them in the future (Rose and Curry, 2010). Writing in the Journal of Surgical Research, surgeons have suggested that the use of PCEs may come to be required practice. They say, "The prospect of fatigued surgeons taking a prescription drug, such as modafinil, to allow them to operate for longer, and possibly to a higher standard, is perhaps not as far-fetched as some may suggest. This drug has already been trialed in emergency physicians, when performing non-medical-related tasks at the end of a nightshift." (Warren et al., 2009, p. 168).

Further, the authors note that there are "useful and warranted forms of coercion" (p. 170) such as forcing surgeons to undertake hygiene practices such as handwashing prior to and during surgery. Given that this *coercion* is acceptable, they go on to ask, "What will our employers feel about a drug that makes us less prone to error, able to work longer hours, or to operate more efficiently? Employers are able to request certain behavioral standards from their employees, dictate rest periods, and insist on abstinence from certain drugs to ensure that their doctors perform well—will a day arise where they can recommend or even insist on surgeons being artificially enhanced? This may seem fanciful, but recent work has suggested that a mixture of napping and caffeine attenuates fatigue in interns and thus should be adopted by hospital administration. Why not other types of stimulant?" (p. 171).

The ethical objection often raised in this context is that, although it is thought to be reasonable to require certain things of employees, such as compulsory training and codes of conduct, requiring them to ingest psychoactive substances into their bodies is too demanding a requirement. It would require a compelling justification (perhaps pointing to the severity of harm that would be prevented through requiring enhancement) to trump the value we place on preserving the right individuals have to determine what happens to their bodies and minds (for discussion of the right to mental self-determination in relation to enhancement and other mental manipulation, see Bublitz and Merkel, 2014). As far as possible, this right should be preserved, and this is especially the case where there is not enough evidence about the harms to which an employer would be subjecting his or her employee. Neuroscientific evidence will have a large role to play in understanding the seriousness of any proposed requirement. In addition to the risks posed by individual instances of PCE use, more data on the potential for dependency will be essential for this discussion. Whilst we *might* think it permissible to require some employees to take small, isolated personal risks, requiring them to do something that results in substance dependency would more comprehensively infringe an individual's autonomy. In this connection, although PCEs may become more common in the workplace, one of us has argued elsewhere that for these and other reasons, it is unlikely that there will ever be a legal obligation for a professional like a surgeon to take a PCE (Goold and Maslen, 2014). At present, no employer requires employees to take caffeine. Caffeine is a PCE.

Even if people were not directly coerced to take enhancers it could still be objected that permitting PCE use could result in indirect pressure to use them. The perception that others are taking substances that make them more productive could lead to the belief that taking them is necessary to keep up (Academy of Medical Sciences et al., 2012) and not taking PCEs might render one *de facto* ineligible for certain jobs (Chatterjee, 2004). However, whether indirect pressure to take PCEs would in fact result in their more prevalent use is a question for social science. (For empirical data relating to this question, see Franke et al., 2011 and Maier et al., 2013). Neuroscientific research will have little to contribute to the debate about the limits of acceptable social pressure and restriction on employees' autonomy. However, as noted above, opposition to enforced PCE use is partly motivated by the current lack of evidence on long-term safety and efficacy. What we can legitimately require of people is closely related to what risks we can require them to take. Assessment of the legitimacy of requiring certain individuals to take PCEs will depend in large part on their medical safety and efficacy. If PCEs are very safe and efficacious, their use in life-saving/threatening professions (e.g., surgeons, politicians, truck drivers, airline pilots, etc.) may legitimately be required.

TREATMENT vs. ENHANCEMENT

As noted in the introductory section, there is much disagreement about what should count as enhancement (c.f., Parens, 1998). Sometimes this disagreement is framed as a debate about where *treatment* ends and *enhancement* begins. The distinction often made is that treatments serve to cure illness and preserve health whereas enhancements make people "better than well." For example, Juengst (1998) defines enhancement as the term "usually used in bioethics to characterize interventions designed to improve human form or functioning beyond what is necessary to sustain or restore good health" (p. 29).

However, a common objection to this distinction is that, in many cases, what we define as "healthy" and "normal" is arbitrary.

This objection does not deny that there can be clear failures of function or physiology as a result of pathology which most would agree are inimical to good health, such as the effects of a brain hemorrhage or stroke. Rather, it emphasizes that the boundary between healthy and unhealthy cognition in many cases is a matter of where we choose to draw the line, not based on either statistically significant subfunctioning or pathology. For example, delimiting normal from defective powers of concentration when diagnosing ADHD is necessarily to engage in marking a categorical point on what is otherwise a continuum (c.f. Schermer and Bolt, 2011). The point could be selected further to the left or right on that continuum of functioning. Would selecting a point which increased ADHD diagnosis increase the instances of individuals being treated or would some be receiving enhancement through the back door? Since the point is to some extent arbitrary, the corresponding labels of treatment and enhancement appear less meaningful in this context.

Similarly, it is difficult to know whether to classify substances used to combat age-related cognitive decline as instances of treatment or enhancement. Drawing sharp lines could have the result that a young person with cognitive abilities just above the cut off for being classified as having a mental disability would be "enhanced" by a drug but the elderly person whose abilities slipped to a level still above the young person would be receiving "treatment" if given the same substance (for a similar example, see Sandberg, 2011). Given the slipperiness of the distinction, one of us has argued (Savulescu et al., 2011) that instead of trying to determine whether certain drugs or certain of their effects constitute treatment or enhancement, it is more coherent and useful to think of a continuum of well-being which can be increased or diminished by various interventions.

It might be thought that evidence from neuroscience could adjudicate between instances of treatment and enhancement. If substances have discernable, discrete effects on different groups of people, it could be argued that these discrete effects mark the difference between a treatment and an enhancement. For example, although the way modafinil works is still unknown in detail (Minzenberg and Carter, 2008), neurologists do know that the brain of the narcoleptic is not neurophysiologically equivalent to the brain of the sleep-deprived individual and, correspondingly, it might be hypothesized that the effects of modafinil on the two groups will differ. Most forms of narcolepsy are associated with a deficiency in the hypothalamic neurotransmitter orexin (Mignot, 2010). The average sleep-deprived person, in contrast, does not exhibit such a deficiency. Accordingly, it might be thought that the more differences neuroscience can reveal between the narcoleptic and the non-narcoleptic, the better equipped we will be to distinguish between the treatment and enhancement effects of at least this PCE.

However, such knowledge would still not provide a definitive solution to which effects we should refer to as treatment and which we should call enhancement. Modafinil is also prescribed for shift work sleep disorder (SWSD), which is a product of unusual working patterns affecting circadian rhythms, not of underlying neurophysiology (Åkerstedt and Wright, 2009). This being said, it should be noted that not everyone who does shift work suffers from SWSD. This suggests that there must be some physiological or psychological difference between sufferers and non-sufferers and our lack of knowledge as to the cause of this difference does not make the disorder less of a treatable disorder.

In labeling the prescription of PCEs for SWSD an instance of treatment, a normative or ethical decision is still being made about which conditions and patterns of functionality should attract medical attention and resources. We are also implicitly making an assessment that medical treatment is the just and appropriate course of action for sufferers of the disorder, rather than prioritizing a change away from shift work. Neither the individual's underlying neurophysiology nor the particular mechanism of action of the substance tells us anything about whether this decision is the correct one.

One avenue through which neuroscience might illuminate the treatment vs. enhancement debate is by identifying pathology associated with mental or psychiatric disorders or limitations. So far, accurate tissue or cellular level pathological classification of psychiatric disease or disorder has eluded researchers. However, if psychiatric disorders could be characterized in the same way as neurological disorders, the presence of pathology would separate conditions which are diseases from those which constitute normal human variation.

Given that PCEs are not universally available through the healthcare system, individuals without conditions for which PCEs are approved would currently have to obtain them through other, unauthorized routes. This means that some people will have access to them but others will not. Even if PCEs were available on an open market, there could still be financial or other barriers to their accessibility. We discuss this issue and its potential implications next.

DISTRIBUTIVE JUSTICE

Society-level debates about PCE-related inequality consider *distributive justice*, and are related the question of whether PCEs will exacerbate existing socio-economic inequality. A common argument is that, as with many technologies, the rich and informed will have access to them whilst the poor and uninformed will not (e.g., Fukuyama, 2002). Assuming that cognitive enhancement confers some benefits, this will make those already at an advantage even better off. Whether this would in fact happen would depend on factors such as the affordability and accessibility of PCEs, as well as on the realities of their cognition-improving effects: the affordability and accessibility of PCEs will determine whether people are able to use them; the effects of the substances will determine whether they really put people who do so at an advantage. However, although there is the potential for PCEs to exacerbate unfairness if their distribution is unregulated, as one of us points out elsewhere, this is not a necessary consequence (Sandberg and Savulescu, 2011): if PCEs were distributed according to a principle of justice such as "prioritarianism"—the principle that says that we should give priority to those who are worst off, but also aim to maximize well-being of everyone in society—then PCEs would be most accessible to the worst off, becoming less accessible (but not inaccessible) as need decreases.

Further as we go on to discuss below in relation to competitive fairness, neuroscientific evidence supports the hypothesis that there is a base-line effect of many PCEs: their effects seem to depend on the subject's baseline working memory capacity. Individuals with low working-memory capacity improve while high-span individuals are either not affected or are even impaired (de Jongh et al., 2008). This means that those most in need of PCE would benefit most from it, with those less in need not benefiting at all or even experiencing impairment from the same substance. Given this evidence, it has been suggested that enhancement might actually serve to *reduce* inequality (Bostrom and Sandberg, 2009). However, whilst this could be true in terms of the equality of cognitive capacity, it must be remembered that cognitive capacity and socio-economic status are not always correlated: there would still be people with more opportunities and resources who could improve their prospects further. Whilst policy decisions about access to PCEs will be principally socio-political matters, those making the decisions will need to know how enhancers affect members of the population in order to best serve the interests of justice and equality. If PCEs have differential effects on those who are already worst off, this will be highly relevant to their permissibility and just distribution. Neuroscience research can thus contribute to ethical debate if effects in targeted and specified populations of ethical significance are studied. This would require ethically relevant population stratification.

COMPETITIVE FAIRNESS AND CHEATING

The ethical discussion of whether using cognitive enhancers constitutes *cheating*—perhaps in exams or at work—is more nuanced than the simple question of whether taking enhancers is "against the rules." It can extend beyond considerations of *fairness in competitive contexts* to ask whether personal achievements facilitated by PCEs are devalued for this reason (c.f., Schermer, 2008; Goodman, 2010; Santoni de Sio et al., in press). We suggest that evidence from neuroscience will help to develop the cheating debate in important ways. Below, we argue that three types of empirical inquiry are relevant to the ethical discussion. The first, the phenomenon of the "inverted U"—according to which the enhancing effects of PCEs are often baseline dependent and exhibit non-linear dose response curves —(de Jongh et al., 2008; Husain and Mehta, 2011), is relevant to efficacy questions involved in debates about cheating. The second type of study relevant to the debate is that which seeks to identify the particular neural systems affected by different substances, leading to disparate effects (e.g., Lanni et al., 2008): whether a substance improves creativity or rote learning may matter for some possible conceptions of what constitutes cheating. Similarly, whether a substance improves motivation and task enjoyment vs. memory capacity might matter for those who place a lot of value on success requiring effort. Third, we argue that the neuroscientific evidence pointing to the likelihood of cognitive trade-offs (de Jongh et al., 2008; Husain and Mehta, 2011) adds an underdeveloped dimension to the cheating debate: if the complaint is that achievements facilitated by PCE are devalued because they do not involve enough personal sacrifice, then evidence suggesting that enhancement in some domains comes at the cost of impairments in others offers a challenge to this view.

The inverted U curve and baseline dependency

Neuroscientific research so far shows that the effects of many purported PCEs are base-line dependent and have an inverted U-shaped dose-response curve (de Jongh et al., 2008; Husain and Mehta, 2011). This is important to the cheating debate as it means that some individuals will benefit from taking PCEs whereas others will gain no benefit and might even be impaired: low performing individuals will tend to be on the upward slope of the inverted-U and so benefit from a substance that moves them further up this slope. High performing individuals, on the other hand, will tend to be at the peak of the inverted U and will therefore become impaired by a substance that increases neurotransmitter levels further. If neuroscience were to more precisely identify the neurological profiles of those who are able to benefit from PCEs and those who are not then ethicists would be able to consider in greater detail whether the prospect of some being able to enhance whilst others cannot counts more decisively against PCE in competitive contexts than if all could enhance in these contexts. They would need to consider whether it is the case that enhancement is only fair if everyone could (in principle) avail themselves of it or whether is it permissible given that some are physiologically denied the possibility of improving.

Disparate effects of different PCEs

Although the exact mechanisms of substances like methylphenidate and modafinil are not yet fully understood, researchers have begun to investigate which PCEs affect which underlying systems, and with which effects (Lanni et al., 2008; Smith and Farah, 2011). Although cognitive functions necessarily interact, attempts have been made to ascertain the primary cognitive functions improved by particular PCEs based on their effects on neurotransmitters. Husain and Mehta (2011) explain that "a simple mapping between a specific neurotransmitter and a particular cognitive function—such as [working memory]—[...] seems untenable. However, subtle but important differences in the precise processes modulated might provide some discriminating value: for instance, dopamine has an established role in reinforcement learning in response to rewards, whereas serotonin seems to modulate reinforcement learning for aversive stimuli." (p. 29). Pursuing such discrimination, Lanni et al. (2008) review the neuroscience literature investigating the neuronal circuits, neurotransmitters and molecular events underlying the cognitive domains of memory, attention, and creativity to distinguish the effects of different enhancement substances. Elsewhere, Smith and Farah (2011) review the cognitive neuroscience literature to examine whether (and which) prescription stimulants improve learning, working memory, cognitive control, and other executive functions.

If neuroscientific research were able to distinguish between the effects of different PCEs this could have some implications for discussions about cheating. This is again effect stratification. Combined with population stratification, neuroscience research could bring us closer to understanding what effect this particular PCE will have in this person. This reflects the move to "personalized medicine" and might be dubbed "personalized enhancement." Only when we can predict the *personal* benefits and costs of enhancement can policy be truly informed and ethical.

It might be thought that the enhancement of some cognitive functions is more unfair than the enhancement of others. For example, the enhancement of creative thinking might be thought to constitute more significant cheating than improving wakefulness or even memory capacity. Imagine someone who says "when I take enhancers my work is no better, I can just do more of the same for longer" vs. someone who says "when I taken enhancers my work is much better than I can do without them." Having links with the debate about authenticity, it is as if the former individual is enabled to make better use of his or her own cognitive resources, whereas the latter is given new cognitive resources upon which he or she can draw. Those who think PCE use is unfair because the achievement is not a reflection of the person's natural abilities to solve and create might be less concerned by a PCE that simply allowed more efficient work of the standard the person could naturally achieve. A PCE that promoted wakefulness might allow an individual to work for longer but it will not come up with ideas on his or her behalf. Of course, it is important to remember that a PCE that improved creativity still has its effects on and through the individual's own brain. What will be interesting for ethicists to discuss is whether "assistance" with time management and efficiency is relevantly different to "assistance" with the content of ideas (if, indeed, we want to characterize the respective effects in this way).

Practical consequences might be to consider certain substances unfair for certain types of tests or for entry into certain types of employment: employers might only be troubled by the use of PCEs, the effects of which are *necessary* to carry out the job. This would be a practical consideration: could the employee continue to work without the PCE? For example, an architect who could only perform satisfactorily when taking a substance like modafinil that seems to improves spatial planning and visual pattern recognition memory (Turner et al., 2003) might be thought to be a higher risk employee than one who uses a memory enhancer which enables him or her to remember the names of building materials that he could look up without problem in the absence of the substance.

Further, neuroscientific research that could distinguish between substances that enhance the *effectiveness* of cognitive capacities, such as working memory, from those that instead (or additionally) increase *motivation* could also have implications for the competitive fairness debate. In the ethical literature, the point is sometimes made that it is effort and striving that makes achievements intelligible and valuable. For example, Fox (2005) argues that "[b]ecause they act directly on the human body and mind, biotechnological enhancements tempt us to shirk individual striving and struggle" (p. 1150).

A common rebuttal to this type of argument is that, whilst PCEs can make efforts more effective, they do not replace the need for dedicated, sustained study—striving and struggle is still required in order to achieve. For example, Greely (2010) notes that "the more plausible cognitive enhancements would not eliminate the need to study; they would just make studying more effective" (p. 6).

If, however, there were a significant enough effect of a PCE on motivation and/or task enjoyment, then it would be open to ethicists to argue that this *does* in some sense reduce the amount of effort that the person puts in. The drive to work or achieve no longer emanates from the individual and no struggle is encountered.

On the motivating effects of prescription stimulants, Smith and Farah (2011) write: "Another empirical question concerns the effects of stimulants on motivation, which can affect academic and occupational performance independent of cognitive ability. Volkow et al. (2004) showed that [methylphenidate] increased participants' self-rated interest in a relatively dull mathematical task. This is consistent with student reports that prescription stimulants make schoolwork seem more interesting (e.g., DeSantis et al., 2008). To what extent are the motivational effects of prescription stimulants distinct from their cognitive effects, and to what extent might they be more robust to differences in individual traits, dosage and task? Are the motivational effects of stimulants responsible for their usefulness when taken by normal healthy individuals for cognitive enhancement?" (p. 735).

If particular PCEs were shown to significantly improve motivation and/or task enjoyment whilst others only improve effectiveness, ethicists would need to consider whether there is any relevant difference between enhancing motivation and enhancing effectiveness and, if so, what the implications would be for the value of resulting achievements.

Enhancement is likely to involve trade-offs

Research suggests that enhancing one domain of cognition might come at the cost of impairing another. de Jongh et al. (2008) review evidence suggesting trade-offs between long-term memory and working memory; between stability and flexibility of long-term memory; between stability and flexibility of working memory; and perhaps, they conjecture, between cognition and mood. If a PCE comes at a cost—and, especially, a mental cost—this could also add a new dimension to the debate about cheating and the value of achievements.

In terms of gaining an unfair advantage over others in exams and other competitive tasks, the trade-offs would be relevant if the test required exercise of *both* the enhanced and the impaired capacity. Whilst the individual gains some advantage in some parts of the test, he or she would be disadvantaged in other parts. More generally, neuroscientific evidence of trade-offs are interesting to the debate about fairness and the value of achievements because some of the objections rest heavily on the idea that using PCEs means that no sacrifice—usually conceived as sacrifice of time, energy or other opportunities—is made by the individual.

For example, Kass (2003) says: "Yet in those areas of human life in which excellence has until now been achieved only by discipline and effort, the attainment of those achievements by means of drugs, genetic engineering, or implanted devices looks to be "cheating" or "cheap." We believe—or until only yesterday believed—that people should work hard for their achievements. "Nothing good comes easily."" (p. 21).

If enhancement of one domain of cognition comes at the cost of another then it does seem that some sort of sacrifice has been made. We might conceive of an individual who chooses to enhance his or her working memory such that he or she can solve complicated puzzles quickly. This same individual might accept that this enhancement comes at the cost of him or her finding it harder to recall facts and experiences from longer ago. Accordingly, whilst the physical act of ingesting a substance might be easy, there is a sense in which the enhanced capacity did not come easily—it did not come without personal cost. Whilst the conceptually most interesting trade-offs will involve impairments to cognitive capacities—like for like—it should also be noted that the more general side effects of PCEs (discussed in relation to medical safety above) also constitute an additional sort of "cost" to enhancement. The evidence on medical safety reviewed in section Medical Safety and Effectiveness suggests that PCE use will always come at a cost and may involve multiple costs of different kinds. The number and nature of these unavoidable costs constitute further challenge to the view that achievements facilitated by enhancement involve no sacrifice.

Important to note is that these costs of a trade-off are not like financial costs, which can be trivial and will constitute diminishment only insofar as they prevent the individual from making other purchases important to him or her. Rather, the costs of an enhancement trade-off are often mental costs—like for like—and are of a kind much more likely to constitute diminishment. Thus, neuroscientific research poses questions for those engaged in the cheating debate about whether there are relevant differences between different various costs of achievement—effort, opportunity, physiological side effects, cognitive trade-offs—and which (if any) are required for achievements to involve a sufficient level of sacrifice.

CONCLUSION

We have reviewed six of the main issues debated by ethicists working on PCE. Often, their purpose in debating these issues is to clarify concepts and normative positions, which then serve as a basis for recommending how society—and especially those tasked with its regulation—should respond to the emergence of PCEs. We have argued that whilst some of these issues are mostly political (coercion) or metaphysical (what constitutes authenticity), others have much to gain from emerging neuroscientific research. As well as providing data on safety and effectiveness, neuroscience will also allow a more fine-grained debate about whether the effects of some PCEs are more unfair than others in competitive contexts and whether employers should be more wary of employee reliance on some PCEs than on others. Further, due to emerging evidence on trade-offs, those who object to PCE on the ground that it facilitates individual gain without any attendant pain will have to explain why accepting an associated impairment in exchange for an enhancement is not a relevant sacrifice. Although we anticipate that ethicists will be far from stumped by this challenge, we hope to have demonstrated that it will, in large part, be though responding to emerging scientific evidence that normative accounts become more refined, complete and practically relevant.

In general, neuroscience can contribute to the formation of ethical policy on PCEs by adopting a "personalized" approach: personalized enhancement. Fine grained and stratified research should seek to identify specific risks, benefits, and trade-offs in small ethically relevant populations, or ideally in individuals. In doing this, according to the ethical values principles and criteria we choose, we can form policy on who should access which PCEs in which ways.

ACKNOWLEDGMENTS

This work was supported by the Wellcome Trust [086041/Z/08/Z]; the Oxford Martin School; and the Uehiro Foundation on Ethics and Education.

REFERENCES

Academy of Medical Sciences, Royal Society, British Academy, and Royal Academy of Engineering. (2012). *Human Enhancement and the Future of Work* (Report from Joint Workshop). Available online at: http://www.acmedsci.ac.uk/p47prid102.html#downloads (Accessed 22 May 2013).

Advokat, C. (2010). What are the cognitive effects of stimulant medication? Emphasis on adults with attentiondeficit/hyperactivity disorder. *Neurosci. Biobehav. Rev.* 34, 1256–1266. doi: 10.1016/j.neubiorev.2010.03.006

Åkerstedt, T., and Wright, K. P. Jr. (2009). Sleep loss and fatigue in shift work and shift work disorder. *Sleep Med. Clin.* 4, 257–271. doi: 10.1016/j.jsmc.2009.03.001

Beglinger, L. J., Gaydos, B. L., Kareken, D. A., Tangphao-Daniels, O., Siemers, E. R., and Mohs, R. C. (2004). Neuropsychological test performance in healthy volunteers before and after donepezil administration. *J. Psychopharmacol.* 18, 102–108. doi: 10.1177/0269881104040248

Beglinger, L. J., Tangphao-Daniels, O., Kareken, D. A., Zhang, L., Mohs, R., and Siemers, E. R. (2005). Neuropsychological test performance in healthy elderly volunteers before and after donepezil administration: a randomized, controlled study. *J. Clin. Psychopharmacol.* 25, 159–165. doi: 10.1097/01.jcp.0000155822.51962.b4

Bolt, I., and Schermer, M. (2009). Psychopharmacological enhancers: enhancing identity? *Neuroethics* 2, 103–111. doi: 10.1007/s12152-008-9031-7

Boot, B. P., Partridge, B., and Hall, W. (2012). Letter to the editor: better evidence for safety and efficacy is needed before neurologists prescribe drugs for neuroenhancement to healthy people. *Neurocase* 18, 181–184. doi: 10.1080/13554794.2011.588174

Bostrom, N., and Sandberg, A. (2009). Cognitive enhancement: methods, ethics, regulatory challenges. *Sci. Eng. Ethics* 15, 311–341. doi: 10.1007/s11948-009-9142-5

Bublitz, J. C., and Merkel, R. (2009). Autonomy and authenticity of enhanced personality traits. *Bioethics* 23, 360–374. doi: 10.1111/j.1467-8519.2009.01725.x

Bublitz, J. C., and Merkel, R. (2014). Crimes against minds: on mental manipulations, harms and a human right to mental self-determination. *Crim. Law and Philos.* 8, 51–77. doi: 10.1007/s11572-012-9172-y

Butler, A. C., Chapman, J. E., Forman, E. M., and Beck, A. T. (2006). The empirical status of cognitive-behavioral therapy: a review of meta-analyses. *Clin. Psychol. Rev.* 26, 17–31. doi: 10.1016/j.cpr.2005.07.003

Caldwell, J. A. and Caldwell, J. L. (2005). Fatigue in military aviation: an overview of us military-approved pharmacological countermeasures. *Aviat. Space Environ. Med.* 76(7 Suppl.), C39–C51.

Chatterjee, A. (2004). Cosmetic neurology the controversy over enhancing movement, mentation, and mood. *Neurology* 63, 968–974. doi: 10.1212/01.WNL.0000138438.88589.7C

DeGrazia, D. (2005). *Human Identity and Bioethics.* Cambridge: Cambridge University Press.

de Jongh, R., Bolt, I., Schermer, M., and Olivier, B. (2008). Botox for the brain: enhancement of cognition, mood and pro-social behavior and blunting of unwanted memories. *Neurosci. Biobehav. Rev.* 32, 760–776. doi: 10.1016/j.neubiorev.2007.12.001

DeSantis, A. D., Webb, E. M., and Noar, S. M. (2008). Illicit use of prescription ADHD medications on a college campus: a multimethodological approach. *J. Am. Coll. Health* 57, 315–324. doi: 10.3200/JACH.57.3.315-324

Drabiak-Syed, K. (2011). Reining in the pharmacological enhancement train: we should remain vigilant about regulatory standards for prescribing controlled substances. *J. Law Med. Ethics* 39, 272–279. doi: 10.1111/j.1748-720X.2011.00596.x

Dresler, M., Sandberg, A., Ohla, K., Bublitz, C., Trenado, C., Mroczko-Wasowicz, A., et al. (2012). Non-pharmacological cognitive enhancement. *Neuropharmacology* 64, 529–543. doi: 10.1016/j.neuropharm.2012.07.002

Elliott, C. (1999). *A Philosophical Disease: Bioethics, Culture and Identity*. Psychology Press.

Elliott, R., Sahakian, B. J., Matthews, K., Bannerjea, A., Rimmer, J., and Robbins, T. W. (1997). Effects of methylphenidate on spatial working memory and planning in healthy young adults. *Psychopharmacology* 131, 196–206. doi: 10.1007/s002130050284

European Medicines Agency. (2010). *Questions and Answers on the Review of Medicines Containing Modafinil. EMA/CHMP/460496/2010*. Available online at: http://www.ema.europa.eu/ema/index.jsp?curl=pages/medicines/human/referrals/Modafinil/human_referral_000236.jsp

Farah, M. J., Smith, M. E., Ilieva, I., and Hamilton, R. H. (2014). Cognitive enhancement. *Wiley Interdiscipl. Rev. Cogn. Sci.* 5, 95–103. doi: 10.1002/wcs.1250

Faulmüller, N., Maslen, H., and Santoni de Sio, F. (2013). The indirect psychological costs of cognitive enhancement. *Am. J. Bioeth.* 13, 45–47. doi: 10.1080/15265161.2013.794880

Fox, D. (2005). *Safety, Efficacy, and Authenticity: The Gap between Ethics and law in FDA Decisionmaking*. Available online at: http://heinonline.org/HOL/Page?handle=hein.journals/mslr2005&div=44&g_sent=1&collection=journals#1147

Franke, A. G., Bonertz, C., Christmann, M., Huss, M., Fellgiebel, A., Hildt, E., et al. (2011). Non-medical use of prescription stimulants and illicit use of stimulants for cognitive enhancement in pupils and students in Germany. *Pharmacopsychiatry* 44, 60–66. doi: 10.1055/s-0030-1268417

Fukuyama, F. (2002). *Our Post human Future: Consequences of the Biotechnology Revolution*. New York, NY: Farrar, Straus and Giroux.

Goodman, R. (2010). Cognitive enhancement, cheating, and accomplishment. *Kennedy Inst. Ethics J.* 20, 145–160. doi: 10.1353/ken.0.0309

Goold, I., and Maslen, H. (2014). Must the surgeon take the pill? Negligence duty in the context of cognitive enhancement. *Mod. Law Rev.* 77, 60–86. doi: 10.1111/1468-2230.12056

Greely, H., Sahakian, B., Harris, J., Kessler, R. C., Gazzaniga, M., Campbell, P., et al. (2008). Towards responsible use of cognitive-enhancing drugs by the healthy. *Nature* 456, 702–705. doi: 10.1038/456702a

Greely, H. T. (2010). "Enhancing brains: what are we afraid of?" in *Cerebrum: the Dana Forum on Brain Science*, Vol. 2010 (Dana Foundation). Available online at: http://dana.org/news/cerebrum/detail.aspx?id=28786

Gron, G., Kirstein, M., Thielscher, A., Riepe, M. W., and Spitzer, M. (2005). Cholinergic enhancement of episodic memory in healthy young adults. *Psychopharmacology* 182, 170–179. doi: 10.1007/s00213-005-0043-2

Hall, W. D., and Lucke, J. C. (2010). Enhancement uses of neuropharmaceuticals: more caution and skepticism needed. *Addiction* 105, 2041–2043. doi: 10.1111/j.1360-0443.2010.03211.x

Husain, M., and Mehta, M. A. (2011). Cognitive enhancement by drugs in health and disease. *Trends Cogn. Sci.* 15, 28–36. doi: 10.1016/j.tics.2010.11.002

Juengst, E. T. (1998). "What does enhancement mean?," in *Enhancing Human Traits: Ethical and Social Implications*, ed E. Parens (Georgetown University press), 29–47.

Juth, N. (2011). "Enhancement, autonomy, and authenticity," in *Enhancing Human Capacities*, eds J. Savulescu, R. ter Meulen, and G. Kahane (Oxford: Wiley-Blackwell), 34–48.

Kahane, G., and Savulescu, J. (2013). Normal human variation: refocussing the enhancement debate. *Bioethics*. doi: 10.1111/bioe.12045. [Epub ahead of print].

Kass, L. (2003). Ageless bodies, happy souls. *New Atlantis* 1, 9–28.

Kroutil, L. A., Van Brunt, D. L., Herman-Stahl, M. A., Heller, D. C., Bray, R. M., and Penne, M. A. (2006). Nonmedical use of prescription stimulants in the United States. *Drug Alcohol Depend.* 84, 135–143. doi: 10.1016/j.drugalcdep.2005.12.011

Lanni, C., Lenzken, S. C., Pascale, A., Del Vecchio, I., Racchi, M., Pistoia, F., et al. (2008). Cognition enhancers between treating and doping the mind. *Pharmacol. Res.* 57, 196–213. doi: 10.1016/j.phrs.2008.02.004

Maher, B. (2008). Poll results: look who's doping. *Nature* 452, 674–675. doi: 10.1038/452674a

Mehta, M. A., Owen, A. M., Sahakian, B. J., Mavaddat, N., Pickard, J. D., and Robbins, T. W. (2000). Methylphenidate enhances working memory by modulating discrete frontal and parietal lobe regions in the human brain. *J. Neurosci.* 20:RC65.

Mignot, E. (2010). "Narcolepsy: genetic predisposition and pathophysiology," in *Narcolepsy: A Clinical Guide*, eds M. Goswami, S. R. Pandi-Perumal, and M. J. Thorpy (New York, NY: Springer), 3–21. doi: 10.1007/978-1-4419-0854-4_1

Minzenberg, M. J., and Carter, C. S. (2008). Modafinil: a review of neurochemical actions and effects on cognition. *Neuropsychopharmacology* 33, 1477–1502. doi: 10.1038/sj.npp.1301534

Maier, L. J., Liechti, M. E., Herzig, F., and Schaub, M. P. (2013). To dope or not to dope: neuroenhancement with prescription drugs and drugs of abuse among Swiss university students. *PLoS ONE* 8:e77967. doi: 10.1371/journal.pone.0077967

Maslen, H., Douglas, T., Cohen Kadosh, R., Levy, N., and Savulescu, J. (2014). The regulation of cognitive enhancement devices: extending the medical model. *J. Law Biosci.* 1, 68–93. doi: 10.1093/jlb/lst003

Maslen, H., Santoni de Sio, F., and Faulmüller, N. (in press). "With cognitive enhancement comes great responsibility?," in *Responsible Innovation*, Vol. 2, eds B. J. Koops et al. (Dordrecht: Springer).

Müller, U., Steffenhagen, N., Regenthal, R., and Bublak, P. (2004). Effects of modafinil on working memory processes in humans. *Psychopharmacology* 177, 161–169. doi: 10.1007/s00213-004-1926-3

Outram, S. M. (2010). The use of methylphenidate among students: the future of enhancement?. *J. Med. Ethics* 36, 198–202. doi: 10.1136/jme.2009.034421

Parens, E. (1998). Is better always good?: the enhancement project. *Hastings Center Rep.* 28, s1–s17. doi: 10.2307/3527981

President's Council on Bioethics. (2003). *Beyond Therapy*. Washington, DC: U.S. Government Printing Office, 253.

Ragan, C. I., Bard, I., and Singh, I. (2013). What should we do about student use of cognitive enhancers? An analysis of current evidence. *Neuropharmacology* 64, 588–595. doi: 10.1016/j.neuropharm.2012.06.016

Repantis, D. (2013). "Psychopharmacological neuroenhancement: evidence on safety and efficacy," in *Cognitive Enhancement*, eds E. Hildt and A. G. Franke (Dordrecht: Springer), 29–38.

Repantis, D., Schlattmann, P., Laisney, O., and Heuser, I. (2010). Modafinil and methylphenidate for neuroenhancement in healthy individuals: a systematic review. *Pharmacol. Res.* 62, 187–206. doi: 10.1016/j.phrs.2010.04.002

Rose, S., and Curry, T. (2010). Fatigue countermeasures, and performance enhancement in resident physicians—reply. *Mayo Clin. Proc.* 85, 301–302. doi: 10.4065/mcp.2009.0704

Sabin, J. E., and Daniels, N. (1994). Determining "medical necessity" in mental health practice. *Hastings Center Rep.* 24, 5–13. doi: 10.2307/3563458

Sandberg, A. (2011). "Cognition enancement: upgrading the brain," in *Enhancing Human Capacities*, eds J. Savulescu, R. ter Meulen, and G. Kahane (Oxford: Wiley-Blackwell), 71–91.

Sandberg, A., and Savulescu, J. (2011). "The social and economic impacts of cognitive enhancements," in *Enhancing Human Capacities*, eds J. Savulescu, R. ter Meulen, and G. Kahane (Oxford: Wiley-Blackwell), 93–112.

Santoni de Sio, F., Faulmüller, N., Savulescu, J., and Vincent, N. A. (in press). "Why less praise for enhanced performance? Moving beyond responsibility-shifting, authenticity, and cheating to a nature of activities approach," in *Cognitive Enhancement: Ethical and Policy Implications in International Perspectives*, eds F. Jotterand and V. Dubljevic (Oxford: Oxford University Press).

Savulescu, J., Sandberg, A., and Kahane, G. (2011). "Well-being and enhancement," in *Enhancing Human Capacities*, J. Savulescu, R. ter Meulen, and G. Kahane (Oxford: Wiley-Blackwell), 3–18.

Schelle, K. J., Faulmüller, N., Caviola, L., and Hewstone, M. (2014). Attitudes towards pharmacological cognitive enhancement – a review. *Front. Syst. Neurosci.* 8:53. doi: 10.3389/fnsys.2014.00053

Schermer, M. (2008). Enhancements, easy shortcuts, and the richness of human activities. *Bioethics* 22, 355–363. doi: 10.1111/j.1467-8519.2008.00657.x

Schermer, M., and Bolt, I. (2011). "What's in a name? ADHD and the gray area between treatment and enhancement," in *Enhancing Human Capacities*, eds J. Savulescu, R. ter Meulen, and G. Kahane (Oxford: Wiley-Blackwell), 179–193.

Singh, I. (2005). Will the "real boy" please behave: dosing dilemmas for parents of boys with ADHD. *Am. J. Bioeth.* 5, 34–47. doi: 10.1080/15265160590945129

Smith, M. E., and Farah, M. J. (2011). Are prescription stimulants "smart pills"? The epidemiology and cognitive neuroscience of prescription stimulant use by normal healthy individuals. *Psychol. Bull.* 137, 717–741. doi: 10.1037/a0023825

Taylor, C. (1991). *The Ethics of Authenticity*. Cambridge, MA: Harvard University Press.

Thomas, R. J., and Kwong, K. (2006). Modafinil activates cortical and subcortical sites in the sleep-deprived state. *Sleep* 29, 1471–1481.

Tricco, A. C., Soobiah, C., Berliner, S., Ho, J. M., Ng, C. H., Ashoor, H. M., et al. (2013). Efficacy and safety of cognitive enhancers for patients with mild cognitive impairment: a systematic review and meta-analysis. *Can. Med. Assoc. J.* 185, 1393–1401. Doi: 10.1503/cmaj.130451

Turner, D. C., Robbins, T. W., Clark, L., Aron, A. R., Dowson, J., and Sahakian, B. J. (2003). Cognitive enhancing effects of modafinil in healthy volunteers. *Psychopharmacology* 165, 260–269. doi: 10.1007/s00213-002-1250-8

Volkow, N. D., Wang, G. J., Fowler, J. S., Telang, F., Maynard, L., Logan, J., et al. (2004). Evidence that methylphenidate enhances the saliency of a mathematical task by increasing dopamine in the human brain. *Am. J. Psychiatry.* 161, 1173–1180. doi: 10.1176/appi.ajp.161.7.1173

Warren, O. J., Leff, D. R., Athanasiou, T., Kennard, C., and Darzi, A. (2009). The neurocognitive enhancement of surgeons: an ethical perspective. *J. Surg. Res.* 152, 167–172. doi: 10.1016/j.jss.2007.12.761

Wesensten, N. J., Killgore, W. D., and Balkin, T. J. (2005). Performance and alertness effects of caffeine, dextroamphetamine, and modafinil during sleep deprivation. *J. Sleep Res.* 14, 255–266. doi: 10.1111/j.1365-2869.2005.00468.x

White, B. P., Becker-Blease, K. A., and Grace-Bishop, K. (2006). Stimulant medication use, misuse, and abuse in an undergraduate and graduate student sample. *J. Am. Coll. Health* 54, 261–268. doi: 10.3200/JACH.54.5.261-268

Yesavage, J. A., Mumenthaler, M. S., Taylor, J. L., Friedman, L., O'Hara, R., Sheikh, J., et al. (2002) Donepezil and flight simulator performance: effects on retention of complex skills. *Neurology* 59, 123–125. doi: 10.1212/WNL.59.1.123

8

Sleep for cognitive enhancement

Susanne Diekelmann*

Institute of Medical Psychology and Behavioral Neurobiology, University Tübingen, Tübingen, Germany

Edited by:
Mikhail Lebedev, Duke University, USA

Reviewed by:
Jessica Payne, University of Notre Dame, USA
Daniel Bendor, University College London, UK
Ivan N. Pigarev, Russian Academy of Sciences, Russia

***Correspondence:**
Susanne Diekelmann, Institute of Medical Psychology and Behavioral Neurobiology, University Tübingen, Otfried-Müller-Str. 25, CIN Building, 72076 Tübingen, Germany
e-mail: susanne.diekelmann@uni-tuebingen.de

Sleep is essential for effective cognitive functioning. Loosing even a few hours of sleep can have detrimental effects on a wide variety of cognitive processes such as attention, language, reasoning, decision making, learning and memory. While sleep is necessary to ensure normal healthy cognitive functioning, it can also enhance performance beyond the boundaries of the normal condition. This article discusses the enhancing potential of sleep, mainly focusing on the domain of learning and memory. Sleep is known to facilitate the consolidation of memories learned before sleep as well as the acquisition of new memories to be learned after sleep. According to a widely held model this beneficial effect of sleep relies on the neuronal reactivation of memories during sleep that is associated with sleep-specific brain oscillations (slow oscillations, spindles, ripples) as well as a characteristic neurotransmitter milieu. Recent research indicates that memory processing during sleep can be boosted by (i) cueing memory reactivation during sleep; (ii) stimulating sleep-specific brain oscillations; and (iii) targeting specific neurotransmitter systems pharmacologically. Olfactory and auditory cues can be used, for example, to increase reactivation of associated memories during post-learning sleep. Intensifying neocortical slow oscillations (the hallmark of slow wave sleep (SWS)) by electrical or auditory stimulation and modulating specific neurotransmitters such as noradrenaline and glutamate likewise facilitates memory processing during sleep. With this evidence in mind, this article concludes by discussing different methodological caveats and ethical issues that should be considered when thinking about using sleep for cognitive enhancement in everyday applications.

Keywords: sleep, cognitive enhancement, memory, learning, reactivation, brain stimulation, pharmacology, ethics

INTRODUCTION

Sleep is vital to ensure normal human cognitive performance. Not obtaining enough sleep diminishes a wide variety of cognitive functions such as attention, language, reasoning, decision making, learning and memory (for reviews see Durmer and Dinges, 2005; Killgore, 2010; Jackson et al., 2013). Acute sleep deprivation of one or more nights without sleep can slow down reaction times (Van Dongen et al., 2003), increase perseveration (Retey et al., 2006), reduce focused attention (Thomas et al., 2000), impair risk assessment (Killgore et al., 2006) and strategic planning (Harrison and Horne, 1999), and deteriorate divergent thinking (Harrison and Horne, 2000) as well as language and communication skills (Harrison and Horne, 1998). Yet, does an impairment of cognition due to the loss of sleep in turn indicate that sleep *enhances* cognition? The answer is no. Evidence for deleterious effects of sleep loss demonstrates that sleep is necessary to enable normal healthy cognitive functioning. Cognitive enhancement, however, is defined as "the amplification or extension of core capacities of the mind" that go beyond the normal healthy condition (Sandberg, 2011). In this way, enhancement contrasts with therapy, which is understood as the treatment and prevention of diseases with the goal to restore or maintain the normal healthy condition (Bostrom and Roache, 2008). A number of methods have proven effective to enhance cognition in the state of wakefulness, such as pharmaceutical drugs, brain stimulation and meditation practices. Sleep is a state of the organism that differs fundamentally from the wake state with regard to the neurochemical milieu, brain activity patterns and mental states. This article reviews evidence for methods of cognitive enhancement during sleep. Sleep-specific manipulations have been found to effectively boost cognitive functions beyond the boundaries of the normal condition.

Cognition is not a unitary process but involves different functions and components. Sleep is effective in facilitating several of these functions such as language processing (Dumay and Gaskell, 2007), working memory (Kuriyama et al., 2008), creativity (Ritter et al., 2012) and decision making (Pace-Schott et al., 2012a). The largest amount of research on enhancing cognition during sleep, however, has focused on the domain of learning and memory (Rasch and Born, 2013). Memory is one of the most essential cognitive functions involved in almost all other cognitive processes. The ability to remember past experiences is not only critical for appropriate behavior in the present but it also allows us to anticipate and predict future events and situations. Our individual memories and our ability to learn new things are an integral part of our identity and influence our prospects of a successful and happy life. Considering that memory is of critical importance for individuals as well as for societies (e.g., in education, professional occupation, economic productivity, personal relationships), the possibility of enhancing memory has received increasing attention (Alberini and Chen, 2012; Collingridge et al., 2013; Stern and Alberini, 2013). Although sleep is widely neglected in the discussion of memory enhancement, the sleep state might be particularly well suited as a target for the enhancement of memory capacities.

Sleep is well known to facilitate memory consolidation, that is, the strengthening and stabilization of new memories acquired before sleep (Maquet, 2001; Walker and Stickgold, 2006; Rasch and Born, 2013). Subjects who are allowed to sleep after learning typically perform better on a subsequent retrieval test than subjects who spend a comparable amount of time awake following learning. Sleep actively promotes the reprocessing of fresh memories as well as their integration into the pre-existing network of long-term memories (Diekelmann and Born, 2010; Lewis and Durrant, 2011; Stickgold and Walker, 2013). Apart from its beneficial effect on the consolidation of previously learned memories, sleep also benefits the subsequent acquisition of new learning material (Van Der Werf et al., 2009). Even a short period of sleep prior to learning can enhance the capacity to encode new information (Mander et al., 2011).

Two main theories have been proposed to explain the beneficial effect of sleep for learning and memory. According to the active system consolidation theory, new memories become reactivated and reorganized on the system-level during sleep, with selected neuronal representations being potentiated and thereby strengthened (Lewis and Durrant, 2011; Inostroza et al., 2013; Rasch and Born, 2013). The synaptic homeostasis hypothesis, on the other hand, assumes that synaptic connections become widely depotentiated during sleep, whereby selected memory representations are depotentiated less or are spared from depotentiation so that these memories come out relatively stronger (Tononi and Cirelli, 2006, 2014). Both theories are well supported by experimental evidence and, importantly, are not mutually exclusive. Although this article is principally biased towards the active system consolidation theory, the reviewed evidence for cognitive enhancement during sleep is largely independent of mechanistic considerations and is also consistent with the synaptic homeostasis hypothesis in its most recent version (Tononi and Cirelli, 2014).

There are two ways in which sleep can be used to facilitate memory. First, sleep can be timed in relation to learning in such a way as to optimally support encoding and memory consolidation processes. In this way, the normal healthy function of sleep for memory can be optimized. For example, introducing short naps before learning of new information fosters the initial acquisition and encoding of new memory traces (Mander et al., 2011). Likewise, sleep episodes that follow shortly after the encoding session benefit the consolidation of fresh memories to preserve these memories for the long-term and protect them from subsequent interfering inputs (Gais et al., 2006b; Ellenbogen et al., 2009; Payne et al., 2012a,b). The second and more intriguing way to actually enhance memory during sleep (in the sense of augmenting memory beyond the normal condition) is to manipulate memory and/or sleep directly. Such manipulations target either the processing of specific memory representations during sleep or particular sleep features that are known to be implicated in memory processing. Additionally, pharmacological interventions can be applied to modulate the processing of memories during sleep.

The following sections Manipulation of Memory Reactivation During Sleep, Manipulation of Sleep-Specific Brain Oscillations and Manipulation of Neurotransmitter Systems outline examples of how memory representations and sleep processes can be directly or indirectly manipulated to enhance memory. Section Considerations and Caveats discusses possible considerations and caveats relating to methodological and ethical issues in the potential use of sleep for cognitive enhancement. Finally, section Conclusions presents general conclusions and an outlook on possible future research directions and practical applications.

MANIPULATION OF MEMORY REACTIVATION DURING SLEEP

The beneficial effect of sleep on memory is believed to rely on the neuronal reactivation of activity patterns that were present during the initial learning experience (Diekelmann and Born, 2010; Lewis and Durrant, 2011; Rasch and Born, 2013). In rats, firing sequences of hippocampal place cells that are observed during training, spontaneously re-express ("replay") in a coordinated fashion during subsequent sleep periods (Wilson and McNaughton, 1994; Skaggs and McNaughton, 1996). Such replay mainly occurs during slow wave sleep (SWS; Lee and Wilson, 2002), sometimes at a faster firing rate than that of the original pattern (Nádasdy et al., 1999), and happens also in other brain regions such as the ventral striatum, visual cortex and prefrontal cortex (Euston et al., 2007; Ji and Wilson, 2007; Lansink et al., 2008). Reactivation of learning-associated brain activation patterns during sleep is also observed in humans, for example following training on a spatial navigation task (Peigneux et al., 2004) as well as a procedural serial reaction time task (Maquet et al., 2000). It is believed that these sleep reactivations strengthen the underlying memory traces and integrate them into long-term associative memory networks.

Intriguingly, memory reactivation does not only occur spontaneously during sleep but can be induced and/or intensified using externally applied reminder cues, a procedure that has been termed "targeted memory reactivation" (Oudiette and Paller, 2013). A ground-breaking study by Rasch et al. showed that memories for object locations can be reactivated during sleep by re-exposing subjects to odor cues that were previously associated with the learned object locations (Rasch et al., 2007). In this study, subjects learned to associate everyday objects and their locations in a 2D object location task, a task also commonly known as the game "concentration". Throughout learning, subjects were presented with puffs of the scent of roses. Subjects went to bed after learning and during ensuing SWS the odor was presented again. When tested on their memory for the object locations in the next morning, subjects showed superior memory for the object locations when they had slept with the odor compared to another night in which they did not receive the odor during sleep (**Figure 1**). Odor re-exposure during rapid eye movement (REM) sleep as well as during wakefulness was not effective in enhancing memory performance. Also, presenting odor cues during SWS without prior odor exposure during learning had no effect on memory. Subsequent studies showed that odor-induced

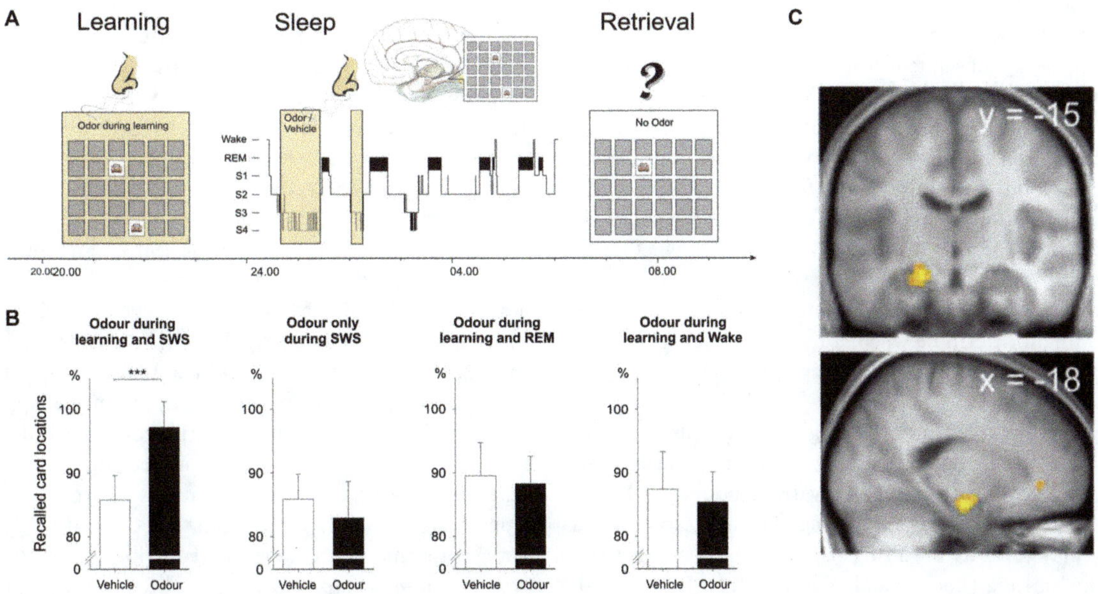

FIGURE 1 | Cueing reactivation during sleep by odors enhances memory. (A) Subjects learned card pair locations in the presence of an odor. The same odor or an odor-less vehicle was then presented during subsequent slow wave sleep (SWS). **(B)** Recall of card pair locations in the next morning was significantly better when subjects had received the odor during SWS. Odor presentation during REM sleep and during wakefulness remained ineffective. Memory was also not enhanced when the odor was omitted during learning. **(C)** Presentation of the learning-associated odor during SWS activated hippocampal regions (activation in the left anterior hippocampus shown here). From Rasch et al. (2007). Reprinted with permission from the American Association for the Advancement of Science.

reactivation during SWS does not only strengthen memories but also transforms them into a more stable form making them resistant to subsequent interfering inputs (Diekelmann et al., 2011). Furthermore, memory reactivation triggered by external odor cues accelerates memory consolidation processes leading to stable memory representations after a short sleep interval of only 40 min—a process that takes roughly double that time without odor cueing (Diekelmann et al., 2012).

Triggering reactivation during sleep to enhance memory performance not only works with odor cues; auditory stimuli seem to be comparably effective. Although auditory memory cues have the disadvantage that they can potentially disrupt sleep patterns, they also provide an important advantage: while odors represent rather broad context cues that presumably reactivate the entire learning experience, tones and sounds are more specific and can be used to reactivate individual memory contents. Rudoy et al. presented pictures at specific locations that were paired with corresponding sounds (Rudoy et al., 2009). Subjects learned the location for each picture (e.g., cat) and listened to the associated sound (e.g., meow) during training. Half of the sounds were then presented again during a nap following the training session. After sleep, subjects were asked to place each picture in its original position. Subjects performed significantly better for those pictures whose associated sounds they had heard during sleep compared to the pictures for which sounds were not presented during sleep. Recent evidence suggests that similar memory enhancing effects can be obtained by cueing vocabulary during sleep. Schreiner et al. presented half of a previously learned set of Dutch-German vocabulary to their participants during post-learning SWS. In the next morning participants correctly remembered more of the words that had been cued during sleep compared to the vocabulary that had not been cued (Schreiner et al., submitted manuscript).

External reactivation during sleep can also enhance procedural memories of sequential finger tapping skills. In a study by Antony et al. subjects were trained to tap two different sequences repeatedly on a keyboard. The tapped sequences corresponded to a melody of specific tones presented simultaneously during sequence tapping training. During a post-training nap of about 90 min the melody of one of the sequences was presented again in SWS. When tested on both sequences after the nap participants showed better tapping performance in the sequence for which the corresponding melody had been played during sleep (Antony et al., 2012). Interestingly, this cueing effect is strongly specific for the individual tones presented during sleep. Cueing only parts of the trained melody sequence results in very specific enhancements of performance in the respective cued sequence finger transitions (Schönauer et al., 2014).

Triggering memory reactivation during sleep cannot only improve subsequent retrieval performance for desired memories but can also help to forget undesired memories. In a study by Hauner et al. human subjects underwent a contextual fear conditioning procedure in which pictures of faces were paired with mild electric shocks while specific odors were presented as contextual background. Presenting one of the contextual odor cues again during subsequent sleep reduced fear responses to the face images in the next morning (Hauner et al., 2013). A similar study in mice used an odor as conditioned stimulus that was systematically paired with foot shocks (Rolls et al., 2013). However, when mice were re-exposed to the odor during post-training sleep, subsequent fear responses to the odor were increased rather than decreased. Injection of a protein synthesis inhibitor in the amygdala before presentation of the odor during sleep resulted in fear extinction, i.e., reduced fear responses to the conditioned odor stimulus. These results demonstrate that subtle methodological differences in the experimental procedure can produce very different outcomes. For example, whether the reminder that is presented during sleep represents a context cue (as in Hauner et al.) or the conditioned stimulus itself (as in Rolls et al.) might determine whether fear memories are reduced or strengthened by reactivation during sleep (Oudiette et al., 2014).

Although the exact neurophysiological mechanisms underlying the effects of targeted memory reactivation during sleep are largely unknown, a seminal study by Bendor and Wilson indicates that external memory cueing during sleep can bias neuronal replay towards the firing patterns that were observed during prior learning (Bendor and Wilson, 2012). In this study, rats were trained on a linear track to run to the left side in response to sound L or to the right side in response to sound R. During subsequent sleep the sounds were presented again and sound L was found to elicit hippocampal firing patterns similar to those observed previously when the rats had been running to the left side during training, while sound R induced firing patterns similar to those observed when the rats had been running to the right side. Similarly, in humans the presentation of learning-associated cues during sleep activated task-specific brain regions in functional magnetic resonance imaging (fMRI). Re-exposure of a memory-associated odor during SWS activated hippocampal and neocortical brain regions (Rasch et al., 2007; Diekelmann et al., 2011), and presenting memory-related sounds during SWS increased activation in the parahippocampal cortex which predicted subsequent recall performance (van Dongen et al., 2012). Furthermore, epileptic patients who suffer from sclerosis in both hippocampi did not show a memory cueing effect with sounds during sleep, while in healthy controls as well as in patients with one functional hippocampus sound cueing enhanced memory consolidation (Fuentemilla et al., 2013). Thus, external memory reactivation biases neuronal replay and essentially depends on the integrity of the hippocampus. A recent study found that external memory cues (odors in this case) also alter sleep-specific brain oscillations presumably associated with memory replay. Odor cues presented during SWS increased slow wave activity (1–4 Hz) and fast spindle activity (13–15 Hz) and induced steeper slopes of slow oscillations, the latter being associated with memory improvement (Rihm et al., 2014).

MANIPULATION OF SLEEP-SPECIFIC BRAIN OSCILLATIONS

Considering that specific field potential oscillations in the sleeping brain have been associated with memory consolidation during sleep, targeting these phenomena directly is another promising road to enhance memory. Several lines of research have implicated SWS as the sleep stage that is most prominently involved in memory consolidation (since the role of REM sleep and stage 2 sleep for memory is less clear, these sleep stages will not be considered here, but see for example Genzel et al., 2013; Ackermann and Rasch, 2014). Neocortical slow oscillations, thalamo-cortical spindles and hippocampal ripples are the hallmark oscillations of SWS that are associated with memory processing. Slow oscillations (<1 Hz) are characterized by global up-states (neuronal firing) and down-states (neuronal silence) and are believed to orchestrate the dialogue between hippocampus and neocortex for long-term memory storage (Sirota and Buzsaki, 2005). Specifically, spindles and ripples occur preferentially during the slow oscillation up-state (Steriade, 2006), which is a state of widespread neuronal activity. Spindles are characteristic waxing and waning oscillations (~10–15 Hz) that seem to prime cortical networks for neuronal plasticity. Hippocampal ripples, on the other hand, are high-frequency oscillations of ~100–300 Hz that accompany memory replay in the hippocampal networks and are believed to carry the actual "memory information". The fine-tuned temporal interplay between slow oscillations, spindles and ripples presumably mediates the redistribution of new memories from the hippocampus, serving as a temporary store, to neocortical regions for longer-term storage (Diekelmann and Born, 2010).

A seminal study by Marshall et al. found that intensifying slow oscillations by electrical transcranial direct current stimulation (tDCS) enhances memory consolidation (Marshall et al., 2006). Subjects studied a list of word pairs in the evening and during subsequent sleep an electrical current that oscillated at the peak frequency of the endogenous slow oscillations (i.e., ~0.75 Hz) was applied to the subjects' forehead. This electrical stimulation boosted endogenous slow oscillation activity and produced superior word recall in the next morning compared to a sleep condition without electrical stimulation (**Figure 2**). Importantly, the stimulation-induced memory improvement is specific for stimulation with the slow oscillation frequency: tDCS oscillating at 5 Hz (i.e., within the theta range) applied during SWS decreases slow oscillations and impairs memory consolidation (Marshall et al., 2011). Inducing slow oscillations can also be achieved with short auditory stimuli presented at the same frequency as endogenous slow oscillations (Ngo et al., 2013a). Presenting such an auditory stimulation closed-loop with endogenous slow oscillation up-states enhances memory consolidation of previously learned word pairs (Ngo et al., 2013b).

The stimulation of slow oscillations during sleep does not only enhance the consolidation of previously learned memories but can also augment the subsequent acquisition of new information. Antonenko et al. applied the previously described electrical slow oscillation stimulation during a midday nap in humans and tested their capacity to learn new word pairs, word lists and pictures thereafter (Antonenko et al., 2013). When subjects had slept with the slow oscillation stimulation, they were able to learn more new words and pictures after the nap compared to a nap without stimulation. Similar findings were observed in rats: electrical stimulation of slow oscillations via tDCS over several days improved the acquisition of task-inherent rules in a radial arm maze task (Binder et al., 2014). Intensifying slow oscillations might speed up processes that enable new learning in the hippocampus, possibly by down-scaling saturated neuronal networks or by shifting old

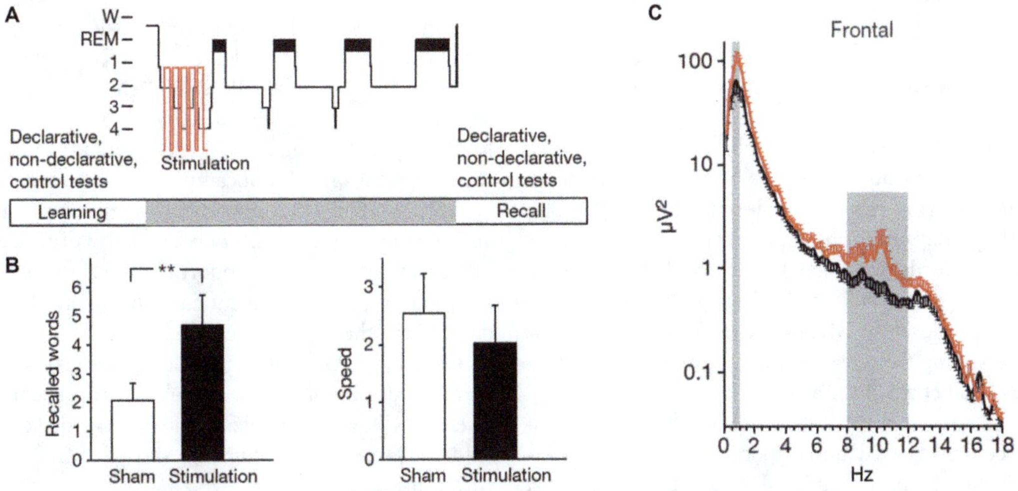

FIGURE 2 | Stimulating slow oscillations during sleep enhances memory. (A) Following learning of word pairs and finger sequence tapping, subjects received electrical stimulation of slow oscillations (tDCS at 0.75 Hz) during ensuing sleep. **(B)** Compared to a sham condition, subjects remembered more word pairs after slow oscillation stimulation. Speed in finger sequence tapping was not affected by the stimulation. **(C)** The stimulation increased activity in the slow oscillation (0.5–1 Hz) and the slow spindle frequency band (8–12 Hz) at frontal sites. Reprinted by permission from Macmillan Publishers Ltd.: Marshall et al. (2006).

memories from hippocampal to neocortical sites for long-term storage thereby freeing space for new memories.

Although spindles have frequently been associated with memory consolidation during sleep, it is unclear whether sleep spindles can be externally manipulated. There are numerous studies showing that spindle activity as well as spindle density increase following learning (e.g., Gais et al., 2002; Schabus et al., 2004; Schmidt et al., 2006) and the number and activity of sleep spindles correlates with subsequent memory performance (e.g., Clemens et al., 2005; Nishida and Walker, 2007). Furthermore, reactivating memories with learning-associated odors enhances spindle activity during odor cue presentation in SWS (Rihm et al., 2014). Increasing slow oscillations by electrical and auditory stimulation likewise induces a concurrent increase in spindle activity (Marshall et al., 2006; Ngo et al., 2013b). Yet, whether the relationship between spindles and memory is a causal one is unclear. It remains to be elucidated whether spindles can be externally triggered and whether such triggered spindles prove effective in enhancing memory.

Like sleep spindles, hippocampal ripple events are commonly associated with memory consolidation during sleep. During SWS in rats, ripples are observed during the replay of hippocampal neuron ensembles (Wilson and McNaughton, 1994; Peyrache et al., 2009) and their occurrence increases following learning (Eschenko et al., 2008). Moreover, during a nap in humans the number of ripples correlated with the consolidation of previously learned picture memories (Axmacher et al., 2008). Suppressing hippocampal ripples by electrical stimulation during post-learning sleep impairs memory for previously learned tasks in rats (Girardeau et al., 2009; Ego-Stengel and Wilson, 2010). However, it is hitherto unknown whether ripples can be induced or increased by external stimulation and whether this would enhance memory consolidation and/or acquisition.

MANIPULATION OF NEUROTRANSMITTER SYSTEMS

A number of different neurotransmitters and hormones modulates and influences the formation of memories. Most of these neurotransmitters and hormones are differentially regulated during sleep and wakefulness. SWS in particular is characterized by a decrease in levels of acetylcholine, noradrenaline and cortisol as well as by a distinct increase in growth hormone concentrations compared to periods of wakefulness (Marrosu et al., 1995; Born and Fehm, 2000). Other neurotransmitters such as glutamate, dopamine and GABA exhibit changes in concentrations across the sleep-wake cycle as well (Sowers and Vlachakis, 1984; Dash et al., 2009; Vanini et al., 2012). The exact mechanisms underlying the specific role of neurotransmitters in memory processing during sleep are not well understood. It is believed that the different levels of the respective neurotransmitters allow for and mediate the replay of firing patterns in neuronal circuits as well as the associated electrophysiological brain oscillations during sleep.

Several neurotransmitters have been found suitable for memory enhancement during sleep. For example, increasing the availability of noradrenaline during sleep with the noradrenaline reuptake inhibitor reboxetine enhances performance in an odor recognition task (Gais et al., 2011). In this study, subjects learned a set of odors and received reboxetine or placebo before a night of sleep. Two days later subjects recognized more of the previously learned odors when they had received reboxetine as compared to the night with placebo administration. In another study, reboxetine enhanced the consolidation of procedural memories in a finger sequence tapping task, which was associated with an increase in the number of sleep spindles (Rasch et al., 2009). The role of noradrenaline in sleep-dependent memory consolidation is further supported by findings showing that reducing the availability of noradrenaline by administering the α2-autoreceptor agonist clonidine blocks the improvement of memory for odors

(Gais et al., 2011) as well as the enhancement of emotional over neutral memories that is typically observed after sleep (Groch et al., 2011).

Enhancing glutamatergic neurotransmission during sleep likewise boosts the consolidation of previously acquired memories. Feld et al. performed a study in which subjects learned a set of word pairs in the evening and received the NMDA receptor coagonist D-cycloserine during subsequent sleep (Feld et al., 2013a). At retrieval testing 1 day later subjects remembered significantly more of the learned words when they had received D-cycloserine during sleep compared to a night of sleep without substance administration. D-cycloserine is assumed to facilitate synaptic plastic changes resulting from reactivation of glutamatergic neuronal ensembles (Feld et al., 2013a).

Other substances that target different neurotransmitter systems can enhance the consolidation of particular memories during sleep. For instance, the dopamine D2-like receptor agonist pramipexole enhances the consolidation of memories that had been associated with low reward during learning before sleep but does not affect memories associated with a high reward (Feld et al., in press). The cytokine interleukin-6, administered intranasally shortly before sleep, increases slow wave activity and enhances the consolidation of emotional but not neutral memories (Benedict et al., 2009). And while reboxetine increases the consolidation of finger sequence tapping skills it does not affect mirror tracing performance (Rasch et al., 2009).

Studies on the effect of GABA for memory enhancement during sleep revealed mixed results (Hall-Porter et al., 2014). Increasing spindle density with the $GABA_A$ positive modulator zolpidem enhances memory for word pairs and emotionally negative pictures but impairs perceptual learning and has no effect on finger sequence tapping and memory for emotionally neutral pictures (Kaestner et al., 2013; Mednick et al., 2013). Intensifying SWS and slow wave activity with the GABA reuptake inhibitor tiagabine did not have an enhancing effect on memory consolidation (Feld et al., 2013b), which was possibly due to a non-functional increase of slow oscillations that was accompanied by a decrease in spindle activity phase-locked to slow oscillations. Growth hormone, another important neuromodulator, had long been suspected to play a role in sleep-dependent memory consolidation as it is mainly secreted during SWS and is involved in hippocampal memory formation (Nyberg and Hallberg, 2013). Yet, effectively blocking growth hormone release during SWS by infusion of somatostatin left memory consolidation unaffected (Gais et al., 2006a). Whether it is possible to enhance memory by increasing the availability of growth hormone during sleep is unclear.

Low levels of the neurotransmitter acetylcholine are known to be critical for SWS-dependent memory consolidation (Buzsáki, 1986; Hasselmo, 1999). Increasing cholinergic activity during SWS by administering the choline esterase inhibitor physostigmine impairs memory consolidation (Gais and Born, 2004). It is unclear, however, whether a reduction of cholinergic activity during SWS can further boost memory. Findings of studies that manipulated the stress hormone cortisol during SWS suggest otherwise. Cortisol shows secretion patterns very similar to those of acetylcholine, with very low concentration levels during SWS. Similar to acetylcholine, increasing cortisol during SWS by infusion of hydrocortisone or dexamethasone blocks the beneficial effect of sleep for memory consolidation (Plihal and Born, 1999; Plihal et al., 1999; Wilhelm et al., 2011). Yet, further decreasing cortisol levels during SWS with the cortisol synthesis inhibitor metyrapone did not enhance but paradoxically reduced the consolidation of hippocampus-dependent memories (Wagner et al., 2005). Thus, the neurochemical milieu of neurotransmitters and hormones during sleep, particularly during SWS, might be intricately optimized to support memory consolidation such that pharmacological manipulations of this finely tuned balance often do not have the expected results.

Overall, manipulating neurotransmitter systems to enhance memory during sleep has revealed inconsistent results. Future research will have to replicate and specify the key findings in this field. At present, these findings should therefore be interpreted with caution.

CONSIDERATIONS AND CAVEATS

Several different manipulations of sleep and memory have been proven effective to enhance learning and memory consolidation. Yet, there are a number of central questions that are still unknown, both in the experimental study of sleep to enhance memory as well as for possible applications of these new methods in everyday life. Among these questions are important issues relating to methodological intricacies, such as possible boundary conditions, potential unintended effects, the actual effect size of the improvement, as well as the practicability for everyday use. Besides these methodological problems, the possibility of enhancing cognitive functions during sleep raises certain ethical questions. Apart from the ethical questions that are discussed in relation to cognitive enhancement in general, applying cognition-altering manipulations during sleep—a state of unconsciousness, reduced voluntary control, and heightened vulnerability of the individual—might pose additional ethical concerns.

METHODOLOGY

Although we know that normal sleep facilitates learning and memory and that specific manipulations of memory during sleep can further boost this effect, we still don't understand the exact conditions under which the memory enhancement occurs (Diekelmann et al., 2009; Diekelmann, 2013). Memory cueing, stimulation of sleep oscillations as well as pharmacological interventions enhance some memories but not others depending on the particular methods used. For example, using odors as context cues to reactivate associated memories during sleep enhances declarative memories for object locations but not procedural memories in the finger sequence tapping task (Rasch et al., 2007). Stimulating slow oscillations via tDCS likewise enhances declarative word pair memories but not procedural finger sequence tapping (Marshall et al., 2006). Yet, cueing memories for finger sequence tapping directly by tones associated with specific finger movements does in fact enhance finger tapping performance (Antony et al., 2012; Schönauer et al., 2014).

Furthermore, increasing the availability of noradrenaline during sleep by reboxetine enhances odor memory (Gais et al., 2011) and finger sequence tapping (Rasch et al., 2009) but does not enhance memory for word pairs and performance in a mirror tracing task (Rasch et al., 2009). Intranasal interleukin-6 improves memory for emotional stories but not for neutral stories, object locations and finger sequence tapping (Benedict et al., 2009). And while the modulation of GABA transmission with zolpidem enhances emotional picture memory and verbal memory, it does not affect neutral picture memory and motor memory, and it even impairs perceptual learning.

Considering that some memories can be enhanced during sleep under some conditions but not under others suggests that there are certain boundary conditions for the enhancing effect of sleep. For cueing memory reactivation with odors, for example, it was found that the same odor needs to be presented during learning and subsequent sleep to enhance memory; presenting a different odor during sleep than during learning remains ineffective (Rihm et al., 2014). Generally, it is unclear how many different odors can be associated with different memories and how many times a single odor can be associated with new learning material before it produces interference rather than enhancement. Olfactory cues presumably represent general context cues that reactivate the entire learning context when presented during sleep, increasing the risk of interference when different memories are learned in the same context. In order to target individual memories, auditory cues might be better suited; yet these cues have the disadvantage to change the natural sleep cycle by inducing arousals and awakenings if the sound level is not optimally adjusted. The effectiveness of memory cueing during sleep might generally depend on whether or not the learning information is relevant for the individual, which can be signaled for example by associated low or high rewards (Oudiette et al., 2013). Furthermore, when trying to reduce undesired memories by cueing during sleep, different methods can produce fundamentally different results. Whether fear memories are weakened or even strengthened during sleep, for instance, depends on methodological subtleties such as contingencies in the conditioning procedure and the nature of the reactivation cue (Oudiette et al., 2014).

Similar boundary conditions are presumably relevant in the stimulation of sleep-specific brain oscillations as well as in pharmacological manipulations of neurotransmitters and hormones. Importantly, sleep oscillations, neurotransmitter concentrations and memory replay during sleep are intricately interlinked. Targeting one or the other component of this interwoven net of factors might produce unexpected adverse effects and can even be harmful to memory. For example, the GABA agonist tiagabine increases slow wave activity but does not enhance memory consolidation, possibly due to a concurrent decrease in functionally coupled spindle activity (Feld et al., 2013b). Likewise, low levels of cortisol during SWS are known to be essential for memory consolidation processes, yet further decreasing cortisol concentrations paradoxically impairs memory rather than further enhancing it (Wagner et al., 2005). These examples show that it is essential to consider the functional role of single components and processes in sleep-dependent memory consolidation as well as their inter-dependencies when trying to manipulate particular aspects of this complex system. However, the way in which the different processes and components interact is not well understood.

Apart from its enhancing effect on memory, manipulations of memory processing during sleep can have side effects and unintended effects. It has been shown, for instance, that the reprocessing and integration of information during sleep can qualitatively change memories. Although in many cases this a positive effect, for example generating insight (Wagner et al., 2004), drawing relational inferences (Ellenbogen et al., 2007) and abstracting schemas (Lewis and Durrant, 2011), it can also lead to the generation of memory distortions and false memories (Payne et al., 2009; Diekelmann et al., 2010). Up to now it is unclear whether and how external manipulations of memory during sleep affect the veridicality of memories. Furthermore, there might be a trade-off between different memories: enhancing one memory could come at the cost of impairing others. For example, sleep increases memory for emotional components of a scene but concurrently decreases memory for the neutral background (Payne et al., 2008, 2012a; Payne and Kensinger, 2010, 2011). Although trade-off effects in sleep-dependent memory consolidation have not been studied directly, indirect evidence suggests that there might be a limited capacity for memory replay during sleep such that increasing reactivation of one memory decreases reactivation of other memories (Antony et al., 2012; Bendor and Wilson, 2012; Kelemen and Born, 2012). It is generally unknown how targeted manipulations of memory during sleep are. The discussed manipulations might not only affect other memories but also other cognitive functions and even other bodily functions. Slow oscillation stimulation with tDCS, for example, was found to improve mood, though the mechanisms for this effect are unclear (Marshall et al., 2006; Göder et al., 2013). Also pharmacological treatments for memory enhancement during sleep are typically "dirty" interventions that affect numerous other functions and can also produce unwanted side effects.

Although the effects of memory enhancement during sleep are reproducible and statistically significant, the practical significance of these effects is unclear. In humans, the estimated performance improvement in studies manipulating memory during sleep (either by cueing memory replay, stimulating sleep oscillations or applying pharmacological substances) is usually in the margins of 5–15% compared to sleep conditions without treatment. Considering that natural sleep without any manipulations produces a memory improvement of about 10–20% compared to wakefulness, the combined improvement of sleep with external manipulations adds up to an enhancement of 15–35% as compared to wake intervals without manipulations. Even taking into account that this number might eventually turn out to be smaller, considering that effect sizes are typically overestimated in the first studies of a new field of research, the true effect size might still be high enough to warrant practical applications. Experimental studies on sleep and memory usually test for enhancing effects of sleep manipulations during one night of sleep only. The long-term effects of using sleep applications for cognitive enhancement on a regular basis are presently unclear. Generally, the effect of sleep and the need for sleep is rather variable between individuals. Considering that current activity schedules, in schools and at work, do not provide an ideal environment for adequate sleep, the most straight forward method to optimize normal cognitive function by sleep in a first step may be a policy change towards more flexible timing of activity and rest.

The practicability of memory enhancing methods during sleep for applications in everyday life depends on the type of method. Odors are relatively easy to apply during learning and subsequent sleep in the home environment. For auditory cues, home applications are likewise relatively easy to conceive. Stimulation of sleep-specific brain oscillations and pharmacological substance administration, however, is more difficult to do in everyday life. Although apparatuses for home use of tDCS in the wake state are already available on the market, their potential for the stimulation of specific sleep oscillations is unclear. Also safety and potential side effects of long-term tDCS treatment is completely unknown. The optimal stimulation of sleep-specific brain oscillations as well as the application of odors and sounds to reactivate memories during specific sleep stages is further complicated by the lack of easy-to-use sleep recording systems for the home environment. Finally, the pharmacological substances that (so far) have been shown to enhance memory during sleep are not available for use outside their medical indication at the moment.

ETHICAL ISSUES

On the one hand, ethical questions regarding the use of sleep for cognitive enhancement relate to the general ethical issues that are discussed in the context of cognitive enhancement and biomedical enhancement at large (for overview see for example Farah et al., 2004; Buchanan, 2011). The enhancement of cognitive capacities can potentially have substantial positive effects for individuals as well as for societies by increasing productivity and overall quality of life through more personally and financially rewarding occupations, more fulfilling personal relationships, and less suffering from cognitively impairing diseases (Buchanan, 2008, 2011; Bostrom and Roache, 2011). Yet, cognitive enhancement might also have direct or indirect negative consequences. Just to name a few, through the enhancement of our cognitive capabilities we could lose our sense of giftedness (Sandel, 2007), we might no longer appreciate the effort to achieve something, we could become inauthentic by changing central features of our identity such as our memories, we might be coerced to use cognitive enhancers if others do it, the use of cognitive enhancers might be seen as cheating, and an unfair access to cognitive enhancers could potentially increase social injustice.

Ethical issues that are specific to manipulations of cognitive capacities by targeting sleep relate to the specific nature of sleep as an exceptional state of the organism. Sleep is characterized by immobility and muscle relaxation, greatly diminished processing and perception of external stimuli as well as greatly limited or even absent voluntary control. These characteristics make the sleeping individual particularly vulnerable for all kinds of external influences. Manipulations of cognitive processes during sleep are designed in such a way that the individual does not notice the treatment. In studies using memory cueing during sleep, subjects typically report not to have noticed any presentation of the cues. Likewise, following stimulation of brain oscillations during sleep as well as after the administration of pharmacological substances, participants usually cannot tell whether they received the treatment or not. Thus, subjects not only have no control over such manipulations but they don't even know whether they have been manipulated at all. This constellation can give rise to a certain misuse potential. In Aldous Huxley's science fiction novel "Brave new world", indoctrination of infants and children during sleep is used to shape how these children will think, feel and behave as members of their respective caste. Huxley calls this procedure "hypnopaedia" and describes it as "the greatest moralizing and socializing force of all time". Although it is unclear whether sleep goes along with an enhanced suggestibility, Huxley's fictitious idea illustrates that sleep is a highly sensitive state in which we are relatively unprotected against external influences.

Such worries and premonitions are legitimate and important to discuss in the context of cognitive enhancement during sleep. However, they do not provide conclusive reasons against the use of sleep for cognitive enhancement. What is needed is a balanced account to weigh possible risks against the benefits to allow for a well-informed and all-things-considered judgment about the responsible use of sleep for cognitive enhancement (Buchanan, 2011). Even if negative consequences were to be expected, the numerous positive effects could be so desirable as to outweigh possible negative effects. The question is not whether or not to use sleep for cognitive enhancement—cognitive enhancers of all sorts are already there and their use will increase even more in the near future—the question is rather how to enhance cognitive capacities responsibly, how to deal with issues of distributive justice and how to prevent misuse and malpractice.

CONCLUSION

This article has focused on the function of sleep to augment cognitive capacities, a function that will arguably receive more and more attention in the next few years, both in research as well as in practical applications. The reviewed evidence shows that targeted manipulations of memory processing during sleep can be used to enhance learning and memory. Sleep can thereby be considered a cognitive enhancer as this state provides optimal conditions to augment memory capacities above and beyond the normal level. It is important to note that the discussed effects of manipulations to enhance memory during sleep are specific for the sleep state. Identical methods applied during wakefulness have no enhancing effect on memory or can even impair memory processing. For instance, reactivating memories by odors during wakefulness does not affect memory for object locations (Rasch et al., 2007) or even renders these memory representations unstable making them more vulnerable for disruptive interfering inputs (Diekelmann et al., 2011). Manipulating sleep-specific brain oscillations is naturally confined to the sleep state. Except for ripples, which also occur during wakefulness (O'Neill et al., 2010), slow oscillations and sleep spindles selectively occur during sleep. Interestingly, stimulating the brain during wakefulness with frequencies oscillating in the slow oscillation range has no effect on memory consolidation but increases theta activity resulting in better encoding of new information (Kirov et al., 2009). Furthermore, the neurochemical milieu of neurotransmitters and hormones is very different during sleep and wakefulness such that administration of certain substances can have fundamentally different effects on memory. For example, while an infusion of cortisol impairs memory consolidation during sleep it facilitates consolidation processes when administered in the wake state (Wilhelm et al., 2011).

Importantly, memory enhancement in the context of cognitive enhancement should not be confused with the term "enhancement" that has sometimes been used in the sleep and memory literature to describe actual sleep-dependent gains in performance. Initial research on memory consolidation during sleep, particularly with respect to procedural memory, showed that performance levels after sleep can exceed performance levels observed before sleep (Walker, 2005). We know now that this is not true (see for example Rickard et al., 2008). Even external manipulations of memory during sleep cannot produce anything that was not previously encoded; rather sleep as well as memory manipulations during sleep enhance memory in the sense of less forgetting (to the point of no forgetting) and higher memory stability (i.e., resistance to subsequent interference). Related to this, only a very few reports show that conditioned responses can be acquired during sleep (Arzi et al., 2012), but new learning of declarative and procedural memories during sleep seems to be impossible. Nevertheless, sleep can produce new knowledge from previously encoded memories through processes of generalization, integration, schema abstraction, and conversion of implicit into explicit knowledge (Wagner et al., 2004; Gomez et al., 2006; Ellenbogen et al., 2007; Durrant et al., 2011; Wilhelm et al., 2013).

It is of note that sleep is not only effective as a cognitive enhancer to boost memory performance, but it can also be applied in clinical settings to restore normal cognitive functioning. A number of disorders and diseases are accompanied by changes in sleep patterns and dysfunctions of memory, such as depression (Steiger et al., 2013), post-traumatic stress disorder (Germain, 2013), Alzheimer's disease (Wang et al., 2011) and schizophrenia (Lu and Goder, 2012). In patients with schizophrenia, stimulation of slow oscillations with tDCS during sleep was found to improve memory for words (Göder et al., 2013). Furthermore, administration of the atypical antipsychotic olanzapine increased SWS, and the GABA agonist eszopiclone enhanced the number of sleep spindles in schizophrenia; yet both treatments failed to normalize memory consolidation in these patients (Göder et al., 2008; Wamsley et al., 2013). Future studies will have to test new methods for the treatment of memory dysfunctions during sleep in different clinical settings, which could also potentially improve the outcome of standard therapeutic treatments. For the treatment of spider phobia, for example, sleep after exposure therapy was found to increase therapeutic effectiveness (Pace-Schott et al., 2012b; Kleim et al., 2013). It remains to be elucidated whether manipulations of memory processing during sleep, such as memory reactivation or sleep oscillation stimulation, can boost this effect further.

Manipulating memory during sleep is a very new field of research and we are only beginning to understand which methods are best suited to use sleep for memory enhancement. Much more research is needed to determine the optimal procedures to unravel this effect and to understand its underlying mechanisms and principles. Future research will have to extend the knowledge obtained from findings in the domain of learning and memory to other cognitive functions such as creativity, executive functions and decision making. This research could not only provide us with new means to augment our cognitive capabilities in different domains but could also help to change the image of sleep as a useless waste of time to being a beneficial state that supports our wake performance.

ACKNOWLEDGMENTS

The author would like to thank Jan Born and Gordon Feld for helpful discussions and comments on an earlier draft of this article. This work was funded by the Deutsche Forschungsgemeinschaft (DFG, TR-SFB 654).

REFERENCES

Ackermann, S., and Rasch, B. (2014). Differential effects of non-REM and REM sleep on memory consolidation? *Curr. Neurol. Neurosci. Rep.* 14:430. doi: 10.1007/s11910-013-0430-8

Alberini, C. M., and Chen, D. Y. (2012). Memory enhancement: consolidation, reconsolidation and insulin-like growth factor 2. *Trends Neurosci.* 35, 274–283. doi: 10.1016/j.tins.2011.12.007

Antonenko, D., Diekelmann, S., Olsen, C., Born, J., and Molle, M. (2013). Napping to renew learning capacity: enhanced encoding after stimulation of sleep slow oscillations. *Eur. J. Neurosci.* 37, 1142–1151. doi: 10.1111/ejn.12118

Antony, J. W., Gobel, E. W., O'Hare, J. K., Reber, P. J., and Paller, K. A. (2012). Cued memory reactivation during sleep influences skill learning. *Nat. Neurosci.* 15, 1114–1116. doi: 10.1038/nn.3152

Arzi, A., Shedlesky, L., Ben-Shaul, M., Nasser, K., Oksenberg, A., Hairston, I. S., et al. (2012). Humans can learn new information during sleep. *Nat. Neurosci.* 15, 1460–1465. doi: 10.1038/nn.3193

Axmacher, N., Elger, C. E., and Fell, J. (2008). Ripples in the medial temporal lobe are relevant for human memory consolidation. *Brain* 131, 1806–1817. doi: 10.1093/brain/awn103

Bendor, D., and Wilson, M. A. (2012). Biasing the content of hippocampal replay during sleep. *Nat. Neurosci.* 15, 1439–1444. doi: 10.1038/nn.3203

Benedict, C., Scheller, J., Rose-John, S., Born, J., and Marshall, L. (2009). Enhancing influence of intranasal interleukin-6 on slow-wave activity and memory consolidation during sleep. *FASEB J.* 23, 3629–3636. doi: 10.1096/fj.08-122853

Binder, S., Rawohl, J., Born, J., and Marshall, L. (2014). Transcranial slow oscillation stimulation during NREM sleep enhances acquisition of the radial maze task and modulates cortical network activity in rats. *Front. Behav. Neurosci.* 7:220. doi: 10.3389/fnbeh.2013.00220

Born, J., and Fehm, H. L. (2000). The neuroendocrine recovery function of sleep. *Noise Health* 2, 25–38.

Bostrom, N., and Roache, N. (2008). "Ethical issues in human enhancement," in *New Waves in Applied Ethics*, eds J. Ryberg, T. Petersen and C. Wolf (Basingstoke: Palgrave Macmillan), 120–152.

Bostrom, N., and Roache, N. (2011). "Smart policy: cognitive enhancement and the public interest," in *Enhancing Human Capacities*, eds J. Savulescu, R. ter Muelen and G. Kahane (Oxford: Wiley-Blackwell), 138–152.

Buchanan, A. (2008). Enhancement and the ethics of development. *Kennedy Inst. Ethics J.* 18, 1–34. doi: 10.1353/ken.0.0003

Buchanan, A. (2011). *Beyond Humanity? The Ethics of Biomedical Enhancement.* New York: Oxford University Press.

Buzsáki, G. (1986). Hippocampal sharp waves: their origin and significance. *Brain Res.* 398, 242–252. doi: 10.1016/0006-8993(86)91483-6

Clemens, Z., Fabo, D., and Halasz, P. (2005). Overnight verbal memory retention correlates with the number of sleep spindles. *Neuroscience* 132, 529–535. doi: 10.1016/j.neuroscience.2005.01.011

Collingridge, G. L., Volianskis, A., Bannister, N., France, G., Hanna, L., Mercier, M., et al. (2013). The NMDA receptor as a target for cognitive enhancement. *Neuropharmacology* 64, 13–26. doi: 10.1016/j.neuropharm.2012.06.051

Dash, M. B., Douglas, C. L., Vyazovskiy, V. V., Cirelli, C., and Tononi, G. (2009). Long-term homeostasis of extracellular glutamate in the rat cerebral cortex across sleep and waking states. *J. Neurosci.* 29, 620–629. doi: 10.1523/jneurosci.5486-08.2009

Diekelmann, S. (2013). Open questions in sleep and memory research. *Somnologie* 17, 21–27. doi: 10.1007/s11818-013-0600-6

Diekelmann, S., Biggel, S., Rasch, B., and Born, J. (2012). Offline consolidation of memory varies with time in slow wave sleep and can be accelerated by cuing memory reactivations. *Neurobiol. Learn. Mem.* 98, 103–111. doi: 10.1016/j.nlm.2012.07.002

Diekelmann, S., and Born, J. (2010). The memory function of sleep. *Nat. Rev. Neurosci.* 11, 114–126. doi: 10.1038/nrn2762

Diekelmann, S., Born, J., and Wagner, U. (2010). Sleep enhances false memories depending on general memory performance. *Behav. Brain Res.* 208, 425–429. doi: 10.1016/j.bbr.2009.12.021

Diekelmann, S., Buchel, C., Born, J., and Rasch, B. (2011). Labile or stable: opposing consequences for memory when reactivated during waking and sleep. *Nat. Neurosci.* 14, 381–386. doi: 10.1038/nn.2744

Diekelmann, S., Wilhelm, I., and Born, J. (2009). The whats and whens of sleep-dependent memory consolidation. *Sleep Med. Rev.* 13, 309–321. doi: 10.1016/j.smrv.2008.08.002

Dumay, N., and Gaskell, M. G. (2007). Sleep-associated changes in the mental representation of spoken words. *Psychol. Sci.* 18, 35–39. doi: 10.1111/j.1467-9280.2007.01845.x

Durmer, J. S., and Dinges, D. F. (2005). Neurocognitive consequences of sleep deprivation. *Semin. Neurol.* 25, 117–129. doi: 10.1055/s-2005-867080

Durrant, S. J., Taylor, C., Cairney, S., and Lewis, P. A. (2011). Sleep-dependent consolidation of statistical learning. *Neuropsychologia* 49, 1322–1331. doi: 10.1016/j.neuropsychologia.2011.02.015

Ego-Stengel, V., and Wilson, M. A. (2010). Disruption of ripple-associated hippocampal activity during rest impairs spatial learning in the rat. *Hippocampus* 20, 1–10. doi: 10.1002/hipo.20707

Ellenbogen, J. M., Hu, P. T., Payne, J. D., Titone, D., and Walker, M. P. (2007). Human relational memory requires time and sleep. *Proc. Natl. Acad. Sci. U S A* 104, 7723–7728. doi: 10.1073/pnas.0700094104

Ellenbogen, J. M., Hulbert, J. C., Jiang, Y., and Stickgold, R. (2009). The sleeping brain's influence on verbal memory: boosting resistance to interference. *PLoS One* 4:e4117. doi: 10.1371/journal.pone.0004117

Eschenko, O., Ramadan, W., Molle, M., Born, J., and Sara, S. J. (2008). Sustained increase in hippocampal sharp-wave ripple activity during slow-wave sleep after learning. *Learn. Mem.* 15, 222–228. doi: 10.1101/lm.726008

Euston, D. R., Tatsuno, M., and McNaughton, B. L. (2007). Fast-forward playback of recent memory sequences in prefrontal cortex during sleep. *Science* 318, 1147–1150. doi: 10.1126/science.1148979

Farah, M. J., Illes, J., Cook-Deegan, R., Gardner, H., Kandel, E., King, P., et al. (2004). Neurocognitive enhancement: what can we do and what should we do? *Nat. Rev. Neurosci.* 5, 421–425. doi: 10.1038/nrn1390

Feld, G. B., Besedovsky, L., Kaida, K., Münte, T. F., and Born, J. (in press). Dopamine D2-like receptor activation wipes out preferential consolidation of high over low reward memories in human sleep. *J. Cogn. Neurosci.*

Feld, G. B., Lange, T., Gais, S., and Born, J. (2013a). Sleep-dependent declarative memory consolidation–unaffected after blocking NMDA or AMPA receptors but enhanced by NMDA coagonist D-cycloserine. *Neuropsychopharmacology* 38, 2688–2697. doi: 10.1038/npp.2013.179

Feld, G. B., Wilhelm, I., Ma, Y., Groch, S., Binkofski, F., Molle, M., et al. (2013b). Slow wave sleep induced by GABA agonist tiagabine fails to benefit memory consolidation. *Sleep* 36, 1317–1326. doi: 10.5665/sleep.2954

Fuentemilla, L., Miro, J., Ripolles, P., Vila-Ballo, A., Juncadella, M., Castaner, S., et al. (2013). Hippocampus-dependent strengthening of targeted memories via reactivation during sleep in humans. *Curr. Biol.* 23, 1769–1775. doi: 10.1016/j.cub.2013.07.006

Gais, S., and Born, J. (2004). Low acetylcholine during slow-wave sleep is critical for declarative memory consolidation. *Proc. Natl. Acad. Sci. U S A* 101, 2140–2144. doi: 10.1073/pnas.0305404101

Gais, S., Hullemann, P., Hallschmid, M., and Born, J. (2006a). Sleep-dependent surges in growth hormone do not contribute to sleep-dependent memory consolidation. *Psychoneuroendocrinology* 31, 786–791. doi: 10.1016/j.psyneuen.2006.02.009

Gais, S., Lucas, B., and Born, J. (2006b). Sleep after learning aids memory recall. *Learn. Mem.* 13, 259–262. doi: 10.1101/lm.132106

Gais, S., Molle, M., Helms, K., and Born, J. (2002). Learning-dependent increases in sleep spindle density. *J. Neurosci.* 22, 6830–6834.

Gais, S., Rasch, B., Dahmen, J. C., Sara, S., and Born, J. (2011). The memory function of noradrenergic activity in non-REM sleep. *J. Cogn. Neurosci.* 23, 2582–2592. doi: 10.1162/jocn.2011.21622

Genzel, L., Ahrberg, K., Roselli, C., Niedermaier, S., Steiger, A., Dresler, M., et al. (2013). Sleep timing is more important than sleep length or quality for medical school performance. *Chronobiol. Int.* 30, 766–771. doi: 10.3109/07420528.2012.763132

Germain, A. (2013). Sleep disturbances as the hallmark of PTSD: where are we now? *Am. J. Psychiatry* 170, 372–382. doi: 10.1176/appi.ajp.2012.12040432

Girardeau, G., Benchenane, K., Wiener, S. I., Buzsaki, G., and Zugaro, M. B. (2009). Selective suppression of hippocampal ripples impairs spatial memory. *Nat. Neurosci.* 12, 1222–1223. doi: 10.1038/nn.2384

Göder, R., Baier, P. C., Beith, B., Baecker, C., Seeck-Hirschner, M., Junghanns, K., et al. (2013). Effects of transcranial direct current stimulation during sleep on memory performance in patients with schizophrenia. *Schizophr. Res.* 144, 153–154. doi: 10.1016/j.schres.2012.12.014

Göder, R., Fritzer, G., Gottwald, B., Lippmann, B., Seeck-Hirschner, M., Serafin, I., et al. (2008). Effects of olanzapine on slow wave sleep, sleep spindles and sleep-related memory consolidation in schizophrenia. *Pharmacopsychiatry* 41, 92–99. doi: 10.1055/s-2007-1004592

Gomez, R. L., Bootzin, R. R., and Nadel, L. (2006). Naps promote abstraction in language-learning infants. *Psychol. Sci.* 17, 670–674. doi: 10.1111/j.1467-9280.2006.01764.x

Groch, S., Wilhelm, I., Diekelmann, S., Sayk, F., Gais, S., and Born, J. (2011). Contribution of norepinephrine to emotional memory consolidation during sleep. *Psychoneuroendocrinology* 36, 1342–1350. doi: 10.1016/j.psyneuen.2011.03.006

Hall-Porter, J. M., Schweitzer, P. K., Eisenstein, R. D., Ahmed, H. A., and Walsh, J. K. (2014). The effect of two benzodiazepine receptor agonist hypnotics on sleep-dependent memory consolidation. *J. Clin. Sleep Med.* 10, 27–34. doi: 10.5664/jcsm.3352

Harrison, Y., and Horne, J. A. (1998). Sleep loss impairs short and novel language tasks having a prefrontal focus. *J. Sleep Res.* 7, 95–100. doi: 10.1046/j.1365-2869.1998.00104.x

Harrison, Y., and Horne, J. A. (1999). One night of sleep loss impairs innovative thinking and flexible decision making. *Organ. Behav. Hum. Decis. Process.* 78, 128–145. doi: 10.1006/obhd.1999.2827

Harrison, Y., and Horne, J. A. (2000). The impact of sleep deprivation on decision making: a review. *J. Exp. Psychol. Appl.* 6, 236–249. doi: 10.1037/1076-898x.6.3.236

Hasselmo, M. E. (1999). Neuromodulation: acetylcholine and memory consolidation. *Trends Cogn. Sci.* 3, 351–359. doi: 10.1016/s1364-6613(99)01365-0

Hauner, K. K., Howard, J. D., Zelano, C., and Gottfried, J. A. (2013). Stimulus-specific enhancement of fear extinction during slow-wave sleep. *Nat. Neurosci.* 16, 1553–1555. doi: 10.1038/nn.3527

Inostroza, M., Binder, S., and Born, J. (2013). Sleep-dependency of episodic-like memory consolidation in rats. *Behav. Brain Res.* 237, 15–22. doi: 10.1016/j.bbr.2012.09.011

Jackson, M. L., Gunzelmann, G., Whitney, P., Hinson, J. M., Belenky, G., Rabat, A., et al. (2013). Deconstructing and reconstructing cognitive performance in sleep deprivation. *Sleep Med. Rev.* 17, 215–225. doi: 10.1016/j.smrv.2012.06.007

Ji, D., and Wilson, M. A. (2007). Coordinated memory replay in the visual cortex and hippocampus during sleep. *Nat. Neurosci.* 10, 100–107. doi: 10.1038/nn1825

Kaestner, E. J., Wixted, J. T., and Mednick, S. C. (2013). Pharmacologically increasing sleep spindles enhances recognition for negative and high-arousal memories. *J. Cogn. Neurosci.* 25, 1597–1610. doi: 10.1162/jocn_a_00433

Kelemen, E., and Born, J. (2012). Sleep tight, wake up bright. *Nat. Neurosci.* 15, 1327–1329. doi: 10.1038/nn.3227

Killgore, W. D. (2010). Effects of sleep deprivation on cognition. *Prog. Brain Res.* 185, 105–129. doi: 10.1016/b978-0-444-53702-7.00007-5

Killgore, W. D., Balkin, T. J., and Wesensten, N. J. (2006). Impaired decision making following 49 h of sleep deprivation. *J. Sleep Res.* 15, 7–13. doi: 10.1111/j.1365-2869.2006.00487.x

Kirov, R., Weiss, C., Siebner, H. R., Born, J., and Marshall, L. (2009). Slow oscillation electrical brain stimulation during waking promotes EEG theta activity and memory encoding. *Proc. Natl. Acad. Sci. U S A* 106, 15460–15465. doi: 10.1073/pnas.0904438106

Kleim, B., Wilhelm, F. H., Temp, L., Margraf, J., Wiederhold, B. K., and Rasch, B. (2013). Sleep enhances exposure therapy. *Psychol. Med.* doi: 10.1017/s0033291713001748. [Epub ahead of print].

Kuriyama, K., Mishima, K., Suzuki, H., Aritake, S., and Uchiyama, M. (2008). Sleep accelerates the improvement in working memory performance. *J. Neurosci.* 28, 10145–10150. doi: 10.1523/jneurosci.2039-08.2008

Lansink, C. S., Goltstein, P. M., Lankelma, J. V., Joosten, R. N., McNaughton, B. L., and Pennartz, C. M. (2008). Preferential reactivation of motivationally relevant information in the ventral striatum. *J. Neurosci.* 28, 6372–6382. doi: 10.1523/jneurosci.1054-08.2008

Lee, A. K., and Wilson, M. A. (2002). Memory of sequential experience in the hippocampus during slow wave sleep. *Neuron* 36, 1183–1194. doi: 10.1016/s0896-6273(02)01096-6

Lewis, P. A., and Durrant, S. J. (2011). Overlapping memory replay during sleep builds cognitive schemata. *Trends. Cogn. Sci.* 15, 343–351. doi: 10.1016/j.tics.2011.06.004

Lu, W., and Goder, R. (2012). Does abnormal non-rapid eye movement sleep impair declarative memory consolidation?: Disturbed thalamic functions in sleep and memory processing. *Sleep Med. Rev.* 16, 389–394. doi: 10.1016/j.smrv.2011.08.001

Mander, B. A., Santhanam, S., Saletin, J. M., and Walker, M. P. (2011). Wake deterioration and sleep restoration of human learning. *Curr. Biol.* 21, R183–R184. doi: 10.1016/j.cub.2011.01.019

Maquet, P. (2001). The role of sleep in learning and memory. *Science* 294, 1048–1052. doi: 10.1016/b978-012370509-9.00181-9

Maquet, P., Laureys, S., Peigneux, P., Fuchs, S., Petiau, C., Phillips, C., et al. (2000). Experience-dependent changes in cerebral activation during human REM sleep. *Nat. Neurosci.* 3, 831–836. doi: 10.1038/77744

Marrosu, F., Portas, C., Mascia, M. S., Casu, M. A., Fa, M., Giagheddu, M., et al. (1995). Microdialysis measurement of cortical and hippocampal acetylcholine release during sleep-wake cycle in freely moving cats. *Brain Res.* 671, 329–332. doi: 10.1016/0006-8993(94)01399-3

Marshall, L., Helgadottir, H., Molle, M., and Born, J. (2006). Boosting slow oscillations during sleep potentiates memory. *Nature* 444, 610–613. doi: 10.1038/nature05278

Marshall, L., Kirov, R., Brade, J., Molle, M., and Born, J. (2011). Transcranial electrical currents to probe EEG brain rhythms and memory consolidation during sleep in humans. *PLoS One* 6:e16905. doi: 10.1371/journal.pone.0016905

Mednick, S. C., McDevitt, E. A., Walsh, J. K., Wamsley, E., Paulus, M., Kanady, J. C., et al. (2013). The critical role of sleep spindles in hippocampal-dependent memory: a pharmacology study. *J. Neurosci.* 33, 4494–4504. doi: 10.1523/jneurosci.3127-12.2013

Nádasdy, Z., Hirase, H., Czurko, A., Csicsvari, J., and Buzsaki, G. (1999). Replay and time compression of recurring spike sequences in the hippocampus. *J. Neurosci.* 19, 9497–9507.

Ngo, H. V., Claussen, J. C., Born, J., and Molle, M. (2013a). Induction of slow oscillations by rhythmic acoustic stimulation. *J. Sleep Res.* 22, 22–31. doi: 10.1111/j.1365-2869.2012.01039.x

Ngo, H. V., Martinetz, T., Born, J., and Molle, M. (2013b). Auditory closed-loop stimulation of the sleep slow oscillation enhances memory. *Neuron* 78, 545–553. doi: 10.1016/j.neuron.2013.03.006

Nishida, M., and Walker, M. P. (2007). Daytime naps, motor memory consolidation and regionally specific sleep spindles. *PLoS One* 2:e341. doi: 10.1371/journal.pone.0000341

Nyberg, F., and Hallberg, M. (2013). Growth hormone and cognitive function. *Nat. Rev. Endocrinol.* 9, 357–365. doi: 10.1038/nrendo.2013.78

O'Neill, J., Pleydell-Bouverie, B., Dupret, D., and Csicsvari, J. (2010). Play it again: reactivation of waking experience and memory. *Trends Neurosci.* 33, 220–229. doi: 10.1016/j.tins.2010.01.006

Oudiette, D., Antony, J. W., Creery, J. D., and Paller, K. A. (2013). The role of memory reactivation during wakefulness and sleep in determining which memories endure. *J. Neurosci.* 33, 6672–6678. doi: 10.1523/jneurosci.5497-12.2013

Oudiette, D., Antony, J. W., and Paller, K. A. (2014). Fear not: manipulating sleep might help you forget. *Trends Cogn. Sci.* 18, 3–4. doi: 10.1016/j.tics.2013.10.003

Oudiette, D., and Paller, K. A. (2013). Upgrading the sleeping brain with targeted memory reactivation. *Trends Cogn. Sci.* 17, 142–149. doi: 10.1016/j.tics.2013.01.006

Pace-Schott, E. F., Nave, G., Morgan, A., and Spencer, R. M. (2012a). Sleep-dependent modulation of affectively guided decision-making. *J. Sleep Res.* 21, 30–39. doi: 10.1111/j.1365-2869.2011.00921.x

Pace-Schott, E. F., Verga, P. W., Bennett, T. S., and Spencer, R. M. (2012b). Sleep promotes consolidation and generalization of extinction learning in simulated exposure therapy for spider fear. *J. Psychiatr. Res.* 46, 1036–1044. doi: 10.1016/j.jpsychires.2012.04.015

Payne, J. D., Chambers, A. M., and Kensinger, E. A. (2012a). Sleep promotes lasting changes in selective memory for emotional scenes. *Front. Integr. Neurosci.* 6:108. doi: 10.3389/fnint.2012.00108

Payne, J. D., and Kensinger, E. A. (2010). Sleep's role in the consolidation of emotional episodic memories. *Curr. Dir. Psychol. Sci.* 19, 290–295. doi: 10.1177/0963721410383978

Payne, J. D., and Kensinger, E. A. (2011). Sleep leads to changes in the emotional memory trace: evidence from FMRI. *J. Cogn. Neurosci.* 23, 1285–1297. doi: 10.1162/jocn.2010.21526

Payne, J. D., Schacter, D. L., Propper, R. E., Huang, L. W., Wamsley, E. J., Tucker, M. A., et al. (2009). The role of sleep in false memory formation. *Neurobiol. Learn. Mem.* 92, 327–334. doi: 10.1016/j.nlm.2009.03.007

Payne, J. D., Stickgold, R., Swanberg, K., and Kensinger, E. A. (2008). Sleep preferentially enhances memory for emotional components of scenes. *Psychol. Sci.* 19, 781–788. doi: 10.1111/j.1467-9280.2008.02157.x

Payne, J. D., Tucker, M. A., Ellenbogen, J. M., Wamsley, E. J., Walker, M. P., Schacter, D. L., et al. (2012b). Memory for semantically related and unrelated declarative information: the benefit of sleep, the cost of wake. *PLoS One* 7:e33079. doi: 10.1371/journal.pone.0033079

Peigneux, P., Laureys, S., Fuchs, S., Collette, F., Perrin, F., Reggers, J., et al. (2004). Are spatial memories strengthened in the human hippocampus during slow wave sleep? *Neuron* 44, 535–545. doi: 10.1016/j.neuron.2004.10.007

Peyrache, A., Khamassi, M., Benchenane, K., Wiener, S. I., and Battaglia, F. P. (2009). Replay of rule-learning related neural patterns in the prefrontal cortex during sleep. *Nat. Neurosci.* 12, 919–926. doi: 10.1038/nn.2337

Plihal, W., and Born, J. (1999). Memory consolidation in human sleep depends on inhibition of glucocorticoid release. *Neuroreport* 10, 2741–2747. doi: 10.1097/00001756-199909090-00009

Plihal, W., Pietrowsky, R., and Born, J. (1999). Dexamethasone blocks sleep induced improvement of declarative memory. *Psychoneuroendocrinology* 24, 313–331. doi: 10.1016/s0306-4530(98)00080-8

Rasch, B., and Born, J. (2013). About sleep's role in memory. *Physiol. Rev.* 93, 681–766. doi: 10.1152/physrev.00032.2012

Rasch, B., Buchel, C., Gais, S., and Born, J. (2007). Odor cues during slow-wave sleep prompt declarative memory consolidation. *Science* 315, 1426–1429. doi: 10.1126/science.1138581

Rasch, B., Pommer, J., Diekelmann, S., and Born, J. (2009). Pharmacological REM sleep suppression paradoxically improves rather than impairs skill memory. *Nat. Neurosci.* 12, 396–397. doi: 10.1038/nn.2206

Retey, J. V., Adam, M., Gottselig, J. M., Khatami, R., Durr, R., Achermann, P., et al. (2006). Adenosinergic mechanisms contribute to individual differences in sleep deprivation-induced changes in neurobehavioral function and brain rhythmic activity. *J. Neurosci.* 26, 10472–10479. doi: 10.1523/jneurosci.1538-06.2006

Rickard, T. C., Cai, D. J., Rieth, C. A., Jones, J., and Ard, M. C. (2008). Sleep does not enhance motor sequence learning. *J. Exp. Psychol. Learn. Mem. Cogn.* 34, 834–842. doi: 10.1037/0278-7393.34.4.834

Rihm, J., Diekelmann, S., Born, J., and Rasch, B. (2014). Reactivating memories during sleep by odors: odor-specificity and associated changes in sleep oscillations. *J. Cogn. Neurosci.* doi: 10.1162/jocn_a_00579. [Epub ahead of print].

Ritter, S. M., Strick, M., Bos, M. W., van Baaren, R. B., and Dijksterhuis, A. (2012). Good morning creativity: task reactivation during sleep enhances beneficial effect of sleep on creative performance. *J. Sleep Res.* 21, 643–647. doi: 10.1111/j.1365-2869.2012.01006.x

Rolls, A., Makam, M., Kroeger, D., Colas, D., de Lecea, L., and Heller, H. C. (2013). Sleep to forget: interference of fear memories during sleep. *Mol. Psychiatry* 18, 1166–1170. doi: 10.1038/mp.2013.121

Rudoy, J. D., Voss, J. L., Westerberg, C. E., and Paller, K. A. (2009). Strengthening individual memories by reactivating them during sleep. *Science* 326:1079. doi: 10.1126/science.1179013

Sandberg, A. (2011). "Cognition enhancement: upgrading the brain," in *Enhancing Human Capacities*, eds J. Savulescu, R. ter Muelen and G. Kahane (Oxford: Wiley-Blackwell), 71–91.

Sandel, M. (2007). *The Case Against Perfection: Ethics in the Age of Genetic Engineering*. Cambridge, MA: Harvard University Press.

Schabus, M., Gruber, G., Parapatics, S., Sauter, C., Klosch, G., Anderer, P., et al. (2004). Sleep spindles and their significance for declarative memory consolidation. *Sleep* 27, 1479–1485.

Schmidt, C., Peigneux, P., Muto, V., Schenkel, M., Knoblauch, V., Munch, M., et al. (2006). Encoding difficulty promotes postlearning changes in sleep spindle activity during napping. *J. Neurosci.* 26, 8976–8982. doi: 10.1523/jneurosci.2464-06.2006

Schönauer, M., Geisler, T., and Gais, S. (2014). Strengthening procedural memories by reactivation in sleep. *J. Cogn. Neurosci.* 26, 143–153. doi: 10.1162/jocn_a_00471

Sirota, A., and Buzsaki, G. (2005). Interaction between neocortical and hippocampal networks via slow oscillations. *Thalamus Relat. Syst.* 3, 245–259. doi: 10.1017/s1472928807000258

Skaggs, W. E., and McNaughton, B. L. (1996). Replay of neuronal firing sequences in rat hippocampus during sleep following spatial experience. *Science* 271, 1870–1873. doi: 10.1126/science.271.5257.1870

Sowers, J. R., and Vlachakis, N. (1984). Circadian variation in plasma dopamine levels in man. *J. Endocrinol. Invest.* 7, 341–345.

Steiger, A., Dresler, M., Kluge, M., and Schussler, P. (2013). Pathology of sleep, hormones and depression. *Pharmacopsychiatry* 46(Suppl. 1), S30–S35. doi: 10.1055/s-0033-1337921

Steriade, M. (2006). Grouping of brain rhythms in corticothalamic systems. *Neuroscience* 137, 1087–1106. doi: 10.1016/j.neuroscience.2005.10.029

Stern, S. A., and Alberini, C. M. (2013). Mechanisms of memory enhancement. *Wiley Interdiscip. Rev. Syst. Biol. Med.* 5, 37–53. doi: 10.1002/wsbm.1196

Stickgold, R., and Walker, M. P. (2013). Sleep-dependent memory triage: evolving generalization through selective processing. *Nat. Neurosci.* 16, 139–145. doi: 10.1038/nn.3303

Thomas, M., Sing, H., Belenky, G., Holcomb, H., Mayberg, H., Dannals, R., et al. (2000). Neural basis of alertness and cognitive performance impairments during sleepiness. I. Effects of 24 h of sleep deprivation on waking human regional brain activity. *J. Sleep Res.* 9, 335–352. doi: 10.1046/j.1365-2869.2000.00225.x

Tononi, G., and Cirelli, C. (2006). Sleep function and synaptic homeostasis. *Sleep Med. Rev.* 10, 49–62. doi: 10.1016/j.smrv.2005.05.002

Tononi, G., and Cirelli, C. (2014). Sleep and the price of plasticity: from synaptic and cellular homeostasis to memory consolidation and integration. *Neuron* 81, 12–34. doi: 10.1016/j.neuron.2013.12.025

Van Der Werf, Y. D., Altena, E., Schoonheim, M. M., Sanz-Arigita, E. J., Vis, J. C., De Rijke, R. W., et al. (2009). Sleep benefits subsequent hippocampal functioning. *Nat. Neurosci.* 12, 122–123. doi: 10.1038/nn.2253

Van Dongen, H. P., Maislin, G., Mullington, J. M., and Dinges, D. F. (2003). The cumulative cost of additional wakefulness: dose-response effects on neurobehavioral functions and sleep physiology from chronic sleep restriction and total sleep deprivation. *Sleep* 26, 117–126.

van Dongen, E. V., Takashima, A., Barth, M., Zapp, J., Schad, L. R., Paller, K. A., et al. (2012). Memory stabilization with targeted reactivation during human slow-wave sleep. *Proc. Natl. Acad. Sci. U S A* 109, 10575–10580. doi: 10.1073/pnas.1201072109

Vanini, G., Lydic, R., and Baghdoyan, H. A. (2012). GABA-to-ACh ratio in basal forebrain and cerebral cortex varies significantly during sleep. *Sleep* 35, 1325–1334. doi: 10.5665/sleep.2106

Wagner, U., Degirmenci, M., Drosopoulos, S., Perras, B., and Born, J. (2005). Effects of cortisol suppression on sleep-associated consolidation of neutral and emotional memory. *Biol. Psychiatry* 58, 885–893. doi: 10.1016/j.biopsych.2005.05.008

Wagner, U., Gais, S., Haider, H., Verleger, R., and Born, J. (2004). Sleep inspires insight. *Nature* 427, 352–355. doi: 10.1038/nature02223

Walker, M. P. (2005). A refined model of sleep and the time course of memory formation. *Behav. Brain Sci.* 28, 51–64. doi: 10.1017/s0140525x05000026

Walker, M. P., and Stickgold, R. (2006). Sleep, memory and plasticity. *Annu. Rev. Psychol.* 57, 139–166. doi: 10.1146/annurev.psych.56.091103.070307

Wamsley, E. J., Shinn, A. K., Tucker, M. A., Ono, K. E., McKinley, S. K., Ely, A. V., et al. (2013). The effects of eszopiclone on sleep spindles and memory consolidation in schizophrenia: a randomized placebo-controlled trial. *Sleep* 36, 1369–1376. doi: 10.5665/sleep.2968

Wang, G., Grone, B., Colas, D., Appelbaum, L., and Mourrain, P. (2011). Synaptic plasticity in sleep: learning, homeostasis and disease. *Trends Neurosci.* 34, 452–463. doi: 10.1016/j.tins.2011.07.005

Wilhelm, I., Rose, M., Imhof, K. I., Rasch, B., Buchel, C., and Born, J. (2013). The sleeping child outplays the adult's capacity to convert implicit into explicit knowledge. *Nat. Neurosci.* 16, 391–393. doi: 10.1038/nn.3343

Wilhelm, I., Wagner, U., and Born, J. (2011). Opposite effects of cortisol on consolidation of temporal sequence memory during waking and sleep. *J. Cogn. Neurosci.* 23, 3703–3712. doi: 10.1162/jocn_a_00093

Wilson, M. A., and McNaughton, B. L. (1994). Reactivation of hippocampal ensemble memories during sleep. *Science* 265, 676–679. doi: 10.1126/science.8036517

9

Performance enhancement in the workplace: why and when healthy individuals should disclose their reliance on pharmaceutical cognitive enhancers

Mirko D. Garasic[1]* and Andrea Lavazza[2]

[1] *The Federmann School of Public Policy and Government Campus, The Hebrew University of Jerusalem, Jerusalem, Israel*
[2] *Centro Universitario Internazionale, Arezzo, Italy*

Edited by:
Manuel Fernando Casanova, University of Louisville, USA

Reviewed by:
Vittorio Alessandro Sironi, Research Center on History of Biomedical Thought, Italy
Markus Christen, University of Zurich, Switzerland

****Correspondence:***
Mirko D. Garasic, The Federmann School of Public Policy and Government Campus, The Hebrew University of Jerusalem, Mount Scopus Jerusalem, 9190501 Jerusalem, Israel
e-mail: mdgarasic@fulbrightmail.org

The use of pharmaceuticals cognitive enhancers (PCE) has been stirring growing interest, not only in the scientific domain but also in the popular media, and has probably had some increase recently in academic, professional and military quarters. So this phenomenon is deemed as a normal procedure aimed at improving the performance of an individual as well as the overall standards of an organization. Although the vast majority of countries have some kind of restrictions to reduce the wide non-medical usage of PCE, these can be overcome quite easily. In arguing for our explicit claim that, in many contexts, the use of cognitive enhancers should be disclosed—as a moral and socially relevant duty—we maintain that PCE present typical, or at least not rare, properties. The features are the following: (a) the enhancer has acute and/or chronic effects. In the first case, shortly after taking the drug the performance is significantly better than average; in the second case, there is a growing or lasting effect, which, however, is poised to diminish when one stops taking the drug; (b) those effects are significant (there is a difference in the outcome considered between taking and not taking the drug) and sometimes dramatic; and (c) a third feature, not directly related to enhancers as such, is their varying safety, availability, and legal permissibility, which might either induce people to take them or refrain them from doing so. We will consider the issue of fairness due to "unenhanced" people as well as the potentially dysfunctional social consequences of an undisclosed PCE use.

Keywords: pharmaceutical cognitive enhancers, privacy, fairness, autonomy, performance-enhancing substances, moral duty, social duty

INTRODUCTION

In recent years, the use of pharmaceuticals cognitive enhancers (PCE) has been stirring growing interest, not only in the scientific domain but also in the popular media, and has probably had some increase in academic, professional and military quarters, although such increase is very difficult to assess (McCabe et al., 2005, 2007; Teter et al., 2005; Sahakian and Morein-Zamir, 2007; Russo et al., 2008; Franke et al., 2014). PCE can be tentatively defined as drugs which have been shown to improve to some degree some features of human cognition, namely attention, executive functioning (planning, inhibition, and problem-solving), memory and learning, via altering specific neurotransmitters. The most investigated and probably used PEC are off-label drugs primarily aimed at treating neurodegenerative diseases, ADHD, or narcolepsy, which are taken by the healthy to enhance their performance (Greely et al., 2008; Lanni et al., 2008; Marchant et al., 2009; Advokat and Scheithauer, 2013; Mereu et al., 2013; Sattler et al., 2013; Wood et al., 2013; Urban and Gao, 2014) across university campuses (Babcock and Byrne, 2000; Shillington et al., 2006; DeSantis et al., 2008; here we talk about "academic doping", see Cakic, 2009) as well as other competitive contexts (Sahakian and Morein-Zamir, 2007; Chandler, 2012). For reason of space, arguments related to the current restrictions in place (Smith and Farah, 2011) concerning the purchase of these "smart drugs" (Mehlman, 2004)[1]—and their very limited impact—(Farah et al., 2004; Herman-Stahl et al., 2007) will not be discussed here. Instead, this paper aims at analyzing a specific problem related to PCE use. In particular, it is our goal to show the tension between the *local effect* (the enhancement of the individual performance) and the *global effects* (the unwanted social results deriving from the spreading of the use of PCE). Those effects are to be related to two distinct concepts, which— in that case—are at odds: (1) autonomy, and consequently privacy, due to people in their choice of enhancing themselves; and (2) fairness, which is a socially appreciated value. In the following sections we shall considered them separately, starting with the former and later considering its implications on the latter.

LOCAL EFFECT AS PRIVACY

In arguing for our explicit claim that the use of cognitive enhancers should be disclosed, we maintain that such enhancers

[1] Maxwell Mehlman provides a useful account of the use, effects and contexts of these drugs (Mehlman, 2004).

present typical, or at least not rare, properties. The features are the following: (a) the enhancer has acute and/or chronic effects. In the first case, shortly after taking the drug the performance is significantly better than average; in the second case, there is a growing or lasting effect, which, however, is poised to diminish when one stops taking the drug; and (b) those effects are significant (the outcome is different depending on whether the drug was taken or not) and sometimes dramatic; (c) a third feature, not directly related to enhancers as such, is their varying safety, availability, and legal permissibility, which might either induce people to take them or refrain them from doing so. Some recent review studies (Lucke et al., 2011; Smith and Farah, 2011) show that a number of scholars are inclined to say that today's enhancers present those features in a small percentage. Yet, recent developments in the public acknowledgement of PCE use in workplaces put doubts over the accuracy of these statements.[2]

Since some scholars argue that current enhancers have little effect on cognition, it is helpful to highlight their overall effects. A recent qualitative study conducted by Scott Vrecko showed that Ritalin and Adderall do affect intellectual capacities (such as executive functions, working memory and information process), but they *also* heavily affect the user's emotional states. "Such alterations appear to be an important dimension of the drug effects that users perceive to enable improved academic performance" (Vrecko, 2013). Participants said that the perception of better emotional or affective states was the most important feature of the enhancers, leading to improvements in the sense of having augmented skills in doing academic work. Emotional dynamics are a salient dimension of the use of stimulant-based medications. Altered emotional states caused by cognitive enhancers are "part of what makes stimulant drugs useful in relation to academic work". This explains why the specifically cognitive effect appears limited. Instead, Ritalin and Adderall have an important action on the dopaminergic system: they affect the attention, the system of pleasure and that of emotions, including a euphoric effect (Racine and Forlini, 2010; Volkow et al., 2012). Therefore, if, as it seems, enhancers are increasingly spreading among intellectual professionals, it means that the users expect a positive and significant effect, at least at the level of subjective perception. Yet, even though research in the field is at the outset, psychostimulants seem to have very complex, dose and context-dependent effects (Konrad et al., 2004; Wood et al., 2013). The role of age, gender, and ethnic groups in drug efficacy is not clear as well, and such factors play a role in creating differences in neurotransmitter systems of individuals. Thus, the effectivity of PCE is deemed to be unreliable. People relying on PCE for their ordinary or extraordinary performances cannot adequately assess the effects of taking different doses of PCE in different contexts and they would often think they are better than they actually are. And that turns in further reason for disclosing the use of PCE beyond those we expose below.

There are no doubts however, that one of the issues that appear more problematic about the idea of disclosing one's use of PCE is that of entering the private sphere of one's (moral) conduct. As Warren and Brandeis famously put it (Warren and Brandeis, 1890), privacy is part of a more general right to immunity of the person and—through the principle of "inviolate personality"—it preserves a space of non-interference by others. The right to privacy seems to suggest that creating publicly embarrassing or accusatory situations against the individual should not be tolerated (Prosser, 1960). The enhancement of individual performances through legal drugs seems to pertain to such a scenario. If we are to accept a "public intrusion" in such a choice of lifestyle, it is thus necessary to provide a counterbalancing moral reason that could legitimize the request for a disclosure of such information. When is it possible to identify, then, a moral duty or a social interest that goes against individual privacy in the case of PCE? We shall look into this question in the next section.

GLOBAL EFFECTS AS UNFAIRNESS

Interestingly, indeed, it has been recently suggested that PCE might represent a shortcut to the redistribution of (cognitive) wealth (Kohn, 2014). Starting from another study conducted by Mullainathan and Shafir (2013) (in which they underlined that external inputs related to the participants' income substantially affect their cognitive response in the experiment), Marek Kohn argues that—while not being an ideal solution—taking a pill to reduce the impact of the external variables related to the contingent economical disparities between individuals might be the way to go. We will focus on fairness in competitive contexts. As we shall see, in general those situations are such that some researchers, workers or students who use PCE can be considered more skilled and better at performing their task than they really are. But this is not the main problem *per se*. The potentially dysfunctional social consequences are due to the undisclosedness of the PCE use. If one does not have her drug dose available, she will not be capable of the same performance as usual and, in some professions, might even put her colleagues at risk. If standards are set based on PCE-using workers, this may lead to an organizational dysfunction. Some brief examples can present realistic scenarios in which the principle of the duty of disclosure seems perfectly suitable and reasonable. These examples will highlight the argument for the moral and socially relevant duty to disclose the use of cognitive enhancers, insofar as it is sufficiently harmful or unfair to third parties, though not sufficiently harmful or unfair to justify a legal or organizational ban.

John and Susan are researchers in the same university department. They are good friends but are now competing to get a new position opening up in the department. The university committee has decided to put them to a test to prepare for which they are given 2 weeks off work. What they do not know is that the committee will be evaluating both the *content* of their answers, and the time they will take to complete the test. John chooses to take a 15-mg Adderall tablet, so as to increase his capacity to concentrate and maximize the efforts of his studies. To be fair to Susan, he offers her the same tablet, but she refuses, claiming that it would be unfair to alter her performance for the sole purpose of passing the test. In the end, John gets the

[2]In a recent interview for example, an Australian Public Servant admitted that in May 2014 there was an extensive (and widespread) use of modafinil in order to complete the Federal Budget on time (Farr, 2014).

job. Although he gave one correct answer less than Susan, he did so in a much shorter time, and so the committee opted for him: they want knowledge, but *also* efficiency. In discovering this, Susan regards the results as clearly unfair: had she taken Adderall as well—she believes—her reaction time in answering the questions would have been comparable to John's. In this way, she would have won for the higher number of correct answers. She thus approaches John urging him to publicly acknowledge that he took Adderall before the test. He refuses to do so for two reasons: first, he *did* give her the chance to have "completely equal" starting conditions, it was only *her choice* not to take the tablet. Second, there is no official requirement to acknowledge the use of any legal substance: why did she not state that she had three coffees that morning?[3] Susan objects that, first, the starting conditions would have been unfair in any case because—unless they decided to take Adderall for the rest of their lives—their performance would still not correspond to their real, normal capacities. Second, coffee is well known by the committee, and they probably assume that people under examination would take some. On the contrary, Adderall's effects are little known, and they vary for each person.

Now consider Robert. He wishes to help his community and has decided to become a professional nurse in the emergency unit of the local hospital. As he approaches the day of the entrance test, he becomes more and more nervous: he knows that if he could only concentrate fully during the written test, he would have a very good chance to pass. He is told by a friend that Ritalin, a legal drug, would increase his alertness, so he decides to give it a try. On the day of the test, he takes his "smart pill" and enters the room of the written exam. After having performed in a way that he deems very close to perfect, he discovers that the practical test is going to follow in 1 h. Given that he still has a few pills left, he takes another one. Even in this context, he can tell that his performance has improved. In line with what he expected, Robert is accepted as a nurse in the emergency unit. Wanting to "help more", however, he decides that he will take Ritalin regularly when in service. He does so for 6 months, until he runs out of tablets. This happens just on the evening when the local stadium in town crumples down. At both the psychological and the psychical level, Robert is shaken by this "deprivation" and his colleagues have to help him stay focused a few times during the night: this has never happened before. Luckily the wounded are taken care of properly and in a relatively short time, and Robert's "under-performance" does not cause any particular damage. However, his boss notices the change and asks him what happened. Having a clean conscience and thinking he had done nothing wrong, Robert tells the truth. His boss is extremely angry at his words: notwithstanding the moral questionability of taking PCE for the tests, the main issue is that he needs to know who can perform what, and under what circumstances. They are dealing with life and death: anything preventing him from having the actual picture of the people working under him potentially jeopardizes the success of their medical assistance. For this reason, Robert's boss asks him to resign. Robert is shocked and objects that he only thought he was going to be more useful, and certainly he did not perceive this as a "secret". It simply never came out in a conversation.[4]

With short notice, the Ministry of Education occasionally sample tests high school students. The goal is to assess the quality of education, in order to have quantitative data to make comparisons between different towns and regions, identifying effective methods to improve the performance of both teachers and students where needed. Let us assume that standardized student assessment tests are also submitted to those who are old enough to legally take PCE. Even if the tests are anonymous, situations could arise in which students take PCE to improve their results, perhaps encouraged by the teachers themselves, who are likely to aspire to high rankings for their classes. In this way, certain classes or schools in certain towns and regions may end up having very high scores, which, however, would have nothing to do with the teaching methods used or with the students' abilities. This would cause evident biases in the interpretation of the results and lead to inefficient decisions (let us not forget that we are dealing with sample tests, and that a handful of classes, picked using statistically valid methods, can be used as indicators for vast geographic areas). On the basis of the analysis of the data collected, school authorities may well think that, in those classes in which students took PCE, the quality of the education was higher due to the teaching methods used, and decide to experiment with these methods elsewhere as well. This would result in a waste of public resources and hinder research on truly better teaching methods. Additionally, it could hide actual differences between geographic areas, resulting in a lack of intervention where school performance is actually poor.

In all the cases considered, there would appear to be both a moral duty and a social interest in reporting the use of PCE. Indeed, the use of PCE could be deemed fully legitimate and in fact, if openly reported, it could become an additional element in the assessment of ways to improve one's performance. To focus on this last case, by knowing what classes, in what geographic areas, took cognitive enhancers, it will be possible to assess their effectiveness without introducing biases in the overall results. This is certainly of social interest as it helps with the efficient allocation of resources. Yet, there also seems to be a moral duty, since teachers who encouraged their students to take PCE without reporting it might be trying to hide their shortcomings as educators. In other contexts, instead, taking PCE unbeknownst to evaluators may result in the failure to identify situations of economic or cultural distress, because school performance has improved only thanks to the use of cognitive enhancers.

LOCAL VS. GLOBAL EFFECTS

The duty to disclose the use of cognitive enhancers (and maybe also of mood affecting drugs) is not just intended to prevent *local effects* from prevailing on *global effects*—with undesirable social

[3]It should be noted that this argument is often used by bio-liberals: given that caffeine is also a cognitive enhancing substance, why should we limit the use of one enhancer over another? For a more precise analysis see Julien (2001), especially pages 145–164.

[4]A similar motivation could be applied to the renowned cases of cocaine use among surgeons around the world. However, our intention is to focus on PCE precisely because—unlike cocaine—they are *not* illegal drugs.

outcomes deriving from unpredictable composition effects. This is certainly the most important consequentialist reasoning that can justify the duty of disclosure. What is at stake, however, is also an ethical principle of fairness that seems to prevail over the right to privacy as we described it earlier. In fact, those who make use of cognitive enhancers in single occasions or non-repeatable competitive situations seem to be required to report the sudden difference that has arisen in their abilities without this enhancement depending on something they can be credited for. Suppose a candidate for a test, on her way to the university, finds the answer sheet that the examiner has lost from her pocket; or that the computer on which a test is run is defective and shows the correct answers together with the questions; or that, even a single time, one gets help from a renowned scientist in conducting a difficult experiment (but claiming full credit for it); or that a junior broker can rely on the advice of a knowledgeable friend who is well introduced in the sphere of finance.

These are situations in which fairness in the competition is lost without violating any rules or prohibitions, but in which the performance has little to do with the actual skills that a candidate may manifest later and with what he has done to improve them. Therefore, fairness in respecting the equality of the starting conditions as a principle of respect for the others leads to reveal aspects related to chance or to the sporadic and extrinsic improvement of one's skills. It is a much needed principle, weaker than the prohibition to resort to means extraneous to the competition or the duty to waive potential favorable conditions (the latter principle would severely limit individual autonomy). As our first example shows, if all relevant information is made available, the competition is fair and everyone can choose how to act within the framework of the existing legislation.

The duty to disclose the use of PCE has a final consequence that one should consider. We have talked mainly about a moral duty to disclose, but such a duty could also carry a legal obligation and a number of consequences. For example, would that disclosure justify that a person is not hired for a position? We think that a simple answer is not available. In some cases, the hirer could judge that the person is perfectly suitable for the position and the variability of her performance based also on PCE is always satisfactory. In other cases, if the person's performance with PCE is near the lower threshold of the minimum performance, considering the dose and context-dependent effects, it could be a risk to rely on her, so the hirer would have good reasons not to hire her. In light of these considerations, there might be a question about the effective incentives (perhaps stressing the moral praiseworthiness of disclosing) to declare the use of PCE. Such incentives deserve attention, but they cannot be analyzed here.

CONCLUSION

The aim of this paper—including the use of realistic examples—has been to shed light over the existing (but overlooked) tension between the *local* and *global effects* of the use of PCE. Even if it is perhaps problematic to accept in a liberal society at first, a partial reduction of our right to privacy might be necessary in order to preserve the equally important principle of fairness (as well as social safety and efficiency) that an unregulated use of PCE could threaten. The legitimacy of this step derives from other values deeply entrenched in liberal societies, such as the restriction of individual autonomy if this puts in jeopardy that of others. Reasons related to equity and social interests, therefore, can suggest that there is a moral duty to publicly acknowledge the use of PCE in order to limit the potential damages. There have already been a number of scientific and moral assessments of PCE in the literature, and we do not expect to have provided an exhaustive account on how to legislate further on PCE with this work, but we do hope to have offered some innovative ways of conceptualizing the debate evolving around the increasing use of PCE.

REFERENCES

Advokat, C., and Scheithauer, M. (2013). Attention-deficit hyperactivity disorder (ADHD) stimulant medications as cognitive enhancers. *Front. Neurosci.* 7:82. doi: 10.3389/fnins.2013.00082

Babcock, Q., and Byrne, T. (2000). Student perceptions of methylphenidate abuse at a public liberal arts college. *J. Am. Coll. Health* 49, 143–145. doi: 10.1080/07448480009596296

Cakic, V. (2009). Smart drugs for cognitive enhancement: ethical and pragmatic considerations in the era of cosmetic neurology. *J. Med. Ethics* 35, 611–615. doi: 10.1136/jme.2009.030882

Chandler, J. A. (2012). "Obligatory Technologies": explaining why people feel compelled to use certain technologies. *Bull. Sci. Technol. Soc.* 32, 255–264. doi: 10.1177/0270467612459924

DeSantis, D. A., Webb, E. M., and Noar, S. M. (2008). Illicit use of prescription ADHD medications on a college campus: a multimethodological approach. *J. Am. Coll. Health* 57, 315–323. doi: 10.3200/JACH.57.3.315-324

Farah, M. J., Illes, J., Cook-Deegan, R., Gardner, H., Kandel, E., King, P., et al. (2004). Neurocognitive enhancement: what can we do and what should we do?. *Nat. Rev. Neurosci.* 5, 421–425. doi: 10.1038/nrn1390

Farr, M. (2014). Public servants used drug, modafinil, to stay awake to complete the federal budget on time. *The Courier Mail.* Available online at: http://www.couriermail.com.au/news/national/public-servants-used-drug-modafinil-to-stay-awake-to-complete-the-federal-budget-on-time/story-fnihslxi-1226932640759. Accessed on 27 May 2014.

Franke, A. G., Bagusat, C., Rust, S., Engel, A., and Lieb, K. (2014). Substances used and prevalence rates of pharmacological cognitive enhancement among healthy subjects. *Eur. Arch. Psychiatry Clin. Neurosci.* 264, S83–S90. doi: 10.1007/s00406-014-0537-1

Greely, H., Sahakian, B., Harris, J., Kessler, R. C., Gazzaniga, M., Campbell, P., et al. (2008). Towards responsible use of cognitive enhancing drugs by the healthy. *Nature* 456, 702–705. doi: 10.1038/456702a

Herman-Stahl, M. A., Krebs, C. P., Kroutil, L. A., and Heller, D. C. (2007). Risk and protective factors for methamphetamine use and nonmedical use of prescription stimulants among young adults aged 18 to 25. *Addict. Behav.* 32, 1003–1015. doi: 10.1016/j.addbeh.2006.07.010

Julien, R. M. (2001). *A Primer of Drug Action.* New York, NY: Holt.

Kohn, M. (2014). Smart and smarter drugs. *Mosaic: The Science of Life.* Available online at: http://mosaicscience.com/story/smart-and-smarter-drugs

Konrad, K., Gunther, T., Hanisch, C., and Herpertz-Dahlmann, B. (2004). Differential effects of methylphenidate on attentional functions in children with attention-deficit/hyperactivity disorder. *J. Am. Acad. Child Adolesc. Psychiatry* 43, 191–198. doi: 10.1097/00004583-200402000-00015

Lanni, C., Lenzken, S. C., Pascale, A., Del Vecchio, I., Racchi, M., Pistoia, F., et al. (2008). Cognition enhancers between treating and doping the mind. *Pharmacol. Res.* 57, 196–213. doi: 10.1016/j.phrs.2008.02.004

Lucke, J. C., Bell, S., Partridge, B., and Hall, W. D. (2011). Deflating the neuroenhancement bubble. *Am. J. Bioeth. Neurosci.* 2, 38–43. doi: 10.1080/21507740.2011.611122

Marchant, N. L., Kamel, F., Echlin, K., Grice, J., Lewis, M., and Rusted, J. M. (2009). Modafinil improves rapid shifts of attention. *Psychopharmacology (Berl)* 202, 487–495. doi: 10.1007/s00213-008-1395-1

McCabe, S. E., Knight, J. R., Teter, C. J., and Wechsler, H. (2005). Non-medical use of prescription stimulants among US college students: prevalence and correlates from a national survey. *Addiction* 100, 96–106. doi: 10.1111/j.1360-0443.2005.00944.x

McCabe, S. E., West, B. T., and Wechsler, H. (2007). Trends and college-level characteristics associated with the non-medical use of prescription drugs among US college students from 1993 to 2001. *Addiction* 102, 455–465. doi: 10.1111/j.1360-0443.2006.01733.x

Mehlman, M. J. (2004). Cognition-enhancing drugs. *Milbank Q.* 82, 483–506. doi: 10.1111/j.0887-378X.2004.00319.x

Mereu, M., Bonci, A., Newman, A. H., and Tanda, G. (2013). The neurobiology of modafinil as an enhancer of cognitive performance and a potential treatment for substance use disorders. *Psychopharmacology (Berl)* 229, 415–434. doi: 10.1007/s00213-013-3232-4

Mullainathan, S., and Shafir, E. (2013). *Scarcity: Why Having Too Little Means So Much.* New York: Times Book.

Prosser, W. (1960). Privacy. *Calif. Law Rev.* 48, 383–423. doi: 10.2307/3478805

Racine, E., and Forlini, C. (2010). Cognitive enhancement, lifestyle choice or misuse of prescription drugs? *Neuroethics* 3, 1–4. doi: 10.1007/s12152-008-9023-7

Russo, M. B., Arnett, M. V., Thomas, M. L., and Caldwell, J. A. (2008). Ethical use of cogniceuticals in the militaries of democratic nations. *Am. J. Bioeth.* 8, 39–41. doi: 10.1080/15265160802015016

Sahakian, B. J., and Morein-Zamir, S. (2007). Professor's little helper. *Nature* 450, 1157–1159. doi: 10.1038/4501157a

Sattler, S., Sauer, C., Mehlkop, G., and Graeff, P. (2013). The rationale for consuming cognitive enhancement drugs in university students and teachers. *PLoS One* 8:e68821. doi: 10.1371/journal.pone.0068821

Shillington, A. M., Reed, M. B., Lange, J. E., Clapp, J. D., and Henry, S. (2006). College undergraduate ritalin abusers in southwestern california: protective and risk factors. *J. Drug Issues* 36, 999–1014. doi: 10.1177/002204260603600411

Smith, M. E., and Farah, M. J. (2011). Are prescription stimulants "smart pills"? The epidemiology and cognitive neuroscience of prescription stimulant use by normal healthy individuals. *Psychol. Bull.* 137, 717–741. doi: 10.1037/a0023825

Teter, C. J., McCabe, S. E., Cranford, J. A., Boyd, C. J., and Guthrie, S. K. (2005). Prevalence and motives for illicit use of prescription stimulants in an undergraduate student sample. *J. Am. Coll. Health* 53, 253–262. doi: 10.3200/jach.53.6.253-262

Urban, K. R., and Gao, W. J. (2014). Performance enhancement at the cost of potential brain plasticity: neural ramifications of nootropic drugs in the healthy developing brain. *Front. Syst. Neurosci.* 8:38. doi: 10.3389/fnsys.2014.00038

Volkow, N. D., Wang, G. J., Tomasi, D., Kollins, S. H., Wigal, T. L., Newcorn, J. H., et al. (2012). Metylphenidate-elicited dopamine increases in ventral striatum are associated with long-term symptom improvements in adults with attention deficit hyperactivity disorder. *J. Neurosci.* 32, 841–849. doi: 10.1523/JNEUROSCI.4461-11.2012

Vrecko, S. (2013). Just how cognitive is "cognitive enhancement"? On the significance of emotions in university students' experiences with study drugs. *AJOB Neurosci.* 4, 4–12. doi: 10.1080/21507740.2012.740141

Warren, S. D., and Brandeis, L. D. (1890). The right to privacy. *Harv. Law Rev.* 4, 193–220. doi: 10.2307/1321160

Wood, S., Sage, J. R., Shuman, T., and Anagnostaras, S. G. (2013). Psychostimulants and cognition: a continuum of behavioral and cognitive activation. *Pharmacol. Rev.* 66, 193–221. doi: 10.1124/pr.112.007054

10

How cognitive enhancement can change our duties

Filippo Santoni de Sio[1]*, Nadira Faulmüller[1,2] and Nicole A Vincent[1,3]

[1] *Department Values, Technology and Innovation, Faculty Technology, Policy and Management, Delft University of Technology, Delft, Netherlands*
[2] *Department of Experimental Psychology, University of Oxford, Oxford, UK*
[3] *Department of Philosophy, Georgia State University, Atlanta, GA, USA*

Edited by:
Mikhail Lebedev, Duke University, USA

Reviewed by:
Fabrice Jotterand, Regis University, USA
Michael Linderman, Norconnect Inc., USA
Jan Christoph Bublitz, University of Hamburg, Germany

*Correspondence:
Filippo Santoni de Sio, Department Values, Technology and Innovation, Faculty Technology, Policy and Management, Delft University of Technology, Postbus 5015, Delft, 2600 GA, Netherlands
e-mail: f.santonidesio@tudelft.nl

This theoretical paper draws the scientific community's attention to how pharmacological cognitive enhancement may impact on society and law. Namely, if safe, reliable, and effective techniques to enhance mental performance are eventually developed, then this may under some circumstances impose *new duties* onto people in high-responsibility professions—e.g., surgeons or pilots—to use such substances to minimize risks of adverse outcomes or to increase the likelihood of good outcomes. By discussing this topic, we also hope to encourage scientists to bring their expertise to bear on this current public debate.

Keywords: cognitive enhancement, neuroenhancement, modafinil, methylphenidate, mental capacity, ethics, law, professional duties

INTRODUCTION

Whereas techniques for the augmentation of brain function are usually seen as beneficial when used as a form of medical treatment, both amongst the general public (Schelle et al., 2014) and in academia (e.g., Sandel, 2009) some concerns have been raised about the possible negative moral and social impacts of the use of these techniques in healthy people. For example, concerns about such so called "cognitive enhancement" include seeing it as a threat to the fairness and meaningfulness of competitive activities, or as a potential threat to a meaningful human life. Even though "cognitive enhancement" may refer to different brain intervention techniques like genetic modification, pharmacological substances, Transcranial Magnetic Stimulations (TMS), or Transcranial Direct Current Stimulation (tDCS; Bostrom and Sandberg, 2009), in this paper we focus on *pharmacological* cognitive enhancers such as methylphenidate and modafinil. These substances have been reported to modestly improve wakefulness, attention, concentration, learning and retention of memory, not only when taken by people diagnosed with mental deficits or disorders, but also when taken by healthy individuals (Repantis et al., 2010; Husain and Mehta, 2011; Coffman et al., 2014; Gilleena et al., 2014; Meinzer et al., 2014).

In what follows, we discuss a seldom-recognized but crucial way in which pharmacological cognitive enhancement may impact on our society's moral and legal norms: the availability of such enhancers might evoke *new duties* for certain people. In particular, it may impact on the *professional duties* of people engaged in jobs where the lives of other people are directly at risk (e.g., surgeons and pilots)—i.e., it may impact on what we can (legally) *demand* these professionals to do. By exploring this issue, we want to offer some insights into a particular way in which scientific work on brain function augmentation may impact on society: by enhancing our cognitive capacities, neuroscientific progress may change our duties to one another (for in-depth discussion see Vincent, 2011, 2013; Enck, 2014; Goold and Maslen, 2014; Santoni de Sio et al., 2014).

HOW PHARMACOLOGICAL COGNITIVE ENHANCEMENT CAN CREATE NEW DUTIES

Our main question may be framed in the following way: assuming that a certain kind of pharmacological enhancement proves to be relatively safe and effective at reducing risks of negative outcomes, may some people, in virtue of what is at stake in the performance of their professional roles (e.g., surgeons or pilots), be sometimes *legitimately expected* to cognitively enhance themselves even if they would rather not do so? Even though this question may sound counterintuitive at present, we think there are good reasons to assume that such an expectation might be a realistic scenario in the future. In particular, we think that the professional duty to use pharmacological enhancers may sooner or later be raised in tort cases at least under restricted circumstances, for instance in emergencies, when less invasive and at least as effective alternatives are not available. If this happens, judges will take a decision mainly through analogical reasoning. We thus think it is important to anticipate how such reasoning is likely to run. By having a clearer picture of such a possible future scenario, the scientific community and the public more generally will be able to think ahead about whether any pre-emptive steps need to be taken to forestall the development of foreseeable undesirable social, political, and legal consequences involved in such a scenario.

In the following we present three main points in support of our claim that a duty to enhance, as circumscribed above, may arise in the future.

Firstly, scientific and technological progress has already affected professional duties in the past. Surgeons, for instance, are nowadays expected to deploy many measures that enhance their performance and/or reduce the risks of fatal outcomes. Historically, this professional duty to take measures has gradually emerged over time, and progress in scientific and technological knowledge has been one decisive element in the creation of the duty. When, for instance, basic antiseptic procedures which are common today—e.g., cleansing hands with carbolic acid—were originally developed, their efficacy was not yet established, their risks for the user were unknown, they were available only in select research laboratories and medical practitioners were not expected to deploy them. But today, now that the clinical value of these techniques is widely recognized, and they are relatively inexpensive, largely free of risk, and ubiquitously available (Gawande, 2012), medical practitioners cannot legitimately reject the request to employ these techniques. The discovery of the antiseptic efficacy of carbolic acid, as it were, brought with it the creation of a duty to use it.

Of course, the analogy between cognitive enhancement medications and carbolic acid is far from perfect—while the former is highly invasive to an important domain, namely brain functioning, the latter is not even skin-deep. Therefore, one should not expect this analogy to be sufficient to make a case for the professional duty to use pharmacological enhancers. However, this analogy is arguably sufficient to make a more general point: when it comes to professions with a high societal value like those aimed at healing people or warranting their safety, it may be legitimate for society to demand professionals to not follow their individual preferences but rather the rules of good practice that are proven to lead to optimal results, including those requiring them to undertake particular treatments of their body. Even in the most democratic society, the value of individual freedom of choice of professionals is not protected unconditionally. For instance, at present we already expect medical or legal professionals to engage in continuing education programs. Often this is quite an invasion on people's lives since they must set aside time from an often already busy schedule to attend classes after hours, often losing sleep, and certainly losing personal time. But yet we do not think that this imposition on their freedom is an unreasonable one. We think that this is a sacrifice that we are entitled to expect professionals to make for the benefit of their patients and clients. The underlying thinking is that what's gained in terms of outcomes is presumed to be more important than the sacrifices that others have to make to secure those outcomes.

Secondly, it may certainly be insisted that things are different with pharmacological enhancers, and that no matter what happens with the compulsory use of non-invasive technologies or with compulsory non-pharmacological enhancement programs, the use of medical substances that directly affect the brain can never be imposed on professionals against their will. However, even as things currently stand we already sometimes expect some people to use medical substances that directly affect their brain for the benefit of others—namely, when we expect people who wish to operate motor vehicles but who are diagnosed with conditions like epilepsy and diabetes to take medical substances to prevent the negative effects of these conditions from adversely affecting others (*Knoxville Optical Supply, Inc. v Thomas*, 1993 WL 574 (TennCtApp Jan 04, 1993)). Naturally, a good reason for them to take these medications is simply the benefits to their own health. But it has to be noted that the argument which justifies legal coercion to use those substances in the case of the epileptic and diabetic motor vehicle drivers is not that the medical substances will benefit *them*—in a liberal democracy paternalism is rarely accepted as a valid justification for infringements on freedom—but rather that their not taking those medications would impose an unacceptable risk to *others* (if they should take to the roads un-medicated).

We offer the above example in support of two points. Firstly, there is already an existing and accepted practice of expecting one group of people to take brain-invasive medications for the benefit of other groups of people. Secondly, it makes little difference that these examples involve the use of medications to *treat* rather than to *enhance*, because the persons concerned are expected to take the medications not for their own benefit, but for the benefit of others. In fact, Queensland Health, the medical regulatory body of the North-East Australian state, has recently followed a similar reasoning pattern in relation to fatigue management. In their Queensland Health (2009), it is suggested that in order to cope with fatigue-related risks, surgeons could take up to "400 mg of caffeine [which is the] equivalent to about 5–6 cups of coffee" (78) because "[c]ompared with other psychoactive drugs (e.g., modafinil), caffeine is... more readily available and less expensive" (79). Given that the report explicitly cites modafinil, and that it only cites availability and cost as considerations that favor the use of caffeine over modafinil, we think it is perfectly conceivable that a future report may recommend such drugs to be used (cf. Maslen et al., in press). To be sure, one may still insist that this is not a desirable scenario, and that the protection of minds from external interference should be recognized as a human right. However, as a matter of fact, the right to "cognitive liberty" (Bublitz, 2013) is not (yet) protected by international human rights in the same way in which bodily integrity is, so that the scenario that we propose remains realistic.

Finally, one may wonder whether concerns about safety will in the end prevent the imposition of a duty to enhance in every situation imaginable. Admittedly, the long-terms possible negative effects of the use of cognitive enhancers are not sufficiently known (Madras et al., 2006; Volkow et al., 2009), and a greater scientific understanding of these substances is needed before normative conclusions can be confidently drawn (Maslen et al., 2014). However, it is also a fact that methylphenidate has been prescribed to children to treat the symptoms of attention deficit and hyperactivity disorder for well over two decades. We cite this example only to illustrate that there is at present already consensus about the relative safety of these drugs to prescribe them to the most vulnerable part of the population—namely, to children. This point is salient because if, as a society, we deem the costs or risks of particular cognitive enhancement technologies to be sufficiently low, then this may lead us, together with the other considerations mentioned above, to impose a duty to use these medications onto some people at least in some emergency situations, namely when other more common forms of intervention like napping or being replaced by another worker who is not fatigued are not available.

A GLANCE INTO THE FUTURE

Admittedly, we are not (yet) in the scenario that we just described. The efficacy of pharmacological cognitive enhancement techniques in reducing the rate of fatal mistakes and thus enhancing the quality of performance of professionals like surgeons and airline pilots has not been established yet (Förstl, 2009; Repantis et al., 2010), and they are not even easily accessible. It is therefore not surprising that the law has not yet demanded any professionals to enhance themselves nor have lay people advanced such a demand.

As for the law, Goold and Maslen (2014) have offered a detailed legal analysis on the issue of whether surgeons who are at risk of making fatigue-related errors during patient care might be considered legally obliged to pharmacologically enhance themselves, i.e., if, at least under certain circumstances, there can be a *legal duty to enhance* for surgeons. Their conclusion is that, at the moment, such a legal duty *cannot* be imposed (at least in England and Wales). However, once one considers the reasons behind their conclusion, it becomes clear that Goold and Maslen's statement about the current legal situation is not necessarily incompatible with our claim about the future. Their case against the imposition of a legal duty to enhance on surgeons, in fact, critically depends on their reasonable doubts about the efficacy of current enhancers, and the possible negative side-effects of these substances. Moreover, this conclusion does not affect the validity of our theoretical point. In fact, as Goold and Maslen themselves explicitly state, in a *hypothetical* scenario in which efficacious and relatively safe cognitive enhancers were available, surgeons *might* be burdened with a duty to take pharmacological cognitive enhancers to reduce the risks of fatal fatigue-related error, at least under some emergency circumstances, namely when other, less invasive, options like napping or being replaced by another surgeons are not available. And it is *this* kind of hypothetical scenario that our reasoning has taken into account, and that future judges may have to decide upon.

As for lay people, they also seem to believe that no obligation to enhance should ever be imposed on professionals or other subjects (Maslen et al., in press). Many are indeed skeptical even about the moral *permissibility* of the use of pharmacological enhancers in any circumstance (Santoni de Sio et al., in press). Again, this is reasonable and understandable. Lay reasoning widely reflects the current state of affairs of scientific progress. From this perspective, lay reasoning is somehow similar to that of the above-mentioned legal scholars: because pharmacological cognitive enhancement is currently neither uncontroversially efficacious nor safe, people are legitimately wary and suspicious of it and reluctant to expect anyone to use it. However, lay reasoning may also reflect less rational and justified concerns. Medical enhancement substances are perceived negatively compared to other "natural" enhancers, and as a consequence the use of pharmacological cognitive enhancement might be stigmatized also in an irrational way (Faulmüller et al., 2013).

CONCLUSION

Reflections on the social impact of scientific and technological progress can come in different forms. On the one hand, we may reflect on how *current* technologies and techniques are already impacting on society. However, we may also wish to reflect on how the social, political, legal, and moral landscape may change due to pressure from reasonably expected *future* advances in science and technology, and think ahead about whether any pre-emptive steps need to be taken to forestall the development of foreseeable undesirable social, political, legal, and moral consequences. Adopting this latter "socially responsible innovation" approach (Moor, 2008; van den Hoven, 2013) which has recently been embraced also by the European Commission (2011), our paper has discussed the possible impact on society of future advances in pharmacological cognitive enhancement. We have argued that the availability of techniques that can enhance performance may in the future impose *new duties* on certain people under certain circumstances.

REFERENCES

Bostrom, N., and Sandberg, A. (2009). Cognitive enhancement: methods, ethics, regulatory challenges. *Sci. Eng. Ethics* 15, 311–341. doi: 10.1007/s11948-009-9142-5

Bublitz, J. C. (2013). "My mind is mine?! cognitive liberty as a legal concept," in *Cognitive Enhancement: An Interdisciplinary Perspective*, eds E. Hildt and A. G. Franke (Dordrecht: Springer), 233–264.

Coffman, B. A., Clark, V. P., and Parasuraman, R. (2014). Battery powered thought: enhancement of attention, learning and memory in healthy adults using transcranial direct current stimulation. *Neuroimage* 85, 895–908. doi: 10.1016/j.neuroimage.2013.07.083

Enck, G. G. (2014). Pharmaceutical enhancement and medical professionals. *Med. Health Care Philos.* 17, 23–28. doi: 10.1007/s11019-013-9507-z

European Commission. (2011). *Horizon 2020—The Framework Programme for Research and Innovation.* Brussels: European Commission. http://ec.europa.eu/research/horizon2020/pdf/proposals/communication_from_the_commission_-_horizon_2020_-_the_framework_programme_for_research_and_innovation.pdf

Faulmüller, N., Maslen, H., and de Sio, F. S. (2013). The indirect psychological costs of cognitive enhancement. *Am. J. Bioeth.* 13, 45–47. doi: 10.1080/15265161.2013.794880

Förstl, H. (2009). Neuro-enhancement. Brain doping. *Nervenarzt* 80, 840–846. doi: 10.1007/s00115-009-2801-6

Gawande, A. (2012). Two hundred years of surgery. *N. Engl. J. Med.* 366, 1716–1723. doi: 10.1056/NEJMra1202392

Gilleena, J., Michalopouloua, P. G., Reichenberg, A., Drake, R., Wykes, T., Lewis, S. W., et al. (2014). Modafinil combined with cognitive training is associated with improved learning in healthy volunteers—A randomised controlled trial. *Eur. Neuropsychopharmacol.* 24, 529–539. doi: 10.1016/j.euroneuro.2014.01.001

Goold, I., and Maslen, H. (2014). Must the surgeon take the pill? Negligence duty in the context of cognitive enhancement. *Mod. Law Rev.* 77, 60–86. doi: 10.1111/1468-2230.12056

Husain, M., and Mehta, M. A. (2011). Cognitive enhancement by drugs in health and disease. *Trends Cogn. Sci.* 15, 28–36. doi: 10.1016/j.tics.2010.11.002

Madras, B. K., Xie, Z., Xie, Z., Lin, Z., Jassen, A., Panas, H., et al. (2006). Modafinil occupies dopamine and norepinephrine transporters in vivo and modulates the transporters and trace amine activity in vitro. *J. Pharmacol. Exp. Ther.* 319, 561–569. doi: 10.1124/jpet.106.106583

Maslen, H., Faulmüller, N., and Savulescu, J. (2014). Pharmacological cognitive enhancement—how neuroscientific research could advance ethical debate. *Front. Syst. Neurosci.* 8:107. doi: 10.3389/fnsys.2014.00107

Maslen, H., Santoni de Sio, F., and Faulmüller, N. (in press). "With cognitive enhancement comes great responsibility?," in *Responsible Innovation* (Vol. 2), ed B. J. Koops (Dordrecht: Springer Verlag).

Meinzer, M., Jähnigen, S., Copland, D. A., Darkow, R., Grittner, U., Avirame, K., et al. (2014). Transcranial direct current stimulation over multiple days improves learning and maintenance of a novel vocabulary. *Cortex* 50, 137–147. doi: 10.1016/j.cortex.2013.07.013

Moor, J. H. (2008). "Why we need better ethics for emerging technologies," in *Information Technology and Moral Philosophy*, eds J. van den Hoven and J. Weckert (New York: Cambridge University Press), 26–39.

Queensland Health. (2009). *Fatigue Risk Management System: Resource Pack*. Brisbane, QLD, Australia. http://www.health.qld.gov.au/qhpolicy/docs/imp/qh-imp-358-1.pdf

Repantis, D., Schlattmann, P., Laisney, O., and Heuser, I. (2010). Modafinil and methylphenidate for neuroenhancement in healthy individuals: a systematic review. *Pharmacol. Res.* 62, 187–206. doi: 10.1016/j.phrs.2010.04.002

Sandel, M. J. (2009). *The Case Against Perfection*. Cambridge, MA: Harvard University Press.

Santoni de Sio, F., Faulmüller, N., Savulescu, J., and Vincent, N. A. (in press). "Why less praise for enhanced performance? Moving beyond responsibility-shifting, authenticity and cheating to a nature of activities approach," in *Cognitive Enhancement: Ethical and Policy Implications in International Perspectives*, eds F. Jotterand and V. Dubljevic (Oxford: Oxford University Press).

Santoni de Sio, F., Robichaud, P., and Vincent, N. A. (2014). Who should enhance? Conceptual and normative dimensions of cognitive enhancement. *Humanamente J. Philos. Stud.* 26, 179–197.

Schelle, K. J., Faulmüller, N., Caviola, L., and Hewstone, M. (2014). Attitudes towards pharmacological cognitive enhancement—a review. *Front. Syst. Neurosci.* 8:53. doi: 10.3389/fnsys.2014.00053

van den Hoven, J. (2013). "Value sensitive design and responsible innovation," in *Responsible Innovation—Managing the Responsible Emergence of Science and Innovation in Society*, eds R. Owen, J. Bessant and M. Heintz (West Sussex: John Wiley), 75–84.

Vincent, N. (2011). "The challenges posed to private law by emerging cognitive enhancement technologies," in *The Law of the Future and The Future of Law*, eds S. Muller, S. Zouridis, M. Frishman and L. Kistemaker (Oslo: Torkel Opsahl Academic EPublisher), 511–521. http://www.fichl.org/fileadmin/fichl/documents/FICHL_11_Web.pdf

Vincent, N. (2013). "Enhancing responsibility," in *Neuroscience and Legal Responsibilty*, ed N. A. Vincent (New York, NY: Oxford University Press), 305–336.

Volkow, N. D., Fowler, J. S., Logan, J., Alexoff, D., Zhu, W., Telang, F., et al. (2009). Effects of modafinil on dopamine and dopamine transporters in the male human brain: clinical implications. *JAMA* 301, 1148–1154. doi: 10.1001/jama.2009.351

11

On the need to better specify the concept of "control" in brain-computer-interfaces/neurofeedback research

Guilherme Wood[1,2]*, Silvia Erika Kober[1,2], Matthias Witte[1,2] and Christa Neuper[1,2]

[1] *Department of Psychology, Karl-Franzens-University Graz, Graz, Austria*
[2] *BioTechMed, Graz, Austria*

Edited by:
Mikhail Lebedev, Duke University, USA

Reviewed by:
Andrea Kübler, University of Würzburg, Germany
Kenji Kansaku, Research Institute of National Rehabilitation Center for Persons with Disabilities, Japan
Annette Sterr, University of Surrey, UK

Correspondence:
Guilherme Wood, Department of Neuropsychology, Institute of Psychology, University of Graz, Brandhofgasse 5 (Palais Apfaltrem), A-8010 Graz, Austria
e-mail: guilherme.wood@uni-graz.at

Aiming at a better specification of the concept of "control" in brain-computer-interfaces (BCIs) and neurofeedback (NF) research, we propose to distinguish "self-control of brain activity" from the broader concept of "BCI control", since the first describes a neurocognitive phenomenon and is only one of the many components of "BCI control". Based on this distinction, we developed a framework based on dual-processes theory that describes the cognitive determinants of self-control of brain activity as the interplay of automatic vs. controlled information processing. Further, we distinguish between cognitive processes that are necessary and sufficient to achieve a given level of self-control of brain activity and those which are not. We discuss that those cognitive processes which are not necessary for the learning process can hamper self-control because they cannot be completely turned-off at any time. This framework aims at a comprehensive description of the cognitive determinants of the acquisition of self-control of brain activity underlying those classes of BCI which require the user to achieve regulation of brain activity as well as NF learning.

Keywords: BCI, neurofeedback, executive functions, dual-process theory, rumination, meta-cognition, cognitive strategies

INTRODUCTION

Brain computer interfaces (BCIs) make possible the direct communication pathway between the brain and an external device. BCIs are often directed at assisting, augmenting, or repairing human cognitive or sensory-motor functions. Individuals learn how to induce certain patterns of brain activity, which can be detected and transcoded into some form of action or feedback in the external device. One special case of BCI is neurofeedback (NF), in which the aim is not to control an external device but rather to use external feedback to modulate specific aspects of physiological signal intrinsic to the brain. Both human and nonhuman animals are able to learn to use BCI/NF with a short amount of training (Sterman, 1977; Nicolelis and Lebedev, 2009; Phillippens and Vanwersch, 2010).

Generally, the term "BCI control" has been used interchangeably to refer to two different processes. On the one side, "BCI control" refers to the ability to control an external device and can be seen mainly as a complex problem of neuroengineering (Donoghue, 2008). This definition simultaneously involves neuro-bio-psychological, data analytical and ergonomical aspects (see Kübler et al., 2011). On the other side, "BCI control" may refer to the much more specific ability of an individual to control some aspects of his/her own brain activity (Hinterberger et al., 2003; Halder et al., 2011), which is clearly a neurocognitive topic that is central but not restricted to BCI/NF. Broadly speaking, not only BCI/NF but many other processes such as meditation techniques (Tang et al., 2014), emotion regulation (Thayer and Lane, 2000) and even psychotherapy (Beauregard, 2007) also induce some form of self-control of brain activity. Since the definition of "BCI control" from either a neuroengineering perspective or from a neurocognitive perspective fundamentally differs, it is necessary to disentangle both views. The topic of the present article is "BCI control" as self-regulation of neuronal activity and, for the sake of transparency, it will be called hereafter "self-control of brain activity".

With the aim of better understanding BCI/NF learning, the first step to characterize "self-control of brain activity" is to specify the cognitive mechanisms responsible for learning control. The more popular models of BCI/NF discuss "operant conditioning" and a "motor skill learning" as these mechanisms (Hammer et al., 2012). However, many studies indicate that other cognitive mechanisms such as locus of control towards technology (Burde and Blankertz, 2006; Ninaus et al., 2013; Witte et al., 2013), aptitude towards BCI (Hammer et al., 2012; Halder et al., 2013), motivation (Kleih et al., 2010) and spontaneous strategies (Kober et al., 2013) also influence BCI or NF learning. As a consequence, these predictors may either constitute a secondary correlate of self-control of brain activity or may represent key cognitive processes in addition to conditioning and skill learning. Given the high variety of cognitive and emotional processes apparently associated with self-control of brain activity and BCI learning, it is particularly useful to define a simple but comprehensible framework to evaluate the common and unique contributions of each one of these processes.

A dual-processes theory has been related to BCI/NF learning (Lacroix, 1986; Hammer et al., 2012). In the following, we shortly point out how this theory can be employed to better understand how the processes mentioned above might determine self-control of brain activity.

TWO TYPES OF MENTAL ACTIVITY

The dual-processes theory categorizes the whole mental activity into two main types of processing: more automatic and capacity-free processes (i.e., type I processes) vs. more controlled and capacity-limited processes (i.e., type II processes). Type I processes reflect the automatic, capacity-free, effortless and context-specific information processing such as for instance trying to open the office door with the home key because one has been thinking about dinner. Moreover, type I processes are usually unconscious and difficult to control by self-instruction. Type II processes reflect the activity of a supervisory attention system, specialized in monitoring and regulating the activity in other cognitive systems (Shallice and Cooper, 2011). Type II processes are usually in the center of our focus of attention (but see Horga and Maia, 2012 for an exception), are regulated mainly by self-instruction and are fundamental for executive functions and metacognitive abilities (Bewick et al., 1995). Accordingly, control beliefs are much more related to the function of the type II processes while the heuristics regulating most of our cognitive activity and behavior are type I processes.

A central aspect of the dual-processes theory is that both automatic and controlled processes have control of behavior as well as of different aspects of cognition (Alos Ferrer, 2013) but both learn from and react to different aspects of the task at hand. Automatic systems learn only through cumulative reward while controlled systems are more flexible, context-oriented and learn fast from instructions. It is beyond the scope of this perspective article to review every single manifestation of automatic vs. controlled processing to each one of the predictors of self-control of brain activity. Instead, we present one example regarding motivation, which may suffice to make our point: motivation consists of a more controlled component called intrinsic motivation, which is highly sensitive to self-instruction and self-efficacy beliefs, and a more automatic component called extrinsic motivation, which is more sensitive to the current amount of reward received (Ryan and Deci, 2000). Accordingly, as long as some reward can be obtained during BCI/NF learning, automatic processing will predominate. Controlled processing will be engaged when negative feedback predominates over longer periods of time and will have a larger impact, if the participant shows high levels of intrinsic motivation. In summary, dual-process models such as Lacroix (1986) make clear that self-regulation is not a unitary process but rather the result of the conjoint action of type I and type II processes.

A FRAMEWORK OF SELF-CONTROL OF BRAIN ACTIVITY

Automatic and controlled processes determine self-control of brain activity in very different ways. Even more, not every cognitive process is necessary and sufficient to perform a specific BCI/NF task, but instead a small subset may play a key role. The remaining mental activity -that is neither necessary nor sufficient for a specific BCI/NF task -will act on BCI/NF learning in one of two ways: firstly, this activity can interfere with the learning process, if it hampers self-control of the specific aspect of brain activity being targeted in a specific BCI/NF task. Secondly, activations can promote the learning process indirectly, if they do not interfere with the activity in that small subset of both automatic and controlled processes necessary and sufficient to perform the BCI/NF task at hand. Although in some BCI classes such as those employing electrocorticogram or other kinds of stable and specific brain signals such as SSVEP the influence of unspecific processes signal is barely important, cognitive BCIs (Astrand et al., 2014) or BCI classes based on cognitive tasks such as mental calculation and motor imagery (Halder et al., 2011; Hammer et al., 2012) should be more subjected to the effects of different forms of self-control over brain activity. Based on the differentiation between automatic vs. controlled processing as well as necessary vs. unnecessary processes, we define a framework of self-control of brain activity.

We start with the automatic and controlled processes both necessary and sufficient to perform BCI/NF tasks: both are subsumed under *local control network*. The more the feedback provided by BCI/NF reflects the activity in these networks, the more efficient is the learning process. The role of automatic and controlled processes in the *local control network* is complementary: automatic processes are driven directly by the amount and quality of feedback obtained whereas controlled processes are driven by the verbalizations and self-instruction (Lacroix, 1986), that are largely under conscious control of the individual and subjected to beliefs and expectations. While automatic learning is very insensitive to verbal instructions and only takes place when some pattern of reaction is systematically rewarded, controlled processes are mainly driven by direct verbal instructions. Efficient BCI/NF learning reflects the timely combination of both processes depending on the present learning rates: when a steep learning curve is forming, automatic processes take the lead, when the learning curve temporarily flattens, controlled processes correct the course by means of self-instruction (Lacroix, 1986). The optimal level of self-control of brain activity in the *local control network* is achieved under two main conditions: (i) avoidance of irrelevant associations between internal states and external reward; and (ii) staying engaged and focused on the task at hand without distractions. As we will discuss below, condition (i) can be achieved when activity in the *organismic control network* is reduced to a minimum and condition (ii), when the *central control network* frees the most of its limited resources for the *local control network*.

We define a framework of three concentric circles (**Figure 1**) representing three sources of self-control. First, the outmost and thus most unspecific level of response to feedback reflects basically automatic processes. Second, the middle circle depicts central control networks performing controlled processing. Finally, in the innermost level, we describe networks responding specifically to the BCI/NF learning protocol. This local control relies on both automatic and controlled processes.

We define those *automatic* processes unnecessary to perform a given BCI/NF task as the *organismic control network*. We call them organismic control because it reflects the activity of the

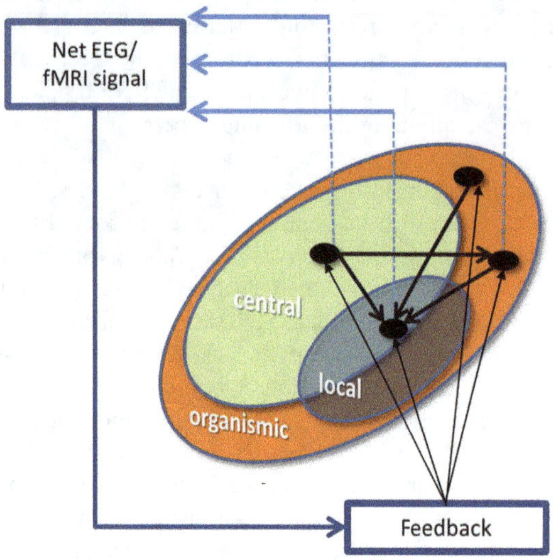

FIGURE 1 | A schema of different types of self-control of the brain activity. Specific cognitive processes such as for instance motivation, mood, attention and executive functions are represented by black dots. Black arrows connecting the dots represent the interactions between the different cognitive functions. Two dots are depicted over the domain of organismic control network to illustrate that these processes are largely independent from one another. The contribution of the three types of self-control to physiological signals is represented by the dashed lines linking the specific cognitive processes to the physiological signals being recorded for BCI/NF learning.

thousands of automatic and unconscious mental processes regulating the largest part of cognitive activity (Dijksterhuis and Nordgren, 2006). The interference of these processes is high when unnecessary automatic reactions to feedback are triggered, which compete with the learning process taking place in the *local control network*. Rumination, for instance, describes the intrusion of negative feelings about past experiences in the stream of thoughts and emerges primarily during relaxation (Nolen-Hoeksema et al., 2008). The intrusion of ruminative thoughts is an example of the negative impact of the *organismic control network* on self-control of brain activity during BCI/NF learning. Cognitive processes subsumed under *organismic control network* are not easily influenced by direct instructions and mostly not even conscious to the participant. Therefore, it may be very important to monitor any signs of negative influences originating in organismic control networks. This unwanted activity should be fed back in a timely manner during training. As a consequence, processes like increased anxiety or intrusive thoughts are accessible to BCI/NF users and can trigger appropriate learning mechanisms capable to control or suppress these processes.

Finally, we define the *central control network* as those *controlled* processes not strictly necessary to perform a given BCI/NF task. Controlled processes have limited capacity, so that every bit of irrelevant information being employed in the *central control network* will be missed by the *local control network*. The negative impact of *central control network* is high when improper strategies, self-instruction, over-instruction or excessive attention to the self (Leary et al., 2006) withdraw resources from the *local control network* and hamper the regulation of the learning process in a similar way as a dual-task (Logan and Gordon, 2001) drains resources. In contrast to the *organismic control network*, controlled processing is largely under conscious control and can be modulated directly by instructions (Dijksterhuis and Nordgren, 2006).

In summary, the aim of any BCI/NF learning is to magnify the signal produced by *local control networks* and suppress as much as possible the activity elsewhere. To do that, it is in our view necessary to take into consideration the specificities of two types of cognitive activity subsumed under *organismic control networks* and *central control networks*, since they imply very different learning mechanisms sensitive to different types of cues and reward. On the one side, participants should learn to decouple irrelevant from those relevant automatic processes. One way to achieve this is to monitor the automatic processes regulating for instance negative emotional reactions and anxiety as well as with a more selective schedule of reward and punishment. On the other side, participants should learn to use the *central control networks* to suppress irrelevant cognitive activity operating under conscious control such as excessive attention to the self (Leary et al., 2006). This can be achieved by direct instruction or self-instruction. Once this balance is achieved, the outcome of BCI/NF learning should be improved. Among many other possibilities, one simple experiment to investigate how the suppression of irrelevant cognitive activity could improve BCI/NF learning would involve the monitoring of inner speech (Perrone-Bertolotti et al., 2014). Extra feedback requiring focus on the concrete task is presented when an increase in the levels of inner speech is detected in combination with a local flattening of the learning curve. As suggested by Leary et al. (2006), this extra feedback should help to reduce excessive attention to the self and improve learning.

FINAL REMARKS

We propose that self-regulation of brain activity should be distinguished from the more general process of "BCI learning", since the latter one is more of a neuroengineering problem whereas the former is mainly a neurocognitive problem. To better understand how self-regulation of brain activity works, we propose to look at the cognitive predictors of BCI/NF performance from the point of view of a framework which organizes them according to the main type of cognitive processing required: more automatic or more controlled processing. Further on, we distinguish between cognitive resources necessary and sufficient for BCI/NF learning and other cognitive processes, which should be suppressed or down-regulated to improve learning. Finally, we argue that our framework can be very useful to optimize BCI learning, since it predicts the most suitable tools to modulate the activation generated by automatic and controlled cognitive processes.

ACKNOWLEDGMENTS

This work is supported by the European STREP Program—Collaborative Project no. FP7-287320—CONTRAST. Possible inaccuracies of information are under the responsibility of the project team. The text reflects solely the views of its authors. The European Commission is not liable for any use that may be made of the information contained therein.

REFERENCES

Alos Ferrer, C. (2013). "Think, but not too much: a dual-process model of willpower and self-control," in *Annual Conference 2013 (Duesseldorf): Competition Policy and Regulation in a Global Economic Order 80019* (Verein für Socialpolitik/German Economic Association).

Astrand, E., Wardak, C., and Ben Hamed, S. (2014). Selective visual attention to drive cognitive brain-machine interfaces: from concepts to neurofeedback and rehabilitation applications. *Front. Syst. Neurosci.* 8:144. doi: 10.3389/fnsys.2014.00144

Beauregard, M. (2007). Mind does really matter: evidence from neuroimaging studies of emotional self-regulation, psychotherapy and placebo effect. *Prog. Neurobiol.* 81, 218–236. doi: 10.1016/j.pneurobio.2007.01.005

Bewick, K. C., Raymond, M. J., Malia, K. B., and Bennett, T. L. (1995). Metacognition as the ultimate executive: techniques and tasks to facilitate executive functions. *NeuroRehabilitation* 5, 367–375. doi: 10.3233/NRE-1995-5411

Burde, W., and Blankertz, B. (2006). "Is the locus of control of reinforcement a predictor of brain-computer interface performance?," in *Proceedings of the 3rd International Brain-Computer Interface Workshop and Training Course* (Graz, Austria), 76–77.

Dijksterhuis, A., and Nordgren, L. F. (2006). A theory of unconscious thought. *Perspect. Psychol. Sci.* 1, 95–109. doi: 10.1111/j.1745-6916.2006.00007.x

Donoghue, J. P. (2008). Bridging the brain to the world: a perspective on neural interface systems. *Neuron* 60, 511–521. doi: 10.1016/j.neuron.2008.10.037

Halder, S., Agorastos, D., Veit, R., Hammer, E. M., Lee, S., Varkuti, B., et al. (2011). Neural mechanisms of brain-computer interface control. *Neuroimage* 55, 1779–1790. doi: 10.1016/j.neuroimage.2011.01.021

Halder, S., Hammer, E. M., Kleih, S. C., Bogdan, M., Rosenstiel, W., Birbaumer, N., et al. (2013). Prediction of auditory and visual p300 brain-computer interface aptitude. *PLoS One* 8:e53513. doi: 10.1371/journal.pone.0053513

Hammer, E. M., Halder, S., Blankertz, B., Sannelli, C., Dickhaus, T., Kleih, S., et al. (2012). Psychological predictors of SMR-BCI performance. *Biol. Psychol.* 89, 80–86. doi: 10.1016/j.biopsycho.2011.09.006

Hinterberger, T., Veit, R., Strehl, U., Trevorrow, T., Erb, M., Kotchoubey, B., et al. (2003). Brain areas activated in fMRI during self-regulation of slow cortical potentials (SCPs). *Exp. Brain Res.* 152, 113–122. doi: 10.1007/s00221-003-1515-4

Horga, G., and Maia, T. V. (2012). Conscious and unconscious processes in cognitive control: a theoretical perspective and a novel empirical approach. *Front. Hum. Neurosci.* 6:199. doi: 10.3389/fnhum.2012.00199

Kleih, S. C., Nijboer, F., Halder, S., and Kübler, A. (2010). Motivation modulates the P300 amplitude during brain-computer interface use. *Clin. Neurophysiol.* 121, 1023–1031. doi: 10.1016/j.clinph.2010.01.034

Kober, S. E., Witte, M., Ninaus, M., Neuper, C., and Wood, G. (2013). Learning to modulate one's own brain activity: the effect of spontaneous mental strategies. *Front. Hum. Neurosci.* 7:695. doi: 10.3389/fnhum.2013.00695

Kübler, A., Blankertz, B., Müller, K. R., and Neuper, C. (2011). "A model of BCI control," in *Proceedings of the 5th International Brain-Computer Interface Conference, September 22–24 2011*, eds G. R. Müller-Putz, R. Scherer, M. Billinger, A. Kreilinger, V. Kaiser and C. Neuper (Austria: Graz University of Technology), 100–103.

Lacroix, J. M. (1986). "Mechanisms of biofeedback control: on the importance of verbal (conscious) processing," in *Consciousness and Self-Regulation: Vol. 4, Chapter Mechanisms of Biofeedback Control*, eds R. J. Davidson, G. E. Schwartz and D. Shapiro (New York: Plenum), 137–162.

Leary, M. R., Adams, C. E., and Tate, E. B. (2006). Hypo-egoic self-regulation: exerting self-control by diminishing the influence of the self. *J. Pers.* 74, 1803–1832. doi: 10.1111/j.1467-6494.2006.00429.x

Logan, G. D., and Gordon, R. D. (2001). Executive control of visual attention in dual-task situations. *Psychol. Rev.* 108, 393–434. doi: 10.1037//0033-295x.108.2.393

Nicolelis, M. A., and Lebedev, M. A. (2009). Principles of neural ensemble physiology underlying the operation of brain-machine interfaces. *Nat. Rev. Neurosci.* 10, 530–540. doi: 10.1038/nrn2653

Ninaus, M., Kober, S. E., Witte, M., Koschutnig, K., Stangl, M., Neuper, C., et al. (2013). Neural substrates of cognitive control under the belief of getting neurofeedback training. *Front. Hum. Neurosci.* 7:914. doi: 10.3389/fnhum.2013.00914

Nolen-Hoeksema, S., Wisco, B. E., and Lyubomirsky, S. (2008). Rethinking rumination. *Perspect. Psychol. Sci.* 3, 400–424. doi: 10.1111/j.1745-6924.2008.00088.x

Perrone-Bertolotti, M., Rapin, L., Lachaux, J. P., Baciu, M., and Loevenbruck, H. (2014). What is that little voice inside my head? Inner speech phenomenology, its role in cognitive performance and its relation to self-monitoring. *Behav. Brain Res.* 261, 220–239. doi: 10.1016/j.bbr.2013.12.034

Phillippens, I. H. C. H. M., and Vanwersch, R. A. P. (2010). Neurofeedback training on sensorimotor rhythm in marmoset monkeys. *Neuroreport* 21, 328–332. doi: 10.1097/wnr.0b013e3283360ba8

Ryan, R., and Deci, E. L. (2000). Intrinsic and extrinsic motivations: classic definitions and new directions. *Contemp. Educ. Psychol.* 25, 54–67. doi: 10.1006/ceps.1999.1020

Shallice, T., and Cooper, R. (2011). *The Organisation of Mind.* Oxford: Oxford University Press.

Sterman, M. B. (1977). Sensorimotor EEG operant conditioning: experimental and clinical effects. *Pavlov. J. Biol. Sci.* 12, 63–92.

Tang, Y. Y., Posner, M. I., and Rothbart, M. K. (2014). Meditation improves self-regulation over the life span. *Ann. N Y Acad. Sci.* 1307, 104–111. doi: 10.1111/nyas.12227

Thayer, J. F., and Lane, R. D. (2000). A model of neurovisceral integration in emotion regulation and dysregulation. *J. Affect. Disord.* 61, 201–216. doi: 10.1016/s0165-0327(00)00338-4

Witte, M., Kober, S. E., Ninaus, M., Neuper, C., and Wood, G. (2013). Control beliefs can predict the ability to up-regulate sensorimotor rhythm during neurofeedback training. *Front. Hum. Neurosci.* 7:478. doi: 10.3389/fnhum.2013.00478

12

The vestibular implant: frequency-dependency of the electrically evoked vestibulo-ocular reflex in humans

Raymond van de Berg[1,2]*, Nils Guinand[3], T. A. Khoa Nguyen[4], Maurizio Ranieri[3], Samuel Cavuscens[3], Jean-Philippe Guyot[3], Robert Stokroos[1], Herman Kingma[1,2] and Angelica Perez-Fornos[3]

[1] *Division of Balance Disorders, Department of Otorhinolaryngology and Head and Neck Surgery, Faculty of Health Medicine and Life Sciences, School for Mental Health and Neuroscience, Maastricht University Medical Center, Maastricht, Netherlands*
[2] *Faculty of Physics, Tomsk State University, Tomsk, Russia*
[3] *Service of Otorhinolaryngology and Head and Neck Surgery, Department of Clinical Neurosciences, Geneva University Hospitals, Geneva, Switzerland*
[4] *Translational Neural Engineering Lab, Center for Neuroprosthetics, Interfaculty Institute of Bioengineering, École Polytechnique Fédérale de Lausanne, Lausanne, Switzerland*

Edited by:
Mikhail Lebedev, Duke University, USA

Reviewed by:
Bernard Cohen, Mount Sinai School of Medicine, USA
Hans VanDerSteen, Erasmus Medical Center, Netherlands
Stefano Ramat, Università degli Studi di Pavia, Italy
Maria Cervera De La Rosa, Universidad Carlos III de Madrid, Spain

****Correspondence:***
Raymond van de Berg, Department of Otorhinolaryngology and Head and Neck Surgery, Maastricht University Medical Center, Postbus 5800, 6202 AZ Maastricht, Netherlands
e-mail: raymond.vande.berg@mumc.nl

The vestibulo-ocular reflex (VOR) shows frequency-dependent behavior. This study investigated whether the characteristics of the electrically evoked VOR (eVOR) elicited by a vestibular implant, showed the same frequency-dependency. Twelve vestibular electrodes implanted in seven patients with bilateral vestibular hypofunction (BVH) were tested. Stimuli consisted of amplitude-modulated electrical stimulation with a sinusoidal profile at frequencies of 0.5, 1, and 2 Hz. The main characteristics of the eVOR were evaluated and compared to the "natural" VOR characteristics measured in a group of age-matched healthy volunteers who were subjected to horizontal whole body rotations with equivalent sinusoidal velocity profiles at the same frequencies. A strong and significant effect of frequency was observed in the total peak eye velocity of the eVOR. This effect was similar to that observed in the "natural" VOR. Other characteristics of the (e)VOR (angle, habituation-index, and asymmetry) showed no significant frequency-dependent effect. In conclusion, this study demonstrates that, at least at the specific (limited) frequency range tested, responses elicited by a vestibular implant closely mimic the frequency-dependency of the "normal" vestibular system.

Keywords: vestibular implant, vestibular prosthesis, neural prosthesis, bilateral vestibular areflexia, bilateral vestibulopathy, vestibulo-ocular reflex

INTRODUCTION

Bilateral vestibular hypofunction (BVH) is most often a chronic condition in which patients can suffer from blurred vision (oscillopsia), impaired spatial orientation and postural instability (Brandt et al., 2010; van de Berg et al., 2011; Hain et al., 2013). These and other symptoms lead to an important decrease in physical activity, social functioning and vitality that dramatically impact the patients' quality of life (Guinand et al., 2012; Ward et al., 2013). The prognosis of BVH is poor and more than 80% of the patients do not improve (Zingler et al., 2008; McCall and Yates, 2011). Until now, treatment options are limited and with low yield (Porciuncula et al., 2012).

A vestibular implant, in a concept analogous to that of the cochlear implant, has been postulated as a possible therapeutic alternative. This idea is currently investigated by research groups in Europe and the United States. Research both from animal and human studies have demonstrated that electrical stimulation is an effective means to activate the vestibular system (Fridman et al., 2010; Guyot et al., 2011; Lewis et al., 2013; Golub et al., 2014). Considerable research efforts have been devoted to the investigation of the electrically evoked vestibulo-ocular reflex (eVOR). Promisingly, results showed that it is possible to elicit a VOR which corresponds to the plane of the canal which is innervated by the electrically stimulated nerve branch (Gong and Merfeld, 2002; Della Santina et al., 2007; Merfeld et al., 2007; Wall et al., 2007; Fridman et al., 2010; van de Berg et al., 2011; Perez Fornos et al., 2014). Current efforts focus on optimizing stimulation paradigms (Davidovics et al., 2011, 2012), on improving the alignment of the eVOR (Migliaccio et al., 2011; Dai et al., 2013; Davidovics et al., 2013), and on investigating the adaptive properties of the eVOR (Merfeld et al., 2006, 2007; Lewis et al., 2010; Guyot et al., 2011; Dai et al., 2013). Important efforts are also undertaken to improve surgical techniques (Feigl et al., 2009; Dai et al., 2011a; Bierer et al., 2012; Rubinstein et al., 2012; van de Berg et al., 2012) and to solve biomechanical issues (Wall et al., 2003; Hayden et al., 2011; van de Berg et al., 2011; Fridman and Della Santina, 2013).

The Geneva-Maastricht group has recently demonstrated that it is possible to restore the VOR in patients with BVH, using a chronically implanted vestibular implant prototype (Perez Fornos et al., 2014). During these experiments, some frequency dependent effects were observed. Frequency-dependency is a well-known feature of the vestibular system. Gain of the semicircular canals (peak eye velocity/peak head velocity) is high for middle frequencies, but decreases with lower and higher frequencies, consistent with the mechanical properties of the semicircular canals

(Barnes, 1993). Interestingly, these middle frequency movements are often encountered by individuals in daily life, for example during voluntary head movements and locomotor activities (Barnes, 1993; Crane and Demer, 1997). Therefore, it is important to further investigate the frequency dependent behavior of the eVOR and how it compares to the frequency dependent characteristics of the "natural" VOR in healthy subjects. This was the main objective of this study.

MATERIALS AND METHODS

IMPLANTED PATIENTS

Between 2007 and 2013, 11 volunteers with BVH received a vestibular implant prototype consisting of a modified cochlear implant (MED-EL, Innsbruck, Austria) with extra-cochlear branches for vestibular stimulation (Guinand et al., Submitted). The devices, inclusion criteria, and surgical techniques have been described in detail previously (Perez Fornos et al., 2014; Guinand et al., Submitted). Seven of them were available for this study (age 46–68 years; mean age 61.4 years; see **Table 1**). Twelve electrodes at different anatomical locations were tested: four electrodes implanted in the vicinity of the superior ampullary nerve (SAN), three electrodes implanted in the vicinity of the lateral ampullary nerve (LAN) and five electrodes implanted in the vicinity of the posterior ampullary nerve (PAN).

HEALTHY SUBJECTS

Seven age-matched healthy volunteers with a blank history for vestibular disorders were selected for the comparison experiments. These tests involved three men and four women (age 59–69 years; mean age 62.7 years).

ELECTRICAL STIMULATION

Electrical stimulation was delivered exclusively to one vestibular electrode at a time. The activation procedure has been previously described (Guyot et al., 2011; Perez Fornos et al., 2014). Briefly, the generation of bi-directional eye movements (e.g., both leftwards and rightwards for stimulation of the LAN) with unilateral electrical stimulation requires first that a "baseline stimulation" (i.e., constant amplitude) is delivered by the vestibular electrode. Then, up- and down-modulation of this "baseline stimulation" effectively results in the generation of smooth, bi-directional eye movements.

Stimulation consisted of amplitude modulated, charge-balanced, cathodic-first, biphasic pulses (200 µs/phase) presented at a pulse rate of 400 pulses/sec. "Baseline stimulation" amplitudes corresponded to the middle of each patient's dynamic range (see Perez Fornos et al., 2014; Guinand et al., Submitted; for details on the determination of thresholds, upper comfortable level and resulting dynamic range). Modulation strengths for each patient/electrode were selected to correspond to 50–75% of the corresponding dynamic range and were kept constant throughout the experiments. **Figure 1** illustrates this electrical stimulation procedure.

STUDY DESIGN

All tests were conducted in a controlled laboratory setting and performed in complete darkness. All participants (from both groups) were instructed to sit still, look in front of them and keep their eyes open during the trials. If necessary, alerting tasks were given to improve concentration and general level of arousal, in order to obtain as reproducible results as possible.

In order to test the eVOR as specifically as possible without any influences of other inputs like residual vestibular function, the eVOR-experiments were conducted in stationary conditions (e.g., without any head or body movement). Patients sat comfortably in a stationary chair while the implant was activated. Each electrode was separately tested with a fixed sequence of approximately 60 sinusoidal cycles of amplitude modulated electrical stimulation (see details in Section Electrical Stimulation). The strength (i.e., intensity) of modulation was kept constant throughout experimental trials and 3 modulation frequencies (0.5, 1, and 2 Hz) were tested. Lower modulation frequencies were intentionally excluded, since previous investigations (in exactly the same conditions) showed only very small eVOR responses at these frequencies (Perez Fornos et al., 2014). Furthermore, 60-cycle trials at low modulation frequencies below 0.5 Hz resulted in very long sessions, which severely compromised the attention of the patients for the rest of the testing session (Perez Fornos et al., 2014). All tests for a given electrode were performed on the same day.

Modulation of the frequency of the electrical stimulus would correspond in real life to modulation of the frequency of the head velocity stimulus in dynamic situations. Therefore, the eVOR obtained by electrical stimulation in patients with BVH was compared to the "natural" VOR obtained in healthy volunteers during velocity controlled whole body rotations. Healthy volunteers were subjected to 60-cycle trials of horizontal whole body rotations in a custom-made, velocity-controlled rotatory chair (Nystagliner Pro; Erich Jaeger Gmbh). Rotations followed the same sinusoidal

Table 1 | Main characteristics of the tested patients with bilateral vestibular hypofunction.

Subject	Sex	Tested electrode(s)	Age at implantation	Etiology	Year of implantation	Surgical approach
BVH1	M	SAN; LAN	67	DFNA-9	2012	Intra-labyrinthine
BVH2	F	PAN	48	Meningitis	2012	Intra-labyrinthine
BVH3	M	SAN; LAN; PAN	66	DFNA-9	2013	Intra-labyrinthine
BVH4	F	SAN; PAN	68	DFNA-9	2013	Intra-labyrinthine
BVH5	F	SAN; LAN	67	Traumatic	2013	Intra-labyrinthine
BVH6	M	PAN	46	Idiopathic	2008	Extra-labyrinthine
BVH7	M	PAN	68	Idiopathic	2007	Extra-labyrinthine

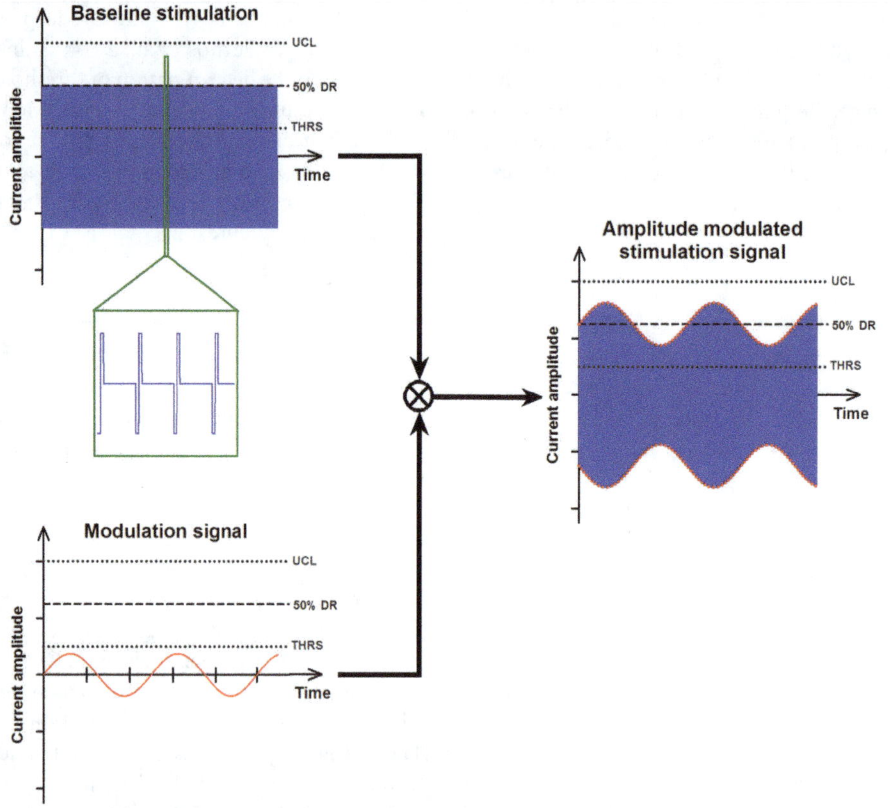

FIGURE 1 | Illustration of the electrical stimulation paradigm. Stimulation was delivered to one vestibular electrode at a time. Patients first received baseline electrical stimulation that consisted of constant amplitude trains of biphasic, cathodic-first pulses (upper-left panel). Baseline stimulation was presented at a fixed pulse rate of 400 pulses per second. Its intensity corresponded to 50% of each electrode's previously measured dynamic range (DR; current range between the vestibular threshold -THRS- and the upper comfortable level -UCL-). Once patients were in "adapted" state, the baseline stimulation could be modulated in amplitude using a signal with a sinusoidal profile (see lower-left panel). The strength (i.e., intensity) of the modulation was kept constant and its frequency was varied between 0.5 and 2 Hz. The right panel shows an example of such an amplitude modulated stimulation signal (blue trace). The envelope of the modulation signal (red dotted lines) has been highlighted for clarity.

profile as electrical stimuli (same frequency range of 0.5, 1, and 2 Hz) and had a peak velocity of 30°/s.

EYE MOVEMENT RECORDING AND ANALYSIS

Bidimensional eye movements (i.e., horizontal and vertical eye position, no torsion) were recorded with the EyeSeeCam system (EyeSeeCam VOG; Munich, Germany) (Bartl et al., 2009; Perez Fornos et al., 2014). Motivation for this choice, as well as the data-processing using cycle-by-cycle analysis and calculation of gain were described previously (Perez Fornos et al., 2014; Guinand et al., Submitted). An example of eye movement data processing is presented in **Figure 2**. Analysis was performed on as many valid cycles (free of saccades and blinks) as possible (minimum 43, maximum 60).

Total peak eye velocity was calculated as the square root of the sums of the squares of horizontal and vertical peak eye velocity. To facilitate the analysis of the frequency-dependent behavior of peak eye velocities of different magnitudes, peak eye velocities per modulation frequency were normalized to the highest measured peak eye velocity per electrode. Angle of the (e)VOR (with respect to the horizontal axis) was defined as the angle between the horizontal and vertical peak eye velocity (Guinand et al., Submitted). The habituation-index was determined by the mean peak eye velocities of the last 10 cycles, divided by the mean peak eye velocities of the first 10 cycles. The asymmetry-index (ratio of excitatory/inhibitory half cycle gain) of the most prominent component (horizontal or vertical) was calculated as (excitatory half cycle gain—inhibitory half cycle gain)/(excitatory half cycle gain + inhibitory half cycle gain) (Dai et al., 2011b) and converted into an absolute value.

STATISTICS

Since normality tests conducted on individual results often failed the normality assumption, individual results (per subject/electrode) are presented as median values, as well as the 25th–75th percentiles. Group results conformed to normal distributions and are therefore presented as mean values ± standard error of the mean (SEM).

Statistics were performed using analysis of variance (ANOVA) modules from IBM SPSS Statistics v22 (IBM Corporation, New York, United States of America). Raw scores were used as input for comparative tests regarding angle, habituation-index and

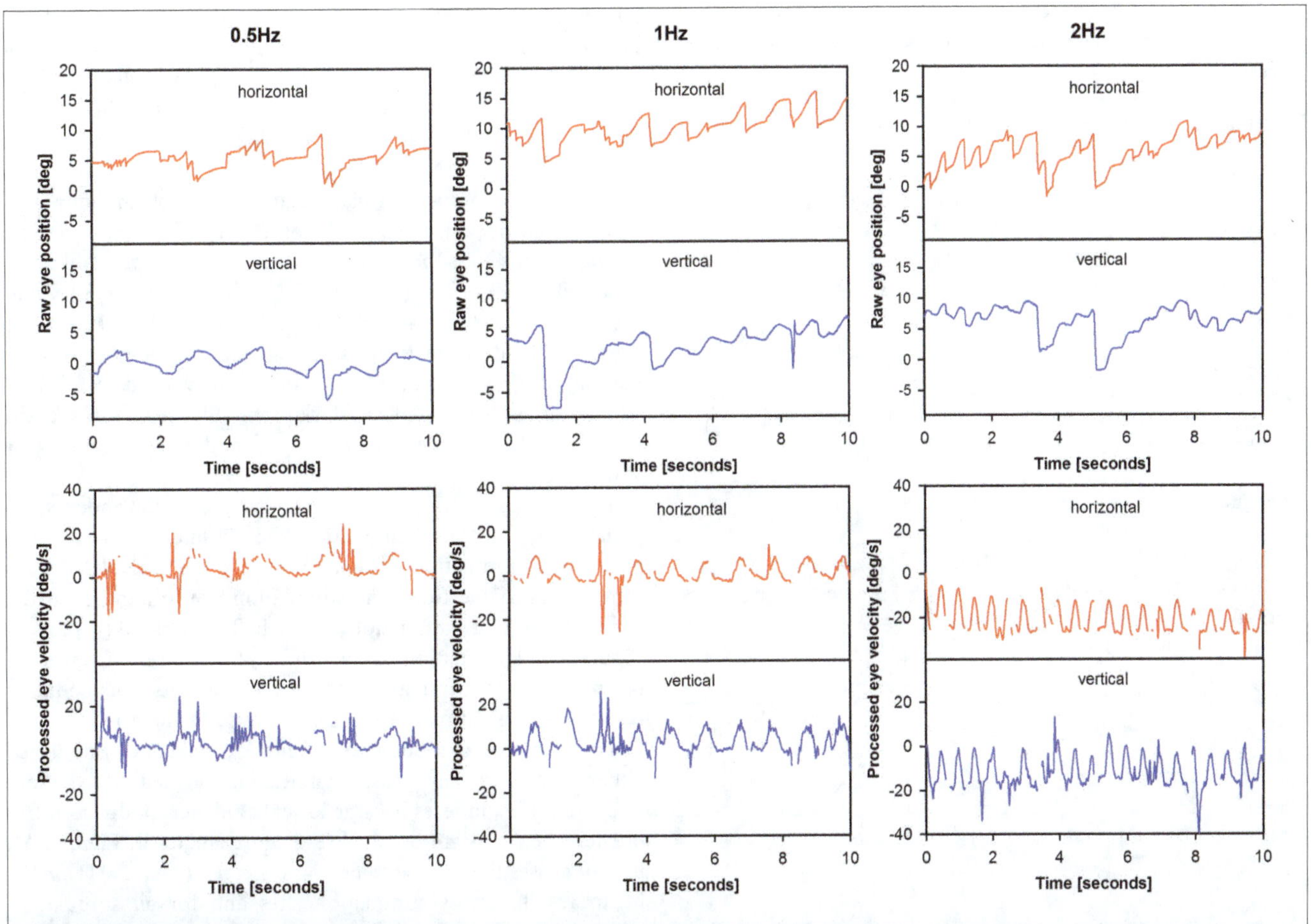

FIGURE 2 | Illustration of eye movement data processing. The figure presents eye movement data tracings for patient BVH1-LAN. Two steps are illustrated for each modulation frequency: raw eye position (e.g., before any processing was performed) and processed eye velocity data.

asymmetry-index. For total peak eye velocity, variance differed between the groups. Therefore, data were first normalized before proceeding to statistical analysis. A significance level of 0.05 was chosen to detect significant differences within and across groups.

ETHICAL CONSIDERATIONS

This study was in accordance with the Declaration of Helsinki (amended version 2013). The testing protocol was approved by the ethical committees of the Maastricht University Medical Center (NL36777.068.11/METC 11-2-031) and the Geneva University Hospital (NAC 11-080).

RESULTS

CHARACTERISTICS OF THE eVOR

The first objective of this paper was to describe the main characteristics of eVOR-responses. Four main characteristics were studied: total peak eye velocity, angle of the eVOR (with respect to the horizontal axis), the habituation-index over 60 cycles, and the asymmetry (ratio of excitatory/inhibitory half cycle gain) of the response.

Total peak eye velocity results obtained per electrode are presented in **Table 2**. Consistent with previous observations (Guinand et al., Submitted), inter-subject variability was high. The medians of the total peak eye velocity for the electrodes ranged from 0.6°/s (BVH4-PAN, 0.5 Hz) up to 21.5°/s (BVH5-SAN, 2 Hz).

To facilitate comparison of the results across patients and across frequencies, total peak eye velocity results were normalized to the highest values per electrode. Individual and pooled results revealed a clear frequency-dependent behavior for the three stimulation sites (**Figure 3**). In general, the lowest peak eye velocities were obtained with a modulation frequency of 0.5 Hz. Peak eye velocities progressively increased with increasing modulation frequency, reaching a maximum at 2 Hz. Note however that interestingly, patient BVH2 showed an opposite behavior (stimulation of the PAN). There was a statistically significant effect of modulation frequency [$F_{(2, 27)} = 16.25$, $p < 0.001$] but not for stimulation site. *Post-hoc* pairwise comparisons (Tukey) indicated that the difference in mean normalized peak eye velocities was statistically significant ($p < 0.05$; 0.5 Hz: 0.53 ± 0.08; 1 Hz: 0.72 ± 0.05; 2 Hz: 0.98 ± 0.02).

Figure 4A shows individual angle results (with respect to the horizontal axis) for each stimulation site. Results for each stimulation site were very variable across subjects. No clear effect of modulation frequency could be distinguished either. For example, stimulation of the SAN in BVH3 (dark green triangles in

Table 2 | Medians, 25th percentiles, and 75th percentiles of total peak eye velocity (°/s) for all electrodes, per modulation frequency (perc. = percentile).

Electrode	Frequency (Hz)	Median	25th perc.	75th perc.
BVH1-SAN	0.5	4.2	2.4	5.3
	1	5.4	3.3	7.6
	2	6.9	5.2	9.1
BVH1-LAN	0.5	6.9	5.3	8.6
	1	9.1	7.1	10.4
	2	9.3	7.3	11.4
BVH2-PAN	0.5	8.5	6.4	9.8
	1	8.3	7.8	9.0
	2	6.9	6.2	7.7
BVH3-SAN	0.5	1.1	0.9	1.5
	1	3.9	3.1	5.0
	2	5.6	4.6	7.2
BVH3-LAN	0.5	0.9	0.6	1.2
	1	1.8	1.4	2.5
	2	3.6	2.2	4.8
BVH3-PAN	0.5	2.0	1.5	2.5
	1	5.7	5.2	6.4
	2	8.6	8.0	9.7
BVH4-SAN	0.5	0.8	0.5	1.1
	1	1.4	1.0	1.7
	2	3.6	2.4	4.4
BVH4-PAN	0.5	0.6	0.5	0.8
	1	1.0	0.6	1.3
	2	1.5	1.0	2.3
BVH5-SAN	0.5	12.4	10.8	14.1
	1	13.5	10.8	17.4
	2	21.5	16.6	24.9
BVH5-LAN	0.5	6.8	6.0	8.1
	1	8.0	6.8	9.5
	2	11.1	9.0	12.9
BVH6-PAN	0.5	10.2	8.1	13.5
	1	12.5	10.6	14.7
	2	12.0	9.8	14.6
BVH7-PAN	0.5	4.0	3.5	4.4
	1	4.0	2.8	5.0
	2	5.7	4.6	7.5

Figure 4A) showed, as expected, angles with a predominantly vertical component ranging from 59 to 83°. The eye movement response progressively shifted toward the vertical axis (the angle increased) as modulation frequency increased. However, results for the same stimulation site were completely different in the case of patient BVH5 (purple triangles in **Figure 4A**). Surprisingly, this patient showed median angles with a predominantly horizontal component, ranging from 12 to 14° during stimulation of the SAN. Furthermore, median angles remained relatively stable across modulation frequencies for this patient. Similar inter-subject variability was observed for stimulation of the LAN and the PAN.

Mean results across stimulation sites (gray plots in **Figure 4B**) showed that overall, the stimulation site with the most vertical eVOR response was the PAN (58.6 ± 5.5°). There were only very small differences in angles between stimulation of the SAN and the LAN (respectively 46.8 ± 6.1° and 40.4 ± 7.1°). Differences across modulation frequencies were small, both when each stimulation site was considered separately and when data from all stimulation sites was pooled (black plot in **Figure 4B**). There was no statistically significant main effect of modulation frequency or stimulation site.

Figure 5A shows individual median habituation-indexes per patient and for each stimulation site. Results across subjects and across stimulation sites were again quite variable. Results were very variable from one stimulation site to another in the same patient (e.g., results for patient BVH3, dark green plots in **Figure 5A**). Habituation could also be very different when comparing the same stimulation site between patients (e.g., compare results for stimulation of the PAN, squares in **Figure 5A**).

No clear effect of modulation frequency could be distinguished either. While in some cases habituation seemed to be more important (i.e., indexes became lower) at higher modulation frequencies (e.g., BVH4-SAN, olive green triangles in **Figure 5A**), in other cases the inverse trend was observed (e.g., BVH1-SAN). Mean results across stimulation sites and for all stimulation sites together showed a clearer picture (**Figure 5B**). Habituation-indexes for stimulation of the PAN were in general higher (1.08 ± 0.09), reflecting less adaptation than stimulation of the SAN and the LAN (respectively 0.72 ± 0.11 and 0.78 ± 0.12). This difference was only statistically significant between stimulation of the SAN and the PAN ($p < 0.05$). Another interesting observation from pooled results was that in general, habituation was more important for the 2 Hz modulation frequency than for 0.5 and 1 Hz. However, the effect of modulation frequency, as well as the interaction effect between modulation frequency and stimulation site, were not statistically significant.

Figure 6 displays asymmetry-indexes for each patient and each stimulation site. Values were <0.3 in all cases. The patient showing the most asymmetrical responses was BVH5 (purple plots in **Figure 6A**) and the one with the most symmetrical responses was BVH4 (olive green plots in **Figure 6A**), particularly for stimulation of the SAN. No systematic frequency-dependent behavior was observed in individual results. Group results (**Figure 6B**) confirmed that asymmetry was in general low, and some variability between stimulation sites was also observed. There were no significant effects of modulation frequency or stimulation site. The interaction effect between modulation frequency and stimulation site was not statistically significant either.

THE eVOR vs. THE "NATURAL" VOR

The second goal of this study was to compare the previously described eVOR-characteristics with those of the "natural" VOR

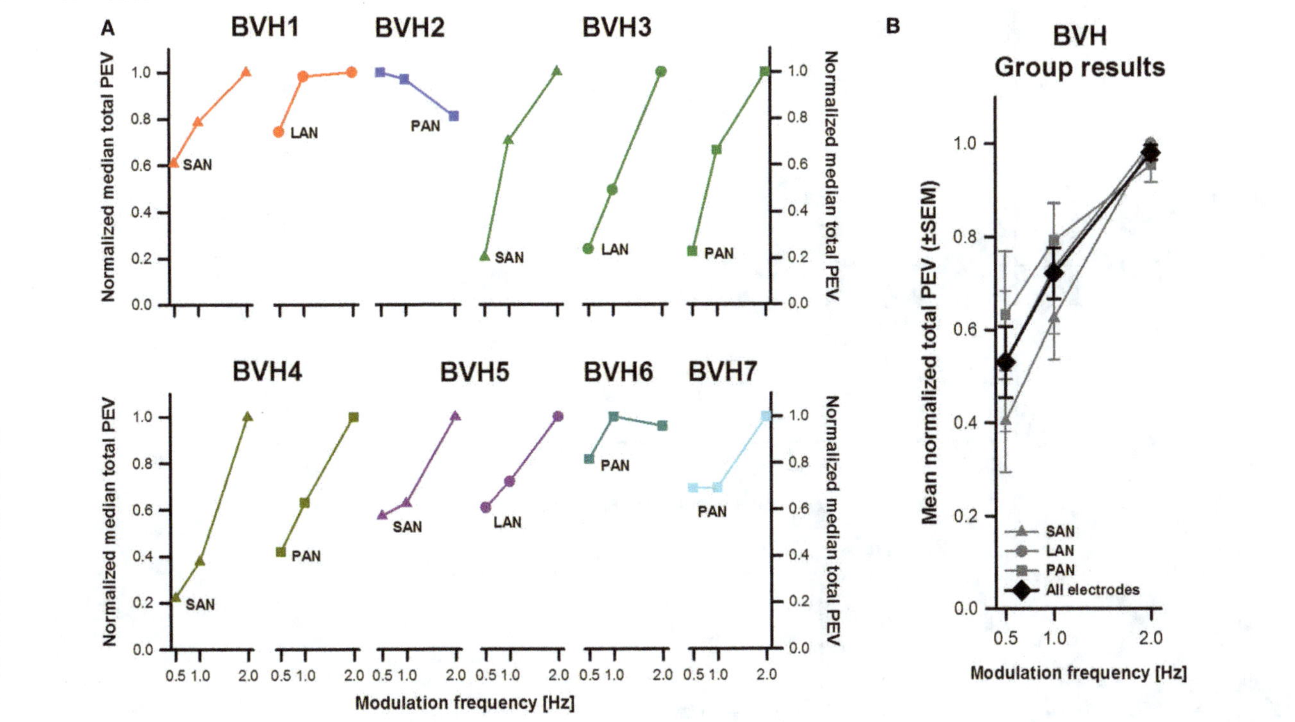

FIGURE 3 | Normalized total peak eye velocity (PEV) vs. modulation frequency. (A) Each panel represents individual results obtained during stimulation for each stimulation site (SAN, LAN, PAN). **(B)** Mean results (±SEM) calculated across patients for each stimulation site (gray plots) and for all electrodes together (black plot).

observed in the group of healthy volunteers. The results of this comparison are summarized in **Figure 7**.

Figure 7A compares the frequency-dependent behavior of the normalized total peak eye velocity of the eVOR to that of the "natural" VOR. From this figure it is clear that both show a strikingly similar frequency-dependent behavior, with the lower peak eye velocities measured at 0.5 Hz (0.53 ± 0.08 for the BVH-group and 0.54 ± 0.05 for the group of healthy volunteers). Peak eye velocities increase progressively with increasing frequency reaching a maximum at 2 Hz (BVH-group: 0.72 ± 0.06 at 1 Hz and 0.98 ± 0.01 at 2 Hz; Group of healthy volunteers: 0.73 ± 0.08 at 1 Hz and 0.99 ± 0.003 at 2 Hz). A Two-Way between-groups ANOVA confirmed a significant effect of frequency [$F_{(2,\ 51)} = 29.39$, $p < 0.001$], but no significant difference between both groups. The interaction between both variables was not significant either.

Figure 7B compares eVOR angles to those of the "natural" VOR. The angles of the "natural" VOR are close to zero (i.e., practically horizontal) and remained relatively stable across modulation frequencies, consistent with the direction of applied whole body rotations. As described previously, mean eVOR angles were much higher, with a predominantly vertical component and also remained relatively stable across modulation frequencies. A Two-Way between-groups ANOVA confirmed a significant difference between both groups [$F_{(1,\ 51)} = 84.91$, $p < 0.001$], but no significant effect of frequency. The interaction effect was not significant either.

Figure 7C compares the habituation-index of the eVOR to that of the "natural" VOR. Habituation-indexes were close to one (i.e., meaning very little adaptation) for both groups at 0.5 and 1 Hz and only slightly decreased at 2 Hz. There was no significant difference between groups or across modulation frequencies. The interaction effect was not significant either.

Finally, **Figure 7D** compares the asymmetry-indexes of the eVOR to those of the "natural" VOR. Mean asymmetry for the eVOR ranged between 0.10 (0.5 Hz) and 0.13 (2 Hz). Mean asymmetry for the "natural" VOR was much lower and close to 0, although values slightly increased at 2 Hz. A Two-Way between-groups ANOVA confirmed a significant difference between both groups [$F_{(1,\ 51)} = 37.64$, $p < 0.001$], but no significant effect of modulation frequency. The interaction effect was not significant either.

DISCUSSION

The goal of this study was to investigate how the characteristics of the eVOR change as a function of modulation frequency in the first group of patients implanted with a vestibular implant prototype, and to compare these results to the "natural" VOR responses obtained in healthy age-matched volunteers.

These results demonstrate that at least in this specific (limited) frequency range, the vestibular implant closely mimics the natural frequency-dependency of the vestibular system. Frequency showed a significant effect on the total peak eye velocity: total peak eye velocity increased with increasing frequency for both groups, without any significant effect between the groups. No significant frequency-dependent changes were observed in angle, habituation-index or asymmetry. This behavior was similar in the eVOR and in the "natural" VOR.

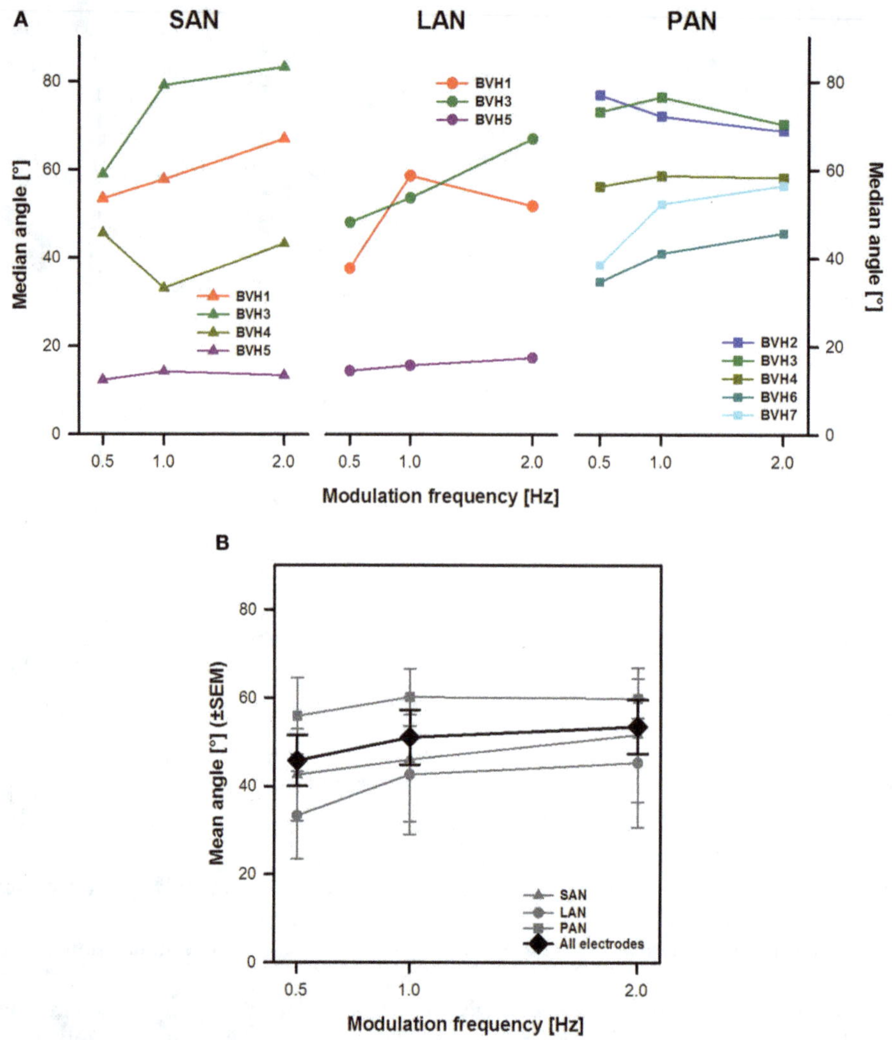

FIGURE 4 | Angle of eye movements vs. modulation frequency. (A) Each panel represents individual results obtained during stimulation for each stimulation site (SAN, LAN, PAN). **(B)** Mean results (±SEM) calculated across patients for each stimulation site (gray plots) and for all electrodes together (black plot).

The increase of peak eye velocity with frequency has already been well documented in normal subjects (Barnes, 1993), but it had never been systematically evaluated in human patients with a vestibular implant. It is reasonable to hypothesize that this effect probably reflects the properties of vestibular afferents, which are the main target of electrical stimulation by a vestibular implant (Goldberg et al., 1984; Kim et al., 2011). However, it cannot be excluded that a small residual population of hair cells and more central connections can contribute to this effect (Aw et al., 2008).

The eVOR angle (with respect to the horizontal axis) was very variable across the BVH-group for the whole tested frequency range. The resulting misalignment has already been described in animals as well as humans and is attributed mainly to current spread or imprecise electrode placement (Fridman et al., 2010; Lewis et al., 2010, 2013; Dai et al., 2011c, 2013; Davidovics et al., 2011; van de Berg et al., 2011; Guinand et al., Submitted). Current spread is particularly relevant in the case of the LAN and the SAN (**Figure 4A**) because of their close anatomical position relative to each other (van de Berg et al., 2012). Many strategies to minimize misalignment have been investigated, such as different stimulus waveforms, precompensation (vector summation), current steering and improving electrode design, but none of these seem totally infallible (Fridman et al., 2010; Dai et al., 2011c, 2013; Davidovics et al., 2013). Fortunately, chronic stimulation experiments in animals have shown that the brain is very adaptive: it is able to significantly improve eVOR alignment, making it possible to develop an ocular response which is aligned with the axis of head motion, even when stimulating the nerve branch of a canal that is orthogonal to the axis of motion. This phenomon is called "cross-axis adaptation." (Lewis et al., 2003, 2010, 2013; Della Santina et al., 2007; Dai et al., 2011c; van de Berg et al., 2011; Guinand et al., Submitted). Therefore, taking the adaptability of the brain into account, it should still be determined to which extent complex stimulation strategies to improve eVOR alignment will have to be incorporated into a device suited for human clinical use.

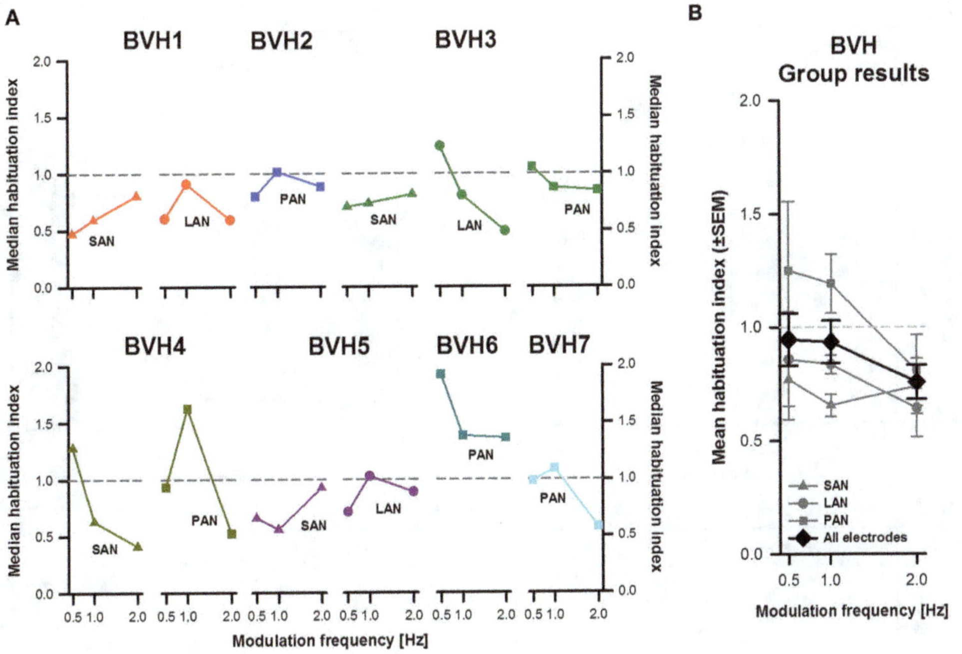

FIGURE 5 | Habituation-index vs. modulation frequency. (A) Each panel represents individual results obtained during stimulation for each stimulation site (SAN, LAN, PAN). **(B)** Mean results (±SEM) calculated across patients for each stimulation site (gray plots) and for all electrodes together (black plot).

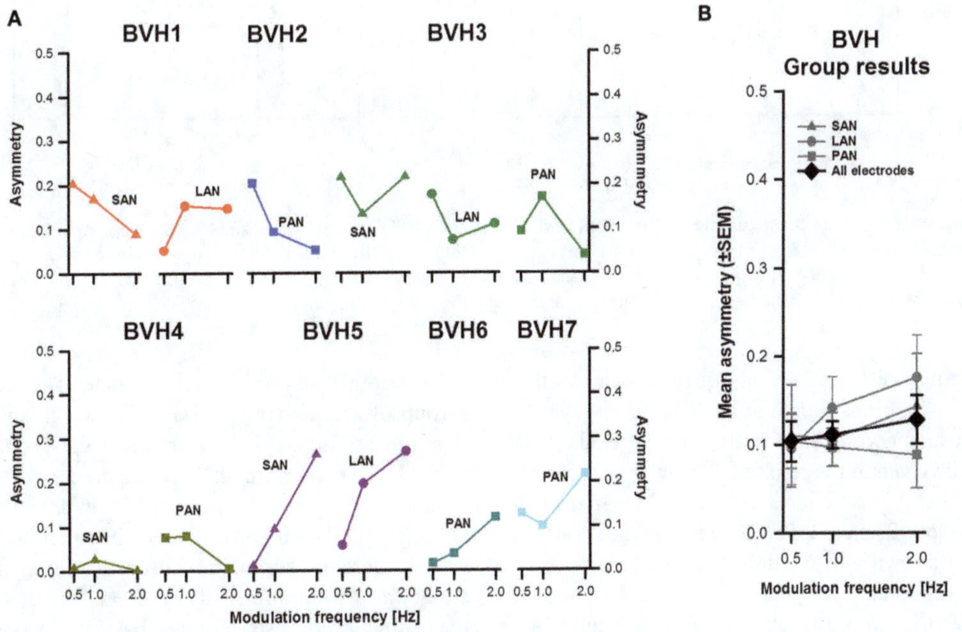

FIGURE 6 | Asymmetry-index vs. modulation frequency. (A) Each panel represents individual results obtained during stimulation for each stimulation site (SAN, LAN, PAN). **(B)** Mean results (±SEM) calculated across patients for each stimulation site (gray plots) and for all electrodes together (black plot).

Repeated exposure to the same sinusoidal stimulus can cause a long-lasting decrease in VOR gain in animals and humans. This habituation can be frequency-specific (Dow and Anastasio, 1999). While significant habituation has been observed for low-frequency stimuli (Buettner et al., 1981; Jäger and Henn, 1981a,b; Dow and Anastasio, 1997, 1999; Clément et al., 2002), repeated stimulation at higher modulation frequencies shows little or no change in VOR gain (Ito et al., 1974; Jäger and Henn,

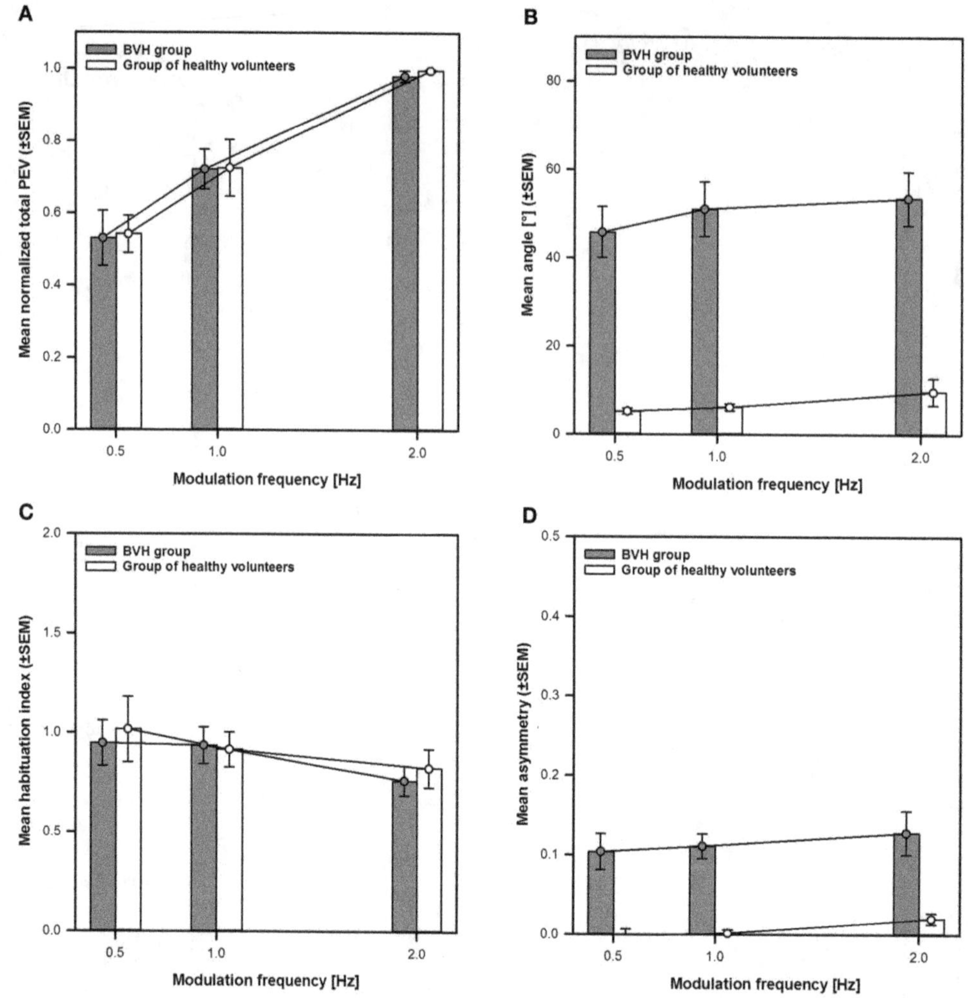

FIGURE 7 | Comparison of the main characteristics of the eVOR to the "natural" VOR. The eVOR is represented as mean group results of the BVH-group (gray bars and circles ±SEM). The "natural" VOR is represented as mean group results of the group of healthy volunteers (white bars and circles ±SEM). **(A)** Normalized total peak eye velocity (PEV) vs. modulation frequency. **(B)** Angle of the VOR responses vs. modulation frequency. **(C)** Habituation-index vs. modulation frequency. **(D)** Asymmetry-index vs. modulation frequency.

1981a; Dow and Anastasio, 1999). Consequently, some authors suggest sinusoidal oscillations should be limited to a few cycles or having a delay between two series of tests (Clément et al., 2002). Other key factors involved in the result of vestibular tests are general level of arousal and instruction set (Wall and Furman, 1989; Weissman et al., 1989; Barnes, 1993; Zee and Leigh, 2006). For example, it is well known and documented that results can be compromised during long testing trials. In this study, low modulation frequencies that would result in long testing times were excluded. Sixty-cycle trials were used and a delay between tests was obeyed. In these testing conditions, no significant habituation was observed. It is therefore reasonable to assume that habituation does not constitute a limiting factor in the tested frequency range.

No significant frequency-dependent changes in asymmetry were observed. However, the BVH-group showed significantly more asymmetry than the group of healthy volunteers. This could be expected, since acute unilateral vestibular stimulation (BVH-group) was compared to bilateral vestibular stimulation (group of healthy volunteers). However, it is interesting to note that the asymmetry index in the BVH-group remained relatively low (maximum 0.27) compared with previous data in unilaterally implanted monkeys (Dai et al., 2013; Guinand et al., Submitted). The major difference between both studies was the level of baseline stimulation used. Baseline stimulation in this study was set supranormally at 50% of the dynamic range, while the animal study used a lower baseline in order to mimic the physiology of normal rhesus monkey vestibular afferent fibers (Sadeghi et al., 2007; Dai et al., 2013). With a supranormal baseline, the decrease in excitatory response is counterbalanced by the increase in inhibitory response, which should improve the symmetry of the response. In other words, using a supranormal baseline corresponding to 50% of the total dynamic range, allows an equal range of stimulation currents to code head movements toward the implanted side and toward the unimplanted side. Consequently, head compensation in all directions should be enhanced (Davidovics et al., 2012). At this point it is important to point out that it is still not clear yet whether asymmetry will be an issue of clinical relevance for vestibular implants. Results on patients with a unilateral vestibular loss show that response asymmetry is generally well compensated (Curthoys and Halmagyi, 1995; Black et al., 1996; van de Berg et al., 2011). It is therefore reasonable to hypothesize that even an asymmetric eVOR might be enough to restore useful vestibular function.

Knowing the minor frequency effects on angle, habituation and asymmetry could open doors for future research. It allows these eVOR-parameters to be determined at only specific frequencies, without the need for testing the whole frequency range. This is likely to result in more precise measurements, since (1) some modulation frequencies which have specific drawbacks (i.e., low gain for low-frequencies or challenging head stabilization during rotatory tests at higher-frequencies) could be left out of the analysis and (2) time is saved in the already long testing sessions, resulting in improved patients' concentration which has to be optimal for all tests.

The fact that a vestibular implant can closely mimick the "natural" frequency-dependency of the vestibular system, is also a promising finding for device development. Since the VOR is appropriately compensated in a frequency range which is important for every-day activities (Crane and Demer, 1997), there might be no need of implementing complex stimulus processing strategies that consider frequency-dependent characteristics.

ADDITIONAL CONSIDERATIONS

In this study, the threshold for vestibular activation was the current where the first vestibular symptom was reported or observed (Guinand et al., Submitted). This could be a change in nystagmus slow peak eye velocity or a clearly vestibular related sensation that could be below the threshold of activation of the VOR-pathway. This latter case suggests that other pathways can be activated before the VOR-pathway. These sub-VOR-threshold perceptions deserve to be investigated more in the future (Guinand et al., Submitted).

Some healthy volunteers were unable to adequately stabilize their heads at 2 Hz. This resulted in an increase in the vertical peak eye velocity component, which is in accordance with clinical experience that effectively stabilizing the head above a certain rotation frequency becomes challenging. A bite bar could be added to improve head stabilization. However, it was decided not to use a bite bar since we considered that this would impose an additional unnecessary burden to subjects. Furthermore, adding a bite bar would hinder communication with subjects. Both these considerations are particularly relevant for our long, repeated testing sessions performed in complete darkness.

Finally, a potential caveat of this study is that results are based on a small number of subjects. This suggests that results of statistical tests should be interpreted with caution. Nevertheless, the trends reported were similar across subjects and inter-subject variability was smaller than the observed effects. In these conditions, adding more subjects to the study would certainly give more statistical power to the results, but it would not fundamentally change the observed trends.

CONCLUSION

A strong and significant frequency-dependency effect in total peak eye velocity was observed in the tested frequency range (0.5–2 Hz). This effect was comparable to the one observed for the "natural" VOR. (e)VOR-angle, habituation-index and asymmetry showed no significant frequency-dependent effect in any group. This study demonstrates that, at least in the specific (limited) frequency range tested, the vestibular implant closely mimics the natural frequency-dependency of the vestibular system.

ACKNOWLEDGMENTS

We would like to thank Dr. Eric Vuurman for his assistance with the statistical analysis and with the description of statistical details.

REFERENCES

Aw, S. T., Todd, M. J., Aw, G. E., Weber, K. P., and Halmagyi, G. M. (2008). Gentamicin vestibulotoxicity impairs human electrically evoked vestibulo-ocular reflex. *Neurology* 71, 1776–1782. doi: 10.1212/01.wnl.0000335971.43443.d9

Barnes, G. R. (1993). Visual-vestibular interaction in the control of head and eye movement: the role of visual feedback and predictive mechanisms. *Prog. Neurobiol.* 41, 435–472. doi: 10.1016/0301-0082(93)90026-O

Bartl, K., Lehnen, N., Kohlbecher, S., and Schneider, E. (2009). Head impulse testing using video-oculography. *Ann. N.Y. Acad. Sci.* 1164, 331–333. doi: 10.1111/j.1749-6632.2009.03850.x

Bierer, S. M., Ling, L., Nie, K., Fuchs, A. F., Kaneko, C. R. S., Oxford, T., et al. (2012). Auditory outcomes following implantation and electrical stimulation of the semicircular canals. *Hear. Res.* 287, 51–56. doi: 10.1016/j.heares.2012.03.012

Black, F. O., Wade, S. W., and Nashner, L. M. (1996). What is the minimal vestibular function required for compensation? *Am. J. Otol.* 17, 401–409.

Brandt, T., Huppert, T., Hüfner, K., Zingler, V. C., Dieterich, M., and Strupp, M. (2010). Long-term course and relapses of vestibular and balance disorders. *Restor. Neurol. Neurosci.* 28, 69–82. doi: 10.3233/RNN-2010-0504

Buettner, U. W., Henn, V., and Young, L. R. (1981). Frequency response of the vestibulo-ocular reflex (VOR) in the monkey. *Aviat. Space Environ. Med.* 52, 73–77.

Clément, G., Flandrin, J. M., and Courjon, J. H. (2002). Comparison between habituation of the cat vestibulo-ocular reflex by velocity steps and sinusoidal vestibular stimulation in the dark. *Exp. Brain Res.* 142, 259–267. doi: 10.1007/s00221-001-0930-7

Crane, B. T., and Demer, J. L. (1997). Human gaze stabilization during natural activities: translation, rotation, magnification, and target distance effects. *J. Neurophysiol.* 78, 2129–2144.

Curthoys, I., and Halmagyi, G. M. (1995). Vestibular compensation: a review of the oculomotor, neural, and clinical consequences of unilateral vestibular loss. *J. Vestib. Res.* 5, 67–107. doi: 10.1016/0957-4271(94)00026-X

Dai, C., Fridman, G. Y., Chiang, B., Davidovics, N. S., Melvin, T.-A., Cullen, K. E., et al. (2011c). Cross-axis adaptation improves 3D vestibulo-ocular reflex alignment during chronic stimulation via a head-mounted multichannel vestibular prosthesis. *Exp. Brain Res.* 210, 595–606. doi: 10.1007/s00221-011-2591-5

Dai, C., Fridman, G. Y., Chiang, B., Rahman, M. A., Ahn, J. H., Davidovics, N. S., et al. (2013). Directional plasticity rapidly improves 3D vestibulo-ocular reflex alignment in monkeys using a multichannel vestibular prosthesis. *J. Assoc. Res. Otolaryngol.* 14, 863–877. doi: 10.1007/s10162-013-0413-0

Dai, C., Fridman, G. Y., Davidovics, N. S., Chiang, B., Ahn, J. H., and Della Santina, C. C. (2011b). Restoration of 3D vestibular sensation in rhesus monkeys using a multichannel vestibular prosthesis. *Hear. Res.* 281, 74–83. doi: 10.1016/j.heares.2011.08.008

Dai, C., Fridman, G. Y., and Della Santina, C. C. (2011a). Effects of vestibular prosthesis electrode implantation and stimulation on hearing in rhesus monkeys. *Hear. Res.* 277, 204–210. doi: 10.1016/j.heares.2010.12.021

Davidovics, N. S., Fridman, G. Y., Chiang, B., and Della Santina, C. C. (2011). Effects of biphasic current pulse frequency, amplitude, duration, and interphase gap on eye movement responses to prosthetic electrical stimulation of the vestibular nerve. *IEEE Trans. Neural Syst. Rehabil. Eng.* 19, 84–94. doi: 10.1109/TNSRE.2010.2065241

Davidovics, N. S., Fridman, G. Y., and Della Santina, C. C. (2012). Co-modulation of stimulus rate and current from elevated baselines expands head motion encoding range of the vestibular prosthesis. *Exp. brain Res.* 218, 389–400. doi: 10.1007/s00221-012-3025-8

Davidovics, N. S., Rahman, M. A., Dai, C., Ahn, J., Fridman, G. Y., and Della Santina, C. C. (2013). Multichannel vestibular prosthesis employing modulation of pulse rate and current with alignment precompensation elicits improved VOR performance in monkeys. *J. Assoc. Res. Otolaryngol.* 14, 233–248. doi: 10.1007/s10162-013-0370-7

Della Santina, C. C., Migliaccio, A. A., and Patel, A. H. (2007). A multichannel semicircular canal neural prosthesis using electrical stimulation to restore 3-d vestibular sensation. *IEEE Trans. Biomed. Eng.* 54(6 Pt 1), 1016–1030. doi: 10.1109/TBME.2007.894629

Dow, E. R., and Anastasio, T. J. (1997). Induction of periodic alternating nystagmus in intact goldfish by sinusoidal rotation. *Neuroreport* 8, 2755–2759. doi: 10.1097/00001756-199708180-00022

Dow, E. R., and Anastasio, T. J. (1999). Analysis and modeling of frequency-specific habituation of the goldfish vestibulo-ocular reflex. *J. Comput. Neurosci.* 7, 55–70. doi: 10.1023/A:1008967511172

Feigl, G. C., Fasel, J. H., Anderhuber, F., Ulz, H., Rienmüller, R., Guyot, J.-P., et al. (2009). Superior vestibular neurectomy: a novel transmeatal approach for a denervation of the superior and lateral semicircular canals. *Otol. Neurotol.* 30, 586–591. doi: 10.1097/MAO.0b013e3181ab9164

Fridman, G. Y., Davidovics, N. S., Dai, C., Migliaccio, A. A., and Della Santina, C. C. (2010). Vestibulo-ocular reflex responses to a multichannel vestibular prosthesis incorporating a 3D coordinate transformation for correction of misalignment. *J. Assoc. Res. Otolaryngol.* 11, 367–381. doi: 10.1007/s10162-010-0208-5

Fridman, G. Y., and Della Santina, C. C. (2013). "Safe direct current stimulator 2: concept and design," in *Proceedings of the Annual International Conference of the IEEE Engineering in Medicine and Biology Society* (Osaka), 3126–3129.

Goldberg, J. M., Smith, C. E., and Fernandez, C. (1984). Relation between discharge regularity and responses to externally applied galvanic currents in vestibular nerve afferents of the squirrel monkey. *J. Neurophysiol.* 51, 1236–1256.

Golub, J. S., Ling, L., Nie, K., Nowack, A., Shepherd, S. J., Bierer, S. M., et al. (2014). Prosthetic implantation of the human vestibular system. *Otol. Neurotol.* 35, 136–147. doi: 10.1097/MAO.0000000000000003

Gong, W., and Merfeld, D. M. (2002). System design and performance of a unilateral horizontal semicircular canal prosthesis. *IEEE Trans. Biomed. Eng.* 49, 175–181. doi: 10.1109/10.979358

Guinand, N., Boselie, F., Guyot, J. P., and Kingma, H. (2012). Quality of life of patients with bilateral vestibulopathy. *Ann. Otol. Rhinol. Laryngol.* 121, 471–477. doi: 10.1177/000348941212100708

Guyot, J.-P., Sigrist, A., Pelizzone, M., and Kos, M. I. (2011). Adaptation to steady-state electrical stimulation of the vestibular system in humans. *Ann. Otol. Rhinol. Laryngol.* 120, 143–149. doi: 10.1177/00034894111 2000301

Hain, T. C., Cherchi, M., and Yacovino, D. A. (2013). Bilateral vestibular loss. *Semin. Neurol.* 33, 195–203. doi: 10.1055/s-0033-1354597

Hayden, R., Sawyer, S., Frey, E., Mori, S., Migliaccio, A. A., and Della Santina, C. C. (2011). Virtual labyrinth model of vestibular afferent excitation via implanted electrodes: validation and application to design of a multichannel vestibular prosthesis. *Exp. Brain Res.* 210, 623–640. doi: 10.1007/s00221-011-2599-x

Ito, M., Shiida, T., Yagi, N., and Yamamoto, M. (1974). Visual influence on rabbit horizontal vestibulo-ocular reflex presumably effected via the cerebellar flocculus. *Brain Res.* 65, 170–174. doi: 10.1016/0006-8993(74)90 344-8

Jäger, J., and Henn, V. (1981a). Habituation of the vestibulo-ocular reflex (VOR) in the monkey during sinusoidal rotation in the dark. *Exp. Brain Res.* 41, 108–114. doi: 10.1007/BF00236599

Jäger, J., and Henn, V. (1981b). Vestibular habituation in man and monkey during sinusoidal rotation. *Ann. N.Y. Acad. Sci.* 374, 330–339. doi: 10.1111/j.1749-6632.1981.tb30880.x

Kim, K. S., Minor, L. B., Della Santina, C. C., and Lasker, D. M. (2011). Variation in response dynamics of regular and irregular vestibular-nerve afferents during sinusoidal head rotations and currents in the chinchilla. *Exp. Brain Res.* 210, 643–649. doi: 10.1007/s00221-011-2600-8

Lewis, R. F., Gong, W., Ramsey, M., Minor, L., Boyle, R., and Merfeld, D. M. (2003). Vestibular adaptation studied with a prosthetic semicircular canal. *J. Vestib. Res.* 12, 87–94.

Lewis, R. F., Haburcakova, C., Gong, W., Makary, C., and Merfeld, D. M. (2010). Vestibuloocular reflex adaptation investigated with chronic motion-modulated electrical stimulation of semicircular canal afferents. *J. Neurophysiol.* 103, 1066–1079. doi: 10.1152/jn.00241.2009

Lewis, R. F., Nicoucar, K., Gong, W., Haburcakova, C., and Merfeld, D. M. (2013). Adaptation of vestibular tone studied with electrical stimulation of semicircular canal afferents. *J. Assoc. Res. Otolaryngol.* 14, 331–340. doi: 10.1007/s10162-013-0376-1

McCall, A. A., and Yates, B. J. (2011). Compensation following bilateral vestibular damage. *Front. Neurol.* 2:88. doi: 10.3389/fneur.2011.00088

Merfeld, D. M., Gong, W., Morrissey, J., Saginaw, M., Haburcakova, C., and Lewis, R. F. (2006). Acclimation to chronic constant-rate peripheral stimulation provided by a vestibular prosthesis. *IEEE Trans. Biomed. Eng.* 53, 2362–2372. doi: 10.1109/TBME.2006.883645

Merfeld, D. M., Haburcakova, C., Gong, W., and Lewis, R. F. (2007). Chronic vestibulo-ocular reflexes evoked by a vestibular prosthesis. *IEEE Trans. Biomed. Eng.* 54(6 Pt 1), 1005–1015. doi: 10.1109/TBME.2007.891943

Migliaccio, A. A., Meierhofer, R., and Della Santina, C. C. (2011). Characterization of the 3D angular vestibulo-ocular reflex in C57BL6 mice. *Exp. Brain Res.* 210, 489–501. doi: 10.1007/s00221-010-2521-y

Perez Fornos, A., Guinand, N., van de Berg, R., Stokroos, R., Micera, S., Kingma, H., et al. (2014). Artificial balance: restoration of the vestibulo-ocular reflex in humans with a prototype vestibular neuroprosthesis. *Front. Neurol.* 5:66. doi: 10.3389/fneur.2014.00066

Porciuncula, F., Johnson, C. C., and Glickman, L. B. (2012). The effect of vestibular rehabilitation on adults with bilateral vestibular hypofunction: a systematic review. *J. Vestib. Res.* 22, 283–298. doi: 10.3233/VES-120464

Rubinstein, J. T., Bierer, S., Kaneko, C., Ling, L., Nie, K., Oxford, T., et al. (2012). Implantation of the semicircular canals with preservation of hearing and rotational sensitivity: a vestibular neurostimulator suitable for clinical research. *Otol. Neurotol.* 33, 789–796. doi: 10.1097/MAO.0b013e31825 4ec24

Sadeghi, S. G., Minor, L. B., and Cullen, K. E. (2007). Response of vestibular-nerve afferents to active and passive rotations under normal conditions and after unilateral labyrinthectomy. *J. Neurophysiol.* 97, 1503–1514. doi: 10.1152/jn.00829.2006

van de Berg, R., Guinand, N., Guyot, J.-P., Kingma, H., and Stokroos, R. J. (2012). The modified ampullar approach for vestibular implant surgery: feasibility and its first application in a human with a long-term vestibular loss. *Front. Neurol.* 3:18. doi: 10.3389/fneur.2012.00018

van de Berg, R., Guinand, N., Stokroos, R. J., Guyot, J.-P., and Kingma, H. (2011). The vestibular implant: quo vadis? *Front. Neurol.* 2:47. doi: 10.3389/fneur.2011.00047

Wall, C., and Furman, J. M. (1989). Eyes open versus eyes closed: effect on human rotational responses. *Ann. Otol. Rhinol. Laryngol.* 98, 625–629. doi: 10.1177/000348948909800811

Wall, C., Kos, M. I., and Guyot, J.-P. (2007). Eye movements in response to electric stimulation of the human posterior ampullary nerve. *Ann. Otol. Rhinol. Laryngol.* 116, 369–374. doi: 10.1177/000348940711600509

Wall, C., Merfeld, D. M., Rauch, S. D., and Black, F. O. (2003). Vestibular prostheses: the engineering and biomedical issues. *J. Vestib. Res.* 12, 95–113.

Ward, B. K., Agrawal, Y., Hoffman, H. J., Carey, J. P., and Della Santina, C. C. (2013). Prevalence and impact of bilateral vestibular hypofunction: results from the 2008 US National Health Interview Survey. *JAMA Otolaryngol. Head Neck Surg.* 139, 803–810. doi: 10.1001/jamaoto.2013.3913

Weissman, B. M., DiScenna, A. O., Ekelman, B. L., and Leigh, R. J. (1989). Effect of eyelid closure and vocalization upon the vestibulo-ocular reflex during rotational testing. *Ann. Otol. Rhinol. Laryngol.* 98, 548–550. doi: 10.1177/000348948909800710

Zee, D., and Leigh, J. (2006). "The vestibular-optokinetic system," in *The Neurology of Eye Movements*, eds S. Gilman and W. Herdman (New York, NY: Oxford University Press), 72.

13

The role of expectations, hype and ethics in neuroimaging and neuromodulation futures

Elena Rusconi[1,2,3]* and Timothy Mitchener-Nissen[4]

[1] *Department of Security and Crime Science, University College London, London, UK*
[2] *Division of Psychology, Abertay University, Dundee, UK*
[3] *Department of Neurosciences, University of Parma, Parma, Italy*
[4] *Department of Science and Technology Studies, University College London, London, UK*

Edited by:
Mikhail Lebedev, Duke University, USA

Reviewed by:
Daniela Ovadia, University of Pavia, Italy
Walter Glannon, University of Calgary, Canada
Marleen Eijkholt, Davidson college, USA

****Correspondence:***
Elena Rusconi, Department of Security and Crime Science, University College London, 35 Tavistock Square, London WC1H9EZ, UK
e-mail: elena.rusconi@gmail.com

The production of *expectations* or future-goals for the development of techniques which "read" and modulate brain function, represent an important practical tool for neuroscientists. These visions-of-the-future assist scientists by providing focus for both individual and cross-disciplinary research programs; they encourage the development of new industrial sectors, are used to justify the allocation of government resources and funding, and via the media can help capture the imagination and support of the public. However, such expectations need to be tempered by reality. Over-hyping brain imaging and modulation will lead to disappointment; disappointment that in turn can undermine its potential. Similarly, if neuroscientists focus their attention narrowly on *the science* without concomitant consideration of its future ethical, legal and social implications, then their expectations may remain unrealized. To develop these arguments herein we introduce the theoretical concept of expectations and the practical consequences of expectations. We contextualize these reflections by referring to brain imaging and modulation studies on deception, which encompass the measurement-suppression-augmentation range.

Keywords: expectations, hype, ethics, brain modulation, neuroimaging, deception

INTRODUCING EXPECTATIONS

On May 25th in 1961 during a special address to Congress, a young and charismatic US President J.F. Kennedy presented an incredibly exciting prospect to Congress and the entire nation: a manned moon landing. He was asking Congress to share his vision, and in so doing to invest an astronomical budget in research and development to increase the likelihood of that vision becoming reality. Less than a decade later that vision was achieved with the Apollo 11 mission and the first moon walk: "one small step for man, one giant leap for mankind" (Neil Armstrong, 1969). Kennedy was perfectly aware that the required technology was not yet available in 1961 but he was well informed about its potential and knew a thing or two about the power of expectations.

Proclaiming the start of the Decade of the Brain on 1st January 1990, President Bush senior stated "The cooperation between [...] agencies and the multidisciplinary efforts of thousands of scientists and health care professionals provide powerful evidence of our nation's determination to conquer brain disease". He raised public awareness and brought to the fore a series of targets (e.g., stopping or curing Alzheimer's disease), which have not been quite met yet but the attention and investments brought upon relevant neuroscientific research see us at a clear advantage compared to our colleagues trying to meet the same targets 25 years ago.

When discussing scientific and technological advancement the concept of *expectations* adopts the shape of; goals, promises, visions of a future reality, "wishful enactments of desired futures" (Tutton, 2011, p. 413), and "real-time representations of future technological situations and capabilities" (Borup et al., 2006 p. 286). The value of such expectations, as a powerful precursor to future scientific and technological advances, cannot be underestimated as both a conceptual and a practical tool.

In this paper we begin by setting out the benefits to neuroscientists of employing *expectations.* This positive message is then balanced by a discussion of *hype* and its potential negative connotations for research programs. We finish by positing that if neuroscientists temper their expectations of future scientific and technological advances with social, ethical, and legal concerns, they will be better placed to avoid the drawbacks associated with hype while maintaining their ability to enjoy the benefits expectations can bring.

EXPECTATIONS: CONCEPTUAL AND PRACTICAL BENEFITS

On a conceptual level, expectations (as described above) represent *the potential pre-manifestation* or *genesis* of a future scientific or technical advance which has yet to be attained. To illustrate; neuroscientists envision a future whereby neuroimaging and brain stimulation techniques have been developed which, say, detect deception and/or increase the disposition and the ability to lie and deceive (Karim et al., 2010; Mameli et al., 2010; Karton and Bachmann, 2011), "simply and safely influenc[e] the human will and freedom by interfering with deception" (Priori et al., 2008, p. 455; see also the "deception inhibitor": Bohning et al., 2004). They may also envision military applications whereby the ability of human operators to sense and assess threats in the real world is enhanced by noninvasive brain stimulation (e.g., Parasuraman and Galster, 2013). These particular near-to-medium term expectations are typically based on converging evidence from a small series of original precursor studies on human participants conducted in one or more laboratories around the world. When neuroscientists envision a future whereby in-helmet ultrasound transducers could be used to remotely control brain activity (Tyler, 2010; Sato et al., 2014), or where a time-slowing pill may be used in law enforcement and prisoner incarceration (Heaven, 2012; Anderson, 2014), or "brain prostheses" can be used by the military to enhance memory for complex environments or existing memories can be wiped out from the brain of personnel under capture (Moreno, 2012) they are envisioning medium-to-long term expectations. Here the know-how needed to achieve these particular goals remains largely unavailable and it is claimed that the ethical and legal implications of such enterprise are still relatively imponderable (Attiah and Farah, 2014).

What makes these particular expectations of specific interest to neuroscientists is that through a combination of their training, expertise, accumulated knowledge, and access to funding and specific equipment, neuroscientists find themselves well placed to successfully act and bring these expectations and visions into reality. This is not to claim that they are the *only scientists* capable of fulfilling these expectations; merely that they may enjoy a head start on their competitors when attempting to do so.

Moving beyond the conceptual, it is via its practical benefits that the true power of expectations becomes recognizable; for expectations possess the power to assist turning future-visions into tangible advancements. With similarities to the concept of the *self-fulfilling prophecy* (see Merton, 1948), future expectations have been described as possessing performative or generative powers (Borup et al., 2006) in that they are "crucial to providing the dynamism and momentum upon which so many ventures in science and technology depend" (Brown and Michael, 2003, p. 3). By studying past advancements, it has been recognized that expectations can provide the following benefits (see: van Lente, 1993; Hedgecoe and Martin, 2003; Borup et al., 2006; Konrad, 2006; Pollock and Williams, 2010; Bakker et al., 2012):

- A focal point to guide and drive research activities, as well as a common vision/bridge with which to enhance interdisciplinary interactions and communication.
- A promise of future benefits with which to justify and legitimize the mobilization and allocation of financial resources and other forms of support.
- The means of attracting the attention and engagement of diverse actors and potential collaborators; from scientists to investors, governments, NGOs and policy actors.
- They enable the production of experiments, models, research projects, and calculations.
- The construction of future scenarios for shaping a technology, as well as the formation of a consensus or structure to counterbalance the inherent uncertainty over the potential of a new technology which is highest during the early development stages.
- A means of enlisting public support through the presentation of possible future(s).

Within the life sciences expectations of future medical advancements have repeatedly been employed by specific research areas seeking to benefit from the points listed above. These expectations have included; the promise of lives being saved and the development of new cures for diseases as the result of human embryonic stem cell research (Rubin, 2008); the development of anti-aging treatments which will extend human lives (Mykytyn, 2010); and the expectation that by identifying one's genetic makeup, pharmacogenetics will deliver bespoke, personalized medications (Limdi and Veenstra, 2010).

Within neuroscience, and in particular the study of neuroimaging and brain stimulation, we can readily identify how neuroscientists are employing expectations in their efforts to secure supporters and resources for research, attract collaborators and potential customers for spin-off businesses, and provide focal points with which to guide research. All of this is achieved through the presentation of possible futures where brain imaging and modulation advances have been successfully developed. What follows is a brief description of some of these research programs, accompanied by the envisioned advances (the expectations) they are predicted to produce. While presenting these, we will intentionally embrace such expectations (whether or not we believe they are realistic), as this will help making the points we are raising in the following sections even more obvious.

EXPECTATIONS ABOUT THE FUTURE OF BRAIN IMAGING AND MODULATION: THE CASE OF DECEPTION

Riding a wave of exciting technical developments in neuroimaging, one popular research enterprise that has provided fertile ground for boosting expectations on a global scale is the study of deception. Here deception is defined as the concealment of the truth, which often takes the form of a memory, in order to mislead. On average humans are thought to be badly equipped to detect deception when the person attempting to deceive is unfamiliar to the observer (Bond and DePaulo, 2006). Expectations in this area have included a promise of a future whereby the scientific detection of deceptive claims and behaviors would add a game-changing weapon to the arsenal of forensic sciences, police, the judiciary, and military and security agencies worldwide. Whether that can be ever achieved is still open to speculation.

Historically a multitude of deception detection systems have been invented and employed by public and private bodies with variable success. Few such systems survived in the present; and none has been scientifically proven to solve the deception detection problem in the real world. The most popular system so far has arguably been the polygraph, however, on close inspection, it was deemed unreliable; though since its myth is very hard to debunk, it still has use as a deterrent (NRC (National Research Council), 2003; see also Moreno, 2012). More recently, advances in functional Magnetic Resonance Imaging (fMRI) and neural decoding techniques prompted expectations that mind-reading (or more accurately brain-reading; Gazzaniga, 2005) may soon become reality (Haynes and Rees, 2006). In relation to deception, expectations and research have focused on systems that can accurately detect deceit from brain activation contrasts or pattern analysis, perhaps in connection with other physiological measures (Kozel et al., 2009; Langleben and Moriarty, 2013). These would help reduce uncertainty and provide information otherwise undetectable to the interviewer. By making the interviewee's brain *more accessible* they would artificially augment the interviewer's detection capabilities. Moreover, they would provide essential information about the localization of deception-relevant brain activity for individually targeted deception modulation tools (see e.g., Bohning et al., 2004). It may be easy to create expectations about potential advantages for the criminal justice system and security at large if such an enterprise were to actually succeed. For example, it could be claimed that it will be possible to accurately discriminate between genuine and concocted eyewitness testimony (Azar, 2011), more judiciary decisions could be based on objective evidence, and trials would become more expedite. Culprits would be less likely to elude unmasking and arguably more likely to be found guilty; crime rates may drop; and organized crime which relies on member loyalty could be more penetrated.[1] On its face, and without critical analysis, the benefits cited here might be presented as both obvious and great in number.

Expectations within deception research are by no means limited to the development of reliable lie detectors. Indeed noninvasive brain stimulation (e.g., tDCS and TMS) may soon offer both a new, upgraded alternative to truth serums by enabling the user to interfere with activity in brain regions that are causally related with deception (e.g., Priori et al., 2008; Karton and Bachmann, 2011), as well as its counterpart; a portable deceit enhancer (Karim et al., 2010; Mameli et al., 2010; Karton and Bachmann, 2011; Fecteau et al., 2013). It is easy to imagine the enormous advantages for counterespionage, policing, and diplomacy if a "deception inhibitor" was available. In extreme scenarios, interrogations would become more humane; negating the need for more outrageous practices such as sleep-deprivation, electric shocks, nail pulling, water-boarding, and so forth, to weaken psychophysical defense mechanisms and coerce the disclosure of information (see e.g., Tarabay, 2014, and the documentary Standard Operating Procedure, 2008). In more ordinary cases, this induced cooperation would make criminal justice mechanisms more agile and cost-effective. Potentially more guilty individuals will confess and be rightfully convicted.

Similarly, it is arguable that difficult diplomatic negotiations could benefit from both sides employing "deception inhibitors". These may decrease the capability of either side negotiating in bad-faith by concealing their true thoughts (though it is equally likely such devices may make parties reluctant to enter into negotiations to begin with). Conversely "deception boosters" would conceivably be invaluable in the hands of private and governmental agencies concerned with security, policing, espionage, and diplomacy. Undercover agents might be better able to conceal their true identities, and negotiators better equipped to convincingly promote positions they knew to be false.

[1]See http://www.fbi.gov/about-us/investigate/organizedcrime

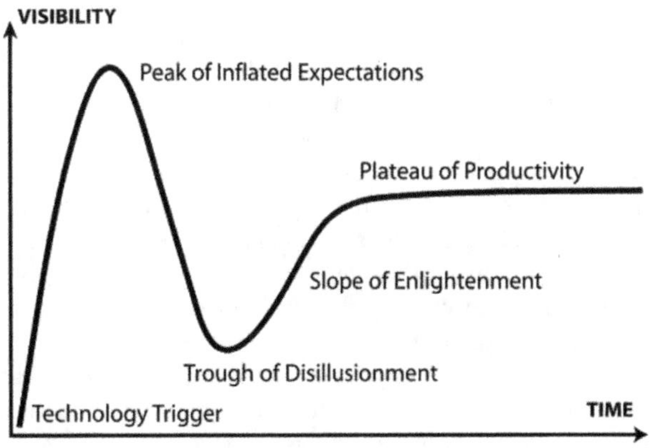

FIGURE 1 | The Gartner Hype Cycle (van Lente et al., 2013).

HYPE: THE DOWNSIDE OF EXPECTATIONS

While expectations such as these play important roles in achieving scientific and technological advancements, we must acknowledge an inherent fundamental limitation: expectations may be unreliable as predictors of the future (Brown and Michael, 2003). Even when high expectations for future advancements are shared by a large multidisciplinary community of scientists enjoying both support and resources, this does not guarantee scientific success (Pollock and Williams, 2010; Tutton, 2011). The failure of a scientific or engineering endeavor to meet its expectations leads to accusations of *hype*. Used in this way hype is referring to unrealistic, unattainable expectations; hence it is often only a distinction in framing that separates expectations from hype. What follows the characterization of (positive) expectations as (negative) hype is usually a period of disappointment or disillusionment. Enthusiasm for the proposed scientific advancement plummets as a result of expectation not being met, possibly followed by a gradual form of recovery. This process is referred to as a hype-disappointment cycle (van Lente et al., 2013). The Gartner hype cycle (see **Figure 1**), employed by the analyst firm Gartner Inc. is probably the most recognized model employing this concept. Note that under this model, the failure of scientific research or technological development to meet its initial expectations does not mean it is automatically and permanently discarded; rather that it is subject to a period of slower development towards more realistic goals.

This process, whereby (what in hindsight proved to be exaggerated) expectations were employed to secure support for research only to be followed by an abrupt collapse, has repeated itself in a multitude of past technologies; including hydrogen-powered cars (Bakker, 2010), nanotechnologies (Ebeling, 2008), and genomics

(Bubela, 2006). No scientific discipline is immune from such outcomes, and some expectations for the promise of brain imaging and modulation will almost inevitably suffer the same result to some extent (see e.g., Walsh, 2013). The likelihood of this occurring is growing as neuroscientists increasingly push the boundaries of what they are presenting as realistic research outcomes in their efforts to secure support and resources for their research. Indeed in Gartner's (2013) Hype Cycle for Emerging Technologies, *human augmentation* (which would include brain augmentation) is specifically identified as a technology currently *on-the-rise* towards its peak of inflated expectations (Gartner, 2013). It has also been suggested that *functional neuroimaging* technologies may be even further advanced along the classic Hype Cycle trajectory than augmentation (Rachul and Zarzeczny, 2012). One example from neuroscience justifying this characterization is the potential use of fMRI in the detection of deception.

More than a decade on since the first peer-reviewed empirical reports on deception detection in fMRI (see e.g., Spence et al., 2001; Langleben et al., 2002; Ganis et al., 2003), the field has seen incremental advances both in the "brain-reading" technique and in the refinement of cognitive testing protocols (see e.g., Sartori et al., 2008; Moreno, 2012; Wright et al., 2012; Park and Friston, 2013). Multiple patent applications have been filed but the envisioned fMRI deception detector looks still far from becoming reality. We have highlighted elsewhere a series of hurdles that an fMRI-based deception detector would need to surmount before it can succeed (Rusconi and Mitchener-Nissen, 2013). These include scientific hurdles such as; the assumptions and inferences underlying fMRI processes, the need to achieve consistent internal validity, manipulation of results by subjects, and the difficulty in moving beyond the laboratory setting. Also included were legal and ethical hurdles, such as; possible human rights violations, the issue of compelled questioning, the probative value of such evidence, and how the right to a fair trial would be impacted. It is open for debate whether or not its stimulation counterpart stands a better chance to translate into an applied deception modulator tool. One obvious advantage is that certain stimulators are both portable and affordable; however the science is probably not mature enough to justify its near-medium term expectations. The reported modulatory effects (facilitation or interference) obtained in controlled laboratory settings are statistically significant but rather minuscule in a standard interrogation context and short-lived, thus as things stand the gains may not eventually justify the efforts. This consideration only applies to applicative expectations—not to the utility and importance of such research within basic science. The in-lab testing protocols have not been validated against real-world situations (Luber et al., 2009), and the relation between modulation of deceits and its effects on other brain functions are still unclear, as is the role of individual differences (see Levasseur-Moreau et al., 2013 for a thorough discussion).

THE DOWNSIDE OF HYPE

The reason why neuroscientists should resist the temptation to over-hype the potential for brain augmentation is the detrimental consequences that can follow once unrealistic expectations are inevitably unmet. These include the following (see Brown, 2003; Ruef and Markard, 2010):

- Unrealistic short-term hype detracts from the long-term value of the basic science.
- Financial losses for corporate investors, and future difficulty in securing resources within fields which have suffered from a collapse of expectations.
- Resources are diverted from more realistically-achievable, yet less exciting, research programs.
- Undermined trust, which can slow or prevent future progress within a field of research.
- The reputations of individuals, companies/institutions, and entire research fields can suffer as past promises fail to materialize in the present.
- Identifiable people can suffer as a result; from individuals who suffer financial loss from investing in unrealistically over-hyped research programs, to patients who suffer emotionally having believed the claims that certain proposed brain augmentation techniques could treat their conditions.

In different combinations, these detrimental consequences arise in the multitude of science and technology examples presented in the annual Gartner hype cycles, as well as the specific case-studies of hydrogen-powered cars, genomics, and nanotechnology discussed above.

Nevertheless, despite all these drawbacks of hype the temptation still remains to present the most ambitious expectations for scientific and technological research as something achievable in the future; be they time-slowing pills to replace prison sentences, portable reliable lie detectors, brain control devices, or extra-memory microchips. Perhaps unsurprisingly the probability of achieving these goals (which may be incredibly small) and the time-frame for doing so (which may be incredibly long) are afforded little discussion. The challenge facing neuroscientists is how to construct and present expectations that are less likely to cross that invisible barrier dividing "hope" from "hype".

ADDRESSING ETHICAL CONCERNS TO PRODUCE BETTER EXPECTATIONS AND THE RISKS OF NOT DOING SO

It is our contention that by reflexively considering the ethical, legal, and social impacts of a potential future technology or field of advancement, neuroscientists can improve the quality of the expectations they disseminate within their own field; thereby developing more nuanced, better expectations. This of course does not replace or neglects but is additional to the need for neuroscientists to educate the media, patients and research subjects about the potential and limits of neuroscience and neuroscientific techniques; to conduct enough studies and generate valid scientific data to know what neuroscience and these techniques can and cannot do. Before we develop this contention below, two points require expansion and clarification here. Firstly, we are characterizing these expectations as "better" if they constitute visions of the future constructed after taking into account existing legal regimes and concepts of human rights, ethical norms, and attitudes of societies into which they are expected to operate. Secondly, it should also be emphasized that the stage we are referring to is the formulation and presentation of initial expectations by the scientists. This stage often precedes wider public/multi-stakeholder engagement and the development of respective communication strategies (for more detailed discussions of such topics see: Jasanoff, 2003; O'Doherty and Einsiedel, 2012; Bucchi and Trench, 2014; Stilgoe et al., 2014).

The concomitant social, legal and ethical implications of a proposed scientific/technological expectation are often neglected at the initial stage of its formulation and proposition. Hence what is often initially presented is the envisioned advancement free from ostensibly non-scientific constraints; i.e., presenting the expectations of a pill that slows one's perception of time or of the portable lie detector device, but doing so free from any contextual discussion. This may occur for a number of reasons, including: (a) because no ethical/legal/social implications exist (highly unlikely for most expectations); (b) those presenting these futures have not considered and/or foreseen such implications; (c) these implications are viewed as either unimportant or not the responsibility of the scientist involved; and/or (d) there is a fear that by acknowledging the existence of such implications, the advancement in question will be viewed less positively thus putting at risk the benefits expectations can bring to a research program.

However, failing to reflexively consider the ethical, legal, and social impacts of a potential future technology or field of advancement does not negate their existence or make them disappear. These factors are going to have to be addressed at some point in the research and development lifecycle of a new technology for scientific advancements do not develop or exist separately to the societies in which they operate (see MacKenzie and Wajcman, 1999). We contend that both the benefits of engaging in this reflexive process early in the development of new expectations, as well as the potential negative implications of failing to do so, make this early consideration of ethical, legal, and social impacts an essential step in their development.

By considering ethical, legal, and social impacts to create "better" expectations, neuroscientists gain a number of advantages. They can act to avoid their expectations becoming characterized as hype. They can identify sources of possible controversy and resistance within their proposed expectations, thereby affording them the opportunity to consciously address such issues both through how they formulate their expectations and how they seek to present them. Also by mitigating the propensity for individuals or societal groups to actively criticize or resist their expectations, the neuroscientist is effectively maximizing their potential network of future supporters.

Failure to create "better" expectations can have specific negative consequences. It can shift expectations into the realm of hype (the inherent negative consequences of such were discussed earlier). It has also been posited that by presenting technological expectations unfettered by non-technical considerations (such as ethics, legality, and social acceptability), critics can more easily create counterarguments by presenting dystopian futures involving them (see Tutton, 2011). Essentially the argument here is that; if the presentation of an expectation devoid of some inherent moral character justifies utopian visions of its future use, then dystopian visions of its future use are also equally valid (see Pickersgill, 2011 for a practical example of this argument in relation to *neuro-law*).

Furthermore, by promoting a real-world version of, and uses for, a future technology absent of a robust consideration of social, legal and ethical issues is to promote a tool that is more easily open to legitimate social, legal and ethical criticism. We believe this advice has resonance for many of the expectations currently being espoused by neuroscientists within the field of neuroimaging and brain modulation; from enhancing the cognitive potential of users, to brain control/manipulation, to increasing/decreasing the capacity of an individual to deceive. An important point here is that each expectation must be individually reflexively examined, for the nature of these social, legal and ethical criticisms will differ depending on the specific application that is being envisaged. This diversity means there are no shortcuts to robust reflexive examinations. For example, in the case of fMRI deception detection in criminal proceedings discussed above, we examined in depth how future expectations of this advancement conflicted with existing legal and human rights regimes, as well as social and ethical norms. This led us to conclude that "[c]ognitive neuroscientists must be careful not to over-play what these technologies can offer criminal courts nor their vision of the potential future role of neuroscience within criminal courts, lest they overplay themselves out of the courtroom altogether" (Rusconi and Mitchener-Nissen, 2013, p. 9). Conversely, the main hurdles of brain reading and modulation may be characterized as: legal and human rights issues over compelled questioning, fair trials, and the probative weight attached to such evidence; as well as the social implications of undermining our naturally evolved capacity to deceive. Whereas those raised by cosmetic enhancement include: the ethicality of altering fundamental elements of self-identity; social justice concerns over the inequitable distribution of cognitive enhancement techniques; the undermining of autonomy; and determining the "proper" role of enhancement technologies in society (Wolpe, 2002; Hamilton et al., 2011). Given the mounting emphasis on "impact", even from government founding agencies that have traditionally encouraged basic research, neuroscientists may need some assistance in this reflexive process. This could be offered in the form of further training and multidisciplinary education opportunities or direct access to professional figures with the relevant expertise. On the other hand, funding agencies and scientific journals could also be required to closely monitor and develop awareness of the more hype-prone research areas, as their endorsement (sometimes motivated by the immediate visibility that inflated expectations can grant) may play a role in amplifying, rewarding and maintaining hype within the scientific community.

CONCLUSION

Expectations are presented as a valuable tool for neuroscientists in acquiring both resources and networks of allies to assist in converting these expectations into reality. However, in applying the often-used adage of caution, that "if a little bit of something is good then a lot is not necessarily better", unrealistic expectations can become synonymous with hype which in turn can threaten the very programs the scientists are seeking to promote. Similarly, promoting the expectation of a scientific or technological advancement free from any social, legal or ethical considerations will not benefit that advancement. For any critical assessment will easily be able to identify these non-technical concerns which neuroscientists have ostensibly ignored; again placing at risk the programs they are seeking to advance.

Provided they are supported by (and are not used as a replacement for) sound research on the safety and efficacy of neuroscientific techniques, expectations *are* a valuable resource for capturing the public's imagination and promoting investment in an area for research. We encourage those neuroscientists working in the field of neuroimaging and brain modulation, with its exciting prospects for the future, to employ this valuable resource as they would any other at their disposal to help further their research goals. We simply caution that when doing so, if they present expectations that are disassociated from any measure of realism, or treat the concomitant legal, social and ethical considerations as optional extras, then hype (and Gartner's *Trough of Disillusionment*) surely awaits.

REFERENCES

Anderson, R. (2014). *Hell on Earth: What Happens to Life Sentences if our Lifespan is Radically Extended? A Philosopher Talks about Future Punishment.* Available online at: http://aeon.co/magazine/living-together/should-biotech-make-life-hellish-for-criminals/. Accessed on July 1, 2014.

Attiah, M. A., and Farah, M. (2014). Minds, motherboards and money: futurism and realism in the neuroethics of BCI technologies. *Front. Syst. Neurosci.* 15:86. doi: 10.3389/fnsys.2014.00086

Azar, B. (2011). The limits of eyewitness testimony. *Monit. Psychol.* 42, 27. doi: 10.1037/e725332011-006

Bakker, S. (2010). The car industry and the blow-out of the hydrogen hype. *Energy Policy* 38, 6540–6544. doi: 10.1016/j.enpol.2010.07.019

Bakker, S., van Lente, H., and Engels, R. (2012). Competition in a technological niche: the cars of the future. *Technol. Anal. Strateg. Manage.* 24, 421–434. doi: 10.1080/09537325.2012.674666

Bohning, D., George, M., and Kozel, F. (2004). *Functional Magnetic Resonance Imaging Guided Transcranial Magnetic Stimulation Deception Inhibitor.* WIPO Patent WO 2004006750 A2.

Bond, C., and DePaulo, B. (2006). Accuracy of deception judgments. *Pers. Soc. Psychol. Rev* 10, 214–234. doi: 10.1207/s15327957pspr1003_2

Borup, M., Brown, N., Konrad, K., and van Lente, H. (2006). The sociology of expectations in science and technology. *Technol. Anal. Strateg. Manage.* 18, 285–298. doi: 10.1080/09537320600777002

Brown, N. (2003). Hope against hype - accountability in biopasts, presents and futures. *Sci. Stud.* 16, 3–21.

Brown, N., and Michael, M. (2003). A sociology of expectations: retrospecting prospects and prospecting retrospects. *Technol. Anal. Strateg. Manage.* 15, 3–18. doi: 10.1080/0953732032000046024

Bubela, T. (2006). Science communication in transition: genomics hype, public engagement, education and commercialization pressures. *Clin. Genet.* 70, 445–450. doi: 10.1111/j.1399-0004.2006.00693.x

Bucchi, M., and Trench, B. (Eds.) (2014). *Routledge Handbook of Public Communication of Science and Technology.* 2nd Edn. New York: Routledge.

Ebeling, M. (2008). Mediating uncertainty: communicating the financial risks of nanotechnology. *Sci. Commun.* 29, 335–361. doi: 10.1177/1075547007312068

Fecteau, S., Boggio, P., Fregni, F., and Pascual-Leone, A. (2013). Modulation of untruthful responses with non-invasive brain stimulation. *Front. Psychiatry* 3:97. doi: 10.3389/fpsyt.2012.00097

Ganis, G., Kosslyn, S., Stose, S., Thompson, W., and Yurgelun-Todd, D. (2003). Neural correlates of different types of deception: an fMRI investigation. *Cereb. Cortex* 13, 830–836. doi: 10.1093/cercor/13.8.830

Gartner. (2013). Hype cycle for emerging technologies maps out evolving relationship between humans and machines [Press Release]. Available online at: http://www.gartner.com/newsroom/id/2575515

Gazzaniga, M. (2005). *The Ethical Brain.* New York: Harper.

Hamilton, R., Messing, S., and Chatterjee, A. (2011). Rethinking the thinking cap. *Neurology* 76, 187–193. doi: 10.1212/WNL.0b013e318205d50d

Haynes, J., and Rees, G. (2006). Decoding mental states from brain activity in humans. *Nat. Rev. Neurosci.* 7, 523–534. doi: 10.1038/nrn1931

Heaven, D. (2012). Brain circuits run their own clock. *New Sci.* 2889, 12.

Hedgecoe, A., and Martin, P. (2003). The drugs don't work: expectations and the shaping of pharmacogenetics. *Soc. Stud. Sci.* 33, 327–364. doi: 10.1177/03063127030333002

Jasanoff, S. (2003). Technologies of humility: citizen participation in governing science. *Minerva* 41, 223–244.

Karim, A., Schneider, M., Lotze, M., Veit, R., Sauseng, P., Braun, C., et al. (2010). The truth about lying: inhibition of the anterior prefrontal cortex improves deceptive behavior. *Cereb. Cortex* 20, 205–213. doi: 10.1093/cercor/bhp090

Karton, I., and Bachmann, T. (2011). Effect of prefrontal transcranial magnetic stimulation on spontaneous truth-telling. *Behav. Brain Res.* 225, 209–214. doi: 10.1016/j.bbr.2011.07.028

Konrad, K. (2006). The social dynamics of expectations: the interaction of collective and actor-specific expectations on electronic commerce and interactive television. *Technol. Anal. Strateg. Manage.* 18, 429–444. doi: 10.1080/09537320600777192

Kozel, F. A., Johnson, K. A., Laken, S. J., Grenesko, E. L., Smith, J. A., Walker, J., et al. (2009). Can simultaneously acquired electrodermal activity improve accuracy of fMRI detection of deception? *Soc. Neurosci.* 4, 510–517. doi: 10.1080/17470910801907168

Langleben, D., and Moriarty, J. (2013). Using brain imaging for lie-detection: where science, law and research policy collide. *Psychol. Public Policy Law* 19, 222–234. doi: 10.1037/a0028841

Langleben, D. D., Schroeder, L., Maldjian, J. A., Gur, R. C., McDonald, S., Ragland, J. D., et al. (2002). Brain activity during simulated deception: an event-related functional magnetic resonance study. *Neuroimage* 15, 727–732. doi: 10.1006/nimg.2001.1003

Levasseur-Moreau, J., Brunelin, J., and Fecteau, S. (2013). Non-invasive brain stimulation can induce paradoxical facilitation. Are these neuroenhancements transferable and meaningful to security services? *Front. Hum. Neurosci.* 7:449. doi: 10.3389/fnhum.2013.00449

Limdi, N., and Veenstra, D. (2010). Expectations, validity and reality in pharmacogenetics. *J. Clin. Epidemiol.* 63, 960–969. doi: 10.1016/j.jclinepi.2009.09.006

Luber, B., Fisher, C., Appelbaum, P. S., Ploesser, M., and Lisanby, S. H. (2009). Non-invasive brain stimulation in the detection of deception: scientific challenges and ethical consequences. *Behav. Sci. Law* 27, 191–208. doi: 10.1002/bsl.860

MacKenzie, D., and Wajcman, J. (Eds.) (1999). *The Social Shaping of Technology.* 2nd Edn. Maidenhead: Open University Press.

Mameli, F., Mrakic-Sposta, S., Vergari, M., Fumagalli, M., Macis, M., Ferrucci, R., et al. (2010). Dorsolateral prefrontal cortex specifically processes general - but not personal - knowledge deception: multiple brain networks for lying. *Behav. Brain Res.* 211, 164–168. doi: 10.1016/j.bbr.2010.03.024

Merton, R. (1948). The self-fulfilling prophecy. *Antioch Rev.* 8, 193–210. doi: 10.2307/4609267

Moreno, J. (2012). *Mind Wars: Brain Science and the Military in the 21st Century.* New York: Bellevue Literary Press.

Mykytyn, C. (2010). A history of the future: the emergence of contemporary anti-ageing medicine. *Sociol. Health Illn.* 32, 181–196. doi: 10.1111/j.1467-9566.2009.01217.x

NRC (National Research Council). (2003). *The Polygraph and Lie Detection.* Washington D.C.: The National Academies Press.

O'Doherty, K., and Einsiedel, E. (Eds.) (2012). *Public Engagement and Emerging Technologies.* Toronto: UBC Press.

Parasuraman, R., and Galster, S. (2013). Sensing, assessing and augmenting threat detection: behavioral, neuroimaging and brain stimulation evidence for the critical role of attention. *Front. Hum. Neurosci.* 7:273. doi: 10.3389/fnhum.2013.00273

Park, H. J., and Friston, K. (2013). Structural and functional brain networks: from connections to cognition. *Science* 342:1238411. doi: 10.1126/science.1238411

Pickersgill, M. (2011). Connecting neuroscience and law: anticipatory discourse and the role of sociotechnical imaginaries. *New Genet. Soc.* 30, 27–40. doi: 10.1080/14636778.2011.552298

Pollock, N., and Williams, R. (2010). The business of expectations: how promissory organizations shape technology and innovation. *Soc. Stud. Sci.* 40, 525–548. doi: 10.1177/0306312710362275

Priori, A., Mameli, F., Cogiamanian, F., Marceglia, S., Tiriticco, M., Mrakic-Sposta, S., et al. (2008). Lie-specific involvement of dorsolateral prefrontal cortex in deception. *Cereb. Cortex* 18, 451–455. doi: 10.1093/cercor/bhm088

Rachul, C., and Zarzeczny, A. (2012). The rise of neuroskepticism. *Int. J. Law Psychiatry* 35, 77–81. doi: 10.1016/j.ijlp.2011.12.008

Rubin, B. (2008). Therapeutic promise in the discourse of human embryonic stem cell research. *Sci. Cult.* 17, 13–27. doi: 10.1080/09505430701872962

Ruef, A., and Markard, J. (2010). What happens after a hype? How changing expectations affected innovation activities in the case of stationary fuel cells. *Technol. Anal. Strateg. Manage.* 22, 317–338. doi: 10.1080/09537321003647354

Rusconi, E., and Mitchener-Nissen, T. (2013). Prospects of functional magnetic resonance imaging as lie detector. *Front. Hum. Neurosci.* 7:594. doi: 10.3389/fnhum.2013.00594

Sartori, G., Agosta, S., Zogmaister, C., Ferrara, S. D., and Castiello, U. (2008). How to accurately detect autobiographical events. *Psychol. Sci.* 19, 772–780. doi: 10.1111/j.1467-9280.2008.02156.x

Sato, T., Tyler, W., Lamb, P., Wetmore, D., Chang, H., and Goldwasser, I. (2014). *Systems and Devices for Coupling Ultrasound Energy to a Body.* WIPO Patent WO 2014036170 A1.

Spence, S. A., Farrow, T. F., Herford, A. E., Wilkinson, I. D., Zheng, Y., and Woodruff, P. W. (2001). Behavioural and functional anatomical correlates of deception in humans. *Neuroreport* 12, 2849–2853. doi: 10.1097/00001756-200109170-00019

Standard Operating Procedure. (2008). *Documentary. Directed by Errol Morris. [DVD].* USA: Sony Pictures.

Stilgoe, J., Lock, S., and Wilsdon, J. (2014). Why should we promote public engagement with science? *Public Underst. Sci.* 23, 4–15. doi: 10.1177/0963662513518154

Tarabay, J. (2014). *Abu Ghraib Closes, Bitter Memories of Torture Remain.* Available online at: http://america.aljazeera.com/articles/2014/4/15/abu-ghraib-s-infamousend.html. Accessed on July 1, 2014.

Tutton, R. (2011). Promising pessimism: reading the futures to be avoided in biotech. *Soc. Stud. Sci.* 41, 411–429. doi: 10.1177/0306312710397398

Tyler, W. J. (2010). Remote control of brain activity using ultrasound (Armed with Science). Available online at: http://science.dodlive.mil/2010/09/01/remote-control-of-brain-activity-using-ultrasound/

van Lente, H. (1993). *Promising Technology: The Dynamics of Expectations in Technological Developments.* Amsterdam: Proefschrift.

van Lente, H., Spitters, C., and Peine, A. (2013). Comparing technological hype cycles: towards a theory. *Technol. Forecast. Soc. Change* 8, 1615–1628. doi: 10.1016/j.techfore.2012.12.004

Walsh, V. Q. (2013). Ethics and social risk in brain stimulation. *Brain Stimul.* 6, 715–717. doi: 10.1016/j.brs.2013.08.001

Wolpe, P. R. (2002). Treatment, enhancement and the ethics of neurotherapeutics. *Brain Cogn.* 50, 387–395. doi: 10.1016/s0278-2626(02)00534-1

Wright, G. R., Berry, C. J., and Bird, G. (2012). "You can't kid a kidder": association between production and detection of deception in an interactive deception task. *Front. Hum. Neurosci.* 6:87. doi: 10.3389/fnhum.2012.00087

14

Brain-machine interfaces can accelerate clarification of the principal mysteries and real plasticity of the brain

Yoshio Sakurai* *

Department of Psychology, Graduate School of Letters, Kyoto University, Kyoto, Japan

Edited by:
Mikhail Lebedev, Duke University, USA

Reviewed by:
Mikhail Lebedev, Duke University, USA
Ioan Opris, Wake Forest University, USA

****Correspondence:***
Yoshio Sakurai, Department of Psychology, Graduate School of Letters, Kyoto University, Yoshida-honmachi, Sakyo-ku, Kyoto 606-8501, Japan
e-mail: ysakurai@bun.kyoto-u.ac.jp

This perspective emphasizes that the brain-machine interface (BMI) research has the potential to clarify major mysteries of the brain and that such clarification of the mysteries by neuroscience is needed to develop BMIs. I enumerate five principal mysteries. The first is "how is information encoded in the brain?" This is the fundamental question for understanding what our minds are and is related to the verification of Hebb's cell assembly theory. The second is "how is information distributed in the brain?" This is also a reconsideration of the functional localization of the brain. The third is "what is the function of the ongoing activity of the brain?" This is the problem of how the brain is active during no-task periods and what meaning such spontaneous activity has. The fourth is "how does the bodily behavior affect the brain function?" This is the problem of brain-body interaction, and obtaining a new "body" by a BMI leads to a possibility of changes in the owner's brain. The last is "to what extent can the brain induce plasticity?" Most BMIs require changes in the brain's neuronal activity to realize higher performance, and the neuronal operant conditioning inherent in the BMIs further enhances changes in the activity.

Keywords: brain-machine interface, neuronal coding, cell assembly, functional localization, ongoing activity, brain-body interaction, brain plasticity

INTRODUCTION

A brain-machine interface (BMI) is used to enable the neuroprosthetic control of external devices by neuronal activity instead of body parts movements (Lebedev and Nicolelis, 2006; Berger et al., 2008; Hatsopoulos and Donoghue, 2009; Nicolelis and Lebedev, 2009; Andersen et al., 2010; Moran, 2010; Green and Kalaska, 2011; Lebedev, 2014). Although the development of invasive BMIs has been making a steady progress and holds promises for future clinical use (Lebedev and Nicolelis, 2011; Lebedev et al., 2011; Nicolelis, 2011; Ethier et al., 2012; Hochberg et al., 2012; Collinger et al., 2013), currently available BMIs are limited in terms of accuracy and efficiency with which they can be controlled. As described in the papers referenced above, it is possible to indicate some technical factors affecting the limited performance of current BMIs. However, as also emphasized in some of the papers (e.g., Nicolelis and Lebedev, 2009; Andersen et al., 2010), improvements in the technical factors alone cannot solve all the problems preventing the realization of an ideal BMI, i.e., a system controlling external neuroprosthetic devices freely as intended by the brain without any special training. The ideal BMI required rich and precise information that depends on the activity and function of the brain. Therefore, as Nicolelis (2003), Baranauskas (2014), and Mandonnet and Duffau (2014) has discussed, knowledge of what the brain is and how it works, the ultimate goals of neuroscience research, are essential for BMI research. To achieve these goals, the present paper enumerates five principal mysteries of the brain that must be clarified. It should be emphasized that BMI research has the potential to clarify these principal mysteries and, at the same time, their clarification by neuroscience research is necessary to realize the ideal BMI.

HOW IS INFORMATION ENCODED IN THE BRAIN?

As the final goal of a BMI is to detect neuronal activity representing information in the brain, BMI research inevitably faces the problem of how is information encoded in the working brain. Neuronal coding (e.g., Calvin, 1996; Abbott and Sejnowski, 1999; Nicolelis, 2001; Nicolelis and Ribeiro, 2006; Holscher and Munk, 2009) is one of the principal mysteries of the brain and may be the ultimate problem of neuroscience, because its final goal is to bridge the mind and brain and detect the mind from brain activity. The early studies of BMIs (Chapin et al., 1999; Wessberg et al., 2000; Nicolelis and Chapin, 2002) have already produced very important and instructive findings demonstrating the nature of the neuronal coding of information. They reported that the activity of only a limited number of neurons randomly sampled from the motor cortex of an animal provided sufficient information to predict arm kinematics during reaching, as well as hand gripping force. In addition, the accuracy of prediction increased as the number of recorded randomly sampled neurons increased. These results indicate that kinematic and kinetic parameters are coded not by the activities of specific motor-related neurons but by the activity of many neurons distributed in the motor cortex. Subsequent BMI studies more or less supported this notion of neuronal coding in the motor cortex (e.g., Carmena et al., 2003). Therefore, as Nicolelis (2003) and Nicolelis and Lebedev (2009) have suggested, a BMI both utilizes population coding by cell assemblies (Hebb, 1949), functionally connected neurons acting as codes representing information in the working brain (Eichenbaum, 1993; Sakurai, 1996b, 1999; Harris, 2005; Sakurai and Takahashi, 2006, 2008; Buzsáki, 2010; Wallace and Kerr, 2010; Sakurai et al., 2013), and provides new insights on this coding. In other words, the theory of cell assembly has been further verified by BMI studies and is approaching an answer to the mystery of neuronal coding.

Although recent neuroscience studies have often reported small populations of neurons related to information processing (e.g., Takahashi and Sakurai, 2009a,b; Opris et al., 2012, 2013) and BMI research has clearly supported the cell assembly theory, the existence of cell assemblies as carriers of neuronal codes has not yet been directly proven, because current BMIs have a bias in the firing rate or amplitude of neuronal activity used as the source signals. This bias may be a factor affecting the limited performance of current BMIs (Sakurai et al., 2014). According to the notion of cell assembly, synchronous and oscillatory activities among many neurons may have the potential to be informative signals for BMIs. It is expected to construct a BMI system which uses ensemble and correlated firing of distributed many neurons, in addition to their firing rates, as neuronal source signals.

HOW IS INFORMATION DISTRIBUTED IN THE BRAIN?

BMI studies have revealed the fact that the neurons whose activity can be used as signals representing information of motor movements are distributed in the motor cortex. Concerning the range of distribution of such neurons, some BMI studies have obtained an optimal basis for brain control of devices by recording the activity of neurons in the precentral (motor) cortical area associated with actual limb movement (Chapin et al., 1999; Taylor et al., 2002; Carmena et al., 2003; Hochberg et al., 2006; Koike et al., 2006; Choi et al., 2009). However, some other studies on BMIs demonstrated their ability to predict movements from neurons in the postcentral (parietal) as well as the precentral cortical areas (Wessberg et al., 2000; Carmena et al., 2003). Although precentral motor neurons can provide accurate predictions of force and displacement even in small numbers (Koike et al., 2006; Choi et al., 2009), many neurons from the parietal and other cortical areas could also have the potential to provide significant predictions. The prediction accuracy increased with the number of neurons included, even when the included neurons were randomly selected from the non-motor area and unrelated to motor movement in nature (Wessberg et al., 2000; Carmena et al., 2003). This indicates that neuronal information on motor movements and forces is widely distributed in cortical areas.

These findings by BMI studies could challenge the classical and conservative view of functional localization based on functional divisions in the brain. Constructing functional divisions is a major problem of neuroscience and many researchers are investigating what functions are localized in what brain areas. The results of BMI studies indicate that the functional boundaries are not definite and fixed but obscure and dynamic. Some BMIs do not necessarily require the selection of functionally specific motor neurons (e.g., Moritz et al., 2008) or, as described above, a specific motor area in the brain to improve their performance in brain control of devices. This notion may be related to the theory of multipotentiality of the brain (John, 1980). This theory suggests that any neuron and region may contribute to the mediation of a diversity of functions and that many neurons and regions contribute to many functions, although it does not imply that different neurons and regions have complete equivalence of functions or that different functions depend equally on diverse neurons and regions. BMI research may again direct the spotlight on the theory of multipotentiality and push back the view of too rigid and too subdivided functional maps. On the other hand, regarding the use of a BMI as a neuroprosthetic system, it is advantageous for it to have the potential to utilize any neuron and any brain region unrelated to the target functions replaced by the BMI.

WHAT IS THE FUNCTION OF THE ONGOING ACTIVITY OF THE BRAIN?

Invasive BMIs will be continuously introduced to use in daily life and should function to voluntarily control moving and resting external devices. Therefore, a principal mystery that BMI research requires present neuroscience to solve is, as Velliste et al. (2014) has discussed, how the brain is active during lengthy periods of behavioral inactivity when no specific tasks are, at least consciously, being performed. This is the problem of the "ongoing" or "intrinsic" activity of the brain (Vincent et al., 2007). Most neuroscience studies have not paid any attention to this problem and have devoted themselves to recording and analyzing neural activity only during the performance of various behavioral tasks. In such recording studies using behavioral tasks, most researchers have implicitly assumed that the spontaneous neural activity prior to the presentation of stimuli or motor responses is an independent random process and have treated it as "baseline activity" or "background noise" unrelated to information processing.

However, this view of spontaneous activity was challenged as early as the 1990s. For example, Arieli et al. (1995) reported that collective ensembles of activity of many neurons of the visual cortex occurred not only during stimulus-evoked periods but also during spontaneous non-stimulus periods. They suggested that the population activity of neurons is not an independent random process even during baseline periods. The correlated activity was detected among neurons comprising a population and among separate populations of neurons. It can be considered that these temporally correlated neurons and populations are cell assemblies, and the ongoing spontaneous activity of cell assemblies may reflect the processing of the context, which affects the processing of incoming sensory stimuli or motor responses (Arieli et al., 1995). The result of Sakurai (1996a) supports this notion, because the correlated activity of hippocampal and auditory cortical neurons, recorded during non-stimulus intertrial intervals, represented the context, i.e., the type of tasks that the animal was currently engaged in. These studies strongly indicate that important mechanisms underlying the higher integrative processing of perception, cognition, attention, and memory depend on the spatiotemporal interactions between ongoing and event-evoked activities of neurons and cell assemblies.

The significant role of the spontaneous activity of neuronal populations may be related to the assumption of "default mode network" suggested by noninvasive imaging (PET, fMRI) studies on human (Raichle, 2010) and monkey (Mantini et al., 2011) brains. The noninvasive images, which represent the activity of large populations of neurons, often show periodic synchronous activation across several close and distant cortical areas during periods of rest with no tasks. Raichle (2010, 2011) suggests that such periodic activation in multiple areas, the "default mode", has a preparatory function to process incoming sensory stimuli or motor responses. Therefore, the default mode and the ongoing activity have the same features and functions and indicate the significant role of the synchronous activity during periods with no tasks. Further clarification of its functional role must contribute to further development of BMIs that can be mounted continuously in daily life.

HOW DOES THE BODILY BEHAVIOR AFFECT THE BRAIN FUNCTION?

The brain controls behavioral functions of the body and, at the same time, the behavior of the body affects the activity of the brain (Chiel and Beer, 1997). In this notion of brain-body interaction, the problem of how bodily movements constrain brain activity is closely related to BMIs, because BMIs require the replacement of bodily movements with machine devices. Typical evidence of the bodily effect on brain activity and function is the "phantom limb" (Ramachandran and Hirstein, 1998). A sudden loss of parts of the body often causes drastic changes in tactile and movement-related perception and generates hallucinations of body images. This confused representation of perceptual information is considered to be due to the reorganization of neuronal networks and the following confused coding of sensory information (Melzack, 1990). Accordingly, a BMI might change functions of the brain, especially the neuronal coding of perceptual information.

The phenomenon of the phantom limb indicates that stable and precise coding in the brain requires stable and precise inputs of sensory information generated from the body. This is not restricted to tactile and movement-related sensations but also applicable to other sensory inputs. "Charles Bonnet syndrome" (Menon et al., 2003) is a typical case of visual hallucinations, i.e., the confused and spontaneous coding of perceptual information caused by the complete and long-lasting deprivation of visual inputs. In addition, isolation experiments cutting off visual, auditory, and tactile sensory inputs, originally discussed by Hebb (1949), showed that several types of hallucination can be generated even in short periods of sensory deprivation (Heron, 1957). If stable and precise sensory inputs are essential for the normal coding of information, the artificial operation of sensory inputs may correct the abnormal hallucinations caused by sensory deprivation. This assumption is supported by the "virtual reality box" experiment (Ramachandran and Hirstein, 1998), in which the artificial presentation of mirror images of lost parts of the body often changes or erases hallucinations that involve body images.

All these findings indicating the importance of sensory inputs consistent with bodily behaviors recommend the further development of BMIs equipped with sensory feedback contingent with the behaviors of brain-controlling devices. Recently, Tabot et al. (2013) have succeeded in restoring tactile feedback using a brain-controlled prosthetic hand. O'Doherty et al. (2011) have developed a BMBI (brain-machine-brain interface), which can provide a monkey with not only visual but also tactile feedback from a brain-controlled device (virtual hand). Further neuroscience research on brain-body interaction will contribute to development of BMBIs, and progress in BMBI research will clarify how the brain interacts with the body, encodes sensory information, and constructs body images (Shokur et al., 2013).

TO WHAT EXTENT CAN THE BRAIN INDUCE PLASTICITY?

This final section further discusses the BMI-induced plasticity of the brain and emphasizes why it is inevitable in all BMIs. Some studies have reported clear changes in the plasticity of neuronal activities and functions induced by the use of BMIs (e.g., Zacksenhouse et al., 2007; Ganguly et al., 2011). Such plastic changes can be thought to be induced to some extent in most BMI experiments, in which the conversion of neuronal signals is aided by appropriate transform algorithms to generate suitable control parameters. The conversion parameters obtained for one set of trials provided increasingly poor predictions of future responses, indicating the drift of neuronal signals over tens of minutes. Therefore, accurate device control under BMI conditions inevitably requires the neuronal activity to be volitionally modulated to become more suitable signals for device control, and the brain surely responds to the request for activity modulation. The BMI-induced changes in neuronal activity are not restricted to the regions from which signals used for device control are recorded. Koralek et al. (2012, 2013) investigated the role of corticostriatal plasticity, usually involved in learning physical skills, in abstract skill learning by a BMI using motor cortical neurons. During the learning of control by the BMI, an alteration of activity was observed in the striatal neurons, and strong correlations, reflected in oscillatory coupling, between the neuronal activity in the motor cortex and the striatum emerged. The authors concluded that temporally precise coherence develops specifically in motor output-related neuronal populations during learning and that the oscillatory activity serves to synchronize widespread brain networks to produce appropriate behaviors.

Discussion of the mechanisms of BMI-induced plastic changes in neuronal activity also requires a psychological view, i.e., operant conditioning. In most BMI situations, the successful control of devices can function as a reward and reinforces the occurrence of volitionally modulated neuronal activity to control the devices. This process of reinforcing the volitional modulation of activity is the operant conditioning of neuronal activity (Fetz, 1969). All BMIs are thought to include this process of conditioning (Fetz, 2007; Sakurai et al., 2014), making plastic changes in neuronal activity inevitable. This leads to the argument that the investigation of neuronal operant conditioning (neurofeedback)

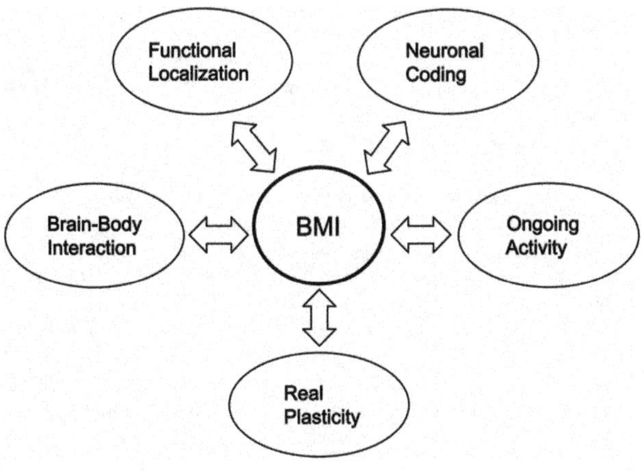

FIGURE 1 | Interactive advancement of researches on BMIs and the principal mysteries of the brain.

will inevitably contribute to the realization of higher-performing BMIs (Fetz, 2007; Moritz et al., 2008; Sakurai et al., 2014). In addition, research on the operant conditioning of synchrony and oscillation of neurons (Engelhard et al., 2013; Fetz, 2013; Sakurai and Takahashi, 2013), i.e., the activity of cell assemblies, will also significantly contribute to the development of BMIs (Sakurai et al., 2014).

It should be noted that the neuronal plasticity inherent in BMI experiments is not always an obstacle for the development of higher-performing BMIs and can be actively applied to research on the extent to which the brain can change and how the brain can be changed efficiently. The former means that BMI studies are able to classify the real plasticity of the brain. The latter suggests that the development of BMIs will lead to the development of better methods of neurorehabilitation to induce changes in neuronal activities and connections for functional compensation (Dobkin, 2007; Fetz, 2007; Jackson and Fetz, 2011; Miller and Weber, 2011).

CONCLUSION

Although research in modern neuroscience has made great progress, BMI research has shown that we still do not fully understand even the major properties of the brain, i.e., the principal mysteries enumerated in the present paper. BMI research has the role of impelling present neuroscience to clarify the major properties, including the real plasticity, of the brain, and further progress in neuroscience in uncovering the properties of the brain contributes to the further development of BMIs (**Figure 1**).

ACKNOWLEDGMENTS

This work was supported by JST Core Research for Evolution Science and Technology (CREST) program and JSPS KAKENHI grant Nos. 24223004 and 24243069 (Yoshio Sakurai).

REFERENCES

Abbott, L., and Sejnowski, T. J. (1999). *Neural Codes and Distributed Representations.* Cambridge: MIT Press.

Andersen, R. A., Hwang, E. J., and Mulliken, G. H. (2010). Cognitive neural prosthetics. *Annu. Rev. Psychol.* 61, 169–190. doi: 10.1146/annurev.psych.093008.100503

Arieli, A., Shoham, D., Hildesheim, R., and Grinvald, A. (1995). Coherent spatiotemporal patterns of ongoing activity revealed by real-time optical imaging coupled with single-unit recording in the cat visual cortex. *J. Neurophysiol.* 73, 2072–2093.

Baranauskas, G. (2014). What limits the performance of current invasive brain machine interfaces? *Front. Sys. Neurosci.* 8:68. doi: 10.3389/fnsys.2014.00068

Berger, T. W., Chapin, J. K., Gerhardt, G. A., McFarland, D. J., Principe, J. C., Soussou, W. V., et al. (2008). *Brain-Computer Interfaces.* New York: Springer.

Buzsáki, G. (2010). Neural syntax: cell assemblies, synapsembles, and readers. *Neuron* 68, 362–385. doi: 10.1016/j.neuron.2010.09.023

Calvin, W. H. (1996). *The Cerebral Code—Thinking a Thought in the Mosaics of the Mind.* Cambridge: MIT Press.

Carmena, J. M., Lebedev, M. A., Crist, R. E., O'Doherty, J. E., Santucci, D. M., Dimitrov, D. F., et al. (2003). Learning to control a brain-machine interface for reaching and grasping by primates. *PLoS Biol.* 1:E42. doi: 10.1371/journal.pbio.0000042

Chapin, J. K., Moxon, K. A., Markowitz, R. S., and Nicolelis, M. A. (1999). Real-time control of a robot arm using simultaneously recorded neurons in the motor cortex. *Nat. Neurosci.* 2, 664–670. doi: 10.1038/10223

Chiel, H. J., and Beer, R. D. (1997). The brain has a body: adaptive behavior emerges from interactions of nervous system, body and environment. *Trends Neurosci.* 20, 553–557. doi: 10.1016/s0166-2236(97)01149-1

Choi, K., Hirose, H., Sakurai, Y., Iijima, T., and Koike, Y. (2009). Prediction of arm trajectory from the neural activities of the primary motor cortex with modular connectionist architecture. *Neural Netw.* 22, 1214–1223. doi: 10.1016/j.neunet.2009.09.003

Collinger, J. L., Wodlinger, B., Downey, J. E., Wang, W., Tyler-Kabara, E. C., Weber, D. J., et al. (2013). High-performance neuroprosthetic control by an individual with tetraplegia. *Lancet* 381, 557–564. doi: 10.1016/s0140-6736(12)61816-9

Dobkin, B. H. (2007). Brain-computer interface technology as a tool to augment plasticity and outcomes for neurological rehabilitation. *J. Physiol.* 579, 637–642. doi: 10.1113/jphysiol.2006.123067

Eichenbaum, H. (1993). Thinking about brain cell assemblies. *Science* 261, 993–994. doi: 10.1126/science.8351525

Engelhard, B., Ozeri, N., Israel, Z., Bergman, H., and Vaadia, E. (2013). Inducing gamma oscillations and precise spike synchrony by operant conditioning via brain-machine interface. *Neuron* 77, 361–375. doi: 10.1016/j.neuron.2012.11.015

Ethier, C., Oby, E. R., Bauman, M. J., and Miller, L. E. (2012). Restoration of grasp following paralysis through brain-controlled stimulation of muscles. *Nature* 485, 368–371. doi: 10.1038/nature10987

Fetz, E. E. (1969). Operant conditioning of cortical unit activity. *Science* 163, 955–958. doi: 10.1126/science.163.3870.955

Fetz, E. E. (2007). Volitional control of neural activity: implications for brain-computer interfaces. *J. Physiol.* 579, 571–579. doi: 10.1113/jphysiol.2006.127142

Fetz, E. E. (2013). Volitional control of cortical oscillations and synchrony. *Neuron* 77, 216–218. doi: 10.1016/j.neuron.2013.01.003

Ganguly, K., Domitrov, D. F., Wallis, J. D., and Carmena, J. M. (2011). Reversible large-scale modification of cortical networks during neuroprosthetic control. *Nat. Neurosci.* 14, 662–667. doi: 10.1038/nn.2797

Green, A. M., and Kalaska, J. F. (2011). Learning to move machines with the mind. *Trends Neurosci.* 34, 61–75. doi: 10.1016/j.tins.2010.11.003

Harris, K. D. (2005). Neural signatures of cell assembly organization. *Nat. Rev. Neurosci.* 6, 399–407. doi: 10.1038/nrn1669

Hatsopoulos, N. G., and Donoghue, J. P. (2009). The science of neural interface systems. *Annu. Rev. Neurosci.* 32, 249–266. doi: 10.1146/annurev.neuro.051508.135241

Hebb, D. O. (1949). *The Organization of Behavior—A Neuropsychological Theory.* New York: Wiley.

Heron, W. (1957). The pathology of boredom. *Sci. Am.* 196, 52–56. doi: 10.1038/scientificamerican0157-52

Hochberg, L. R., Bacher, D., Jarosiewicz, B., Masse, N. Y., Simeral, J. D., Vogel, J., et al. (2012). Reach and grasp by people with tetraplegia using a neurally controlled robotic arm. *Nature* 485, 372–375. doi: 10.1038/nature11076

Hochberg, L. R., Serruya, M. D., Friehs, G. M., Mukand, J. A., Saleh, M., Caplan, A. H., et al. (2006). Neuronal ensemble control of prosthetic devices by a human with tetraplegia. *Nature* 442, 164–171. doi: 10.1038/nature04970

Holscher, C., and Munk, M. (2009). *Information Processing by Neuronal Populations.* New York: Cambridge University Press.

Jackson, A., and Fetz, E. E. (2011). Interfacing with the computational brain. *IEEE Trans. Neural Syst. Rehabil. Eng.* 19, 534–541. doi: 10.1109/tnsre.2011.2158586

John, E. R. (1980). "Multipotentiality: a statistical theory of brain function–evidence and implications," in *The Psychobiology of Consciousness*, ed D. Richard (New York: Springer), 129–146.

Koike, Y., Hirose, H., Sakurai, Y., and Iijima, T. (2006). Prediction of arm trajectory from a small number of neuron activities in the primary motor cortex. *Neurosci. Res.* 55, 146–153. doi: 10.1016/j.neures.2006.02.012

Koralek, A. C., Costa, R. M., and Carmena, J. M. (2013). Temporally precise cell-specific coherence develops in corticostriatal networks during learning. *Neuron* 79, 865–872. doi: 10.1016/j.neuron.2013.06.047

Koralek, A. C., Jin, X., Long, J. D. II., Costa, R. M., and Carmena, J. M. (2012). Corticostriatal plasticity is necessary for learning intentional neuroprosthetic skills. *Nature* 483, 331–335. doi: 10.1038/nature10845

Lebedev, M. A. (2014). Brain-machine interfaces: an overview. *Trans. Neurosci.* 5, 99–110. doi: 10.2478/s13380-014-0212-z

Lebedev, M. A., and Nicolelis, M. A. L. (2006). Brain-machine interfaces: past, present and future. *Trends Neurosci.* 29, 536–546. doi: 10.1016/j.tins.2006.07.004

Lebedev, M. A., and Nicolelis, M. A. L. (2011). Toward a whole body neuroprosthetic. *Prog. Brain Res.* 194, 47–60. doi: 10.1016/b978-0-444-53815-4.00018-2

Lebedev, M. A., Tate, A. J., Hanson, T. L., Li, Z., O'Doherty, J. E., Winans, J. A., et al. (2011). Future developments in brain-machine interface research. *Clinics (Sao Paulo)* 66(Suppl. 1), 25–32. doi: 10.1590/s1807-59322011001300004

Mandonnet, E., and Duffau, H. (2014). Understanding entangled cerebral networks: a prerequisite for restoring brain function with brain-computer interfaces. *Front. Sys. Neurosci.* 8:82. doi: 10.3389/fnsys.2014.00082

Mantini, D., Gerits, A., Neilssen, K., Durand, J.-B., Joly, O., Simone, L., et al. (2011). Default mode of brain function in monkeys. *J. Neurosci.* 31, 12954–12962. doi: 10.1523/JNEUROSCI.2318-11.2011

Melzack, R. (1990). Phantom limbs and the concept of a neuromatrix. *Trends Neurosci.* 13, 88–92. doi: 10.1016/0166-2236(90)90179-e

Menon, G. J., Rahman, I., Menon, S. J., and Dutton, G. N. (2003). Complex visual hallucinations in the visually impaired: the Charles Bonnet Syndrome. *Surv. Ophthalmol.* 48, 58–72. doi: 10.1016/S0039-6257(02)00414-9

Miller, L. E., and Weber, D. J. (2011). Brain training: cortical plasticity and afferent feedback in brain-machine interface system. *IEEE Trans. Neural Syst. Rehabil. Eng.* 19, 465–467. doi: 10.1109/tnsre.2011.2168989

Moran, D. (2010). Evolution of brain-computer interface: action potentials, local field potentials and electrocorticograms. *Cur. Opin. Neurobiol.* 20, 741–745. doi: 10.1016/j.conb.2010.09.010

Moritz, C. T., Perimutter, S. I., and Fetz, E. E. (2008). Direct control of paralysed muscles by cortical neurons. *Nature* 456, 639–642. doi: 10.1038/nature07418

Nicolelis, M. A. L. (2001). *Advances in Neural Population Coding (Progress in Brain Research)* (Vol. 130). New York: Elsevier.

Nicolelis, M. A. L. (2003). Brain–machine interfaces to restore motor function and probe neural circuits. *Nat. Rev. Neurosci.* 4, 417–422. doi: 10.1038/nrn1105

Nicolelis, M. A. L. (2011). Mind out of body. *Sci. Am.* 304, 80–83. doi: 10.1038/scientificamerican0211-80

Nicolelis, M. A. L., and Chapin, J. K. (2002). Controlling robots with the mind. *Sci. Am.* 287, 46–53. doi: 10.1038/scientificamerican1002-46

Nicolelis, M. A. L., and Lebedev, M. A. (2009). Principles of neural ensemble physiology underlying the operation of brain-machine interfaces. *Nat. Rev. Neurosci.* 10, 530–540. doi: 10.1038/nrn2653

Nicolelis, M. A. L., and Ribeiro, S. (2006). Seeking the neural code. *Sci. Am.* 295, 70–77. doi: 10.1038/scientificamerican1206-70

O'Doherty, J. E., Lebedev, M. A., Ifft, P. J., Zhuang, K. Z., Shokur, S., Bleuler, H., et al. (2011). Active tactile exploration enabled by a brain-machine-brain interface. *Nature* 479, 228–231. doi: 10.1038/nature10489

Opris, I., Fuqua, J. L., Huettl, P. F., Gerhardt, G. A., Berger, T. W., Hampson, R. E., et al. (2012). Closing the loop in primate prefrontal cortex: inter-laminar processing. *Front. Neural Circuits* 6:88. doi: 10.3389/fncir.2012.00088

Opris, I., Santos, L., Gerhardt, G. A., Song, D., Berger, T. W., Hampson, R. E., et al. (2013). Prefrontal cortical microcircuits bind perception to executive control. *Sci. Rep.* 3:2285. doi: 10.1038/srep02285

Raichle, M. E. (2010). Two views of brain function. *Trends Cogn. Sci.* 14, 180–190. doi: 10.1016/j.tics.2010.01.008

Raichle, M. E. (2011). The restless brain. *Brain Connect.* 1, 3–12. doi: 10.1089/brain.2011.0019

Ramachandran, V. S., and Hirstein, W. (1998). The perception of phantom limbs. The D. O. Hebb lecture. *Brain* 121, 1603–1630. doi: 10.1093/brain/121.9.1603

Sakurai, Y. (1996a). Hippocampal and neocortical cell assemblies encode memory processes for different types of stimuli in the rat. *J. Neurosci.* 16, 2809–2819.

Sakurai, Y. (1996b). Population coding by cell assemblies—what it really is in the brain. *Neurosci. Res.* 26, 1–16. doi: 10.1016/0168-0102(96)01075-9

Sakurai, Y. (1999). How do cell assemblies encode information in the brain? *Neurosci. Biobehav. Rev.* 23, 785–796. doi: 10.1016/s0149-7634(99)00017-2

Sakurai, Y., and Takahashi, S. (2006). Dynamic synchrony of firing in the monkey prefrontal cortex during working memory tasks. *J. Neurosci.* 26, 10141–10153. doi: 10.1523/jneurosci.2423-06.2006

Sakurai, Y., and Takahashi, S. (2008). Dynamic synchrony of local cell assembly. *Rev. Neurosci.* 19, 425–440. doi: 10.1515/revneuro.2008.19.6.425

Sakurai, Y., and Takahashi, S. (2013). Conditioned enhancement of firing rates and synchrony of hippocampal neurons and firing rates of motor cortical neurons in rats. *Eur. J. Neurosci.* 37, 623–639. doi: 10.1111/ejn.12070

Sakurai, Y., Nakazono, T., Ishino, S., Terada, S., Yamaguchi, K., and Takahashi, S. (2013). Diverse synchrony of firing reflects diverse cell-assembly coding in the prefrontal cortex. *J. Physiol. Paris* 107, 459–470. doi: 10.1016/j.jphysparis.2013.05.004

Sakurai, Y., Song, K., Tachibana, S., and Takahashi, S. (2014). Volitional enhancement of firing synchrony and oscillation by neuronal operant conditioning: interaction with neurorehabilitation and brain-machine interface. *Front. Sys. Neurosci.* 8:11. doi: 10.3389/fnsys.2014.00011

Shokur, S., O'Doherty, J. E., Winans, J. A., Bleuler, H., Lebedev, M. A., and Nicolelis, M. A. L. (2013). Expanding the primate body schema in sensorimotor cortex by virtual touches of an avatar. *Proc. Natl. Acad. Sci. U S A* 110, 15121–15126. doi: 10.1073/pnas.1308459110

Tabot, G. A., Dammann, J. F., Berg, J. A., Tenore, F. V., Boback, J., Vogelstein, R. J., et al. (2013). Restoring the sense of touch with a prosthetic hand through a brain interface. *Proc. Natl. Acad. Sci. U S A* 110, 18279–18284. doi: 10.1073/pnas.1221113110

Takahashi, S., and Sakurai, Y. (2009a). Information in small neuronal ensemble activity in the hippocampal CA1 during delayed non-matching to sample performance in rats. *BMC Neurosci.* 10:115. doi: 10.1186/1471-2202-10-115

Takahashi, S., and Sakurai, Y. (2009b). Sub-millisecond firing synchrony of closely neighboring pyramidal neurons in hippocampal CA1 of rats during delayed non-matching to sample task. *Front. Neural Circuits* 3:9. doi: 10.3389/neuro.04.009.2009

Taylor, D. M., Tillery, S. I., and Schwartz, A. B. (2002). Direct cortical control of 3D neuroprosthetic devices. *Science* 296, 1829–1832. doi: 10.1126/science.1070291

Velliste, M., Kennedy, S. D., Schwartz, A. B., Whitford, A. S., Sohn, J.-W., and McMorland, A. J. C. (2014). Motor cortical correlates of arm resting in the context of a reaching task and implications for prosthetic control. *J. Neurosci.* 34, 6011–6022. doi: 10.1523/jneurosci.3520-13.2014

Vincent, J. L., Patel, G. H., Fox, M. D., Snyder, A. Z., Baker, J. T., Van Essen, D. C., et al. (2007). Intrinsic functional architecture in the anaesthetized monkey brain. *Nature* 447, 83–86. doi: 10.1038/nature05758

Wallace, D. J., and Kerr, J. N. (2010). Chasing the cell assembly. *Curr. Opin. Neurobiol.* 20, 296–305. doi: 10.1016/j.conb.2010.05.003

15

Hypothesis-driven methods to augment human cognition by optimizing cortical oscillations

Jörn M. Horschig[1]*, Johanna M. Zumer[1,2] and Ali Bahramisharif[1]

[1] Radboud University Nijmegen, Donders Institute for Brain, Behaviour and Cognition, Nijmegen, Netherlands
[2] School of Psychology, University of Birmingham, Birmingham, UK

Edited by:
Mikhail Lebedev, Duke University, USA

Reviewed by:
Markus Werkle-Bergner, Max Planck Institute for Human Development, Germany
Sepideh Sadaghiani, University of California Berkeley, USA
Ali Mazaheri, University of Amsterdam, Netherlands

***Correspondence:**
Jörn M. Horschig, Radboud University Nijmegen, Donders Institute for Brain, Behaviour and Cognition, Kapittelweg 29, 6525 EN Nijmegen, Netherlands
e-mail: jm.horschig@donders.ru.nl

Cortical oscillations have been shown to represent fundamental functions of a working brain, e.g., communication, stimulus binding, error monitoring, and inhibition, and are directly linked to behavior. Recent studies intervening with these oscillations have demonstrated effective modulation of both the oscillations and behavior. In this review, we collect evidence in favor of how hypothesis-driven methods can be used to augment cognition by optimizing cortical oscillations. We elaborate their potential usefulness for three target groups: healthy elderly, patients with attention deficit/hyperactivity disorder, and healthy young adults. We discuss the relevance of neuronal oscillations in each group and show how each of them can benefit from the manipulation of functionally-related oscillations. Further, we describe methods for manipulation of neuronal oscillations including direct brain stimulation as well as indirect task alterations. We also discuss practical considerations about the proposed techniques. In conclusion, we propose that insights from neuroscience should guide techniques to augment human cognition, which in turn can provide a better understanding of how the human brain works.

Keywords: neuronal oscillations, working memory, attention, elderly, ADHD, brain stimulation, brain-computer interfacing, brain state dependent tasks

INTRODUCTION

Recent advances in cognitive neuroscience have provided insight into the functional mechanisms of the human brain. Neuroscientists have identified specific brain patterns, for example neuronal oscillations, that co-fluctuate with the task and behavioral performance (Buzsáki, 2006). These fluctuations are not random but depend on the specific task and cognitive settings; these findings have allowed functional hypotheses to be formed, directly tested, and confirmed. Throughout the previous decades, huge progress has been made in understanding how the human brain works, and in understanding differences across age groups, pathologies, and individuals. Applying this in-depth knowledge in practice might therefore be a key to creating brain tools for different target groups to improve different aspects of human cognition.

Cognitive functioning declines with age (Deary et al., 2009) and does not necessarily occur in the presence of a neurological disorder. Healthy elderly suffer from problems with memory and attention more than healthy, young individuals. With an increasing aging population, it has become a societal priority to look into approaches that can delay or prevent functional degeneracy or even augment cognitive abilities in the elderly. Brain tools might have the potential to rejuvenate the functionality of an aging brain.

Many people suffer from cognitive deficiencies in daily activities, but there are population groups in which these problems are more severe. Attention deficit/hyperactivity disorder (ADHD) is a well-studied disorder with problems of attention, hyperactivity, and impulsivity. Although the cause of ADHD is unknown, there have been many attempts to treat it using medication (e.g., Chang et al., 2012). Next to many unknown side-effects of medication, about 30% of the ADHD population do not respond to any medication, which calls for alternative treatments (Kidd, 2000). Brain tools might serve this population by normalizing their brain activities.

Most of our knowledge from cognitive neuroscience about the human brain stems from studies on healthy, young individuals, which have helped to form functional hypotheses about traits of human brain activity. These hypotheses can serve as a benchmark for other populations groups. In addition, also healthy young adults show large task variability in cognitive tasks. Next to individual differences, individuals' performance varies momentarily in cognitive tasks (Kane and Engle, 2002; Paulus et al., 2009). Thus, while constituting a proper control group, we will also discuss our current knowledge on whether young, healthy adults can benefit from cognitive improvements.

The brain is a highly flexible organ which can adapt to different manipulations very quickly (Pascual-Leone et al., 2011). Entrainment of neuronal oscillations to augment human behavior has already been proposed in the past (see e.g., Thut et al., 2011a; Herrmann et al., 2013; Calderone et al., 2014; Enriquez-Geppert et al., 2014). We complement these reviews by proposing different techniques in different target groups to relate the to-be-augmented aspect of cognition to associated neuronal signatures, specifically neuronal oscillations. Identifying the neural signatures of different tasks will allow for proposing protocols for manipulating the brain and thereby the individual's cognitive abilities. Recent studies suggest a causal role of neuronal oscillations in cognitive tasks (Thut and Miniussi, 2009; Romei et al., 2010). Based on this hypothesis and the possibility of manipulating neuronal oscillations in several ways, we propose that by using "hypothesis-driven" approaches, one can augment human cognition by optimizing cortical oscillations. In this paper, we begin with discussing the functional role of neuronal oscillations and their cognitive relevance. We then continue with more details about three target population groups, healthy elderly, patients with ADHD, and healthy young adults, and elaborate on how cognitive improvement can be gained. Next, we go into different ways of manipulating functional oscillations in order to improve cognitive performance in the three target groups. The paper ends with practical considerations and conclusions.

FUNCTIONAL ROLE OF NEURONAL OSCILLATIONS

Spontaneous and goal-related fluctuations of the brain state are reflected in electrophysiological activity that can be measured non-invasively using various techniques like electroencephalography (EEG) and magnetoencephalography (MEG). EEG and MEG measure the strength of the voltage potentials and magnetic fields at the scalp associated with postsynaptic potentials along the dendrites of pyramidal neurons, i.e., the synaptic input to these cells (Nunez, 2000; Niedermeyer and Lopes da Silva, 2005; Wang, 2010; Lopes da Silva, 2013). Non-invasive measurements require strongly synchronized activity across nearby neurons to result in a measurable signal at scalp level. Neuronal oscillations at the scalp level are rhythmic patterns that represent the degree of synchronized neuronal input to the underlying neuronal ensemble (Lopes da Silva, 1991; Buzsáki and Draguhn, 2004), which are reflected as power increases (commonly known as event-related synchronization, ERS) or power decreases (event-related desynchronization, ERD; see Pfurtscheller and Lopes da Silva, 1999).

Neuronal oscillations are commonly divided into different frequency bands. While lower frequencies are often associated with long-range connectivity between cortical regions (von Stein and Sarnthein, 2000), higher frequencies reflect the local firing pattern of neurons (Xing et al., 2012). Furthermore, different neuronal oscillations have been associated with specific neuronal processes (e.g., Engel et al., 2001; Kopell et al., 2010), which have been related to behavioral performance, e.g., in attention and working memory tasks (reviewed in more detail below). In this paper, we will focus on cortical oscillations in three frequency bands: alpha oscillations (8–13 Hz), theta oscillations (5–8 Hz), and gamma oscillations (>30 Hz). In the following, we will introduce these three oscillations, describe the current dominant views on their function, and elucidate their role on qualitative aspects of cognition.[1]

ALPHA OSCILLATIONS (8–13 HZ): FUNCTIONAL INHIBITION OF NEURONAL REGIONS

Human alpha oscillations are the dominant rhythms in EEG and MEG. They were observed almost a century ago (Berger, 1929; Adrian and Matthews, 1934) and, while originally having been associated with the idle state of the visual cortex, the current dominant view has changed towards a functional, inhibitory role, elaborated upon below. Alpha is generated via thalamocortical and cortico-cortical loops (Lopes Da Silva and Storm Van Leeuwen, 1977; Lopes da Silva et al., 1980; Suffczynski et al., 2001; Bollimunta et al., 2011). Cortical alpha has been shown to be modulated by the pulvinar nucleus of the thalamus (Saalmann et al., 2012) as well as by frontal regions (Capotosto et al., 2009). The precise mediation of cortical alpha via the interplay between frontocortical and subcortical mechanisms still requires further investigation. Individual variations of alpha power appear as stable traits. The peak frequency of alpha oscillations has been related to the latent factors of general cognitive abilities, and the frequency and power of alpha oscillations have been shown to change with age (Klimesch, 1999; Grandy et al., 2013).

Alpha oscillations are strongly involved in attention processes. While low alpha activity can be observed in regions that are processing information, sensory regions that are not involved in the current task show high alpha activity. For example, in covert spatial attention studies, selective attention and successful inhibition of the task-irrelevant hemifield are often indexed using the extent of alpha power lateralization. Highly lateralized alpha activity thereby suggests a high inhibition of the task-irrelevant hemifield and has been shown to lead to better task performance (Worden et al., 2000; Thut et al., 2006; Kelly et al., 2009), whereas a weak or reverse alpha lateralization leads to failures in motor inhibition (Bengson et al., 2012). During the retention interval of working memory tasks, it has been shown that the degree of alpha power increase in early sensory regions scales with memory load (Jensen et al., 2002). This effect also holds true for paradigms in non-visual domains, e.g., occipital alpha increases during a somatosensory delayed-match-to-sample task (Haegens et al., 2010; Spitzer and Blankenburg, 2012). Additionally, strong alpha during the immediate rehearsal of an item for long-term memory encoding has been shown to predict the long-term memory encoding success (Meeuwissen et al., 2011). Alpha activity has therefore been suggested to reflect the amount of top-down controlled cortical inhibition (reviewed in Klimesch, 1999, 2012; Klimesch et al., 2007; Jensen and Mazaheri, 2010; Foxe and Snyder, 2011; Jensen et al., 2012).

Alpha oscillations are also strongly involved in the anticipation of upcoming stimuli, which has been convincingly shown by Rohenkohl and Nobre (2011). They showed that when stimulation was temporally anticipated but absent, alpha power decreased to a similar degree compared to when stimulation actually occurred when anticipated, see **Figure 1A**. Moreover, the degree of anticipatory alpha power correlates with subsequent

[1] Note that we focus on power of the oscillation and do not cover its phasic role. Other frequency bands, such as delta (1–3 Hz) or beta (13–30 Hz) oscillations, or slow cortical potentials lie outside the scope of this article. Some alternative approaches are shortly discussed in Section Alternative Aspects of Neuronal Oscillations to Utilize.

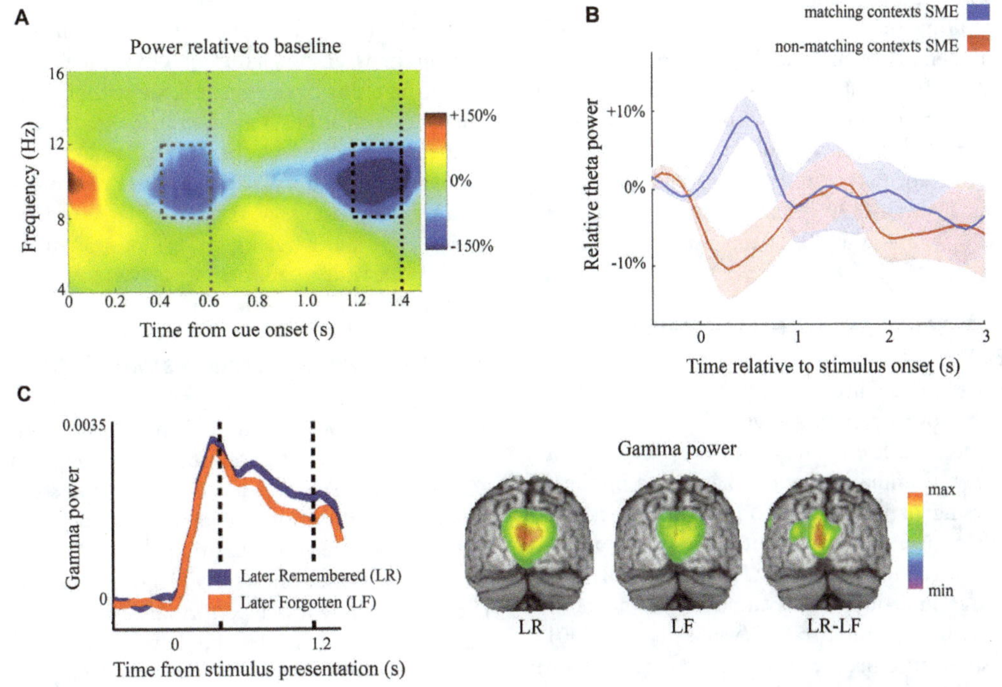

FIGURE 1 | Example of the functional involvement of neuronal oscillations. (A) The time-frequency representation of an anticipation task. The gray dotted line shows the time that the stimulus could have been presented, but was not. The black dotted line indicates the onset of the target. Alpha power decreases in anticipation of a stimulus even without subsequent stimulation. Reproduced with permission from Rohenkohl and Nobre (2011). **(B)** The dynamics of frontal theta power. Depending on the encoding task, both increases and decreases of frontal theta power were found for successful versus unsuccessful remembering. SME = subsequent memory effect. Reproduced with permission from Hanslmayr and Staudigl (2014). **(C)** During visual stimulus encoding, posterior gamma power (60–90 Hz) is predictive of subsequent memory performance in young, healthy adults. The vertical dashed bars indicate the window for significance testing and beamformer application. The left panel shows gamma power from one significant posterior sensor and the right panel is the beamformer projection (Osipova et al., 2006).

behavioral performance in attention tasks (Worden et al., 2000; Thut et al., 2006; Kelly et al., 2009) and correlates with subsequent long-term memory performance (Park et al., 2014). Anticipatory alpha power also scales with stimulation likelihood (Gould et al., 2011; Haegens et al., 2012; Horschig et al., 2014). Upon stimulation, however, alpha oscillations robustly decrease in early sensory regions. Recently, Hanslmayr et al. (2012) suggested an entropy-based explanation for this: the more complex the information is that needs to be encoded, the less structured (i.e., the more de-synchronized) the activity in a network has to be. An alternative explanation, which is not mutually exclusive, is that early sensory regions become disinhibited, i.e., functionally engaged, and therefore show low alpha power.

THETA OSCILLATIONS (5–8 HZ): WORKING MEMORY AND NEURONAL ORGANIZATION

Depending on where in the brain theta oscillations are observed, they can be divided into two groups of hippocampal and cortical theta rhythms (reviewed in Mitchell et al., 2008). In this paper we only focus on the cortical theta rhythms that can be measured non-invasively and are probably generated in hippocampal-cortical feedback loops (Klimesch, 1999). Cortical theta power has been related to encoding, retaining, and retrieving items in working memory (Kahana et al., 2001; Klimesch et al., 2010; Sauseng et al., 2010). The frequency of theta rhythms shows a large inter-individual variability similar to alpha oscillations, and the individual theta peak frequency has been shown to be significantly correlated to the individual alpha peak frequency (Klimesch et al., 1996).

During working memory tasks, theta power increases over temporal sites during encoding, maintenance, and retrieval (Raghavachari et al., 2001; Fell et al., 2011). Over frontal regions, theta power increases proportionally with task demands (Gevins et al., 1997). In working memory tasks, for example, a higher memory load produces stronger frontal theta activity (Jensen and Tesche, 2002). However, both frontal theta increases and decreases have been found to be beneficial for successful memory retrieval (Staudigl and Hanslmayr, 2013; see **Figure 1B**). Hanslmayr and Staudigl (2014) recently suggested that the context of the memory and the probe items is the crucial factor for whether theta increases or decreases upon successful retrieval. Raghavachari et al. (2006), however, argued for local theta generators where frontal theta exerts executive control and parietal theta serves to maintain items in working memory.

Apart from their role in working memory, frontal theta oscillations link prediction errors to behavioral adaptations (Cavanagh et al., 2010). Theta oscillations are also involved in long-range neuronal communication between cortical and subcortical regions including the hippocampus (Mitchell et al., 2008) and nucleus accumbens (Cohen et al., 2009, 2012) as well as for corticocortical communication (reviewed in von Stein and Sarnthein, 2000). In conclusion, contemporary theory posits that theta oscillations are crucially involved in the organization and coordination of information and for memory storage and retrieval (Jensen and Lisman, 1996; Buzsáki and Draguhn, 2004; Lisman, 2005, 2010; Sauseng et al., 2010; Lisman and Jensen, 2013).

GAMMA (>30 HZ): PERCEPTUAL AND MULTISENSORY BINDING AND MEMORY MAINTENANCE

Gamma oscillations are defined as frequencies above 30 Hz, subdivided into the lower gamma range (30–80 Hz) and the higher gamma range (>80 Hz; Buzsáki and Draguhn, 2004; Ray and Maunsell, 2011). Gamma oscillations have been implicated with active processing of information and thus increase with stimulation intensity and amount of attention to stimulation (Engel and Singer, 2001; Engel et al., 2001; Fries et al., 2001; Jensen et al., 2007). A large inter-individual variability in the gamma peak frequency has been demonstrated (van Pelt et al., 2012) as well as a correspondence between the gamma peak frequency and the characteristics of the visual stimuli (van Pelt and Fries, 2013).

Gamma oscillations are also observed during working memory maintenance (Tallon-Baudry et al., 1998; Miltner et al., 1999; Jokisch and Jensen, 2007), possibly reflecting active processing and binding of the to-be-maintained information in frontal and parietal cortices (Polanía et al., 2012b). The degree of gamma power during encoding of visual items has been found to correlate with working memory load (Howard et al., 2003) and predicts successful memory encoding, see **Figure 1C** (Osipova et al., 2006). Also, during successful multisensory integration, an increase of gamma band power has been observed (Schneider et al., 2008; Kanayama et al., 2012), strengthening the idea that gamma band oscillations serve to form a coherent object representation in working memory. Gamma band activity has been suggested to reflect the process of mentally forming and binding objects (Tallon-Baudry et al., 1996; Tallon-Baudry, 1999).

Many studies report a simultaneous decrease of alpha power and increase in gamma power in task relevant brain regions, whereas a number of studies have shown that alpha and gamma power are not always inversely coupled (Haegens et al., 2010; Scheeringa et al., 2011). For example, while alpha power has been shown to decrease in anticipation of a stimulus (Rohenkohl and Nobre, 2011; see **Figure 1A**), gamma activity is induced by stimulation and active maintenance but is not observable in anticipation to stimulation (Hoogenboom et al., 2006). Thus, while alpha decreases may serve to disinhibit a brain region, gamma oscillations reflect the active, ongoing processing and binding of information.

POPULATION TARGET GROUPS AND THEIR NEURONAL SIGNATURES

Many common individual differences in cognition can be traced back to differences in memory or attention processes. In the previous section we outlined the functional role of neuronal oscillations in cognition and presented strong evidence for a relationship between oscillatory power and behavioral performance in specific tasks. In this section, we will outline how optimizing neuronal oscillations might improve cognition in three target groups: the elderly, who commonly have problems with attention and working memory, patients suffering from ADHD, and also healthy, young adults who show remarkable inter-individual differences in cognitive tasks. We will propose that optimizing neuronal oscillations might help to alleviate symptoms and improve cognition.

THE ELDERLY AND THEIR PROBLEMS WITH ATTENTION AND WORKING MEMORY

In the western world, there is a continuous demographic change with an increased percentage of elderly people in the population (Cohen, 2005; Peters et al., 2010). Several studies have statistically assessed the areas of compromised cognition in the elderly. Elderly people have more trouble in task switching paradigms compared to younger adults (Kray and Lindenberger, 2000). The elderly show lower performance in working memory tasks (Salthouse et al., 1991) and have reduced working memory capacity (at least in part) due to problems in binding multiple low-level features (Brockmole and Logie, 2013). Additionally, it has been shown that elderly have trouble inhibiting distracting information in unimodal tasks (Folk and Lincourt, 1996; Groth and Allen, 2000; Gaeta et al., 2001; Tales et al., 2002; Andrés et al., 2006; Fabiani et al., 2006; Rowe et al., 2006; Yang and Hasher, 2007), in cross-modal tasks (Alain and Woods, 1999; Poliakoff et al., 2006; Hugenschmidt et al., 2009b), and multi-modal tasks (Hugenschmidt et al., 2009a). The studies by Hugenschmidt et al. and others suggest that while elderly have trouble ignoring task-irrelevant items, they do show intact attention abilities. For example, elderly showed behavioral cueing effects, even in more complex environments (Hugenschmidt et al., 2009a,b).

In addition, a number of structural and functional changes have been reported in the brain of the elderly. For example, with increasing age, alpha peak frequency and power decrease while theta power increases (Dustman et al., 1993; Grandy et al., 2013) and the amount of evoked gamma band activity is reduced in the elderly compared to young adults (Werkle-Bergner et al., 2009). Recently, Sander et al. (2012a) proposed to disassemble working memory into two components: a global top-down control mechanism and a local perceptual binding mechanism. They further hypothesized that both components are differentially impaired in the elderly. By incorporating the reviewed evidence from the previous section, global top-down control is reflected by the power of frontal theta and posterior alpha oscillations (reviewed in Klimesch, 1999; Klimesch et al., 2007; Jensen and Mazaheri, 2010; Foxe and Snyder, 2011; Jensen et al., 2012; Klimesch, 2012), whereas local binding is reflected by gamma band oscillations (Tallon-Baudry et al., 1996; Tallon-Baudry, 1999). Under this framework, reduced alpha or theta power would suggest a problem with top down control, whereas a reduction in evoked gamma-power would predict a problem with perceptual binding.

A number of studies showed the absence of correlations between behavior and oscillatory activity in the elderly, while present in healthy young adults. For example, a strong increase in frontal theta power with working memory load has been reported in young adults (Jensen and Tesche, 2002), but there was no such relation in the elderly (McEvoy et al., 2001). Also, McEvoy et al. (2001) found that with increasing task difficulty, alpha power in both parietal and frontal cortices decreased in the elderly, whereas in young adults alpha power only decreased over parietal regions. In a similar vein, Gazzaley et al. (2008) showed that frontal theta power scaled with the relevance of the to-be-processed item in young healthy adults, but not in the elderly, see **Figure 2A**. Sander et al. (2012b) showed that in a visual covert attention working memory paradigm, the degree of lateralized alpha power was maximal under high memory load in healthy, young adults, whereas it peaked under medium memory load in the elderly and was nearly absent in the high memory load condition. Despite the absence of this correlation, the elderly were still able to successfully perform well in this task, although worse than the young adults.

All studies in elderly are fraught with the problem that compensatory mechanisms seem to be active (Reuter-Lorenz et al., 2000; Cabeza et al., 2002; Logan et al., 2002; Nielson et al., 2002; Riis et al., 2008). While a reduced amount of activity might highlight the locus of the problem, an increase in activity elsewhere might indicate the compensation. Hence, in the above finding by Sander et al. (2012b) it is likely that a compensatory mechanism took over the functional role of posterior alpha lateralization under high memory load. Identifying such mechanisms and studying whether they are compensatory or competing with normal functioning could help in determining whether this mechanism is causing or resulting in the degraded bottom up sensory processing and binding.

ATTENTION DEFICIT/HYPERACTIVITY DISORDER

ADHD is the most common psychiatric disorder in the western world (Cantwell, 1996; Barry et al., 2003) with an estimated prevalence of 3–6% (Pelham et al., 1992; Polanczyk et al., 2007). Diagnosis of ADHD is characterized by two components: an attention and a hyperactivity component. While some patients show traits of both components (the "combined" subtype), a large proportion of patients show only one component strongly with the other component weaker or absent (Barkley et al., 1990; Lockwood et al., 2001). Here, we will focus on the combined and the inattentive subgroups, i.e., those with attention deficits. However, the combined patient subgroup is characterized by different attention deficits in cognitive tasks than the inattentive subgroup (Weiss et al., 2003; Booth et al., 2007; Adams et al., 2008), leading to the proposition of categorizing patients showing inattentive without hyperactivity symptoms as a patient group distinct from ADHD (Barkley, 2001; Milich et al., 2001; Derefinko et al., 2008). Nonetheless, we will discuss characteristics and possible treatments for attention deficits of both the combined and the inattentive subgroups.

The inattentive subtype is characterized, as the name implies, by problems in engaging and sustaining attention. In behavioral paradigms it has been found that the inattentive subgroup showed either reduced attention resources (Carr et al., 2010) or reduced visual processing power (Weiler et al., 2002). The inattentive subtype also showed a lack of response cueing effect (Lockwood et al., 2001; Derefinko et al., 2008). Behavioral deficits and oscillatory power differences between ADHD patients and

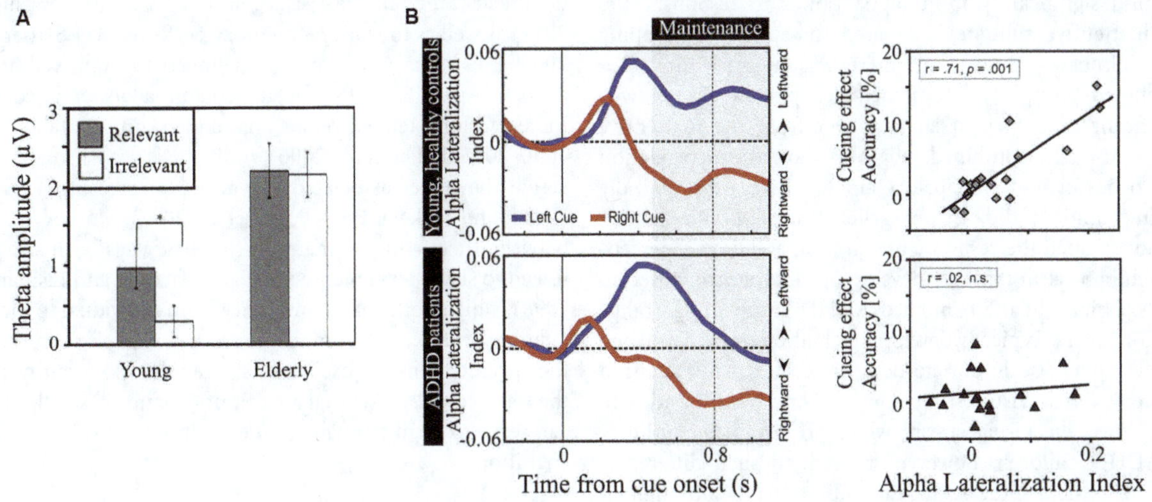

FIGURE 2 | Oscillatory power differences in different task settings in the three discussed population groups. (A) Frontal theta power during stimulus encoding is significantly higher for elderly versus young adults, and scales with relevance of the stimuli in young, healthy adults, but not in the elderly (* $p < 0.001$). Reproduced with permission from Gazzaley et al. (2008). **(B)** During visual spatial covert attention, the degree of alpha lateralization indexes the relative disengagement of the task-irrelevant ipsilateral hemisphere versus the task-relevant contralateral hemisphere. While young, healthy adults are able to modulate their alpha lateralization symmetrically around zero, inattentive ADHD patients show a lack of maintaining a high degree of alpha lateralization to the left side. In addition, there is an absence of correlation between alpha lateralization index and behavioral cueing effect in ADHD patients, whereas there is a strong relationship in healthy, young adults. Reproduced with permission from ter Huurne et al. (2013).

control subjects have been investigated recently. In adolescents, Mazaheri et al. (2013) found that ADHD patients of the inattentive subgroup showed a reduced behavioral cueing effect and weaker suppression of posterior alpha in response to the cue that indicates with which hand to respond. In young adults with the inattentive subtype, ter Huurne et al. (2013) showed an absence of maintaining posterior anticipatory alpha lateralization in response to a left attention cue, but not to a right attention cue. Interestingly, they found the same initial level of alpha lateralization in control and ADHD groups. In both studies, the degree of alpha power modulation with task showed a strong correlation with behavior for the control group but not for the ADHD group; see **Figure 2B**. These studies suggest that inattentive ADHD patients do not only suffer from reduced but also from inefficient integration of posterior alpha power as it does not seem to be beneficial for behavior, whereas it is for healthy people.

Studies on the combined ADHD subgroup and neuronal oscillations in task settings are sparse. Recently Karch et al. (2012) found that young adults suffering from ADHD showed increased frontocentral gamma band activity shortly after auditory stimulation followed by a voluntary motor response. Yordanova et al. (2001) found that ADHD children between 9 and 12 years of age showed increased induced fronto-central gamma band responses for right auditory stimulation compared to normally developing children, but not for left auditory stimulation. Lenz et al. (2008) found that children of the combined ADHD group showed enhanced visual stimulus-induced gamma power. While gamma power correlated with long-term memory performance for typically developing children, it did not for the ADHD children. In addition, Mazaheri et al. (2013) tested children of the inattentive subgroup and the combined subgroup and compared these two groups with typically developing children. They found significantly more alpha power to response cues for the inattentive subtypes compared to typically developing children (discussed above), but there was no such effect for the combined group. The combined group, however, showed no significant difference in alpha power from the inattentive subgroup. Also, the combined subgroup showed no correlation between behavior and anticipatory alpha, whereas the typically developing children did. In an earlier study, Mazaheri et al. (2010) investigated the response preparation ability in a perceptual switching task in typically developing children compared to children classified in the combined ADHD group in age range from 8 to 12 years. Typically developing children showed a strong alpha power increase in parieto-occipital cortex in preparation for auditory versus visual stimulation, in line with the idea of shutting down the visual stream when preparing for auditory input. ADHD children, however, showed no such difference, but a frontal theta increase instead. Additionally, although in typically developing children parieto-occipital alpha power was inversely correlated with the behavioral cueing effect in the visual condition, there was no such correlation for the ADHD children. Recently, Lenartowicz et al. (2014) investigated the neuronal patterns in a group of children between 7 and 14 years of age comprised of both the inattentive and combined subgroups. In a working memory paradigm, they found reduced vigilance attributed to a less pronounced alpha depression during encoding (i.e., higher occipital alpha activity) in ADHD children than in typically developing children, but in return a stronger alpha power synchronization during stimulus maintenance in ADHD children. Frontal theta during the maintenance period was also elevated in ADHD children, which they interpreted as a compensation for the lack of vigilance during encoding.

The above studies indicate a versatile interplay of hyper- and hypo-activity in specific phases during a task. In line with Lenartowicz et al. (2014) we propose that this might be anchored to improper preparation for the task, indicated by a lack of modulating anticipatory alpha activity to stimulation. Higher gamma during stimulation and higher alpha and theta during stimulus maintenance might thus be the product of compensation for this improper preparation.

COGNITION IN HEALTHY, YOUNG ADULTS

Within young healthy adults there is a large spread of inter- and intra-individual differences in both neuronal oscillations and behavior. For example, healthy individuals differ in visual working memory capacity (Luck and Vogel, 2013). Individuals with better working memory capacity have greater frontal theta power during stimulus encoding (Gevins and Smith, 2000). Similarly, individuals with greater pre-stimulus frontal theta power better remembered source context (Addante et al., 2011). Also within subjects, high frontal pre-stimulus theta power was predictive of whether an item was remembered (Addante et al., 2011), as was increased gamma power during stimulus encoding; see **Figure 1C** (Osipova et al., 2006).

The ability to sustain attention varies among individuals. Individual differences in the degree of alpha lateralization have been linked to differential abilities to ignore the task-irrelevant hemifield (Fu et al., 2001; Haegens et al., 2011a; Horschig et al., 2014) as well as to working memory performance (Sauseng et al., 2009b). Gamma power has been linked to improved attention as well. Apart from the fact that gamma power is commonly increased for attended versus unattended stimuli (Tallon-Baudry et al., 2005; Bauer et al., 2006), individuals with stronger gamma activity have been associated with improved perceptual processing (Jokeit and Makeig, 1994; Fründ et al., 2007). Moreover, the ratio between theta and gamma peak frequency has been successfully linked to short-term memory capacity (Jensen and Lisman, 1996, 1998), which both consistently vary from individual to individual (Kamiński et al., 2011). In future studies, explicit perturbation of the specific neuronal oscillations is required to identify whether they are causally involved in cognition and, if so, the findings can serve to form strong hypotheses on how to augment human cognition.

TECHNIQUES TO MANIPULATE NEURONAL OSCILLATIONS

In this section we will discuss how to apply our framework in practice. We will combine the fundamental insights of neuronal oscillations from the second section with the studies on different population groups discussed in the third section to answer which oscillatory components might be suitable for optimization and whether and how this optimization could increase cognitive performance. Since there are oscillations-behavior correlations in healthy adults and oscillations-pathology correlations, optimization of neuronal oscillations could lead to optimized behavior. We will introduce different, non-invasive approaches to manipulate neuronal oscillations, outline how these techniques work, and present studies on what has already been achieved. In addition we will suggest steps to fill the gap in current literature on successful augmentation of human cognition.

TRANSCRANIAL STIMULATION OF THE HUMAN BRAIN

The most direct way to manipulate neuronal firing is by electrical stimulation to manipulate the neuron's membrane potential causing it to de- or hyperpolarize. The two common non-physically-invasive techniques to do so are transcranial magnetic stimulation (TMS) and transcranial current stimulation (tCS). TMS utilizes the fact that a changing current in a wire induces a changing external magnetic field that, if in the presence of a conducting material such as neural tissue, induces a secondary electric current in the opposite direction (Pascual-Leone et al., 1999, 2000). This secondary current then affects local membrane potentials. Although the exact mechanism is still not completely understood, it is assumed that TMS pulses primarily influence the axons of both excitatory and inhibitory neurons and might actively elicit action potentials (Dayan et al., 2013). Two basic TMS approaches are commonly used. The "online" approach applies single, double, or brief bursts of pulses, each lasting a few 100 ms, during the task. The "offline" approach applies repetitive stimulation (rTMS) before a task or other measurement (Huang et al., 2005). Depending on the exact pattern and frequency of rTMS, cortical excitability can be facilitated or inhibited for a period outlasting the stimulation itself from 15 up to 90 min (Thut and Pascual-Leone, 2010). However, it has also been suggested that the frequency of stimulation entrains the neuronal oscillations at the stimulation frequency, which outlasts stimulation for a short period of time (hundreds of milliseconds; Thut and Miniussi, 2009). There is some first direct evidence for rhythmically entraining alpha oscillations in the visual cortex by means of brief bursts of rTMS around 10 Hz (Thut et al., 2011b and **Figure 3A**), yet stimulation not necessarily in the alpha frequency range can induce an alpha power increase (Thut and Pascual-Leone, 2010). Several studies have provided convincing indirect evidence for rTMS entrainment by its impact on behavior (Romei et al., 2010 and **Figure 3B**; Klimesch et al., 2003; Sauseng et al., 2009a).

The basic principle of tCS is that a weak electrical current is established between an anode and cathode, thereby altering neural membrane potentials. Importantly, because of the weak electrical current, tCS cannot trigger action potentials but rather slightly facilitates or inhibits spontaneous neuronal firing, depending on its polarity (Dayan et al., 2013; Reato et al., 2013). Transcranial current stimulation can be applied in two different ways: transcranial alternating current stimulation (tACS) and

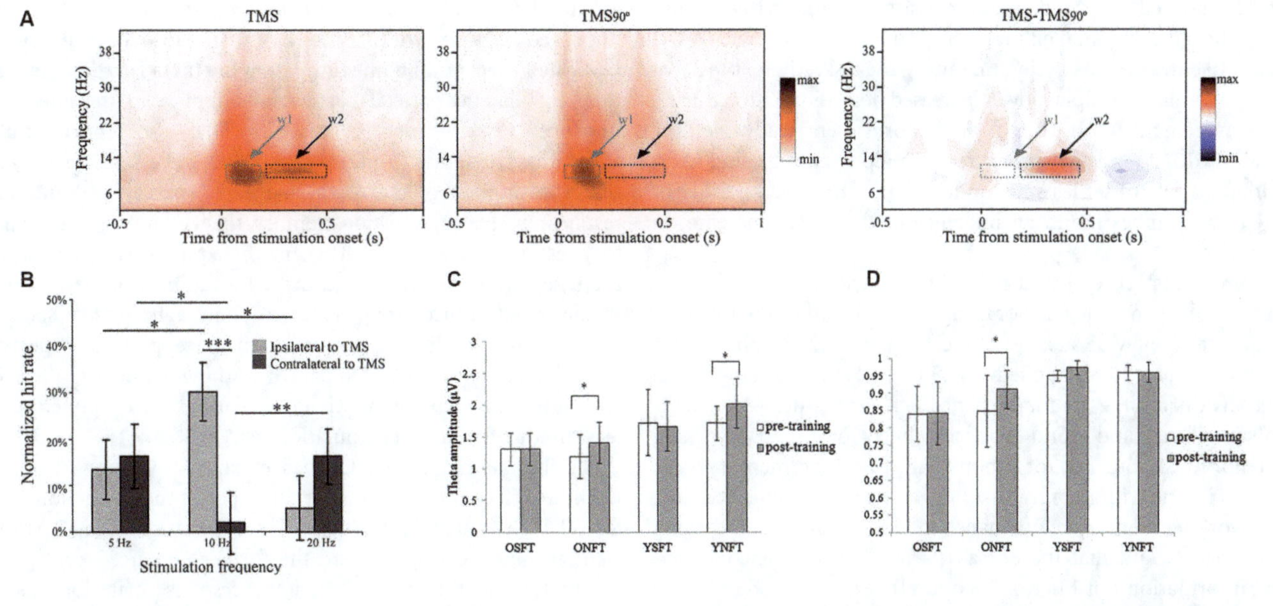

FIGURE 3 | Examples of manipulating neuronal oscillations and their impact on cognition. (A) rTMS stimulation at 10 Hz to right parietal cortex results in alpha oscillations outlasting the stimulation period ($t = 0$ s), compared to the control condition of rotating the TMS coil by 90° (TMS90). The condition contrast with other control conditions confirmed the exclusive effect of rTMS at 10 Hz. w1 = time window of the first two pulses and w2 = time window of the last three pulses. Reproduced with permission from Thut et al. (2011b). **(B)** 10 Hz rTMS stimulation, but not 5 or 20 Hz, of parietal cortex ipsilateral to stimulation results in behavioral improvement, whereas contralateral stimulation results in decreased performance (* $p < 0.05$, ** $p < 0.01$, *** $p < 0.001$). Reproduced with permission from Romei et al. (2010). **(C)** Frontal theta neurofeedback training results in increased frontal theta in both young and old adults. OSFT = old subjects, sham feedback; ONFT = old subjects, neurofeedback group; YSFT = young subjects, sham feedback; YNFT = young subjects, neurofeedback (* $p < 0.01$). Taken with permission from Wang and Hsieh (2013). **(D)** Only old adults receiving neurofeedback on frontal theta increased working memory accuracy in a Sternberg task (depicted on the y-axis). Young adults were already performing at ceiling level. (for acronym, see **panel C**; * $p < 0.01$). Taken with permission from Wang and Hsieh (2013).

transcranial direct current stimulation (tDCS). While with tDCS the polarity between anode and cathode stays constant (see Priori, 2003, for a review), with tACS the polarity constantly changes, thereby producing an alternating flow of current similar to an oscillation (Antal and Paulus, 2013; Herrmann et al., 2013; Reato et al., 2013). Sometimes tACS is used in conjunction with a DC offset. In that case, the polarity between anode and cathode stays fixed, as the current strength oscillates around the DC offset instead of zero. Consequently current only flows in one direction, from the cathode to the anode, which is in contrast to the classical tACS definition, where not only current strength but also direction changes throughout each oscillatory cycle. Here, we will explicitly clarify if we refer to tACS studies with a DC offset.

In the past a number of studies has shown improved cognition or performance in tasks using tCS or TMS (Meinzer et al., 2012, 2013; Snowball et al., 2013; Vollmann et al., 2013; Coffman et al., 2014; Luber and Lisanby, 2014; Schutter, 2014). However, most of these studies did not use tCS or tACS to stimulate neuronal oscillations or concurrently recorded them by EEG or MEG. In the following we will summarize a number of studies that used tACS or TMS to stimulate in the alpha, theta, or gamma range.

Although this is a relatively recent field, a number of studies has demonstrated that stimulating in the alpha range results in sustained alpha power increases in the cortex. Zaehle et al. (2010) showed that applying tACS offline for 10 min at the subject's individual peak alpha frequency over left and right posterior cortex resulted in an increase in alpha power for at least 3 min after the stimulation. Neuling et al. (2012) used tACS with a DC offset to entrain a 10 Hz rhythm during the task. After 3 blocks of 7 min stimulation, alpha power increased post-stimulation during a measurement lasting 3 min. In a more recent study, Neuling et al. (2013) found that the increase in alpha power using tACS without a DC offset lasts for up to 30 min. However, neither of these two studies found an influence of the power increase on behavior.

In contrast, several studies have found effects of entrainment in the alpha band on behavior using TMS, albeit they do not *per se* show that they were successful in changing cortical alpha power. Hamidi et al. (2009) applied rTMS at 10 Hz in parieto-central regions during the 3 s maintenance period in a delayed-match-to-sample task and found beneficial effects for a spatial working memory task, but not for a non-spatial working memory task. This is in line with the idea that high alpha power is needed during working memory maintenance to block additional incoming information and that the dorsal (parietal) regions encode spatial information but inferior (temporal) regions encode identity information (Goodale and Milner, 1992). Interestingly however, while Hamidi et al. (2009) did not find a change in alpha power due to TMS at the group level, they did find an across-subjects correlation of alpha power with behavior. Romei et al. (2010) found that entraining the alpha rhythm ipsilateral to the attended hemifield increased perceptual accuracy, whereas entraining alpha contralaterally decreased accuracy, strongly in line with the idea that strong alpha inhibits processing (**Figure 3B**). However, the effect of TMS stimulations on neuronal oscillations was not concurrently assessed by EEG, so it remains to be investigated whether the stimulation also resulted in changes in cortical oscillations.

Brignani et al. (2013) also tried to increase the ipsilateral alpha rhythm but with tACS to parieto-occipital cortex. Surprisingly, they found no spatially specific effect but a general task impairment during a covert spatial attention task. This might have been caused because the stimulated area using tCS is widespread and not easily inferable from the placement of the anode and cathode (Manoli et al., 2012; Bai et al., 2014). Also in this study, no concurrent EEG recordings were done, so the effect of stimulation on cortical oscillations could not be directly assessed. These studies show that different brain regions are affected differently by different techniques on different target areas and that precise *a priori* hypotheses and knowledge about the brain region to be stimulated are necessary for successful augmentation of human cognition. *A priori* computational modeling of the stimulation protocol using advanced physical models has recently been demonstrated (tCS: Manoli et al., 2012; Bai et al., 2014; TMS: Bijsterbosch et al., 2012; Janssen et al., 2013; Wagner et al., 2014). This could help in applying protocols and stimulation electrodes and thereby aid in studying whether modulation of cortical alpha power in specific regions has behavioral consequences.

Fewer studies are available which attempt to induce theta oscillations. Meiron and Lavidor (2014) applied tACS in the theta range to bilateral frontal cortex during a working memory task and found an improvement in online working memory capacity. Jaušovec and Jaušovec (2014) used tACS in the theta range but around left parietal cortex and showed that this leads to an improved memory working memory span. Jaušovec et al. (2014) replicated their finding on stimulating the theta rhythm, but this time in bilateral parietal cortices and replicated the effect on improved working memory capacity. They also report a null-effect for stimulating frontal cortex. While these findings suggest that entrainment of the theta rhythm is spatially specific and results in increasing working memory, they did not report oscillatory responses to assess whether the theta power was successfully increased over the stimulated area. In addition, none of these studies used control frequencies to show a frequency specific effect. Further studies are required to measure spatial and spectral specificity, disentangle which part of working memory is affected, and show convincingly that theta oscillations are entrained or at least modulated during stimulation.

In the gamma range, Chanes et al. (2013) showed a differential effect on performance in a perceptual detection task for 30 Hz stimulation versus 50 Hz stimulation using TMS to right frontal eye fields, where the former enhanced perceptual sensitivity and the latter shifted the response criterion. Using tACS, Santarnecchi et al. (2013) showed that entraining gamma around 40 Hz at the left mid-frontal gyrus improved performance in conditioning and reasoning tasks. Laczó et al. (2012) showed that gamma stimulation to early visual cortex around 60 Hz but not at 40 or 80 Hz resulted in a lower contrast detection threshold. Importantly, none of the stimulation frequencies resulted in behavioral changes in spatial detection tasks. While showing promising results, studies on rhythmically entraining the gamma range are sparse and differ in exact frequency range and spatial location. Reproductions of these findings are required in order to draw definite conclusions on where and how to stimulate to improve what aspect of perceptual performance by gamma entrainment.

All of the above reviewed literature was on healthy, young adults and not on other target groups. Given the partly incomplete literature and understanding of TMS and tACS, it remains to be tested whether such hypothesis-driven brain stimulation shows success in the elderly and ADHD patients, and whether this results in a reduction of cognitive problems.

HYPOTHESIS-DRIVEN BRAIN COMPUTER INTERFACING AND NEUROFEEDBACK

Brain-computer interfacing (BCI) commonly refers to the technique to use a signal measured from the brain to control a computer or a machine without the use of the peripheral muscle system (Wolpaw et al., 2002). This requires the user's awareness of the ongoing brain activity, which is made perceivable by means of visual, tactile, or auditory feedback (van Gerven et al., 2009a). The original goal of BCI was to provide the user with an additional output channel for the purpose of communication.

Neurofeedback serves a different purpose by similar means. The goal of neurofeedback is to make the users aware of their brain activity to learn to enhance or decrease the fed back aspects, e.g., theta power, and thereby alleviate pathological symptoms, such as in ADHD (Lubar et al., 1995; Fuchs et al., 2003). An unfortunate major criticism in the field of neurofeedback, however, is often the absence of control conditions, significant effects, a scientifically grounded hypothesis, or reproducibility (see Vollebregt et al., 2014). Recently it has been proposed to start using hypothesis-driven BCI to improve subsequent behavior (Jensen et al., 2011), on which we will now elaborate.

Hypothesis-driven BCI (hdBCI) refers to the idea that insights from fundamental and cognitive neuroscience are applied to infer a robust and reliable control signal to improve cognition. Such a control signal must show strong single trial correlation with behavior and must be trainable. As described above, neuronal oscillations have been well studied and show strong correlation with cognition in a multitude of task settings ranging from attention or working memory studies to studies on long-term memory encoding and retrieval. This robustness and reliability allows making a concrete hypothesis to be tested when applying neurofeedback techniques. We suggest using a control signal that shows strong correlations with behavior, for example frontal theta during working memory or alpha lateralization during covert visual spatial attention tasks, and train the subjects to gain awareness and control of that signal. Before and after hdBCI training, a number of behavioral tasks orthogonal to the hdBCI task should be used to assess whether the neurofeedback training translates to subsequent improvements in cognition. The neuronal oscillation and the hdBCI paradigm need to reflect the underlying cognitive mechanism to be trained. For example, we described problems with general attention and reduced ability to suppress distracting stimuli in the elderly or in ADHD patients - a functional role that alpha oscillations are supposed to fulfill. The aim of hdBCI training is to study whether the training effect on oscillatory power brings along changes in behavior, in particular ideally, that has been shown to be correlated to that oscillation. If subsequent behavioral improvements in untrained, but related tasks are found, this would serve as a strong case that neuronal oscillations are causally involved in cognition. In the following we will review studies that can serve as templates for how hdBCI training can be used to study the functional role of neuronal oscillations.

While alpha-based neurofeedback has been shown to modulate not only the alpha power but also performance on a mental rotation task (Hanslmayr et al., 2005b; Zoefel et al., 2011), we link the findings of alpha power's role in inhibition of distracters (see Section Functional Role of Neuronal Oscillations) to hdBCI training with the goal of improving resilience to distraction. No such study has been conducted so far. If successful, one might ask whether the same rationale can be used for treating inattentive symptoms of the elderly or ADHD patients. As a concrete example, one could study whether the alpha lateralization pattern during covert spatial attention can be trained and strengthened. Alpha lateralization has been studied intensively in the past and has been shown to be a reliable control signal for BCI (Kelly et al., 2005; van Gerven and Jensen, 2009; van Gerven et al., 2009b; Bahramisharif et al., 2010; Tonin et al., 2012). In healthy young adults, high memory load coincided with strong alpha lateralization during a covert attention working memory task—an aspect that was missing in the elderly (Sander et al., 2012b). An hdBCI can consist of training alpha lateralization in the elderly asking whether strong alpha lateralization will be of beneficial nature as observed in young adults and whether a correlation between alpha lateralization and high memory load will reemerge. In a similar line a lack of maintaining alpha lateralization has been found in inattentive ADHD patients (ter Huurne et al., 2013). hdBCI training on maintaining a high degree of alpha lateralization could help to restore this ability. Again, a correlation between behavioral performance and degree of alpha lateralization was observed in healthy adults, but lacking in ADHD patients. The most critical question is, if the ability to maintain a high degree of alpha lateralization is restored in inattentive ADHD patients, will the underlying mechanisms leading to the alpha power shifts be beneficial for their performance again? No studies in this direction have been pursued so far, but they would elucidate the functional role of alpha oscillations.

Complementarily, during working memory paradigms it has been shown that frontal theta reflects the memory load in healthy individuals (Jensen and Tesche, 2002), but no such relation was found in the elderly (McEvoy et al., 2001). One might ask whether training the elderly to increase their frontal theta proportional to memory load during a working memory task results in improved working memory performance. Recently, Enriquez-Geppert et al. (2014) and Wang and Hsieh (2013) provide preliminary evidence that frontal theta neurofeedback training does work. The latter shows that both young and old participants learned to increase frontal theta by neurofeedback in contrast to control groups (see **Figures 3C,D**). In addition elderly receiving frontal theta neurofeedback training showed improved performance in a subsequent working memory task in contrast to the control group. However, they do not show whether the neurofeedback training restored the correlation between memory load and frontal theta in the elderly. Also their study was confounded by several other issues, for example young, healthy, adults were performing at ceiling level already before the training, which resulted in a null-effect training for them. Thus, this study is inconclusive on whether frontal theta training increases working memory capacity in young, healthy adults. For ADHD patients it has been found that frontal theta is already relatively high compared to young healthy adults, e.g., during working memory encoding, which might be caused by a lack of proper preparation to the task, quantified by weaker anticipatory alpha oscillations in posterior regions (Lenartowicz et al., 2014; see also Section Population Target Groups and Their Neuronal Signatures). Given all reviewed literature, it seems plausible that an additional increase in frontal theta during encoding or increase in posterior alpha in anticipation of the stimulus would further boost working memory performance.

Neurofeedback on gamma oscillations has been studied by Keizer et al. (2010), who found that successful increases in gamma band power in young, healthy adults correlated with an increase in fluid intelligence and reduced cost of feature binding reflected in the lower reaction times. In line with the current view on feature-binding problems in the elderly (cf. Sander et al., 2012a), Staufenbiel et al. (2014) used neurofeedback training of gamma oscillations in the elderly. Although the neurofeedback training resulted in increased gamma, they failed to show a beneficial nature of this training for fluid intelligence, working memory, and quality of life. However, these studies did not feedback gamma power during stimulation, but during resting state. It might have been beneficial to give feedback of gamma power during stimulation, as the neural sources processing stimuli are likely to differ from resting state sources, when no stimulus is being processed. No studies on training gamma band in ADHD patients have been conducted.

For a more complete overview on neurofeedback studies, the interested reader is referred to Gruzelier (2013). In general, we advise that neurofeedback studies should follow hypotheses and paradigms that are more focused and grounded in insights gained from fundamental and cognitive research conducted in the last decades, in particular using information on the functional role of neuronal oscillations.

BRAIN STATE DEPENDENT TASKS (BSDT): ADAPTING THE ENVIRONMENT TO THE USER'S MENTAL STATE

The former approach aimed at shaping the user's brain activity for optimal stimulus processing or task performance. Recent insight in the field of cognitive neuroscience (see Section Functional Role of Neuronal Oscillations) suggests that we can predict cognitive behavior by neuronal oscillations. This knowledge can be used to adapt the task environment based on the user's current brain activity to allow for optimal performance. Ultimately this could aid the user to develop an optimal brain state more quickly or efficiently. Specifically, the timing and properties of the task would be determined by an online read-out of the current brain state, as quantified by ongoing neuronal oscillatory activity (Hartmann et al., 2011; Jensen et al., 2011). It is even possible to combine this with active brain stimulation (Silvanto and Pascual-Leone, 2008), which was recently demonstrated by Gharabaghi et al. (2014), who applied TMS and provided haptic feedback according to relevant neural oscillatory activity.

Brain state dependent tasks (BSDT) serve two purposes. First, by adapting the environment to the ongoing brain activity, individual cognition could be improved as described below. Second, BSDT informs the user about his ongoing brain state and rewards the user for a "good" brain state in a similar manner as in BCI. BSDT therefore could help the subject's ability to modulate his brain activity to reach a certain mind setting, or brain state. BSDT can be used in two complementary manners. First, stimulus presentation can be triggered to ongoing oscillatory activity. For example, it has been found that strong prestimulus alpha power in task-relevant regions negatively affects subsequent stimulus processing (e.g., Ergenoglu et al., 2004; Hanslmayr et al., 2005a, 2007; van Dijk et al., 2008; Mazaheri et al., 2009). In a BSDT paradigm, stimulus presentation could thus be triggered only when alpha power is relatively low, thereby increasing efficiency of stimulus processing. A reverse rationale applies, where the task is to inhibit some aspect of the environment: stimulate during high alpha power in task-irrelevant brain regions. For example, background speech might be distracting when visually learning vocabularies. Thus, in a BSDT environment one could first reward high temporal alpha by removing some artificially-added, auditory distraction while visually presenting vocabularies and, in a second step, additionally only present vocabularies when posterior alpha power is low. This could lead to increased processing of the visually presented vocabularies and also increased inhibition of the distracting auditory noise. To generalize this idea, training could be provided in a variety of tasks where the direction and location of alpha modulation varies; this way, it is the control of alpha that is important and learned, not just a focal or unidirectional lesson which might interfere with other tasks. The subject thereby learns the skill to consciously modulate brain oscillations in similar manner to neurofeedback.

A second manner for BSDT is the fact that based on the activity during stimulus processing or maintenance, subsequent behavior can be predicted, as already proposed e.g., by Mazaheri et al. (2009). For example, increased alpha activity during visual processing (Park et al., 2014) and during the retention interval (Meeuwissen et al., 2011) has been shown to strongly correlate with long-term memory encoding performance. Based on these findings, one could predict which items are most likely to be forgotten and present these items again to the subject in order to facilitate long-term memory performance. In addition, measures correlating with memory load, e.g., frontal theta or occipital gamma for visual items, can be read out to predict the current load. This could also be used to prevent memory overload (discussed in Huggins et al., 2014). This second manner represents an online adaptation of the environment and cannot necessarily be utilized offline or result in an offline skill.

For young, healthy adults, strong correlations between oscillatory power and cognition have been found as reviewed in Sections Functional Role of Neuronal Oscillations and Techniques to Manipulate Neuronal Oscillations. However, in Section Population Target Groups and Their Neuronal Signatures we also review evidence that this correlation seems to be absent in the elderly and ADHD patients. In these population groups, compensatory mechanisms might have taken over the function that some oscillations usually represent. While brain stimulation techniques aim to restore the beneficial nature of these oscillations, BSDT aims to predict cognition. It remains to be tested whether BSDT is beneficial for the elderly and ADHD patients when utilizing hypotheses based on another population group. Both manners of applying BSDT—waiting with stimulation until a good distribution of oscillatory power and predicting subsequent behavior by the distribution of oscillatory power—might prove useless, without a correlation between oscillation and behavior. We would therefore advise to identify neural signatures of the compensatory mechanisms, and find appropriate hypotheses for these population groups, or to manipulate the neural oscillations as proposed in the previous two subsections before applying BSDT in a patient group.

PRACTICAL CONSIDERATIONS

In the previous section we made some concrete suggestions on how insights from cognitive neuroscience can be applied to augment human behavior. In this section, we will discuss how to define successful interventions, outline practical considerations about our hypothesis that should be regarded when following above suggestions, suggest alternative approaches, and point to possible pitfalls when applying these techniques in the lab, at home, or when valorizing these ideas for commercial use. For ethical considerations, we encourage the reader to read the Nuffield report on neurotechnology (Nuffield Councils on Bioethics, 2013).

DEFINING AND ASSESSING SUCCESS

We have collected supporting evidence for hypothesis-driven approaches to augment human behavior. Although literature on this topic is relatively sparse, studies often differ in crucial aspects such as motivation for the study (i.e., the original hypothesis), methodology (e.g., control conditions, number or duration of training sessions, or the number of hours or days after training to test for long-term effects), and conclusions on how to generalize the findings. The most important question to ask when drawing conclusions about these studies is how best to quantify if the applied technique resulted in augmentation of cognition. This question can be disentangled into two parts.

First, we need to quantify that the augmentation effect is caused by the applied technique and not by confounding other reasons. For example, proper control conditions in neurofeedback settings yield results similar to neurofeedback protocols often used for ADHD treatment (van Dongen-Boomsma et al., 2013; Vollebregt et al., 2014). Thus, special care needs to be taken when attributing the beneficial effect to the applied technique, and that the effect is specific to the modulated frequency-band. As another example, it has been shown that auditory perception of the clicking sound of TMS stimulation alone is sufficient to induce an effect in visual cortex (Romei et al., 2012). Other control conditions aside from sham stimulation, such as cognitive behavioral training (Safren et al., 2010; Strenziok et al., 2014) or physical exercise (Halperin and Healey, 2011; Verret et al., 2012), are often more easily applied than brain stimulation techniques. Furthermore, it is very important to be aware of misleading causes of experimental observations, such as temporal ordering of the tasks; a randomized design order is a crucial part of any paradigm.

Second, we need to define what we mean by augmentation of cognition. We first need to define a baseline level of performance before starting the intervention and we need to show a strong, significant increase from this baseline, above the appropriate control discussed above. Additionally, an improvement in one skill might come at a cost in another skill (Brem et al., 2014; Reinhart and Woodman, 2014). Therefore, one core assertion of successful augmentation of human cognition needs to be measured by transfer learning (Klingberg et al., 2002; Dahlin et al., 2008; Klingberg, 2010), i.e., quantifying how the intervention translates to other domains that were not explicitly trained and tempered by any deficits gained in other domains. In other words, one need to clearly establish the scope of the intervention and what does and does not work.

THE DANGER OF UNDESIRED SIDE EFFECTS

One important aspect to consider when proposing any study with stimulation is to *a priori* think about which brain region to stimulate and for what purpose. In the vast majority of this article, we talked about how to manipulate neuronal oscillations, but for successful augmentation of human cognition one needs to understand that the human brain is organized into different cortical and subcortical structures and each serves multiple, partly overlapping functionalities. When considering augmenting human cognition, one needs to be precise on which part of human cognition. Let us take the example of increased alpha power in task-irrelevant regions. Firstly, one needs to define "task-irrelevant"; for example, in a covert visual spatial attention task, the posterior ipsilateral hemisphere is "task-irrelevant", but not the contralateral hemisphere (Worden et al., 2000; Thut et al., 2006; Kelly et al., 2009). Secondly, the natural region(s) exerting modulation of the task-irrelevant region(s) should be noted; for example, it has been found that the intraparietal sulcus and the frontal eye fields exert top-down control on posterior areas and that stimulating them has consequences for posterior alpha and subsequent behavior (Capotosto et al., 2009, 2012; Sauseng et al., 2011). Thirdly, stimulation of the "wrong" brain region can lead to unexpected, reversed effects, i.e., where stimulation of one brain region is beneficial for one task and impedimental for another task (Romei et al., 2010; Iuculano and Cohen Kadosh, 2013); for example, when conducting a purely auditory task, the whole visual cortex becomes "task-irrelevant". Note that the anatomical precision of non-invasive EEG recordings is not high enough to verify the spatial specificity of the measured oscillations. While source reconstruction techniques can increase spatial certainty beyond sensor level information, invasive recordings are necessary for precise spatial localization.

Additional side effects can arise from improper task settings. For example, one might think to save time by concurrently testing for items in memory while memorizing new items. This, however, has been found to be inefficient and led to deteriorated memory performance (Huijbers et al., 2009). In addition, the functional hypothesis has to be correct and grounded in previous findings. For example, while many studies have convincingly related alpha power with inhibition of task-irrelevant regions, this might not hold true for all brain regions (Mo et al., 2011). Thus the exact experimental paradigm has to be vigorously thought through, which requires intensive knowledge from an expert in the field of cognitive neuroscience and/or brain stimulation or hdBCI techniques. Therefore, one needs to be sure which region requires which treatment (e.g., excitation is distinct from release from inhibition) in order to augment cognition successfully without burdensome side effects.

Non-optimal stimulation protocols and task settings might not be the only cause for side effects. As the mechanism behind electromagnetic brain stimulation is not fully understood, a number of unforeseen side effects can occur. Manufacturers restrict the maximum amplitude in their amplifier to a rather low value to reduce the possible risks (e.g., infrequent reports of inducing seizures, kindling, mood changes and scalp burnings) which can be further minimized by following general guidelines (Wassermann, 1998; Rossi et al., 2009). In addition, effects of long-term electromagnetic brain stimulation are rarely studied and not well understood. As Antal and Paulus (2013) wrote about the motor evoked potential (MEP): "Increasing the duration of tDCS results in a prolongation of the induced aftereffects (Nitsche and Paulus, 2000) up to about 13 min whereas doubling the 13 stimulation to 26 min inverses MEP aftereffects into inhibition (Batsikadze et al., 2013). It is unclear if this can be translated to tACS, too". While an aftereffect reversal is an obvious crucial side-effect and would be undesired, e.g., in the case of attention boosting, even stronger side effects might occur, especially due to the unknown long-term effects on plasticity and anatomical and functional connectivity. Plastic white matter changes in humans have been found following behavioral training (Zatorre et al., 2012; Sampaio-Baptista et al., 2013), and there is some preliminary evidence for white matter changes following electric stimulation (Allendorfer et al., 2012) and neurofeedback (Ghaziri et al., 2013).

INDIVIDUAL DIFFERENCES

Cognitive neuroscience aims to infer general mechanisms of the brain by studying a subgroup of some homogenous population. Significant statistical tests using random effects analysis then allow making inference from the subgroup to the population. However, finding a group level effect does not automatically mean that all individuals show the same effect, or even a significant effect. An example is found in the strength and adaptation of alpha lateralization (e.g., Händel et al., 2011; Horschig et al., 2014). Inter-individual variability has extensively been described as an issue in the field of BCI, where it has been found that about 1/5 of all individuals are unable to gain control over the control signal (Dickhaus et al., 2009; Vidaurre and Blankertz, 2010). A similar kind of inter-subject variability is reported in tCS techniques, which might arise due to a multitude of factors (Horvath et al., 2014; Krause and Cohen Kadosh, 2014). Thus, while we are proposing that these techniques can be used to decrease interindividual variability, it might be that interindividual variability requires different solutions for different subjects, e.g., different frequency bands or a different location of stimulation sites.

ALTERNATIVE ASPECTS OF NEURONAL OSCILLATIONS TO UTILIZE

In this review, we focused on the region-specific power of neuronal oscillations because, as discussed in Section Functional Role of Neuronal Oscillations, they are a robust read-out of the brain state and show strong across-trials correlations with behavior. However, investigating the power of neuronal oscillations is not the only means of quantifying electrophysiological data. The alternatives we discuss below, as well as others not mentioned, may also provide a handle with which to augment cognition via manipulation as discussed in Section Techniques to Manipulate Neuronal Oscillations, if a suitable hypothesis can be formed linking neural activity to behavior. We believe however that our main point has been sufficiently illustrated by the examples (i.e., oscillatory power and patient groups) used.

One natural alternative to power is the phase. In particular, the phase of the alpha and theta oscillations has been studied intensively in the past (Buzsáki and Draguhn, 2004; Montemurro et al., 2008; VanRullen et al., 2014). Recent evidence suggests that specific phases are more optimal for specific tasks (Gho and Varela, 1988; Kruglikov and Schiff, 2003; Mathewson et al., 2009). For example, ignoring a distracter is more successful in a specific phase of alpha oscillations than in its opposed phase (Bonnefond and Jensen, 2012). Interestingly, it has also been shown that tACS can be used to gain control over the phase of an oscillation (Helfrich et al., 2014; Jaegle and Ro, 2014; Strüber et al., 2014; Zanto et al., 2014), which has corresponding, orthogonal behavioral effects. Recent studies also indicate that a visual stimulus regularly flickering at 10 Hz can entrain alpha oscillations in visual cortex outlasting the stimulation period and also that subsequent behavior was modulated in a phasic manner according to the phase of the stimulation flickering (Mathewson et al., 2012; de Graaf et al., 2013; Spaak et al., 2014). In conclusion, studying the phasic nature of oscillations will provide further insight into human perception and provide important, additional information for brain stimulation techniques, hypothesis-driven brain-computer interfaces, and BSDT.

Furthermore another quantification of oscillations includes cross-frequency phase-amplitude coupling, whereby the phase of a slower oscillation is linked to the amplitude of a faster oscillation. For example it has been shown that gamma power waxes and wanes with the phase of alpha or theta oscillations (Canolty et al., 2006; Jensen et al., 2012; Bonnefond and Jensen, 2013; Lisman and Jensen, 2013; Roux and Uhlhaas, 2014). This also has important implications for behavior as, already discussed briefly in Section Functional Role of Neuronal Oscillations, the ratio between a theta cycle and a gamma cycle has been suggested to determine working memory capacity (Jensen and Lisman, 1996, 1998; Kamiński et al., 2011). This knowledge could be used to optimize cross-frequency coupling in order to study its direct effect on behavior.

In addition, we also chose not to focus on connectivity between brain regions, which can be a phase adjustment across regions (Varela et al., 2001; Gross et al., 2004; Fries, 2005; Sauseng and Klimesch, 2008) or a simultaneous power adjustment (e.g., Mazaheri et al., 2009). For example, several studies found a different functional connectivity pattern in the elderly compared to healthy, young adults (Hogan et al., 2011; Onoda et al., 2012;

Geerligs et al., 2013, 2014; Oh and Jagust, 2013; Waring et al., 2013). In children with ADHD compared to typically developing children the pattern of functional connectivity is also different (Murias et al., 2007; Mazaheri et al., 2010). Further evidence for the importance of functional connectivity comes from TMS/tCS studies showing that not only is the activity in the stimulated region modified, but also connectivity of the stimulated region to other regions (Strens et al., 2002; Polanía et al., 2012a; Veniero et al., 2013; Shafi et al., 2014) and in some cases this altered connectivity correlated with task modulations (Vidal-Piñeiro et al., 2014) or improved/altered behavior (Lee and D'Esposito, 2012). As the human brain is a huge network of neurons, it seems logical that an optimization of functional connectivity within and across brain-regions is a crucial aspect to optimize human behavior. However, we have just begun to understand the mechanisms behind inter- and intra-regional coupling (Felleman and Essen, 1991; Varela et al., 2001; Callaway, 2004; Fox et al., 2005; Canolty et al., 2006; Lakatos et al., 2008; Schroeder and Lakatos, 2009; Maier et al., 2010; Haegens et al., 2011b; Spaak et al., 2012), so we still have a long way to go until we fully grasp the effect that artificially manipulating functional connectivity has on the human brain and human cognition.

PROBLEMS OF USAGE AT HOME

Applying some of these techniques at home can be a challenge on its own. The most obvious question to ask is whether the proposed techniques can be used alone at home or whether an expert, e.g., a neuroscientist or a physician with proper training, should be visited. Currently, there is a trend in crowd funding and open source projects, which allow individuals to propose and share ideas. This has led to projects such as OpenrTMS[2] or OpenBCI,[3] which in theory allow everyone to create their own TMS or BCI protocol. As the human brain is overly complex, however, special care has to be taken on this path of neuro-hacking.[4] Obviously side-effects, as discussed above, are likely to occur during improper application. Apart from that, additional problems can be expected when applying the discussed brain augmentation techniques at home, e.g., motivational reasons can cause irregular, inefficient use and eventually lead to stopping the treatment. In addition, environmental noise may influence the measurements at home differently than in a well-controlled laboratory. Studies in the lab under special, controlled circumstances might not easily transfer to use at home or other situations of daily life (see e.g., Vaughan et al., 2006). Therefore and especially due to medical reasons we would propose that, first, more research is required to investigate side-effects and long-term effects. Second, application should only be administered by trained experts. Only in the far future does usage at home seem realistic.

CONSIDERATIONS FOR SUCCESSFUL VALORIZATION AND COMMERCIALIZATION

The above suggestions and hypotheses might seem like a great promise for augmentation of human behavior, so it is natural that commercial companies will pick up on these ideas in the near future. However, when considering augmentation of human behavior from a commercial perspective, there are additional considerations apart from those already discussed, foremost safety issues. Modern advertisements focus on short, catchy messages to attract potential customers (Dahlén and Rosengren, 2005; Kohli et al., 2007). The human brain, however, is a complicated machine and we are just beginning to understand its fundamental mechanisms and functions. Companies have to take responsibility for the products they sell and be wary of linking false promises to their commercial products. Also, companies need to be explicit to the customer on the consequences of not using devices properly as intended. Yet, there is no consensus on proper use of brain stimulation technique. Thus, extreme caution needs to be exercised before bringing a product onto the market. We therefore advise any company with serious perspectives on developing and selling these devices to collaborate strongly with established neuroscientists in the field and ethical committees and to conduct extensive studies on their products.

CONCLUSIONS

In this review, we started from the hypothesis that neuronal oscillations serve as strong neuronal correlates of behavior and are involved in human cognition. We reviewed this hypothesis in light of three target groups: the healthy elderly, ADHD patients, and healthy young adults. Most of the evidence supporting our hypothesis stemmed from studies on healthy young adults showing reliable correlations between the power of the oscillations and cognitive aspects of human behavior, e.g., working memory capacity or detection accuracy. Our hypothesis was corroborated by brain stimulation studies using TMS and tACS showing a strong link between the strength of induced neuronal oscillations and behavioral performance (see Section Techniques to Manipulate Neuronal Oscillations).

This hypothesis has important implications for the realm of cognitive neuroscience: if an oscillation is causally involved in cognition, a manipulation of that oscillation has to lead to a subsequent change in behavior. Such a strong, functional hypothesis helps to drive the field of cognitive neuroscience forward in understanding how the human brain functions.

Further, we hypothesized in Section Population Target Groups and Their Neuronal Signatures that the elderly and ADHD patients suffer from a lack of integrating neuronal oscillations properly, due to an absence of correlation with behavior, and that compensatory mechanisms could have taken over the functional shaping of cognition. We further hypothesized that manipulating neuronal oscillations in these target groups might restore their beneficial nature. This is a far-fetched claim without any empirical evidence and should be further studied. First of all, we need to ask whether the absence of the correlation between neuronal oscillations and behavior still allows the control and modulation of oscillations. Further, if these target groups could increase some neuronal oscillation during tasks, would that have behavioral consequences? Although we hypothesized that there would be, even if there would not be a behavioral benefit, we would gain important, fundamental insight in different neuronal mechanisms to shape human cognition.

[2]http://open-rtms.sourceforge.net/
[3]http://www.openbci.com/
[4]http://en.wikipedia.org/wiki/Neurohacking

In sum, we conclude that many more studies need to be conducted and reproduced, in both young, healthy and other target groups, to elucidate the role of and effects of manipulation of neuronal oscillations on behavior. Further insight from fundamental research into neuronal mechanisms is required to develop robust products for augmenting cognition.

ACKNOWLEDGMENTS

The authors would like to thank Madelon Vollebregt for useful feedback and discussion on Section Attention Deficit/Hyperactivity Disorder, and Til Ole Bergmann for useful feedback and discussion on Section Transcranial Stimulation of the Human Brain. The authors are or have been supported by a VICI grant of the Organization for Scientific Research (NWO) to Prof. Ole Jensen under grant number 453-09-002, and the research program "The healthy brain" funded by the Netherlands Initiative Brain and Cognition (NIHC), a part of NWO, to Prof. Ole Jensen under grant number 056-14-011. All authors declare no conflict of interest or other financial support.

REFERENCES

Adams, Z. W., Derefinko, K. J., Milich, R., and Fillmore, M. T. (2008). Inhibitory functioning across ADHD subtypes: recent findings, clinical implications and future directions. *Dev. Disabil. Res. Rev.* 14, 268–275. doi: 10.1002/ddrr.37

Addante, R. J., Watrous, A. J., Yonelinas, A. P., Ekstrom, A. D., and Ranganath, C. (2011). Prestimulus theta activity predicts correct source memory retrieval. *Proc. Natl. Acad. Sci. U S A* 108, 10702–10707. doi: 10.1073/pnas.1014528108

Adrian, E. D., and Matthews, B. H. C. (1934). The berger rhythm: potential changes from the occipital lobes in man. *Brain* 57, 355–385. doi: 10.1093/brain/57.4.355

Alain, C., and Woods, D. L. (1999). Age-related changes in processing auditory stimuli during visual attention: evidence for deficits in inhibitory control and sensory memory. *Psychol. Aging* 14, 507–519. doi: 10.1037//0882-7974.14.3.507

Allendorfer, J. B., Storrs, J. M., and Szaflarski, J. P. (2012). Changes in white matter integrity follow excitatory rTMS treatment of post-stroke aphasia. *Restor. Neurol. Neurosci.* 30, 103–113. doi: 10.3233/RNN-2011-0627

Andrés, P., Parmentier, F. B. R., and Escera, C. (2006). The effect of age on involuntary capture of attention by irrelevant sounds: a test of the frontal hypothesis of aging. *Neuropsychologia* 44, 2564–2568. doi: 10.1016/j.neuropsychologia.2006.05.005

Antal, A., and Paulus, W. (2013). Transcranial alternating current stimulation (tACS). *Front. Hum. Neurosci.* 7:317. doi: 10.3389/fnhum.2013.00317

Bahramisharif, A., van Gerven, M., Heskes, T., and Jensen, O. (2010). Covert attention allows for continuous control of brain-computer interfaces. *Eur. J. Neurosci.* 31, 1501–1508. doi: 10.1111/j.1460-9568.2010.07174.x

Bai, S., Dokos, S., Ho, K.-A., and Loo, C. (2014). A computational modelling study of transcranial direct current stimulation montages used in depression. *Neuroimage* 87, 332–344. doi: 10.1016/j.neuroimage.2013.11.015

Barkley, R. A. (2001). The Inattentive type of ADHD As a distinct disorder: what remains to be done. *Clin. Psychol. Sci. Pract.* 8, 489–493. doi: 10.1093/clipsy.8.4.489

Barkley, R. A., DuPaul, G. J., and McMurray, M. B. (1990). Comprehensive evaluation of attention deficit disorder with and without hyperactivity as defined by research criteria. *J. Consult. Clin. Psychol.* 58, 775–789. doi: 10.1037//0022-006x.58.6.775

Barry, R. J., Clarke, A. R., and Johnstone, S. J. (2003). A review of electrophysiology in attention-deficit/hyperactivity disorder: I. Qualitative and quantitative electroencephalography. *Clin. Neurophysiol.* 114, 171–183. doi: 10.1016/s1388-2457(02)00362-0

Batsikadze, G., Moliadze, V., Paulus, W., Kuo, M.-F., and Nitsche, M. A. (2013). Partially non-linear stimulation intensity-dependent effects of direct current stimulation on motor cortex excitability in humans. *J. Physiol.* 591, 1987–2000. doi: 10.1113/jphysiol.2012.249730

Bauer, M., Oostenveld, R., Peeters, M., and Fries, P. (2006). Tactile spatial attention enhances gamma-band activity in somatosensory cortex and reduces low-frequency activity in parieto-occipital areas. *J. Neurosci.* 26, 490–501. doi: 10.1523/JNEUROSCI.5228-04.2006

Bengson, J. J., Mangun, G. R., and Mazaheri, A. (2012). The neural markers of an imminent failure of response inhibition. *Neuroimage* 59, 1534–1539. doi: 10.1016/j.neuroimage.2011.08.034

Berger, P. D. H. (1929). Über das Elektrenkephalogramm des Menschen. *Arch. Für Psychiatr. Nervenkrankh.* 87, 527–570.

Bijsterbosch, J. D., Barker, A. T., Lee, K.-H., and Woodruff, P. W. R. (2012). Where does transcranial magnetic stimulation (TMS) stimulate? Modelling of induced field maps for some common cortical and cerebellar targets. *Med. Biol. Eng. Comput.* 50, 671–681. doi: 10.1007/s11517-012-0922-8

Bollimunta, A., Mo, J., Schroeder, C. E., and Ding, M. (2011). Neuronal mechanisms and attentional modulation of corticothalamic α oscillations. *J. Neurosci.* 31, 4935–4943. doi: 10.1523/jneurosci.5580-10.2011

Bonnefond, M., and Jensen, O. (2012). Alpha oscillations serve to protect working memory maintenance against anticipated distracters. *Curr. Biol.* 22, 1969–1974. doi: 10.1016/j.cub.2012.08.029

Bonnefond, M., and Jensen, O. (2013). The role of gamma and alpha oscillations for blocking out distraction. *Commun. Integr. Biol.* 6:e22702. doi: 10.4161/cib.22702

Booth, J. E., Carlson, C. L., and Tucker, D. M. (2007). Performance on a neurocognitive measure of alerting differentiates ADHD combined and inattentive subtypes: a preliminary report. *Arch. Clin. Neuropsychol.* 22, 423–432. doi: 10.1016/j.acn.2007.01.017

Brem, A.-K., Fried, P. J., Horvath, J. C., Robertson, E. M., and Pascual-Leone, A. (2014). Is neuroenhancement by noninvasive brain stimulation a net zero-sum proposition? *Neuroimage* 85(Pt. 3), 1058–1068. doi: 10.1016/j.neuroimage.2013.07.038

Brignani, D., Ruzzoli, M., Mauri, P., and Miniussi, C. (2013). Is transcranial alternating current stimulation effective in modulating brain oscillations? *PLoS One* 8:e56589. doi: 10.1371/journal.pone.0056589

Brockmole, J. R., and Logie, R. H. (2013). Age-related change in visual working memory: a study of 55,753 participants aged 8–75. *Front. Psychol.* 4:12. doi: 10.3389/fpsyg.2013.00012

Buzsáki, G. (2006). *Rhythms of the Brain.* New York, NY: Oxford University Press.

Buzsáki, G., and Draguhn, A. (2004). Neuronal oscillations in cortical networks. *Science* 304, 1926–1929. doi: 10.1126/science.1099745

Cabeza, R., Anderson, N. D., Locantore, J. K., and McIntosh, A. R. (2002). Aging gracefully: compensatory brain activity in high-performing older adults. *Neuroimage* 17, 1394–1402. doi: 10.1006/nimg.2002.1280

Calderone, D. J., Lakatos, P., Butler, P. D., and Castellanos, F. X. (2014). Entrainment of neural oscillations as a modifiable substrate of attention. *Trends Cogn. Sci.* 18, 300–309. doi: 10.1016/j.tics.2014.02.005

Callaway, E. M. (2004). Feedforward, feedback and inhibitory connections in primate visual cortex. *Neural Netw.* 17, 625–632. doi: 10.1016/j.neunet.2004.04.004

Canolty, R. T., Edwards, E., Dalal, S. S., Soltani, M., Nagarajan, S. S., Kirsch, H. E., et al. (2006). High gamma power is phase-locked to theta oscillations in human neocortex. *Science* 313, 1626–1628. doi: 10.1126/science.1128115

Cantwell, D. P. (1996). Attention deficit disorder: a review of the past 10 years. *J. Am. Acad. Child Adolesc. Psychiatry* 35, 978–987. doi: 10.1097/00004583-199608000-00008

Capotosto, P., Babiloni, C., Romani, G. L., and Corbetta, M. (2009). Frontoparietal cortex controls spatial attention through modulation of anticipatory alpha rhythms. *J. Neurosci.* 29, 5863–5872. doi: 10.1523/jneurosci.0539-09.2009

Capotosto, P., Babiloni, C., Romani, G. L., and Corbetta, M. (2012). Differential contribution of right and left parietal cortex to the control of spatial attention: a simultaneous EEG-rTMS study. *Cereb. Cortex* 22, 446–454. doi: 10.1093/cercor/bhr127

Carr, L., Henderson, J., and Nigg, J. T. (2010). Cognitive control and attentional selection in adolescents with ADHD versus ADD. *J. Clin. Child Adolesc. Psychol.* 39, 726–740. doi: 10.1080/15374416.2010.517168

Cavanagh, J. F., Frank, M. J., Klein, T. J., and Allen, J. J. B. (2010). Frontal theta links prediction errors to behavioral adaptation in reinforcement learning. *Neuroimage* 49, 3198–3209. doi: 10.1016/j.neuroimage.2009.11.080

Chanes, L., Quentin, R., Tallon-Baudry, C., and Valero-Cabré, A. (2013). Causal Frequency-specific contributions of frontal spatiotemporal patterns induced by non-invasive neurostimulation to human visual performance. *J. Neurosci.* 33, 5000–5005. doi: 10.1523/JNEUROSCI.4401-12.2013

Chang, Z., Lichtenstein, P., and Larsson, H. (2012). The effects of childhood ADHD symptoms on early-onset substance use: a Swedish twin study. *J. Abnorm. Child Psychol.* 40, 425–435. doi: 10.1007/s10802-011-9575-6

Coffman, B. A., Clark, V. P., and Parasuraman, R. (2014). Battery powered thought: enhancement of attention, learning and memory in healthy adults using transcranial direct current stimulation. *Neuroimage* 85(Pt. 3), 895–908. doi: 10.1016/j.neuroimage.2013.07.083

Cohen, J. E. (2005). Human population grows up. *Sci. Am.* 293, 48–55. doi: 10.1038/scientificamerican0905-48

Cohen, M. X., Axmacher, N., Lenartz, D., Elger, C. E., Sturm, V., and Schlaepfer, T. E. (2009). Nuclei accumbens phase synchrony predicts decision-making reversals following negative feedback. *J. Neurosci.* 29, 7591–7598. doi: 10.1523/jneurosci.5335-08.2009

Cohen, M. X., Bour, L., Mantione, M., Figee, M., Vink, M., Tijssen, M. A. J., et al. (2012). Top-down-directed synchrony from medial frontal cortex to nucleus accumbens during reward anticipation. *Hum. Brain Mapp.* 33, 246–252. doi: 10.1002/hbm.21195

Dahlén, M., and Rosengren, S. (2005). Brands affect slogans affect brands? Competitive interference, brand equity and the brand-slogan link. *J. Brand Manag.* 12, 151–164. doi: 10.1057/palgrave.bm.2540212

Dahlin, E., Neely, A. S., Larsson, A., Bäckman, L., and Nyberg, L. (2008). Transfer of learning after updating training mediated by the striatum. *Science* 320, 1510–1512. doi: 10.1126/science.1155466

Dayan, E., Censor, N., Buch, E. R., Sandrini, M., and Cohen, L. G. (2013). Noninvasive brain stimulation: from physiology to network dynamics and back. *Nat. Neurosci.* 16, 838–844. doi: 10.1038/nn.3422

de Graaf, T. A., Gross, J., Paterson, G., Rusch, T., Sack, A. T., and Thut, G. (2013). Alpha-Band rhythms in visual task performance: phase-locking by rhythmic sensory stimulation. *PLoS One* 8:e60035. doi: 10.1371/journal.pone.0060035

Deary, I. J., Corley, J., Gow, A. J., Harris, S. E., Houlihan, L. M., Marioni, R. E., et al. (2009). Age-associated cognitive decline. *Br. Med. Bull.* 92, 135–152. doi: 10.1093/bmb/ldp033

Derefinko, K. J., Adams, Z. W., Milich, R., Fillmore, M. T., Lorch, E. P., and Lynam, D. R. (2008). Response style differences in the inattentive and combined subtypes of attention-deficit/hyperactivity disorder. *J. Abnorm. Child Psychol.* 36, 745–758. doi: 10.1007/s10802-007-9207-3

Dickhaus, T., Sannelli, C., Müller, K.-R., Curio, G., and Blankertz, B. (2009). Predicting BCI performance to study BCI illiteracy. *BMC Neurosci.* 10:84. doi: 10.1186/1471-2202-10-s1-p84

Dustman, R. E., Shearer, D. E., and Emmerson, R. Y. (1993). EEG and event-related potentials in normal aging. *Prog. Neurobiol.* 41, 369–401. doi: 10.1016/0301-0082(93)90005-d

Engel, A. K., Fries, P., and Singer, W. (2001). Dynamic predictions: oscillations and synchrony in top-down processing. *Nat. Rev. Neurosci.* 2, 704–716. doi: 10.1038/35094565

Engel, A. K., and Singer, W. (2001). Temporal binding and the neural correlates of sensory awareness. *Trends Cogn. Sci.* 5, 16–25. doi: 10.1016/s1364-6613(00)01568-0

Enriquez-Geppert, S., Huster, R. J., Scharfenort, R., Mokom, Z. N., Zimmermann, J., and Herrmann, C. S. (2014). Modulation of frontal-midline theta by neurofeedback. *Biol. Psychol.* 95, 59–69. doi: 10.1016/j.biopsycho.2013.02.019

Ergenoglu, T., Demiralp, T., Bayraktaroglu, Z., Ergen, M., Beydagi, H., and Uresin, Y. (2004). Alpha rhythm of the EEG modulates visual detection performance in humans. *Brain Res. Cogn. Brain Res.* 20, 376–383. doi: 10.1016/j.cogbrainres.2004.03.009

Fabiani, M., Low, K. A., Wee, E., Sable, J. J., and Gratton, G. (2006). Reduced suppression or labile memory? Mechanisms of inefficient filtering of irrelevant information in older adults. *J. Cogn. Neurosci.* 18, 637–650. doi: 10.1162/jocn.2006.18.4.637

Fell, J., Ludowig, E., Staresina, B. P., Wagner, T., Kranz, T., Elger, C. E., et al. (2011). Medial temporal theta/alpha power enhancement precedes successful memory encoding: evidence based on intracranial EEG. *J. Neurosci.* 31, 5392–5397. doi: 10.1523/jneurosci.3668-10.2011

Felleman, D. J., and Essen, D. C. V. (1991). Distributed hierarchical processing in the primate. *Cereb. Cortex* 1, 1–47. doi: 10.1093/cercor/1.1.1

Folk, C. L., and Lincourt, A. E. (1996). The effects of age on guided conjunction search. *Exp. Aging Res.* 22, 99–118. doi: 10.1080/03610739608254000

Fox, M. D., Snyder, A. Z., Vincent, J. L., Corbetta, M., Essen, D. C. V., and Raichle, M. E. (2005). The human brain is intrinsically organized into dynamic, anticorrelated functional networks. *Proc. Natl. Acad. Sci. U S A* 102, 9673–9678. doi: 10.1073/pnas.0504136102

Foxe, J. J., and Snyder, A. C. (2011). The role of alpha-band brain oscillations as a sensory suppression mechanism during selective attention. *Front. Psychol.* 2:154. doi: 10.3389/fpsyg.2011.00154

Fries, P. (2005). A mechanism for cognitive dynamics: neuronal communication through neuronal coherence. *Trends Cogn. Sci.* 9, 474–480. doi: 10.1016/j.tics.2005.08.011

Fries, P., Reynolds, J. H., Rorie, A. E., and Desimone, R. (2001). Modulation of oscillatory neuronal synchronization by selective visual attention. *Science* 291, 1560–1563. doi: 10.1126/science.1055465

Fründ, I., Busch, N. A., Schadow, J., Körner, U., and Herrmann, C. S. (2007). From perception to action: phase-locked gamma oscillations correlate with reaction times in a speeded response task. *BMC Neurosci.* 8:27. doi: 10.1186/1471-2202-8-27

Fu, K. M., Foxe, J. J., Murray, M. M., Higgins, B. A., Javitt, D. C., and Schroeder, C. E. (2001). Attention-dependent suppression of distracter visual input can be cross-modally cued as indexed by anticipatory parieto-occipital alpha-band oscillations. *Brain Res. Cogn. Brain Res.* 12, 145–152. doi: 10.1016/s0926-6410(01)00034-9

Fuchs, T., Birbaumer, N., Lutzenberger, W., Gruzelier, J. H., and Kaiser, J. (2003). Neurofeedback treatment for attention-deficit/hyperactivity disorder in children: a comparison with methylphenidate. *Appl. Psychophysiol. Biofeedback* 28, 1–12. doi: 10.1023/A:1022353731579

Gaeta, H., Friedman, D., Ritter, W., and Cheng, J. (2001). An event-related potential evaluation of involuntary attentional shifts in young and older adults. *Psychol. Aging* 16, 55–68. doi: 10.1037//0882-7974.16.1.55

Gazzaley, A., Clapp, W., Kelley, J., McEvoy, K., Knight, R. T., and D'Esposito, M. (2008). Age-related top-down suppression deficit in the early stages of cortical visual memory processing. *Proc. Natl. Acad. Sci.* 105, 13122–13126. doi: 10.1073/pnas.0806074105

Geerligs, L., Maurits, N. M., Renken, R. J., and Lorist, M. M. (2014). Reduced specificity of functional connectivity in the aging brain during task performance. *Hum. Brain Mapp.* 35, 319–330. doi: 10.1002/hbm.22175

Geerligs, L., Saliasi, E., Renken, R. J., Maurits, N. M., and Lorist, M. M. (2013). Flexible connectivity in the aging brain revealed by task modulations. *Hum. Brain Mapp.* doi: 10.1002/hbm.22437. [Epub ahead of print].

Gevins, A., and Smith, M. E. (2000). Neurophysiological measures of working memory and individual differences in cognitive ability and cognitive style. *Cereb. Cortex* 10, 829–839. doi: 10.1093/cercor/10.9.829

Gevins, A., Smith, M. E., McEvoy, L., and Yu, D. (1997). High-resolution EEG mapping of cortical activation related to working memory: effects of task difficulty, type of processing and practice. *Cereb. Cortex* 7, 374–385. doi: 10.1093/cercor/7.4.374

Gharabaghi, A., Kraus, D., Leao, M. T., Spüler, M., Walter, A., Bogdan, M., et al. (2014). Coupling brain-machine interfaces with cortical stimulation for brain-state dependent stimulation: enhancing motor cortex excitability for neurorehabilitation. *Front. Hum. Neurosci.* 8:122. doi: 10.3389/fnhum.2014.00122

Ghaziri, J., Tucholka, A., Larue, V., Blanchette-Sylvestre, M., Reyburn, G., Gilbert, G., et al. (2013). Neurofeedback training induces changes in white and gray matter. *Clin. EEG Neurosci.* 44, 265–272. doi: 10.1177/1550059413476031

Gho, M., and Varela, F. J. (1988). A quantitative assessment of the dependency of the visual temporal frame upon the cortical rhythm. *J. Physiol. (Paris)* 83, 95–101.

Goodale, M. A., and Milner, A. D. (1992). Separate visual pathways for perception and action. *Trends Neurosci.* 15, 20–25. doi: 10.1016/0166-2236(92)90344-8

Gould, I. C., Rushworth, M. F., and Nobre, A. C. (2011). Indexing the graded allocation of visuospatial attention using anticipatory alpha oscillations. *J. Neurophysiol.* 105, 1318–1326. doi: 10.1152/jn.00653.2010

Grandy, T. H., Werkle-Bergner, M., Chicherio, C., Lövdén, M., Schmiedek, F., and Lindenberger, U. (2013). Individual alpha peak frequency is related to latent factors of general cognitive abilities. *Neuroimage* 79, 10–18. doi: 10.1016/j.neuroimage.2013.04.059

Gross, J., Schmitz, F., Schnitzler, I., Kessler, K., Shapiro, K., Hommel, B., et al. (2004). Modulation of long-range neural synchrony reflects temporal limitations of visual attention in humans. *Proc. Natl. Acad. Sci. U S A* 101, 13050–13055. doi: 10.1073/pnas.0404944101

Groth, K. E., and Allen, P. A. (2000). Visual attention and aging. *Front. Biosci.* 5, D284–D297. doi: 10.2741/Groth

Gruzelier, J. H. (2013). EEG-neurofeedback for optimising performance. I: a review of cognitive and affective outcome in healthy participants. *Neurosci. Biobehav. Rev.* doi: 10.1016/j.neubiorev.2013.09.015

Haegens, S., Händel, B. F., and Jensen, O. (2011a). Top-down controlled alpha band activity in somatosensory areas determines behavioral performance in a discrimination task. *J. Neurosci.* 31, 5197–5204. doi: 10.1523/jneurosci.5199-10.2011

Haegens, S., Luther, L., and Jensen, O. (2012). Somatosensory anticipatory alpha activity increases to suppress distracting input. *J. Cogn. Neurosci.* 24, 677–685. doi: 10.1162/jocn_a_00164

Haegens, S., Nácher, V., Luna, R., Romo, R., and Jensen, O. (2011b). α-Oscillations in the monkey sensorimotor network influence discrimination performance by rhythmical inhibition of neuronal spiking. *Proc. Natl. Acad. Sci. U S A* 108, 19377–19382. doi: 10.1073/pnas.1117190108

Haegens, S., Osipova, D., Oostenveld, R., and Jensen, O. (2010). Somatosensory working memory performance in humans depends on both engagement and disengagement of regions in a distributed network. *Hum. Brain Mapp.* 31, 26–35. doi: 10.1002/hbm.20842

Halperin, J. M., and Healey, D. M. (2011). The influences of environmental enrichment, cognitive enhancement and physical exercise on brain development: can we alter the developmental trajectory of ADHD? *Neurosci. Biobehav. Rev.* 35, 621–634. doi: 10.1016/j.neubiorev.2010.07.006

Hamidi, M., Slagter, H. A., Tononi, G., Postle, B. R., Hamidi, M., Slagter, H. A., et al. (2009). Repetitive transcranial magnetic stimulation affects behavior by biasing endogenous cortical oscillations. *Front. Integr. Neurosci.* 3:14. doi: 10.3389/neuro.07.014.2009

Händel, B. F., Haarmeier, T., and Jensen, O. (2011). Alpha oscillations correlate with the successful inhibition of unattended stimuli. *J. Cogn. Neurosci.* 23, 2494–2502. doi: 10.1162/jocn.2010.21557

Hanslmayr, S., Aslan, A., Staudigl, T., Klimesch, W., Herrmann, C. S., and Bäuml, K.-H. (2007). Prestimulus oscillations predict visual perception performance between and within subjects. *Neuroimage* 37, 1465–1473. doi: 10.1016/j.neuroimage.2007.07.011

Hanslmayr, S., Klimesch, W., Sauseng, P., Gruber, W., Doppelmayr, M., Freunberger, R., et al. (2005a). Visual discrimination performance is related to decreased alpha amplitude but increased phase locking. *Neurosci. Lett.* 375, 64–68. doi: 10.1016/j.neulet.2004.10.092

Hanslmayr, S., Sauseng, P., Doppelmayr, M., Schabus, M., and Klimesch, W. (2005b). Increasing individual upper alpha power by neurofeedback improves cognitive performance in human subjects. *Appl. Psychophysiol. Biofeedback* 30, 1–10. doi: 10.1007/s10484-005-2169-8

Hanslmayr, S., and Staudigl, T. (2014). How brain oscillations form memories–a processing based perspective on oscillatory subsequent memory effects. *Neuroimage* 85(Pt. 2), 648–655. doi: 10.1016/j.neuroimage.2013.05.121

Hanslmayr, S., Staudigl, T., and Fellner, M.-C. (2012). Oscillatory power decreases and long-term memory: the information via desynchronization hypothesis. *Front. Hum. Neurosci.* 6:74. doi: 10.3389/fnhum.2012.00074

Hartmann, T., Schulz, H., and Weisz, N. (2011). Probing of brain states in real-time: introducing the console environment. *Front. Psychol.* 2:36. doi: 10.3389/fpsyg.2011.00036

Helfrich, R. F., Schneider, T. R., Rach, S., Trautmann-Lengsfeld, S. A., Engel, A. K., and Herrmann, C. S. (2014). Entrainment of brain oscillations by transcranial alternating current stimulation. *Curr. Biol.* 24, 333–339. doi: 10.1016/j.cub.2013.12.041

Herrmann, C. S., Rach, S., Neuling, T., and Strüber, D. (2013). Transcranial alternating current stimulation: a review of the underlying mechanisms and modulation of cognitive processes. *Front. Hum. Neurosci.* 7:279. doi: 10.3389/fnhum.2013.00279

Hogan, M., Collins, P., Keane, M., Kilmartin, L., Kaiser, J., Kenney, J., et al. (2011). Electroencephalographic coherence, aging and memory: distinct responses to background context and stimulus repetition in younger, older and older declined groups. *Exp. Brain Res.* 212, 241–255. doi: 10.1007/s00221-011-2726-8

Hoogenboom, N., Schoffelen, J.-M., Oostenveld, R., Parkes, L. M., and Fries, P. (2006). Localizing human visual gamma-band activity in frequency, time and space. *Neuroimage* 29, 764–773. doi: 10.1016/j.neuroimage.2005.08.043

Horschig, J. M., Jensen, O., van Schouwenburg, M. R., Cools, R., and Bonnefond, M. (2014). Alpha activity reflects individual abilities to adapt to the environment. *Neuroimage* 89, 235–243. doi: 10.1016/j.neuroimage.2013.12.018

Horvath, J. C., Carter, O., and Forte, J. D. (2014). Transcranial direct current stimulation: five important issues we aren't discussing (but probably should be). *Front. Syst. Neurosci.* 8:2. doi: 10.3389/fnsys.2014.00002

Howard, M. W., Rizzuto, D. S., Caplan, J. B., Madsen, J. R., Lisman, J., Aschenbrenner-Scheibe, R., et al. (2003). Gamma oscillations correlate with working memory load in humans. *Cereb. Cortex* 13, 1369–1374. doi: 10.1093/cercor/bhg084

Huang, Y.-Z., Edwards, M. J., Rounis, E., Bhatia, K. P., and Rothwell, J. C. (2005). Theta burst stimulation of the human motor cortex. *Neuron* 45, 201–206. doi: 10.1016/j.neuron.2004.12.033

Hugenschmidt, C. E., Mozolic, J. L., and Laurienti, P. J. (2009a). Suppression of multisensory integration by modality-specific attention in aging. *Neuroreport* 20, 349–353. doi: 10.1097/wnr.0b013e328323ab07

Hugenschmidt, C. E., Peiffer, A. M., McCoy, T. P., Hayasaka, S., and Laurienti, P. J. (2009b). Preservation of crossmodal selective attention in healthy aging. *Exp. Brain Res.* 198, 273–285. doi: 10.1007/s00221-009-1816-3

Huggins, J. E., Guger, C., Allison, B., Anderson, C. W., Batista, A., Brouwer, A.-M., et al. (2014). Workshops of the fifth international brain-computer interface meeting: defining the future. *Brain-Comput. Interfaces* 1, 27–49. doi: 10.1080/2326263x.2013.876724

Huijbers, W., Pennartz, C. M., Cabeza, R., and Daselaar, S. M. (2009). When learning and remembering compete: a functional MRI study. *PLoS Biol.* 7:e1000011. doi: 10.1371/journal.pbio.1000011

Iuculano, T., and Cohen Kadosh, R. (2013). The mental cost of cognitive enhancement. *J. Neurosci.* 33, 4482–4486. doi: 10.1523/JNEUROSCI.4927-12.2013

Jaegle, A., and Ro, T. (2014). Direct control of visual perception with phase-specific modulation of posterior parietal cortex. *J. Cogn. Neurosci.* 26, 422–432. doi: 10.1162/jocn_a_00494

Janssen, A. M., Rampersad, S. M., Lucka, F., Lanfer, B., Lew, S., Aydin, U., et al. (2013). The influence of sulcus width on simulated electric fields induced by transcranial magnetic stimulation. *Phys. Med. Biol.* 58, 4881–4896. doi: 10.1088/0031-9155/58/14/4881

Jaušovec, N., and Jaušovec, K. (2014). Increasing working memory capacity with theta transcranial alternating current stimulation (tACS). *Biol. Psychol.* 96, 42–47. doi: 10.1016/j.biopsycho.2013.11.006

Jaušovec, N., Jaušovec, K., and Pahor, A. (2014). The influence of theta transcranial alternating current stimulation (tACS) on working memory storage and processing functions. *Acta Psychol. (Amst)* 146, 1–6. doi: 10.1016/j.actpsy.2013.11.011

Jensen, O., Bahramisharif, A., Oostenveld, R., Klanke, S., Hadjipapas, A., Okazaki, Y. O., et al. (2011). Using brain-computer interfaces and brain-state dependent stimulation as tools in cognitive neuroscience. *Front. Psychol.* 2:100. doi: 10.3389/fpsyg.2011.00100

Jensen, O., Bonnefond, M., and VanRullen, R. (2012). An oscillatory mechanism for prioritizing salient unattended stimuli. *Trends Cogn. Sci.* 16, 200–206. doi: 10.1016/j.tics.2012.03.002

Jensen, O., Gelfand, J., Kounios, J., and Lisman, J. E. (2002). Oscillations in the alpha band (9–12 Hz) increase with memory load during retention in a short-term memory task. *Cereb. Cortex* 12, 877–882. doi: 10.1093/cercor/12.8.877

Jensen, O., Kaiser, J., and Lachaux, J.-P. (2007). Human gamma-frequency oscillations associated with attention and memory. *Trends Neurosci.* 30, 317–324. doi: 10.1016/j.tins.2007.05.001

Jensen, O., and Lisman, J. E. (1996). Novel lists of 7 +/− 2 known items can be reliably stored in an oscillatory short-term memory network: interaction with long-term memory. *Learn. Mem.* 3, 257–263. doi: 10.1101/lm.3.2-3.257

Jensen, O., and Lisman, J. E. (1998). An oscillatory short-term memory buffer model can account for data on the Sternberg task. *J. Neurosci.* 18, 10688–10699.

Jensen, O., and Mazaheri, A. (2010). Shaping functional architecture by oscillatory alpha activity: gating by inhibition. *Front. Hum. Neurosci.* 4:186. doi: 10.3389/fnhum.2010.00186

Jensen, O., and Tesche, C. D. (2002). Frontal theta activity in humans increases with memory load in a working memory task. *Eur. J. Neurosci.* 15, 1395–1399. doi: 10.1046/j.1460-9568.2002.01975.x

Jokeit, H., and Makeig, S. (1994). Different event-related patterns of gamma-band power in brain waves of fast- and slow-reacting subjects. *Proc. Natl. Acad. Sci. U S A* 91, 6339–6343. doi: 10.1073/pnas.91.14.6339

Jokisch, D., and Jensen, O. (2007). Modulation of gamma and alpha activity during a working memory task engaging the dorsal or ventral stream. *J. Neurosci.* 27, 3244–3251. doi: 10.1523/jneurosci.5399-06.2007

Kahana, M. J., Seelig, D., and Madsen, J. R. (2001). Theta returns. *Curr. Opin. Neurobiol.* 11, 739–744. doi: 10.1016/s0959-4388(01)00278-1

Kamiński, J., Brzezicka, A., and Wróbel, A. (2011). Short-term memory capacity (7 ± 2) predicted by theta to gamma cycle length ratio. *Neurobiol. Learn. Mem.* 95, 19–23. doi: 10.1016/j.nlm.2010.10.001

Kanayama, N., Tamè, L., Ohira, H., and Pavani, F. (2012). Top down influence on visuo-tactile interaction modulates neural oscillatory responses. *Neuroimage* 59, 3406–3417. doi: 10.1016/j.neuroimage.2011.11.076

Kane, M. J., and Engle, R. W. (2002). The role of prefrontal cortex in working-memory capacity, executive attention and general fluid intelligence: an individual-differences perspective. *Psychon. Bull. Rev.* 9, 637–671. doi: 10.3758/bf03196323

Karch, S., Segmiller, F., Hantschk, I., Cerovecki, A., Opgen-Rhein, M., Hock, B., et al. (2012). Increased gamma oscillations during voluntary selection processes in adult patients with attention deficit/hyperactivity disorder. *J. Psychiatr. Res.* 46, 1515–1523. doi: 10.1016/j.jpsychires.2012.07.017

Keizer, A. W., Verschoor, M., Verment, R. S., and Hommel, B. (2010). The effect of gamma enhancing neurofeedback on the control of feature bindings and intelligence measures. *Int. J. Psychophysiol.* 75, 25–32. doi: 10.1016/j.ijpsycho.2009.10.011

Kelly, S. P., Gomez-Ramirez, M., and Foxe, J. J. (2009). The strength of anticipatory spatial biasing predicts target discrimination at attended locations: a high-density EEG study. *Eur. J. Neurosci.* 30, 2224–2234. doi: 10.1111/j.1460-9568.2009.06980.x

Kelly, S. P., Lalor, E. C., Reilly, R. B., and Foxe, J. J. (2005). Visual spatial attention tracking using high-density SSVEP data for independent brain-computer communication. *IEEE Trans. Neural. Syst. Rehabil. Eng.* 13, 172–178. doi: 10.1109/tnsre.2005.847369

Kidd, P. M. (2000). Attention deficit/hyperactivity disorder (ADHD) in children: rationale for its integrative management. *Altern. Med. Rev.* 5, 402–428.

Klimesch, W. (1999). EEG alpha and theta oscillations reflect cognitive and memory performance: a review and analysis. *Brain Res. Brain Res. Rev.* 29, 169–195. doi: 10.1016/s0165-0173(98)00056-3

Klimesch, W. (2012). α-band oscillations, attention and controlled access to stored information. *Trends Cogn. Sci.* 16, 606–617. doi: 10.1016/j.tics.2012.10.007

Klimesch, W., Doppelmayr, M., Russegger, H., and Pachinger, T. (1996). Theta band power in the human scalp EEG and the encoding of new information. *Neuroreport* 7, 1235–1240. doi: 10.1097/00001756-199605170-00002

Klimesch, W., Freunberger, R., and Sauseng, P. (2010). Oscillatory mechanisms of process binding in memory. *Neurosci. Biobehav. Rev.* 34, 1002–1014. doi: 10.1016/j.neubiorev.2009.10.004

Klimesch, W., Sauseng, P., and Gerloff, C. (2003). Enhancing cognitive performance with repetitive transcranial magnetic stimulation at human individual alpha frequency. *Eur. J. Neurosci.* 17, 1129–1133. doi: 10.1046/j.1460-9568.2003.02517.x

Klimesch, W., Sauseng, P., and Hanslmayr, S. (2007). EEG alpha oscillations: the inhibition-timing hypothesis. *Brain Res. Rev.* 53, 63–88. doi: 10.1016/j.brainresrev.2006.06.003

Klingberg, T. (2010). Training and plasticity of working memory. *Trends Cogn. Sci.* 14, 317–324. doi: 10.1016/j.tics.2010.05.002

Klingberg, T., Forssberg, H., and Westerberg, H. (2002). Training of working memory in children with ADHD. *J. Clin. Exp. Neuropsychol.* 24, 781–791. doi: 10.1076/jcen.24.6.781.8395

Kohli, C., Leuthesser, L., and Suri, R. (2007). Got slogan? Guidelines for creating effective slogans. *Bus. Horiz.* 50, 415–422. doi: 10.1016/j.bushor.2007.05.002

Kopell, N., Kramer, M. A., Malerba, P., and Whittington, M. A. (2010). Are different rhythms good for different functions? *Front. Hum. Neurosci.* 4:187. doi: 10.3389/fnhum.2010.00187

Krause, B., and Cohen Kadosh, R. (2014). Not all brains are created equal: the relevance of individual differences in responsiveness to transcranial electrical stimulation. *Front. Syst. Neurosci.* 8:25. doi: 10.3389/fnsys.2014.00025

Kray, J., and Lindenberger, U. (2000). Adult age differences in task switching. *Psychol. Aging* 15, 126–147. doi: 10.1037//0882-7974.15.1.126

Kruglikov, S. Y., and Schiff, S. J. (2003). Interplay of electroencephalogram phase and auditory-evoked neural activity. *J. Neurosci.* 23, 10122–10127.

Laczó, B., Antal, A., Niebergall, R., Treue, S., and Paulus, W. (2012). Transcranial alternating stimulation in a high gamma frequency range applied over V1 improves contrast perception but does not modulate spatial attention. *Brain Stimulat.* 5, 484–491. doi: 10.1016/j.brs.2011.08.008

Lakatos, P., Karmos, G., Mehta, A. D., Ulbert, I., and Schroeder, C. E. (2008). Entrainment of neuronal oscillations as a mechanism of attentional selection. *Science* 320, 110–113. doi: 10.1126/science.1154735

Lee, T. G., and D'Esposito, M. (2012). The dynamic nature of top-down signals originating from prefrontal cortex: a combined fMRI-TMS study. *J. Neurosci.* 32, 15458–15466. doi: 10.1523/JNEUROSCI.0627-12.2012

Lenartowicz, A., Delorme, A., Walshaw, P. D., Cho, A. L., Bilder, R. M., McGough, J. J., et al. (2014). Electroencephalography correlates of spatial working memory deficits in attention-deficit/hyperactivity disorder: vigilance, encoding and maintenance. *J. Neurosci.* 34, 1171–1182. doi: 10.1523/JNEUROSCI.1765-13.2014

Lenz, D., Krauel, K., Schadow, J., Baving, L., Duzel, E., and Herrmann, C. S. (2008). Enhanced gamma-band activity in ADHD patients lacks correlation with memory performance found in healthy children. *Brain Res.* 1235, 117–132. doi: 10.1016/j.brainres.2008.06.023

Lisman, J. (2005). The theta/gamma discrete phase code occuring during the hippocampal phase precession may be a more general brain coding scheme. *Hippocampus* 15, 913–922. doi: 10.1002/hipo.20121

Lisman, J. (2010). Working memory: the importance of theta and gamma oscillations. *Curr. Biol.* 20, R490–R492. doi: 10.1016/j.cub.2010.04.011

Lisman, J. E., and Jensen, O. (2013). The θ-γ neural code. *Neuron* 77, 1002–1016. doi: 10.1016/j.neuron.2013.03.007

Lockwood, K. A., Marcotte, A. C., and Stern, C. (2001). Differentiation of attention-deficit/hyperactivity disorder subtypes: application of a neuropsychological model of attention. *J. Clin. Exp. Neuropsychol.* 23, 317–330. doi: 10.1076/jcen.23.3.317.1179

Logan, J. M., Sanders, A. L., Snyder, A. Z., Morris, J. C., and Buckner, R. L. (2002). Under-recruitment and nonselective recruitment: dissociable neural mechanisms associated with aging. *Neuron* 33, 827–840. doi: 10.1016/s0896-6273(02)00612-8

Lopes da Silva, F. (1991). Neural mechanisms underlying brain waves: from neural membranes to networks. *Electroencephalogr. Clin. Neurophysiol.* 79, 81–93. doi: 10.1016/0013-4694(91)90044-5

Lopes da Silva, F. (2013). EEG and MEG: relevance to neuroscience. *Neuron* 80, 1112–1128. doi: 10.1016/j.neuron.2013.10.017

Lopes Da Silva, F. H., and Storm Van Leeuwen, W. (1977). The cortical source of the alpha rhythm. *Neurosci. Lett.* 6, 237–241. doi: 10.1016/0304-3940(77)90024-6

Lopes da Silva, F. H., Vos, J. E., Mooibroek, J., and Van Rotterdam, A. (1980). Relative contributions of intracortical and thalamo-cortical processes in the generation of alpha rhythms, revealed by partial coherence analysis. *Electroencephalogr. Clin. Neurophysiol.* 50, 449–456. doi: 10.1016/0013-4694(80)90011-5

Lubar, J. F., Swartwood, M. O., Swartwood, J. N., and O'Donnell, P. H. (1995). Evaluation of the effectiveness of EEG neurofeedback training for ADHD in a clinical setting as measured by changes in T.O.V.A. scores, behavioral ratings and WISC-R performance. *Biofeedback Self Regul.* 20, 83–99. doi: 10.1007/bf01712768

Luber, B., and Lisanby, S. H. (2014). Enhancement of human cognitive performance using transcranial magnetic stimulation (TMS). *Neuroimage* 85(Pt. 3), 961–970. doi: 10.1016/j.neuroimage.2013.06.007

Luck, S. J., and Vogel, E. K. (2013). Visual working memory capacity: from psychophysics and neurobiology to individual differences. *Trends Cogn. Sci.* 17, 391–400. doi: 10.1016/j.tics.2013.06.006

Maier, A., Adams, G. K., Aura, C., and Leopold, D. A. (2010). Distinct superficial and deep laminar domains of activity in the visual cortex during rest and stimulation. *Front. Syst. Neurosci.* 4:31. doi: 10.3389/fnsys.2010.00031

Manoli, Z., Grossman, N., and Samaras, T. (2012). Theoretical investigation of transcranial alternating current stimulation using realistic head model. *Conf. Proc. IEEE Eng. Med. Biol. Soc.* 2012, 4156–4159. doi: 10.1109/EMBC.2012.6346882

Mathewson, K. E., Gratton, G., Fabiani, M., Beck, D. M., and Ro, T. (2009). To see or not to see: prestimulus alpha phase predicts visual awareness. *J. Neurosci.* 29, 2725–2732. doi: 10.1523/JNEUROSCI.3963-08.2009

Mathewson, K. E., Prudhomme, C., Fabiani, M., Beck, D. M., Lleras, A., and Gratton, G. (2012). Making waves in the stream of consciousness: entraining oscillations in EEG alpha and fluctuations in visual awareness with rhythmic visual stimulation. *J. Cogn. Neurosci.* 24, 2321–2333. doi: 10.1162/jocn_a_0 0288

Mazaheri, A., Coffey-Corina, S., Mangun, G. R., Bekker, E. M., Berry, A. S., and Corbett, B. A. (2010). Functional disconnection of frontal cortex and visual cortex in attention-deficit/hyperactivity disorder. *Biol. Psychiatry* 67, 617–623. doi: 10.1016/j.biopsych.2009.11.022

Mazaheri, A., Fassbender, C., Coffey-Corina, S., Hartanto, T. A., Schweitzer, J. B., and Mangun, G. R. (2013). Differential oscillatory electroencephalogram between attention-deficit/hyperactivity disorder subtypes and typically developing adolescents. *Biol. Psychiatry* doi: 10.1016/j.biopsych.2013.08.023. [Epub ahead of print].

Mazaheri, A., Nieuwenhuis, I. L. C., van Dijk, H., and Jensen, O. (2009). Prestimulus alpha and mu activity predicts failure to inhibit motor responses. *Hum. Brain Mapp.* 30, 1791–1800. doi: 10.1002/hbm.20763

McEvoy, L. K., Pellouchoud, E., Smith, M. E., and Gevins, A. (2001). Neurophysiological signals of working memory in normal aging. *Brain Res. Cogn. Brain Res.* 11, 363–376. doi: 10.1016/s0926-6410(01)00009-x

Meeuwissen, E. B., Takashima, A., Fernández, G., and Jensen, O. (2011). Increase in posterior alpha activity during rehearsal predicts successful long-term memory formation of word sequences. *Hum. Brain Mapp.* 32, 2045–2053. doi: 10. 1002/hbm.21167

Meinzer, M., Antonenko, D., Lindenberg, R., Hetzer, S., Ulm, L., Avirame, K., et al. (2012). Electrical brain stimulation improves cognitive performance by modulating functional connectivity and task-specific activation. *J. Neurosci.* 32, 1859–1866. doi: 10.1523/JNEUROSCI.4812-11.2012

Meinzer, M., Lindenberg, R., Antonenko, D., Flaisch, T., and Flöel, A. (2013). Anodal transcranial direct current stimulation temporarily reverses age-associated cognitive decline and functional brain activity changes. *J. Neurosci.* 33, 12470–12478. doi: 10.1523/JNEUROSCI.5743-12.2013

Meiron, O., and Lavidor, M. (2014). Prefrontal oscillatory stimulation modulates access to cognitive control references in retrospective metacognitive commentary. *Clin. Neurophysiol.* 125, 77–82. doi: 10.1016/j.clinph.2013.06.013

Milich, R., Balentine, A. C., and Lynam, D. R. (2001). ADHD combined type and adhd predominantly inattentive type are distinct and unrelated disorders. *Clin. Psychol. Sci. Pract.* 8, 463–488. doi: 10.1093/clipsy.8.4.463

Miltner, W. H., Braun, C., Arnold, M., Witte, H., and Taub, E. (1999). Coherence of gamma-band EEG activity as a basis for associative learning. *Nature* 397, 434–436. doi: 10.1038/17126

Mitchell, D. J., McNaughton, N., Flanagan, D., and Kirk, I. J. (2008). Frontal-midline theta from the perspective of hippocampal "theta". *Prog. Neurobiol.* 86, 156–185. doi: 10.1016/j.pneurobio.2008.09.005

Mo, J., Schroeder, C. E., and Ding, M. (2011). Attentional modulation of alpha oscillations in macaque inferotemporal cortex. *J. Neurosci.* 31, 878–882. doi: 10. 1523/JNEUROSCI.5295-10.2011

Montemurro, M. A., Rasch, M. J., Murayama, Y., Logothetis, N. K., and Panzeri, S. (2008). Phase-of-firing coding of natural visual stimuli in primary visual cortex. *Curr. Biol.* 18, 375–380. doi: 10.1016/j.cub.2008.02.023

Murias, M., Swanson, J. M., and Srinivasan, R. (2007). Functional connectivity of frontal cortex in healthy and ADHD children reflected in EEG coherence. *Cereb. Cortex* 17, 1788–1799. doi: 10.1093/cercor/bhl089

Neuling, T., Rach, S., and Herrmann, C. S. (2013). Orchestrating neuronal networks: sustained after-effects of transcranial alternating current stimulation depend upon brain states. *Front. Hum. Neurosci.* 7:161. doi: 10.3389/fnhum. 2013.00161

Neuling, T., Rach, S., Wagner, S., Wolters, C. H., and Herrmann, C. S. (2012). Good vibrations: oscillatory phase shapes perception. *Neuroimage* 63, 771–778. doi: 10.1016/j.neuroimage.2012.07.024

Niedermeyer, E., and Lopes da Silva, F. H. (2005). *Electroencephalography: Basic Principles, Clinical Applications and Related Fields.* Philadelphia, PA: Lippincott Williams and Wilkins.

Nielson, K. A., Langenecker, S. A., and Garavan, H. (2002). Differences in the functional neuroanatomy of inhibitory control across the adult life span. *Psychol. Aging* 17, 56–71. doi: 10.1037//0882-7974.17.1.56

Nitsche, M. A., and Paulus, W. (2000). Excitability changes induced in the human motor cortex by weak transcranial direct current stimulation. *J. Physiol.* 527(Pt. 3), 633–639. doi: 10.1111/j.1469-7793.2000.t01-1-00633.x

Nuffield Councils on Bioethics. (2013). Novel neurotechnologies: intervening in the brain. Available at: http://www.nuffieldbioethics.org/sites/default/files/Novel_neurotechnologies_report_PDF_web_0.pdf

Nunez, P. L. (2000). Toward a quantitative description of large-scale neocortical dynamic function and EEG. *Behav. Brain Sci.* 23, 371–398; discussion 399–437. doi: 10.1017/s0140525x00003253

Oh, H., and Jagust, W. J. (2013). Frontotemporal network connectivity during memory encoding is increased with aging and disrupted by beta-amyloid. *J. Neurosci.* 33, 18425–18437. doi: 10.1523/JNEUROSCI.2775-13.2013

Onoda, K., Ishihara, M., and Yamaguchi, S. (2012). Decreased functional connectivity by aging is associated with cognitive decline. *J. Cogn. Neurosci.* 24, 2186–2198. doi: 10.1162/jocn_a_00269

Osipova, D., Takashima, A., Oostenveld, R., Fernández, G., Maris, E., and Jensen, O. (2006). Theta and gamma oscillations predict encoding and retrieval of declarative memory. *J. Neurosci.* 26, 7523–7531. doi: 10.1523/jneurosci.1948-06. 2006

Park, H., Lee, D. S., Kang, E., Kang, H., Hahm, J., Kim, J. S., et al. (2014). Blocking of irrelevant memories by posterior alpha activity boosts memory encoding. *Hum. Brain Mapp.* doi: 10.1002/hbm.22452. [Epub ahead of print].

Pascual-Leone, A., Bartres-Faz, D., and Keenan, J. P. (1999). Transcranial magnetic stimulation: studying the brain-behaviour relationship by induction of "virtual lesions". *Philos. Trans. R. Soc. Lond. B Biol. Sci.* 354, 1229–1238. doi: 10. 1098/rstb.1999.0476

Pascual-Leone, A., Freitas, C., Oberman, L., Horvath, J. C., Halko, M., Eldaief, M., et al. (2011). Characterizing brain cortical plasticity and network dynamics across the age-span in health and disease with TMS-EEG and TMS-fMRI. *Brain Topogr.* 24, 302–315. doi: 10.1007/s10548-011-0196-8

Pascual-Leone, A., Walsh, V., and Rothwell, J. (2000). Transcranial magnetic stimulation in cognitive neuroscience—virtual lesion, chronometry and functional connectivity. *Curr. Opin. Neurobiol.* 10, 232–237. doi: 10.1016/s0959-4388(00)00081-7

Paulus, M. P., Potterat, E. G., Taylor, M. K., Van Orden, K. F., Bauman, J., Momen, N., et al. (2009). A neuroscience approach to optimizing brain resources for human performance in extreme environments. *Neurosci. Biobehav. Rev.* 33, 1080–1088. doi: 10.1016/j.neubiorev.2009.05.003

Pelham, W. E. Jr., Gnagy, E. M., Greenslade, K. E., and Milich, R. (1992). Teacher ratings of DSM-III-R Symptoms for the disruptive behavior disorders. *J. Am. Acad. Child Adolesc. Psychiatry* 31, 210–218. doi: 10.1097/00004583-199203000-00006

Peters, E., Pritzkuleit, R., Beske, F., and Katalinic, A. (2010). [Demographic change and disease rates: a projection until 2050]. *Bundesgesundheitsblatt Gesundheitsforschung Gesundheitsschutz* 53, 417–426. doi: 10.1007/s00103-010-1050-y

Pfurtscheller, G., and Lopes da Silva, F. H. (1999). Event-related EEG/MEG synchronization and desynchronization: basic principles. *Clin. Neurophysiol. Off. J. Int. Fed. Clin. Neurophysiol.* 110, 1842–1857. doi: 10.1016/s1388-2457(99)00141-8

Polanczyk, G., de Lima, M. S., Horta, B. L., Biederman, J., and Rohde, L. A. (2007). The worldwide prevalence of ADHD: a systematic review and metaregression analysis. *Am. J. Psychiatry* 164, 942–948. doi: 10.1176/appi.ajp.164.6.942

Polanía, R., Nitsche, M. A., Korman, C., Batsikadze, G., and Paulus, W. (2012a). The importance of timing in segregated theta phase-coupling for cognitive performance. *Curr. Biol.* 22, 1314–1318. doi: 10.1016/j.cub.2012.05.021

Polanía, R., Paulus, W., and Nitsche, M. A. (2012b). Noninvasively decoding the contents of visual working memory in the human prefrontal cortex within high-gamma oscillatory patterns. *J. Cogn. Neurosci.* 24, 304–314. doi: 10.1162/jocn_a_00151

Poliakoff, E., Ashworth, S., Lowe, C., and Spence, C. (2006). Vision and touch in ageing: crossmodal selective attention and visuotactile spatial interactions. *Neuropsychologia* 44, 507–517. doi: 10.1016/j.neuropsychologia.2005.07.004

Priori, A. (2003). Brain polarization in humans: a reappraisal of an old tool for prolonged non-invasive modulation of brain excitability. *Clin. Neurophysiol.* 114, 589–595. doi: 10.1016/s1388-2457(02)00437-6

Raghavachari, S., Kahana, M. J., Rizzuto, D. S., Caplan, J. B., Kirschen, M. P., Bourgeois, B., et al. (2001). Gating of human theta oscillations by a working memory task. *J. Neurosci.* 21, 3175–3183.

Raghavachari, S., Lisman, J. E., Tully, M., Madsen, J. R., Bromfield, E. B., and Kahana, M. J. (2006). Theta oscillations in human cortex during a working-memory task: evidence for local generators. *J. Neurophysiol.* 95, 1630–1638. doi: 10.1152/jn.00409.2005

Ray, S., and Maunsell, J. H. R. (2011). Different origins of gamma rhythm and high-gamma activity in macaque visual cortex. *PLoS Biol.* 9:e1000610. doi: 10.1371/journal.pbio.1000610

Reato, D., Rahman, A., Bikson, M., and Parra, L. C. (2013). Effects of weak transcranial alternating current stimulation on brain activity—a review of known mechanisms from animal studies. *Front. Hum. Neurosci.* 7:687. doi: 10.3389/fnhum.2013.00687

Reinhart, R. M. G., and Woodman, G. F. (2014). Causal control of medial–frontal cortex governs electrophysiological and behavioral indices of performance monitoring and learning. *J. Neurosci.* 34, 4214–4227. doi: 10.1523/JNEUROSCI.5421-13.2014

Reuter-Lorenz, P. A., Jonides, J., Smith, E. E., Hartley, A., Miller, A., Marshuetz, C., et al. (2000). Age differences in the frontal lateralization of verbal and spatial working memory revealed by PET. *J. Cogn. Neurosci.* 12, 174–187. doi: 10.1162/089892900561814

Riis, J. L., Chong, H., Ryan, K. K., Wolk, D. A., Rentz, D. M., Holcomb, P. J., et al. (2008). Compensatory neural activity distinguishes different patterns of normal cognitive aging. *Neuroimage* 39, 441–454. doi: 10.1016/j.neuroimage.2007.08.034

Rohenkohl, G., and Nobre, A. C. (2011). α oscillations related to anticipatory attention follow temporal expectations. *J. Neurosci.* 31, 14076–14084. doi: 10.1523/JNEUROSCI.3387-11.2011

Romei, V., Gross, J., and Thut, G. (2010). On the role of prestimulus alpha rhythms over occipito-parietal areas in visual input regulation: correlation or causation? *J. Neurosci.* 30, 8692–8697. doi: 10.1523/JNEUROSCI.0160-10.2010

Romei, V., Gross, J., and Thut, G. (2012). Sounds reset rhythms of visual cortex and corresponding human visual perception. *Curr. Biol.* 22, 807–813. doi: 10.1016/j.cub.2012.03.025

Rossi, S., Hallett, M., Rossini, P. M., and Pascual-Leone, A. (2009). Safety, ethical considerations and application guidelines for the use of transcranial magnetic stimulation in clinical practice and research. *Clin. Nerophysiol.* 120, 2008–2039. doi: 10.1016/j.clinph.2009.08.016

Roux, F., and Uhlhaas, P. J. (2014). Working memory and neural oscillations: alpha-gamma versus theta-gamma codes for distinct WM information? *Trends Cogn. Sci.* 18, 16–25. doi: 10.1016/j.tics.2013.10.010

Rowe, G., Valderrama, S., Hasher, L., and Lenartowicz, A. (2006). Attentional disregulation: a benefit for implicit memory. *Psychol. Aging* 21, 826–830. doi: 10.1037/0882-7974.21.4.826

Saalmann, Y. B., Pinsk, M. A., Wang, L., Li, X., and Kastner, S. (2012). The pulvinar regulates information transmission between cortical areas based on attention demands. *Science* 337, 753–756. doi: 10.1126/science.1223082

Safren, S. A., Sprich, S., Mimiaga, M. J., Surman, C., Knouse, L., Groves, M., et al. (2010). Cognitive behavioral therapy vs relaxation with educational support for medication-treated adults with adhd and persistent symptoms: a randomized controlled trial. *JAMA* 304, 875–880. doi: 10.1001/jama.2010.1192

Salthouse, T. A., Babcock, R. L., and Shaw, R. J. (1991). Effects of adult age on structural and operational capacities in working memory. *Psychol. Aging* 6, 118–127. doi: 10.1037/0882-7974.6.1.118

Sampaio-Baptista, C., Khrapitchev, A. A., Foxley, S., Schlagheck, T., Scholz, J., Jbabdi, S., et al. (2013). Motor skill learning induces changes in white matter microstructure and myelination. *J. Neurosci.* 33, 19499–19503. doi: 10.1523/JNEUROSCI.3048-13.2013

Sander, M. C., Lindenberger, U., and Werkle-Bergner, M. (2012a). Lifespan age differences in working memory: a two-component framework. *Neurosci. Biobehav. Rev.* 36, 2007–2033. doi: 10.1016/j.neubiorev.2012.06.004

Sander, M. C., Werkle-Bergner, M., and Lindenberger, U. (2012b). Amplitude modulations and inter-trial phase stability of alpha-oscillations differentially reflect working memory constraints across the lifespan. *Neuroimage* 59, 646–654. doi: 10.1016/j.neuroimage.2011.06.092

Santarnecchi, E., Polizzotto, N. R., Godone, M., Giovannelli, F., Feurra, M., Matzen, L., et al. (2013). Frequency-dependent enhancement of fluid intelligence induced by transcranial oscillatory potentials. *Curr. Biol.* 23, 1449–1453. doi: 10.1016/j.cub.2013.06.022

Sauseng, P., Feldheim, J. F., Freunberger, R., and Hummel, F. C. (2011). Right prefrontal TMS disrupts interregional anticipatory EEG alpha activity during shifting of visuospatial attention. *Front. Psychol.* 2:241. doi: 10.3389/fpsyg.2011.00241

Sauseng, P., Griesmayr, B., Freunberger, R., and Klimesch, W. (2010). Control mechanisms in working memory: a possible function of EEG theta oscillations. *Neurosci. Biobehav. Rev.* 34, 1015–1022. doi: 10.1016/j.neubiorev.2009.12.006

Sauseng, P., and Klimesch, W. (2008). What does phase information of oscillatory brain activity tell us about cognitive processes? *Neurosci. Biobehav. Rev.* 32, 1001–1013. doi: 10.1016/j.neubiorev.2008.03.014

Sauseng, P., Klimesch, W., Gerloff, C., and Hummel, F. C. (2009a). Spontaneous locally restricted EEG alpha activity determines cortical excitability in the motor cortex. *Neuropsychologia* 47, 284–288. doi: 10.1016/j.neuropsychologia.2008.07.021

Sauseng, P., Klimesch, W., Heise, K. F., Gruber, W. R., Holz, E., Karim, A. A., et al. (2009b). Brain oscillatory substrates of visual short-term memory capacity. *Curr. Biol.* 19, 1846–1852. doi: 10.1016/j.cub.2009.08.062

Scheeringa, R., Fries, P., Petersson, K.-M., Oostenveld, R., Grothe, I., Norris, D. G., et al. (2011). Neuronal dynamics underlying high- and low-frequency EEG oscillations contribute independently to the human BOLD signal. *Neuron* 69, 572–583. doi: 10.1016/j.neuron.2010.11.044

Schneider, T. R., Debener, S., Oostenveld, R., and Engel, A. K. (2008). Enhanced EEG gamma-band activity reflects multisensory semantic matching in visual-to-auditory object priming. *Neuroimage* 42, 1244–1254. doi: 10.1016/j.neuroimage.2008.05.033

Schroeder, C. E., and Lakatos, P. (2009). Low-frequency neuronal oscillations as instruments of sensory selection. *Trends Neurosci.* 32, 9–18. doi: 10.1016/j.tins.2008.09.012

Schutter, D. J. (2014). Syncing your brain: electric currents to enhance cognition. *Trends Cogn. Sci.* doi: 10.1016/j.tics.2014.02.011. [Epub ahead of print].

Shafi, M. M., Brandon Westover, M., Oberman, L., Cash, S. S., and Pascual-Leone, A. (2014). Modulation of EEG functional connectivity networks in subjects undergoing repetitive transcranial magnetic stimulation. *Brain Topogr.* 27, 172–191. doi: 10.1007/s10548-013-0277-y

Silvanto, J., and Pascual-Leone, A. (2008). State-dependency of transcranial magnetic stimulation. *Brain Topogr.* 21, 1–10. doi: 10.1007/s10548-008-0067-0

Snowball, A., Tachtsidis, I., Popescu, T., Thompson, J., Delazer, M., Zamarian, L., et al. (2013). Long-term enhancement of brain function and cognition using cognitive training and brain stimulation. *Curr. Biol.* 23, 987–992. doi: 10.1016/j.cub.2013.04.045

Spaak, E., Bonnefond, M., Maier, A., Leopold, D. A., and Jensen, O. (2012). Layer-specific entrainment of gamma-band neural activity by the alpha rhythm in monkey visual cortex. *Curr. Biol.* 22, 2313–2318. doi: 10.1016/j.cub.2012.10.020

Spaak, E., de Lange, F. P., and Jensen, O. (2014). Local entrainment of Alpha oscillations by visual stimuli causes cyclic modulation of perception. *J. Neurosci.* 34, 3536–3544. doi: 10.1523/jneurosci.4385-13.2014

Spitzer, B., and Blankenburg, F. (2012). Supramodal parametric working memory processing in humans. *J. Neurosci.* 32, 3287–3295. doi: 10.1523/jneurosci.5280-11.2012

Staudigl, T., and Hanslmayr, S. (2013). Theta oscillations at encoding mediate the context-dependent nature of human episodic memory. *Curr. Biol.* 23, 1101–1106. doi: 10.1016/j.cub.2013.04.074

Staufenbiel, S. M., Brouwer, A.-M., Keizer, A. W., and van Wouwe, N. C. (2014). Effect of beta and gamma neurofeedback on memory and intelligence in the elderly. *Biol. Psychol.* 95, 74–85. doi: 10.1016/j.biopsycho.2013.05.020

Strens, L. H. A., Oliviero, A., Bloem, B. R., Gerschlager, W., Rothwell, J. C., and Brown, P. (2002). The effects of subthreshold 1 Hz repetitive TMS on cortico-cortical and interhemispheric coherence. *Clin. Neurophysiol.* 113, 1279–1285. doi: 10.1016/s1388-2457(02)00151-7

Strenziok, M., Parasuraman, R., Clarke, E., Cisler, D. S., Thompson, J. C., and Greenwood, P. M. (2014). Neurocognitive enhancement in older adults: comparison of three cognitive training tasks to test a hypothesis of training transfer in brain connectivity. *Neuroimage* 85(Pt. 3), 1027–1039. doi: 10.1016/j.neuroimage.2013.07.069

Strüber, D., Rach, S., Trautmann-Lengsfeld, S. A., Engel, A. K., and Herrmann, C. S. (2014). Antiphasic 40 Hz oscillatory current stimulation affects bistable motion perception. *Brain Topogr.* 27, 158–171. doi: 10.1007/s10548-013-0294-x

Suffczynski, P., Kalitzin, S., Pfurtscheller, G., and Lopes da Silva, F. H. (2001). Computational model of thalamo-cortical networks: dynamical control of alpha rhythms in relation to focal attention. *Int. J. Psychophysiol.* 43, 25–40. doi: 10.1016/s0167-8760(01)00177-5

Tales, A., Troscianko, T., Wilcock, G. K., Newton, P., and Butler, S. R. (2002). Age-related changes in the preattentional detection of visual change. *Neuroreport* 13, 969–972. doi: 10.1097/00001756-200205240-00014

Tallon-Baudry, C. (1999). Oscillatory gamma activity in humans and its role in object representation. *Trends Cogn. Sci.* 3, 151–162. doi: 10.1016/s1364-6613(99)01299-1

Tallon-Baudry, C., Bertrand, O., Delpuech, C., and Pernier, J. (1996). Stimulus specificity of phase-locked and non-phase-locked 40 Hz visual responses in human. *J. Neurosci.* 16, 4240–4249.

Tallon-Baudry, C., Bertrand, O., Hénaff, M.-A., Isnard, J., and Fischer, C. (2005). Attention modulates gamma-band oscillations differently in the human lateral occipital cortex and fusiform gyrus. *Cereb. Cortex* 15, 654–662. doi: 10.1093/cercor/bhh167

Tallon-Baudry, C., Bertrand, O., Peronnet, F., and Pernier, J. (1998). Induced gamma-band activity during the delay of a visual short-term memory task in humans. *J. Neurosci.* 18, 4244–4254.

ter Huurne, N., Onnink, M., Kan, C., Franke, B., Buitelaar, J., and Jensen, O. (2013). Behavioral consequences of aberrant alpha lateralization in attention-deficit/hyperactivity disorder. *Biol. Psychiatry* 74, 227–233. doi: 10.1016/j.biopsych.2013.02.001

Thut, G., and Miniussi, C. (2009). New insights into rhythmic brain activity from TMS–EEG studies. *Trends Cogn. Sci.* 13, 182–189. doi: 10.1016/j.tics.2009.01.004

Thut, G., and Pascual-Leone, A. (2010). A review of combined TMS-EEG studies to characterize lasting effects of repetitive TMS and assess their usefulness in cognitive and clinical neuroscience. *Brain Topogr.* 22, 219–232. doi: 10.1007/s10548-009-0115-4

Thut, G., Nietzel, A., Brandt, S. A., and Pascual-Leone, A. (2006). Alpha-band electroencephalographic activity over occipital cortex indexes visuospatial attention bias and predicts visual target detection. *J. Neurosci.* 26, 9494–9502. doi: 10.1523/jneurosci.0875-06.2006

Thut, G., Schyns, P. G., and Gross, J. (2011a). Entrainment of perceptually relevant brain oscillations by non-invasive rhythmic stimulation of the human brain. *Front. Psychol.* 2:170. doi: 10.3389/fpsyg.2011.00170

Thut, G., Veniero, D., Romei, V., Miniussi, C., Schyns, P., and Gross, J. (2011b). Rhythmic TMS causes local entrainment of natural oscillatory signatures. *Curr. Biol.* 21, 1176–1185. doi: 10.1016/j.cub.2011.05.049

Tonin, L., Leeb, R., and Del R Millán, J. (2012). Time-dependent approach for single trial classification of covert visuospatial attention. *J. Neural Eng.* 9:045011. doi: 10.1088/1741-2560/9/4/045011

van Dijk, H., Schoffelen, J.-M., Oostenveld, R., and Jensen, O. (2008). Prestimulus oscillatory activity in the alpha band predicts visual discrimination ability. *J. Neurosci.* 28, 1816–1823. doi: 10.1523/jneurosci.1853-07.2008

van Dongen-Boomsma, M., Vollebregt, M. A., Slaats-Willemse, D., and Buitelaar, J. K. (2013). A randomized placebo-controlled trial of electroencephalographic (EEG) neurofeedback in children with attention-deficit/hyperactivity disorder. *J. Clin. Psychiatry* 74, 821–827. doi: 10.4088/jcp.12m08321

van Gerven, M. A. J., Farquhar, J., Schaefer, R., Vlek, R., Geuze, J., Nijholt, A., et al. (2009a). The brain–computer interface cycle. *J. Neural Eng.* 6:041001. doi: 10.1088/1741-2560/6/4/041001

van Gerven, M., and Jensen, O. (2009). Attention modulations of posterior alpha as a control signal for two-dimensional brain-computer interfaces. *J. Neurosci. Methods* 179, 78–84. doi: 10.1016/j.jneumeth.2009.01.016

van Gerven, M., Bahramisharif, A., Heskes, T., and Jensen, O. (2009b). Selecting features for BCI control based on a covert spatial attention paradigm. *Neural Netw.* 22, 1271–1277. doi: 10.1016/j.neunet.2009.06.004

van Pelt, S., Boomsma, D. I., and Fries, P. (2012). Magnetoencephalography in twins reveals a strong genetic determination of the peak frequency of visually induced γ-band synchronization. *J. Neurosci.* 32, 3388–3392. doi: 10.1523/jneurosci.5592-11.2012

van Pelt, S., and Fries, P. (2013). Visual stimulus eccentricity affects human gamma peak frequency. *Neuroimage* 78, 439–447. doi: 10.1016/j.neuroimage.2013.04.040

VanRullen, R., Zoefel, B., and Ilhan, B. (2014). On the cyclic nature of perception in vision versus audition. *Philos. Trans. R. Soc. Lond. B Biol. Sci.* 369:20130214. doi: 10.1098/rstb.2013.0214

Varela, F., Lachaux, J. P., Rodriguez, E., and Martinerie, J. (2001). The brainweb: phase synchronization and large-scale integration. *Nat. Rev. Neurosci.* 2, 229–239. doi: 10.1038/35067550

Vaughan, T. M., McFarland, D. J., Schalk, G., Sarnacki, W. A., Krusienski, D. J., Sellers, E. W., et al. (2006). The wadsworth BCI research and development program: at home with BCI. *IEEE Trans. Neural Syst. Rehabil. Eng.* 14, 229–233. doi: 10.1109/tnsre.2006.875577

Veniero, D., Ponzo, V., and Koch, G. (2013). Paired associative stimulation enforces the communication between interconnected areas. *J. Neurosci.* 33, 13773–13783. doi: 10.1523/jneurosci.1777-13.2013

Verret, C., Guay, M.-C., Berthiaume, C., Gardiner, P., and Béliveau, L. (2012). A physical activity program improves behavior and cognitive functions in children with ADHD an exploratory study. *J. Atten. Disord.* 16, 71–80. doi: 10.1177/1087054710379735

Vidal-Piñeiro, D., Martin-Trias, P., Arenaza-Urquijo, E. M., Sala-Llonch, R., Clemente, I. C., Mena-Sánchez, I., et al. (2014). Task-dependent activity and connectivity predict episodic memory network-based responses to brain stimulation in healthy aging. *Brain Stimul.* 7, 287–296. doi: 10.1016/j.brs.2013.12.016

Vidaurre, C., and Blankertz, B. (2010). Towards a cure for BCI illiteracy. *Brain Topogr.* 23, 194–198. doi: 10.1007/s10548-009-0121-6

Vollebregt, M. A., van Dongen-Boomsma, M., Buitelaar, J. K., and Slaats-Willemse, D. (2014). Does EEG-neurofeedback improve neurocognitive functioning in children with attention-deficit/hyperactivity disorder? A systematic review and a double-blind placebo-controlled study. *J. Child Psychol. Psychiatry* 55, 460–472. doi: 10.1111/jcpp.12143

Vollmann, H., Conde, V., Sewerin, S., Taubert, M., Sehm, B., Witte, O. W., et al. (2013). Anodal transcranial direct current stimulation (tDCS) over supplementary motor area (SMA) but not pre-SMA promotes short-term visuomotor learning. *Brain Stimul.* 6, 101–107. doi: 10.1016/j.brs.2012.03.018

von Stein, A., and Sarnthein, J. (2000). Different frequencies for different scales of cortical integration: from local gamma to long range alpha/theta synchronization. *Int. J. Psychophysiol.* 38, 301–313. doi: 10.1016/s0167-8760(00)00172-0

Wagner, T., Eden, U., Rushmore, J., Russo, C. J., Dipietro, L., Fregni, F., et al. (2014). Impact of brain tissue filtering on neurostimulation fields: A modeling study. *Neuroimage* 85(Pt. 3), 1048–1057. doi: 10.1016/j.neuroimage.2013.06.079

Wang, J.-R., and Hsieh, S. (2013). Neurofeedback training improves attention and working memory performance. *Clin. Neurophysiol.* 124, 2406–2420. doi: 10.1016/j.clinph.2013.05.020

Wang, X.-J. (2010). Neurophysiological and computational principles of cortical rhythms in cognition. *Physiol. Rev.* 90, 1195–1268. doi: 10.1152/physrev.00035.2008

Waring, J. D., Addis, D. R., and Kensinger, E. A. (2013). Effects of aging on neural connectivity underlying selective memory for emotional scenes. *Neurobiol. Aging* 34, 451–467. doi: 10.1016/j.neurobiolaging.2012.03.011

Wassermann, E. M. (1998). Risk and safety of repetitive transcranial magnetic stimulation: report and suggested guidelines from the international workshop on the safety of repetitive transcranial magnetic stimulation, June 5–7, 1996. *Electroencephalogr. Clin. Neurophysiol.* 108, 1–16. doi: 10.1016/s0168-5597(97)00096-8

Weiler, M. D., Bernstein, J. H., Bellinger, D., and Waber, D. P. (2002). Information processing deficits in children with attention-deficit/hyperactivity disorder, inattentive type and children with reading disability. *J. Learn. Disabil.* 35, 448–461. doi: 10.1177/00222194020350050501

Weiss, M., Worling, D., and Wasdell, M. (2003). A chart review study of the inattentive and combined types of ADHD. *J. Atten. Disord.* 7, 1–9. doi: 10.1177/108705470300700101

Werkle-Bergner, M., Shing, Y. L., Müller, V., Li, S.-C., and Lindenberger, U. (2009). EEG gamma-band synchronization in visual coding from childhood to old age: evidence from evoked power and inter-trial phase locking. *Clin. Neurophysiol.* 120, 1291–1302. doi: 10.1016/j.clinph.2009.04.012

Wolpaw, J. R., Birbaumer, N., McFarland, D. J., Pfurtscheller, G., and Vaughan, T. M. (2002). Brain-computer interfaces for communication and control. *Clin. Neurophysiol.* 113, 767–791. doi: 10.1016/S1388-2457(02)00057-3

Worden, M. S., Foxe, J. J., Wang, N., and Simpson, G. V. (2000). Anticipatory biasing of visuospatial attention indexed by retinotopically specific alpha-band electroencephalography increases over occipital cortex. *J. Neurosci.* 20:RC63.

Xing, D., Yeh, C.-I., Burns, S., and Shapley, R. M. (2012). Laminar analysis of visually evoked activity in the primary visual cortex. *Proc. Natl. Acad. Sci. U S A* 109, 13871–13876. doi: 10.1073/pnas.1201478109

Yang, L., and Hasher, L. (2007). The enhanced effects of pictorial distraction in older adults. *J. Gerontol. B. Psychol. Sci. Soc. Sci.* 62, P230–P233. doi: 10.1093/geronb/62.4.p230

Yordanova, J., Banaschewski, T., Kolev, V., Woerner, W., and Rothenberger, A. (2001). Abnormal early stages of task stimulus processing in children with attention-deficit hyperactivity disorder—evidence from event-related gamma oscillations. *Clin. Neurophysiol.* 112, 1096–1108. doi: 10.1016/s1388-2457(01)00524-7

Zaehle, T., Rach, S., and Herrmann, C. S. (2010). Transcranial alternating current stimulation enhances individual alpha activity in human EEG. *PLoS One* 5:e13766. doi: 10.1371/journal.pone.0013766

Zanto, T. P., Chadick, J. Z., and Gazzaley, A. (2014). Anticipatory alpha phase influences visual working memory performance. *Neuroimage* 85(Pt. 2), 794–802. doi: 10.1016/j.neuroimage.2013.07.048

Zatorre, R. J., Fields, R. D., and Johansen-Berg, H. (2012). Plasticity in gray and white: neuroimaging changes in brain structure during learning. *Nat. Neurosci.* 15, 528–536. doi: 10.1038/nn.3045

Zoefel, B., Huster, R. J., and Herrmann, C. S. (2011). Neurofeedback training of the upper alpha frequency band in EEG improves cognitive performance. *Neuroimage* 54, 1427–1431. doi: 10.1016/j.neuroimage.2010.08.078

16

The pregnane xenobiotic receptor, a prominent liver factor, has actions in the midbrain for neurosteroid synthesis and behavioral/neural plasticity of female rats

Cheryl A. Frye[1,2,3,4,5,6,7]*, *Carolyn J. Koonce*[1,6,7] and *Alicia A. Walf*[1,6,7]

[1] Department of Psychology, The University at Albany-SUNY, Albany, NY, USA
[2] Department of Biological Sciences, The University at Albany-SUNY, Albany, NY, USA
[3] The Center for Neuroscience Research, The University at Albany-SUNY, Albany, NY, USA
[4] The Center for Life Sciences Research, The University at Albany-SUNY, Albany, NY, USA
[5] Department of Chemistry and Biochemistry, The University of Alaska–Fairbanks, Fairbanks, AK, USA
[6] Institute of Arctic Biology, The University of Alaska–Fairbanks, Fairbanks, AK, USA
[7] IDeA Network of Biomedical Excellence (INBRE), The University of Alaska–Fairbanks, Fairbanks, AK, USA

Edited by:
Mikhail Lebedev, Duke University, USA

Reviewed by:
Raúl G. Paredes, National University of Mexico, Mexico
Mikhail Lebedev, Duke University, USA
Graziano Pinna, University of Illinois at Chicago, USA
Nico Mitro, Università degli Studi di Milano, Italy

***Correspondence:**
Cheryl A. Frye, Department of Chemistry and Biochemistry, Institute of Arctic Biology, The University of Alaska–Fairbanks, 223 Murie Life Sciences Building, 982 Koyukuk Drive, Fairbanks, AK 99775, USA
e-mail: cheryl.a.frye@gmail.com

A novel factor of interest for growth/plasticity in the brain is pregnane xenobiotic receptor (PXR). PXR is a liver factor known for its role in xenobiotic clearance and cholesterol metabolism. It is expressed in the brain, suggesting a potential role for plasticity, particularly involving cholesterol-based steroids and neurosteroids. Mating induces synthesis of neurosteroids in the midbrain Ventral Tegmental Area (VTA) of female rodents, as well as other "plastic" regions of the brain, including the hippocampus, that may be involved in the consolidation of the mating experience. Reducing PXR in the VTA attenuates mating-induced biosynthesis of the neurosteroid, 5α-pregnan-3α-ol-20-one (3α,5α-THP). The 18 kDA translocator protein (TSPO) is one rate-limiting factor for 3α,5α-THP neurosteroidogenesis. The hypothesis tested was that PXR is an upstream factor of TSPO for neurosteroidogenesis of 3α,5α-THP in the VTA for lordosis, independent of peripheral glands. First, proestrous rats were administered a TSPO blocker (PK11195) and/or 3α,5α-THP following infusions of PXR antisense oligonucleotides (AS-ODNs) or vehicle to the VTA. Inhibiting TSPO with PK11195 reduced 3α,5α-THP levels in the midbrain and lordosis, an effect that could be reversed with 3α,5α-THP administration, but not AS-ODN+3α,5α-THP. Second, proestrous, ovariectomized (OVX), or ovariectomized/adrenalectomized (OVX/ADX) rats were infused with a TSPO enhancer (FGIN 1-27) subsequent to AS-ODNs or vehicle to the VTA. PXR AS-ODNs blocked actions of FGIN 1–27 for lordosis and 3α,5α-THP levels among proestrous > OVX > OVX/ADX rats. Thus, PXR may be upstream of TSPO, involved in neurosteroidogenesis of 3α,5α-THP in the brain for plasticity. This novel finding of a liver factor involved in behavioral/neural plasticity substantiates future studies investigating factors known for their prominent actions in the peripheral organs, such as the liver, for modulating brain function and its augmentation.

Keywords: midbrain ventral tegmental area, allopregnanolone, progesterone, cognition, reproduction

INTRODUCTION

Steroid hormones are well-recognized for their role for growth processes in the body. For example, physiological roles of steroids hormones for growth are apparent during puberty, with the onset of the patterned secretion of these steroids from the gonads, and morphological differences (secondary sex characteristics), and during pregnancy, with substantial changes in many systems modulated by steroid hormones (e.g., the progestogens—progesterone and its metabolites), as two examples. In these two examples there are obvious physical changes, but the effects, mechanisms, and brain targets of steroids, such as the progestogens, for cognitive and behavioral processes, in relation to the body, are starting to become better understood. Data from large clinical trials conducted of hormone replacement therapies (HRTs) (which typically include synthetic compounds to mimic hormones lost during menopause, estradiol and progesterone), do not entirely support the basic literature on the beneficial role of these hormones for brain functions, like enhancements in learning/memory (described below) and reduction in stroke- and injury-related pathology (Roof et al., 1992, 1993; Chen et al., 1999; He et al., 2004; Shapiro, 2006; Billeci et al., 2007). Moreover, these trials were halted early due to increased cardiovascular and cancer risks and there was a subsequent backlash against clinical use of HRTs that did not take into account individual patient characteristics and risk (Rossouw et al., 2002; Shumaker et al., 2003; Maki and Henderson, 2012). Together, these examples substantiate the importance of understanding the role and mechanisms of steroids in the body and brain.

In addition to the controversy of whether the potential benefits of hormones outweigh their risks, there has been controversy of the role of progestogens for benefiting brain function *per se.* Historically, the basic experimental design to understand whether a particular hormone was necessary and sufficient for a physiological process was to assess co-variation in the hormone of interest and a process and remove the gland that produced the hormone (extirpation) and replace back the hormone (to see if the process is abrogated and then reinstated, respectively). In rodent models of cognitive function, studies assessing natural increases in progestogens over the estrous cycle, or during and after pregnancy, support the mnemonic effects of these high, physiological levels of progestogens in spatial and object recognition tasks (Lambert et al., 2005; Walf et al., 2006; Kinsley and Lambert, 2008; Paris and Frye, 2008; Macbeth and Luine, 2010). Moreover, ovariectomy (surgical removal of the ovaries) of young, adult female rats produces performance deficits in the object recognition and placement tasks, which can be abrogated with replacement back with progesterone or its neuroactive metabolite, 5α-pregnan-3α-ol-20-one (3α,5α-THP, a.k.a. allopregnanolone; Walf et al., 2006; Frye et al., 2007). However, these beneficial effects of progestogens are not uniformly observed in other studies, using different tasks, or dosing and formulation of progestogens, or involving investigations in aged rodents (Murphy et al., 2002; Toung et al., 2004; see review by Acosta et al., 2013). Together, these data suggest that progestogens' effects for cognitive function may be influenced by task, dosing and formulation of progestogen administered, age and likely many other factors.

Given that there are many factors that can influence responses to progestogens for neural processes, an approach that we have taken is to use the well-characterized behavioral model of reproductive behavior of rodents to investigate progestogens' mechanisms. The notion is that we can begin to understand the mechanisms of progestogens in regions that have been investigated for decades (hypothalamus and midbrain) for this basic, hormone-dependent behavior (lordosis, or mating posture of female rodents), substantiating subsequent studies on such mechanisms in corticolimbic structures underlying complex cognitive processes. Lordosis only occurs in appropriate neuroendocrine and environmental context, with reductions in the response supported by effects of ovariectomy, steroid blockers or environmental stressors (Uphouse et al., 2005, 2013; reviewed in Frye, 2011; Frye et al., 2013). From studies using this approach, the effects of progesterone and/or its metabolite, 3α,5α-THP, in the midbrain ventral tegmental area (VTA), through novel neurotransmitter targets (e.g., GABA, dopamine, glutamate, and second messenger cascades) have been supported (reviewed in Frye and Walf, 2008). Interestingly, there is high expression of factors involved in the metabolism and synthesis of 3α,5α-THP in the VTA (from precursor of all steroids, cholesterol; reviewed in Frye, 2011), suggesting the importance of 3α,5α-THP production and action in this region.

Another consideration is that experience can alter hormone levels (and thereby modify the CNS). An example of this is mating-induced neurosteroid synthesis. Mating induces synthesis of neurosteroids in the midbrain VTA of female rodents, as well as other "plastic" regions of the brain, including the hippocampus and prefrontal cortex, that may be involved in the consolidation of the mating experience in rodents. There can be dynamic changes in 3α,5α-THP production in midbrain and corticolimbic structures following mating or other social and environmental challenges (Purdy et al., 1991; Barbaccia et al., 2001; Agís-Balboa et al., 2007; Pinna et al., 2008; Pinna and Rasmusson, 2012). In further support, midbrain 3α,5α-THP levels are higher after female rats are tested in the paced mating task, compared to standard mating task (which does not involve females temporally controlling the frequency of contacts with males), compared to no mating (reviewed in Frye, 2011). Thus, our model system is to use lordosis as a bioassay to further understand mechanisms involved in 3α,5α-THP synthesis and actions for neural/behavioral plasticity.

Studies focused on mechanistic questions about progestogens' actions and production in the VTA, using lordosis as the bioassay, have been extended to understand novel targets, such as the pregnane xenobiotic receptor (PXR), for these responses. PXR has a well-established role as a ubiquitous and promiscuous nuclear receptor in the liver and other excretory organs (kidneys, intestines) for metabolism and xenobiotic clearance (Geick et al., 2001; Dussault and Forman, 2002; Francis et al., 2002; Kliewer et al., 2002). Its role in the CNS was not understood until more recently. Some of the first studies examining PXR's role were those focused on its function in the blood-brain-barrier, which was similar to other excretory organs in the body (Bauer et al., 2004, 2006; Xu et al., 2005; Harmsen et al., 2007; Ma et al., 2008; Zhang et al., 2008; Ott et al., 2009). However, PXR is also expressed in the brain itself, suggesting a potential role for plasticity, particularly involving steroids (which are cholesterol-based hormones) and neurosteroids (which are produced from metabolism of cholesterol in the central nervous system itself). For example, for synthesis of 3α,5α-THP, cholesterol is transported into the mitochondria by way of the 18-kDa translocator protein (TSPO) on the outer mitochondrial membrane. Inside the mitochondria, cholesterol interacts with steroidogenic acute regulatory protein and cytochrome P450-dependent side chain cleavage (P450scc) enzymes (Mellon and Deschepper, 1993; King et al., 2002; Papadopoulos et al., 2006), as well downstream steroidogenic enzymes (5α-reductase, 3α-hydroxysteroid dehydrogenase) to produce pregnenolone, progesterone, dihydroprogesterone, and, ultimately, 3α,5α-THP. A question is the role of PXR in this pathway. Our interest in PXR as a novel target was supported by a microarray study in which the gene for this receptor was expressed in the midbrain following paced mating of female rodents (reviewed in Frye, 2011). We subsequently characterized the expression of this receptor in the midbrain across the estrous cycle of rats (in which we found higher expression associated with higher progestogen levels; Frye et al., 2012, 2013). Moreover, knocking down PXR expression in the VTA reduces mating-induced biosynthesis of 3α,5α-THP in the VTA. Given that TSPO is one rate-limiting factor for 3α,5α-THP neurosteroidogenesis, a question is whether metabolism at TSPO involves, or requires, PXR for production of 3α,5α-THP. The hypothesis was that PXR is a necessary upstream factor of TSPO for neurosteroidogenesis of 3α,5α-THP in the VTA for lordosis, independent of peripheral glands. We assessed the role of

PXR, and TSPO manipulations in different hormonal contexts (i.e., over the estrous cycle with extirpation of the ovaries and/or adrenal glands). First, proestrous rats were administered a TSPO blocker (PK11195) and/or 3α,5α-THP following infusions of PXR antisense oligonucleotides (AS-ODNs) or vehicle to the VTA in Experiment 1. We aimed to determine the extent to which the TSPO inhibitor may have effects similar to PXR knockdown and whether this may be reversed with 3α,5α-THP replacement. Second, proestrous (Experiment 2), ovariectomized (OVX; Experiment 3), or ovariectomized/adrenalectomized (OVX/ADX; Experiment 4) rats were infused with a TSPO enhancer (FGIN 1–27) subsequent to AS-ODNs or vehicle to the VTA. We aimed to determine the extent to which the TSPO enhancer may reverse effects of PXR knockdown and whether this may be related to hormonal milieu. Results from these experiments supported the notion that PXR (traditionally considered a liver factor), may be upstream of TSPO, acting as a homeostatic regulator involved in neurosteroidogenesis of 3α,5α-THP in the brain and behavioral plasticity.

MATERIALS AND METHODS

SUBJECTS AND HOUSING

Adult, Long–Evans female rats ($n = 236$), approximately 55 days of age, were bred in the Life Sciences Laboratory Animal Care Facility at The University at Albany–SUNY (original stock: Taconic Farms, Germantown, NY, USA) and/or shipped from Taconic. Rats were group-housed in polycarbonate cages with woodchip bedding (45 × 24× 21 cm) in a temperature- (21 ± 1°C) and humidity- (50 ± 5%) controlled room in the Laboratory Animal Care Facility. Rats were maintained on a 12:12 h reversed light cycle (lights off at 0800 hours) with continuous access to Purina Rat Chow and tap water in their home cages.

GENERAL PROCEDURE

Four experiments were run, using a between- and within-subjects design. All experimental rats had stereotaxic surgery to implant cannulae aimed at the VTA, 7 days before drug manipulations were initiated. Experimental rats were randomly-assigned to one treatment condition (between-subjects) within a single experiment, and then were tested in a single battery of behavioral tasks (within-subjects). The general procedure utilized is depicted in **Figure 1**. All experimental techniques in rats were approved by the Institutional Animal Care and Use Committee at the University at Albany, where the experiments were conducted.

SURGICAL MANIPULATIONS

All rats in Experiments 1–4 were stereotaxically implanted with bilateral guide cannulae aimed at the VTA (from bregma: AP = −5.3, ML = ±0.4, DV = −7.0; Paxinos and Watson, 1986) under xylazine (12 mg/kg) and ketamine (80 mg/kg) anesthesia per prior methods (Frye et al., 2013). Immediately following stereotaxic surgery, rats were OVX ($n = 49$; Experiment 3) and/or OVX/ADX ($n = 48$; Experiment 4). For OVX/ADX, dorsal incisions were made between the ribs and hip, so that the ovaries and the adrenals could be isolated. The ovaries were ligated and removed, and the adrenals were isolated and removed. As ADX rats are sodium deficient, all rats received a bottle of 0.9% saline and a bottle of tap water in their home cages to maintain water/salt balance. Following surgery and prior to testing, animals were monitored for loss of weight, righting response, flank stimulation response, and/or muscle tone. Only rats that passed neurological evaluations and gained weight following surgery until behavioral testing commenced were continued in the experiment. All rats that underwent ADX were validated to have complete ADX surgery via *post-hoc* assessment of corticosterone in plasma. Rats were administered ibuprofen (once per oral, and daily in

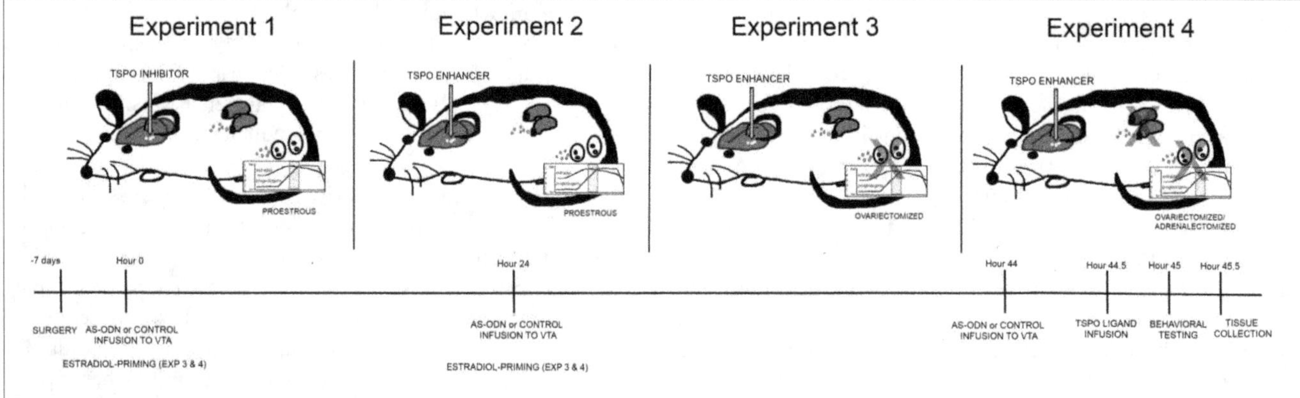

FIGURE 1 | Depicts different hormonal conditions and TSPO ligand infusions in rats (top) and timeline of experimental protocol (bottom). In Experiment 1, all rats were in the proestrous phase of the estrous cycle and administered via infusions to the VTA, placebo or PXR AS-ODNs (at hour 0, 24, and 44), followed by an inhibitor of TSPO (PK11195) or saline vehicle and/or 3α,5α-THP (at hour 44.5). In Experiment 2, all rats were in the proestrous phase of the estrous cycle and administered via infusions to the VTA, placebo or PXR AS-ODNs (at hour 0, 24, and 44), followed by an enhancer of TSPO (FGIN) or saline vehicle (at hour 44.5). In Experiment 3, all rats were ovariectomized (OVX) and administered subcutaneous injections of E_2 at hour 0 and 24 and then administered via infusions to the VTA, placebo or PXR AS-ODNs (at hour 0, 24, and 44), followed by an enhancer of TSPO (FGIN) or saline vehicle (at hour 44.5). In Experiment 4, all rats were OVX and adrenalectomized (OVX/ADX), and administered subcutaneous injections of E_2 at hour 0 and 24 and then administered via infusions to the VTA, placebo or PXR AS-ODNs (at hour 0, 24, and 44), followed by an enhancer of TSPO (FGIN) or saline vehicle (at hour 44.5). All rats were tested at hour 45, and euthanized for tissue collection immediately after behavioral testing was complete. In all experiments, knockdown of PXR expression in the VTA was validated and levels of 3α,5α-THP were measured in the midbrain.

the recovery period in drinking water; 30 mg/kg) as post-surgical analgesia.

ESTROUS CYCLE

Vaginal epithelium of each rat was collected and examined daily under a light microscope (between 0800–1000). Rats were cycled through two normal estrous cycles (4–5 days cycle) prior to testing. Rats were tested on proestrus (epithelium characterized by nucleated cells, 4–5 days after the previous occurrence) for Experiments 1 ($n = 68$) and 2 ($n = 71$).

INFUSIONS

For Experiments 1–4, rats received either sterile saline (0.9% w/v) or PXR AS-ODN infusions. AS-ODNs by (5′ CTTGCGGAAGGGGCACCTCA 3′; made in a concentration of 100 ng/μl; Frye et al., 2012, 2013, 2014, in press) were synthesized and desalted Invitrogen Life Technologies (Carlsbad, CA). This PXR AS-ODN strategy decreases expression of PXR in the midbrain, as measured by quantitative polymerase chain reaction (qPCR) (which was utilized here to validate) and western blotting (Frye, 2011; Frye et al., 2012, 2013). In Experiment 1, PK11195 (Tocris Biosciences, R&D Systems, Minneapolis, MN) was utilized as a TSPO antagonist (compounded by adding crystalline drug to sterile saline at a concentration of 50 ng per μl; Bitran et al., 2000; Frye et al., 2006, 2009). 3α,5α-THP (purchased from Dr. Robert Purdy, Scripps Institute, CA) was prepared to a concentration of 100 ng per μl in β-cyclodextran (with 5% concentration of β-cyclodextran in sterile water; Frye and Rhodes, 2006; Frye et al., 2008a, 2014). In Experiments 2–4, a neurosteroidogenesis enhancer, FGIN 1–27, an agonist of TSPO was utilized (Petralia and Frye, 2005; Frye et al., 2009, used in Experiments 2–4). Crystalline FGIN was compounded in a concentration of 50 ng per μl (Tocris) in sterile saline. Rats received bilateral infusions of each compound or placebo vehicle. This infusion protocol has been utilized without any indication of damaging effects as assessed by behavioral changes, or estradiol levels (given damage can induce aromatase activity, and thereby local estradiol levels; Azcoitia et al., 2003); this was determined by comparing rats that were sham surgerized, had stereotaxic implantation of cannulae to the VTA, but were not administered infusions, and those that were administered infusions of saline vehicle in the same volumes as drugs are administered (Frye et al., 2013).

ESTRADIOL PRIMING

For Experiment 3 and 4, OVX and OVX/ADX rats were primed with subcutaneous administration of estradiol(10 μg in 0.2 cc vegetable oil) at 0 and 24 h before behavioral testing.

BEHAVIORAL MEASURES

Our primary interest was in the role of PXR and TSPO for reproductive responding (as measured in the paced mating task); however, control measures of exploration, anxiety, and social interaction were also collected. Behavioral data were simultaneously collected by using the Any-maze behavioral assessment computer program (Stoelting Inc., Wood Lawn, IL; for open field, elevated plus maze, and social interaction) or a digital video camera (for paced mating) and trained experimenters.

Control measures- exploration, anxiety, non-sexual social interaction

Immediately before assessment in the paced mating task, rats were tested sequentially in the open field for 5 min, the elevated plus maze for 5 min, and the social interaction tasks, as per established methods (see Frye et al., 2013). Across experiments, there were no differences between comparisons groups in rats that were tested for exploratory behavior in the open field, anxiety behavior in the elevated plus maze, or social interaction with a female conspecific.

Paced mating

Paced mating was conducted per previous methods (Erskine, 1985; Frye et al., 2013) in an apparatus (37.5 × 75 × 30 cm) that was divided down the center by a Plexiglas partition. An experimental female has access to both sides of the pacing chamber, while a stimulus male was confined to one side for a 15-min test period. Standard measures of mating behavior (lordosis quotients, proceptivity quotients, and aggression quotients) are being reported herein. Lordosis quotients are the percentage of total number of lordosis responses per total number of sexual contacts by the male. Aggression/rejection (aggression quotients) are defined as behaviors such as boxing and kicking the male during contacts.

TISSUE COLLECTION AND PREPARATION

Immediately after testing, rats were euthanized by rapid decapitation and whole brain and trunk blood was collected, frozen, and stored in a freezer. For brain dissections, punches from the midbrain, around the VTA, were taken from coronal frozen slices (approximately 60 microns thick), made anterior and posterior to the VTA, and used for analyses of PXR expression (described below). At this time of collecting these slices, whether cannulae/infusion tracks were aimed at the VTA was determined (as per Frye et al., 2013, 2014). There were a total of $n = 17$ rats that had placement outside of the VTA; their data was excluded from analyses of the data from rats with placement to the VTA. Not all experimental groups were represented in rats that had missed sites, precluding systematic analyses of the data from these rats to those with placement to the VTA. However, in comparing the data available, the pattern that emerged was that rats with placement outside of the VTA had responses similar to control groups.

VALIDATION OF PXR KNOCKDOWN FOLLOWING PXR AS-ODNs

Standard qPCR methods were utilized on VTA punches to determine whether PXR AS-ODN infusions reduced PXR expression (described in Frye et al., 2013, 2014). Data were analyzed by comparing PXR values to actin control, and PXR expression is described as fold-change of the rats infused with PXR AS-ODNs to those infused with control (saline; Livak and Schmittgen, 2001; Schmittgen and Livak, 2008; Frye et al., 2013, 2014).

STEROID HORMONE MEASUREMENT

Plasma levels of corticosterone, estradiol, and progesterone were measured to validate adequacy of ADX, estrous cycle stage and/or OVX and hormone-priming, respectively. Concentrations of corticosterone, estradiol, progesterone and 3α,5α-THP were assessed using standard steroid extraction and radioimmunoassay (primarily for corticosterone and 3α,5α-THP) or commercially-available enzyme-linked immunosorbent assays (estradiol, progesterone) techniques used by our laboratory (Frye and Bayon, 1999; Frye et al., 2008a, 2013, 2014, in press). Concentrations were determined for each sample based upon concurrent standard curves run in duplicate for each of the assays. Concentrations reflect the approximate concentrations of the volume of plasma, or protein concentrations determined in midbrain homogenate samples measured by a NanoDrop spectrometer.

STATISTICAL ANALYSES

Analyses of variances (ANOVAs) were used to examine effects of PXR AS-ODN condition (control, PXR AS-ODN), PK11195 condition (control, PK11195) and 3α,5α,-THP condition (β-cyclodextrin, 3α,5α,-THP for Experiment 1) and for Experiment 2–4, PXR AS-ODN condition (control, PXR AS-ODN) and FGIN condition (control, FGIN), and/or testing condition (non tested, tested) on behavioral and endocrine measures. The assumptions of homogeneity of variance were supported, suggesting that parametric ANOVA tests be utilized as the most appropriate statistic across experiments. When the α level for statistical significance was reached ($p = 0.05$) for main effects and interactions, Fisher's Least Significant Differences *post-hoc* tests were used to determine group differences.

RESULTS

EXPERIMENT 1: EFFECTS OF TSPO BLOCKER, PK11195, IN PROESTROUS RATS

Validation of PXR AS-ODNs for PXR expression in the midbrain

Rats infused with PXR AS-ODN had 1.5 fold lower PXR expression in the midbrain VTA compared to rats infused with control condition [$F_{(1,29)} = 11.9, P < 0.001$].

3α,5α-THP levels in the midbrain (Figure 2A)

There was significant interaction between PXR AS-ODN condition and 3α,5α-THP condition [$F_{(1, 60)} = 10.7$, $P < 0.002$] for 3α,5α-THP levels in the midbrain VTA, such that control rats infused with 3α,5α-THP had higher levels of 3α,5α-THP levels in the midbrain compared to PXR AS-ODN infusions. There were significant main effects of PXR AS-ODN [$F_{(1, 60)} = 29.7$, $P < 0.0001$], 3α,5α-THP [$F_{(1, 60)} = 13.1$, $P = 0.0007$], and PK11195 [$F_{(1, 60)} = 7.3$, $P = 0.01$] conditions for 3α,5α-THP levels in the midbrain. Infusions of PXR AS-ODNs reduced, 3α,5α-THP increased, and PK11195 reduced 3α,5α-THP levels in midbrain compared to control infusions for each manipulation.

Lordosis quotients (Figure 2B)

There was an interaction between 3α,5α-THP condition and PK11195 condition [$F_{(1, 60)} = 11.4$, $P = 0.001$] for lordosis quotients, such that PK11195 reduced lordosis quotients, but not when co-administered with 3α,5α-THP. There was significant interaction between PXR AS-ODN condition and 3α,5α-THP condition [$F_{(1, 60)} = 4.7$, $P = 0.03$] for lordosis quotients, such that control rats infused with 3α,5α-THP had increased lordosis quotients, but not when co-administered PXR AS-ODNs. There was a significant main effect of PXR AS-ODN condition [$F_{(1, 60)} = 12.5$, $P = 0.0008$] to reduce lordosis quotients compared to those infused with control.

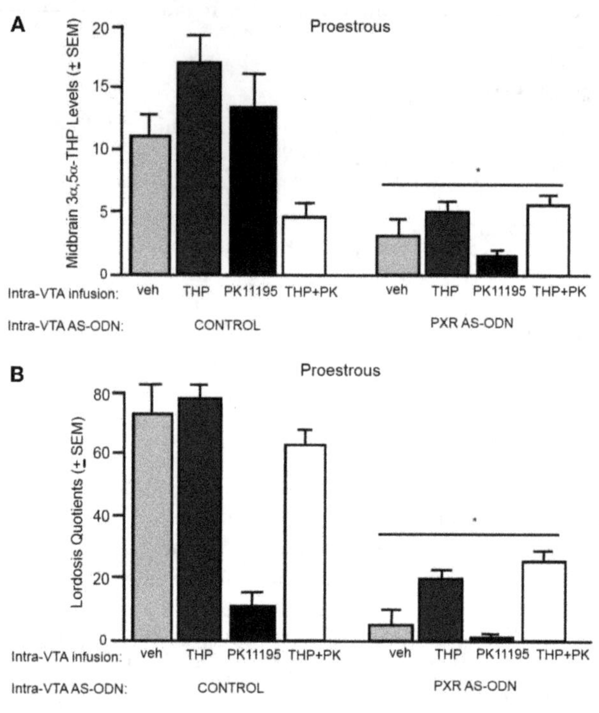

FIGURE 2 | (A) Depicts the mean (+s.e.m.) 3α,5α-THP levels in the midbrain of proestrous rats infused first with control and vehicle (veh, n = 5), 3α,5α-THP ($n = 7$), PK11195 ($n = 12$), PK11195+3α,5α-THP ($n = 11$), or pregnane xenobiotic receptor (PXR) antisense deoxynucleotides (AS-ODNs) and veh ($n = 10$), PXR AS-ODN +3α,5α-THP ($n = 8$), PXR AS-ODN+ PK11195 ($n = 7$), PXR AS-ODN + PK11195+ 3α,5α-THP ($n = 8$) in Experiment 1. **(B)** Depicts the mean (+s.e.m.) lordosis quotient of proestrous rats in these conditions. Rats infused with PXR AS-ODN had a mean 1.5 fold lower PXR expression in the midbrain compared to control infusions in Experiment 1 (data not shown). *above a line indicates a significant effect of PXR AS-ODNs compared to control infusion ($P < 0.05$). *above a bar indicates a significant effect of PK11195 and PK1195+3α,5α-THP compared to vehicle infusions ($P < 0.05$).

Aggression quotients (Table 1)

There was significant main effect of PXR AS-ODN condition [$F_{(1, 60)} = 19.9$, $P = 0.0003$] and PK11195 condition [$F_{(1, 60)} = 3.9$, $P = 0.05$] for aggression quotients. Rats infused with PXR AS-ODN or PK11195 had increased aggression quotients compared to respective control infusions.

EXPERIMENT 2: EFFECTS OF TSPO ENHANCER, FGIN 1–27, IN PROESTROUS RATS

Validation of PXR AS-ODNs for PXR expression in the midbrain

Rats infused with PXR AS-ODN had 1.8 fold lower PXR expression in the midbrain VTA compared to rats administered control infusions [$F_{(1, 37)} = 36.4, P < 0.0001$].

3α,5α-THP levels in the midbrain (Figure 3A)

There was a significant main effect of PXR AS-ODN condition [$F_{(1, 52)} = 14.4$, $P = 0.0004$] for 3α,5α-THP levels in the midbrain. Rats infused with PXR AS-ODN had significantly lower

Table 1 | Depicts mean (± s.e.m.) aggression quotients (AQ) of rats during the paced mating task In Experiments 1–4.

EXPERIMENT 1								
Hormone condition	Proestrous							
AS-ODN condition	Control				PXR AS-ODN			
Infusion condition	Veh	3α,5α-THP	PK11195	PK11195 + 3α,5α-THP	Veh	3α,5α-THP	PK11195	PK11195 + 3α,5α-THP
AQ	33.9 ± 10.6	14.4^ ± 8.8	49.2 ± 9.1	12.5 ± 5.1	51.8* ± 18.2	37.9*^ ± 7.5	58.3* ± 8.3	46.4* ± 9.7
EXPERIMENT 2								
Hormone condition	Proestrous							
AS-ODN condition	Control				PXR AS-ODN			
FGIN condition	Veh		FGIN		Veh		FGIN	
AQ	26.5 ± 9.0		30.9 ± 7.6		34.2 ± 12.6		46.5 ± 9.2	
EXPERIMENT 3								
Hormone condition	OVX, E_2-primed							
AS-ODN condition	Control				PXR AS-ODN			
FGIN condition	Veh		FGIN		Veh		FGIN	
AQ	40.6 ± 11.6		74.2 ± 10.4		75.2 ± 12.1		66.2 ± 7.9	
EXPERIMENT 4								
Hormone condition	OVX/ADX, E_2-primed							
AS-ODN condition	Control				PXR AS-ODN			
FGIN condition	Veh		FGIN		Veh		FGIN	
AQ	39.6 ± 12.9		23.0 ± 10.1		61.1* ± 10.3		66.6* ± 16.0	

**Indicates a significant difference of pregnane xenobiotic receptor (PXR) PXR antisense oliodeoxynucleotides (AS-ODN) from control ($P > 0.05$).*
^Indicates significant interaction between AS-ODN, PK11195, and 3α, 5α-THP ($P > 0.05$).

3α,5α-THP in the midbrain compared to those infused with control; effects of testing and FGIN infusions did not reach statistical significance.

Lordosis Quotients (Figure 4A)

There was a significant interaction between PXR AS-ODN condition and FGIN condition [$F_{(1, 47)} = 3.8$, $P < 0.05$] for lordosis quotients, such that PXR AS-ODNs reduced lordosis, but not when co-administered with FGIN. There was a significant main effect of PXR AS-ODN condition [$F_{(1, 47)} = 3.8$, $P = 0.05$] for lordosis quotients. Rats infused with PXR AS-ODN had significantly lower lordosis quotients compared to those infused with control condition.

Aggression quotients (Table 1)

There were no statistically significant effects of conditions for aggression quotients in this experiment.

EXPERIMENT 3: EFFECTS OF TSPO ENHANCER, FGIN 1–27, IN OVX RATS

Validation of PXR AS-ODNs for PXR expression in the midbrain

Rats infused with PXR AS-ODN had 1.5 fold lower PXR expression in the midbrain VTA compared to control infusions [$F_{(1, 41)} = 14.2$, $P = 0.0005$].

3α,5α-THP levels in the midbrain (Figure 3B)

There was a main effect for testing condition [$F_{(1, 41)} = 16.9$, $P = 0.002$] for 3α,5α-THP levels in the midbrain, such that tested rats had higher levels of 3α,5α-THP inmidbrain compared to non-tested rats; effects of PXR AS-ODN and FGIN infusions did not reach statistical significance.

Lordosis quotients (Figure 4B)

There was a significant main effect of PXR AS-ODN condition [$F_{(1, 24)} = 18.9$, $P = 0.0002$] and FGIN condition [$F_{(1, 24)} = 9.3$, $P = 0.005$] for lordosis quotients. Rats infused with PXR AS-ODN had significantly lower, and those infused with FGIN had significantly higher, lordosis quotients, compared to those infused with respective control conditions.

Aggression quotients (Table 1)

There were no significant main effects for AS-ODN condition or FGIN condition for aggression quotients.

EXPERIMENT 4: EFFECTS OF TSPO ENHANCER, FGIN 1–27, IN OVX/ADX RATS

Validation of PXR AS-ODNs for PXR expression in the midbrain

Rats infused with PXR AS-ODN had 1.4 fold lower PXR expression in the midbrain VTA compared to control infusions [$F_{(1, 24)} = 6.4$, $P = 0.01$].

3α,5α-THP levels in the midbrain (Figure 3C)

There was main effect of testing condition [$F_{(1, 38)} = 10.3$, $P = 0.002$] and PXR AS-ODN condition [$F_{(1, 38)} = 4.4$, $P = 0.04$] for 3α,5α-THP levels in the midbrain. Tested rats had higher levels of 3α,5α-THP in midbrain compared tonon-tested rats, and rats

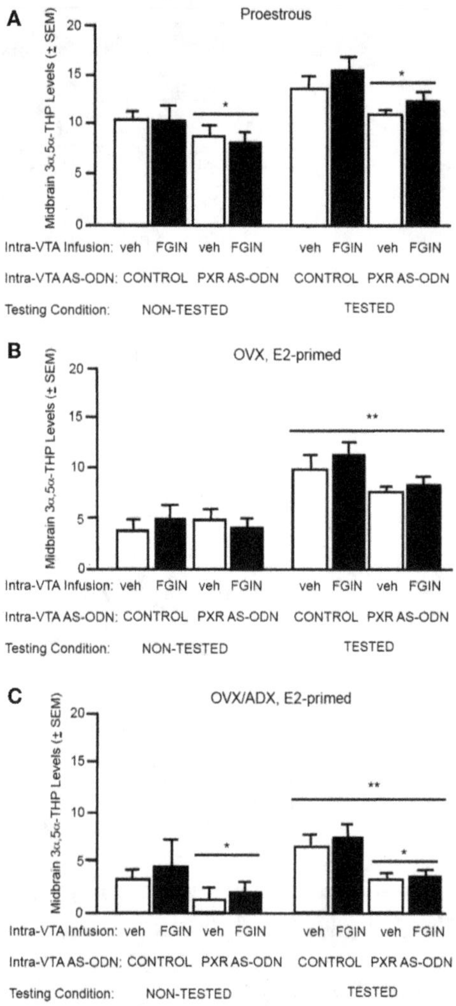

FIGURE 3 | (A) Depicts the mean (±s.e.m.) 3α,5α-THP levels in the midbrain of proestrous non tested rats infused with control and vehicle (veh, $n = 5$) or control+FGIN ($n = 4$), or pregnane xenobiotic receptor (PXR) antisense deoxynucleotides (AS-ODNs) and veh ($n = 6$), or PXR AS-ODN+FGIN ($n = 6$) or behaviorally-tested rats infused with control+veh ($n = 15$), control+FGIN ($n = 15$), PXR AS-ODN+veh ($n = 8$), or PXR AS-ODN+FGIN ($n = 13$) in Experiment 2. Rats infused with PXR AS-ODN had a mean 1.8 fold lower PXR expression in the midbrain compared to control infusions in Experiment 2 (data not shown). **(B)** Depicts the mean (±s.e.m.) 3α,5α-THP levels in the midbrain of ovariectomized (OVX) estradiol (E2)-primed non tested rats infused with control+veh ($n = 5$), control+FGIN ($n = 6$), PXR AS-ODN+veh ($n = 5$), PXR AS-ODN+FGIN ($n = 5$), or behaviorally-tested rats infused with control+veh ($n = 8$), control+FGIN ($n = 7$), PXR AS-ODN+veh ($n = 7$), or PXR AS-ODN+FGIN ($n = 6$) in Experiment 3. Rats infused with PXR AS-ODN had a mean 1.5 fold lower PXR expression in the midbrain compared to control infusions in Experiment 3 (data not shown). **(C)** Depicts the mean (±s.e.m.) 3α,5α-THP levels in the midbrain of OVX/adrenalectomized (ADX), E2-primed rats that were non tested and infused with control+veh ($n = 6$), control+FGIN ($n = 5$), PXR AS-ODN+veh ($n = 5$), PXR AS-ODN+FGIN ($n = 5$), or behaviorally-tested and infused with control+veh ($n = 9$), control+FGIN ($n = 5$), PXR AS-ODN+veh ($n = 8$), or PXR AS-ODN+FGIN ($n = 5$) in Experiment 4. Rats infused with PXR AS-ODN had a mean 1.4 fold lower PXR expression in the midbrain compared to control infusions in Experiment 4 (data not shown). *above a line indicates a significant effect of PXR AS-ODNs compared to control. **above a line indicates significant effect of testing compared to non-tested rats ($P < 0.05$).

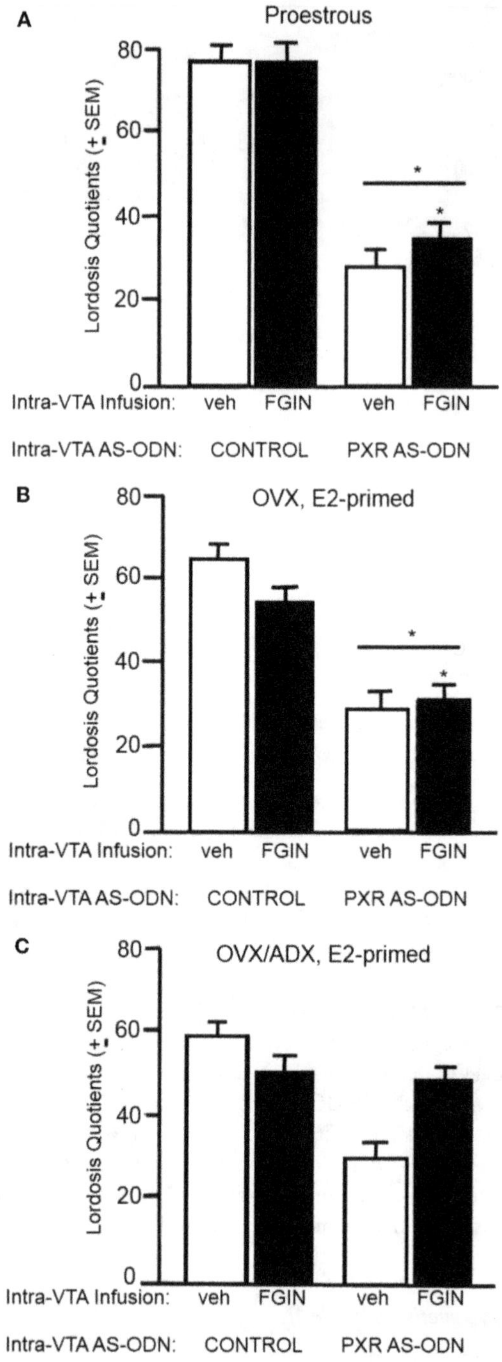

FIGURE 4 | (A) Depicts the mean (±s.e.m.) lordosis quotients of proestrous rats infused with control and vehicle (veh, $n = 15$), control+FGIN ($n = 15$), pregnane xenobiotic receptor (PXR) antisense deoxynucleotides (AS-ODNs)+vehicle ($n = 8$), or PXR AS-ODN+FGIN ($n = 13$) in Experiment 2. **(B)** Depicts the mean (±s.e.m.) lordosis quotients of ovariectomized (OVX) estradiol (E2)-primed rats infused with control+veh ($n = 8$), control+FGIN ($n = 7$), PXR AS-ODN+veh ($n = 7$), or PXR AS-ODN+FGIN ($n = 6$) in Experiment 3. **(C)** Depicts the mean (±s.e.m.) lordosis quotients of OVX/adrenalectomized (ADX), E2-primed rats infused with control+veh ($n = 9$), control+FGIN ($n = 5$), PXR AS-ODN+veh ($n = 8$), or PXR AS-ODN+FGIN ($n = 5$) in Experiment 4. *above a line indicates a significant effect of PXR AS-ODNs compared to control. ($P < 0.05$).

infused with PXR AS-ODNs had lower levels compared to control infusions.

Lordosis quotients (Figure 4C)

There was main effect of PXR AS-ODN condition [$F_{(1, 25)} = 5.8$, $P = 0.02$] for lordosis quotients, such that infusions of PXR AS-ODN decreased lordosis quotients compared to control infusions; effects of FGIN infusions did not reach statistical significance.

Aggression quotients (Table 1)

There was main effect of PXR AS-ODN condition [$F_{(1, 25)} = 4.9$, $P = 0.03$] for aggression quotients, such that infusions of PXR AS-ODN decreased aggression quotients compared to control infusions; effects of FGIN infusions did not reach statistical significance.

DISCUSSION

The data support, in part, the hypothesis tested that PXR is an upstream factor of TSPO for neurosteroidogenesis of 3α,5α-THP in the VTA for lordosis, independent of peripheral glands. First, proestrous rats administered a TSPO blocker (PK11195), subsequent to AS-ODNs to the VTA, had lower 3α,5α-THP levels in the midbrain and lordosis; the effects on lordosis could be reversed with replacement with 3α,5α-THP administration alone, but not when co-administered with PXR AS-ODN. Second, proestrous, OVX, or OVX/ADX rats infused with a TSPO enhancer (FGIN 1–27), subsequent to AS-ODNs to the VTA, had lower 3α,5α-THP levels in the midbrain and lordosis particularly among proestrous rats, compared to those that were OVX or OVX/ADX. Comparisons with removal of the main peripheral sources of steroids, ovaries and adrenals, were completed to address the role of PXR and TSPO for steroid synthesis in the brain. These data with a greater response in proestrous compared to rats with glands surgically removed suggest that there is not complete independence of these peripheral sources for PXR's actions in the midbrain VTA, which are likely upstream of TSPO. Thus, PXR may be acting as a homeostatic regulator, upstream of TSPO in the pathway for production of 3α,5α-THP in the midbrain VTA, and behavioral responses of female rats.

The present data confirm the importance of PXR in the midbrain for 3α,5α-THP and lordosis. Inhibiting PXR with the same AS-ODN approach used here reduces 3α,5α-THP in the midbrain VTA concomitant with reductions in lordosis and enhancements in aggressive responding toward males during paced mating of proestrous rats, or those that were OVX and estradiol-primed (Frye et al., 2013, 2014). Additionally, activating PXR with ligands infused to the midbrain VTA enhances reproductive responding of female rats (Frye, 2011). Moreover, the present data confirm the role of biosynthesis of 3α,5α-THP from cholesterol in the midbrain VTA for lordosis. Inhibitors of TSPO, as well as downstream factors involved in biosynthesis, StAR or P450scc, infused to the midbrain VTA of female rats attenuates progestogen-facilitated lordosis (Petralia et al., 2005; Frye et al., 2008a; Frye, 2009; Frye and Paris, 2011). An opposite effect is observed with TSPO agonist, such as FGIN, when infused to the midbrain VTA as was observed here (Frye et al., 2009; Frye and Paris, 2011).

It should be noted that FGIN infusions in this study did not produce the same pattern of reduction for 3α,5α-THP levels in the midbrain as was observed in lordosis quotients. A consideration is that this experiment was conducted in proestrous rats, with peripheral sources of steroids, as well as typical steroid feedback mechanisms in place; a more robust response may have been observed with this FGIN dosing in OVX and/or OVX/ADX rats. Another consideration is that comparisons with non-tested rats in this experiment may have provided an indication of mating-induced 3α,5α-THP production from metabolism of progesterone from the ovaries, which could account for little difference in 3α,5α-THP levels in the midbrain after mating, albeit low lordosis responding with this manipulation. A third consideration is that measurement of dihydroprogesterone, or other steroids, were not assessed in the midbrain. Indeed, in the group that was co-administered PK11195 and 3α,5α-THP, the enhancements in lordosis were more robust than post-mating levels of 3α,5α-THP on the midbrain that were measured; whether this could have been due to back-conversion of administered 3α,5α-THP or 3α,5α-THP from other sources is not known. Together, these data extends previous findings to suggest that PXR, which is known to act as a transcription factor for P450 enzymes involved in steroid metabolism, such as CYP11A1 (Ma et al., 2008; Zhang et al., 2008), may be another important neuroregulatory factor in the biosynthesis of 3α,5α-THP in the midbrain, upstream of TSPO, and resulting actions on lordosis in the adult. Moreover, the data that there were differences between proestrous, OVX, and OVX/ADX rats suggest that biosynthesis in the brain, as well as metabolism from peripheral sources of progesterone, are involved in PXR's modulation of 3α,5α-THP. Alternatively, the removal of the glands disrupts multiple negative feedback loops of steroids, and thereby disrupts typical responses to steroids for behavior. We have observed that effects of PXR AS-ODN infusions to reduce lordosis and 3α,5α-THP levels in the midbrain of OVX rats only when they were estradiol-primed (Frye et al., 2014). Thus, hormonal milieu provides a significant context for interactions between neuroendocrine and behavioral responses.

The pattern of results here confirms prior studies showing a greater influence of PXR knockdown in the midbrain for behavior in the paced mating task, compared to the other behavioral tasks assessed (even when the order of testing in these tasks is altered as in Frye et al., in press). There were very few animals that received infusions outside the targeted area, and all experimental groups were not represented. The data from these subjects suggest that manipulations to other midbrain sites (e.g., substantia nigra, or central gray) did not produce the same pattern of effects as did infusions to the VTA, but rather produced responses similar to the control groups. Manipulations of 3α,5α-THP from exposure to mating, or infusions of 3α,5α-THP directly to this the midbrain (but not substantia nigra or central gray), increase levels of 3α,5α-THP in corticolimbic structures and reduce anxiety-like responding; however, manipulations of PXR typically produce less robust effects on these other measures, as was observed here. A question for future studies is the expression patterns and actions of PXR beyond the midbrain for reproduction-relevant behaviors, such as cognition, exploration, anxiety, and interactions with conspecifics. Mating-induced neurosteroidogenesis occurs beyond the midbrain to the hippocampus, cortex, and striatum (Frye and Rhodes, 2006; Frye et al., 2009). Indeed, we have observed that manipulating PXR in the midbrain of proestrous rats reduces 3α,5α-THP levels in the midbrain and the hippocampus, as well as a growth factor (brain-derived neurotrophic factor; BDNF) in the hippocampus (Frye et al., 2013, in press). It is plausible that PXR is having effects beyond those involving progestogen-facilitated lordosis through actions in the midbrain.

Beyond facilitating successful mating, progestogens are considered to have organizing effects on the nervous system during gestation/perinatally to influence later adult behaviors that ultimately are adaptive (reducing stress/anxiety, enhancing cognition, and conferring protection to neural insults/aging; Frye, 2009; Brinton, 2013; Brunton et al., 2014; Bali and Jaggi, 2014). We have focused on using lordosis as a bioassay to understand progestogens' mechanisms and effects in the central nervous system; albeit, other models support a role of progestogens for motivated, and cognitive processes. One example is mating-induced conditioned placed preference, where females will change their initial preference to spend time in a context associated with mating (González-Flores et al., 2004; Camacho et al., 2009; Arzate et al., 2011). Beneficial effects of progesterone or 3α,5α-THP administration to ovariectomized rats or mice has been described for spatial and object recognition memory tasks (Sandstrom and Williams, 2001; Tanabe et al., 2004; Walf et al., 2006; Frye et al., 2007, 2013). Furthermore, the capacity for *de novo* steroid synthesis in the prefrontal cortex and hippocampus (Cheng and Karavolas, 1975; Li et al., 1997; Furukawa et al., 1998; Frye, 2001a,b) suggests that PXR may also be a factor to investigate systematically in these regions for behaviors that contribute to successful mating. For example, in recent studies assessing the requirement of PXR for mating-induced 3α,5α-THP synthesis in the midbrain and the hippocampus, knocking down PXR attenuated effects of paced mating experience to increase 3α,5α-THP in these regions, as well as increase BDNF in the hippocampus, of proestrous rats (Frye et al., in press). Given the role of progestogens throughout the lifespan, the importance of PXR-mediated 3α,5α-THP production and other measures of neural plasticity (e.g., BDNF) and behavioral plasticity (e.g., mating) are of continued interest.

In addition to further understanding potential downstream factors, such as TSPO and BDNF, the contributory role of other "liver" factors in the same nuclear receptor super family as PXR, such as liver X receptor (LXR), for neural and behavioral plasticity needs to be explored. Although the present experiment focused on the role of PXR, it would be of interest to consider the respective roles of these factors, which were first described in the liver, but both have received a greater focus on their effects in the nervous system more recently (Mellon et al., 2008). One focus of the effects of these receptors is their role in cholesterol clearance, which is related to diet and cardiovascular function, as well as important for neurodegenerative disorders, such as Alzheimer's disease, and neurodevelopmental disorders, such as Niemann-Pick disease (Whitney et al., 2002; Repa et al., 2007; Ma et al., 2008; Tang et al., 2008). As one example, mouse models of Niemann-Pick disease show deficits in cholesterol metabolism and 3α,5α-THP production in the brain, and such deficits could be reversed with administration of PXR ligands, one of them being 3α,5α-THP (Frye and Rhodes, 2006; Frye, 2009; Brinton, 2013).

Early developmental effects of LXR in the brain have also been described. For example, protective effects similar to those described for PXR have been noted with LXR modulation in a Niemann-Pick disease mouse model (Repa et al., 2007) as well as promoting neurosteroidogenesis and protective effects in animal models of diabetic neuropathy and multiple sclerosis (Cermenati et al., 2010, 2012; Mitro et al., 2012). As well, the role of LXR in typical neurodevelopmental processes, such as neurogenesis, in the VTA of mice, using an *in vitro* model, has been recently described (Theofilopoulos et al., 2013). Additionally, knockout of the beta form of LXR that is highly expressed in the central nervous system increases anxiety-like responding of female mice and alters GABA in the cortex (Tan et al., 2012). In the present study, the role of PXR in the VTA for 3α,5α-THP production from cholesterol and subsequent behavioral effects was assessed. A consideration for future studies is elucidating how PXR and LXR may act synergistically for efficient cholesterol metabolism and clearance in neurons and glia, respectively, supporting neural and behavioral plasticity. Another important question is the role of PXR for neurosteroidogenesis in males; production of androstane neurosteroids, such as 3α-androstanediol, occurs after mating of male rodents and has robust behavioral actions (Edinger and Frye, 2007; Frye et al., 2008b). Although proestrous female rats have higher expression of PXR in the midbrain than do males (Frye et al., 2013), the expression of PXR in males and females in other brain regions with high capacity for neurosteroidogenesis is not completely known. Together, these results involving liver factors, such as PXR, substantiate further studies of an interaction between peripheral and brain factors for behavior.

In summary, inhibiting TSPO with PK11195 reduced 3α,5α-THP levels in the midbrain and lordosis, an effect that could be reversed with 3α,5α-THP administration, but not AS-ODN+3α,5α-THP. PXR AS-ODNs blocked actions of FGIN 1–27 for lordosis and 3α,5α-THP levels among proestrous > OVX > OVX/ADX rats. Together, these data suggest the liver factor, PXR, may be upstream of TSPO, acting as a homeostatic regulator involved in neurosteroidogenesis of 3α,5α-THP in the brain for behavior. Understanding these basic mechanisms of how steroids are involved, and what factors are necessary for their production, for behavioral/neural plasticity supports future work on how a prominent peripheral factor, such as PXR, may have actions in the brain and, ultimately, find use in brain augmentation approaches.

AUTHOR CONTRIBUTIONS

All authors on this paper substantially contributed to the work described herein. Carolyn J. Koonce was involved in acquisition, analysis, and interpretation of data, and drafting of figures for paper and Results and Methods section. Alicia A.Walf was involved in acquisition, analysis, and interpretation of data, and drafting and revising of all sections of the paper. Cheryl A. Frye was involved in the conception and study design, acquisition, analysis, and interpretation of data, reviewing drafts of the work, and giving final approval of the paper to be submitted.

ACKNOWLEDGMENTS

This research was supported by grants from the National Institute of Mental Health (MH0676980; RMH067698B). Technical assistance, provided by Drs. Paris and Rusconi, and Anthony Santarelli, Jennifer Torgersen, and Zhenhong Zhao, is greatly appreciated. Experiments described herein comply with the current laws of the United States. All authors report that they have no conflicts of interest (financial or otherwise) that would bias them to the outcome of these experiments.

REFERENCES

Acosta, S. A., Tajiri, N., Shinozuka, K., Ishikawa, H., Grimmig, B., Diamond, D., et al. (2013). Long-term upregulation of inflammation and suppression of cell proliferation in the brain of adult rats exposed to traumatic brain injury using the controlled cortical impact model. *PLoS ONE* 8:e53376. doi: 10.1371/journal.pone.0053376

Agís-Balboa, R. C., Pinna, G., Pibiri, F., Kadriu, B., Costa, E., and Guidotti, A. (2007). Down-regulation of neurosteroid biosynthesis in corticolimbic circuits mediates social isolation-induced behavior in mice. *Proc. Natl. Acad. Sci. U.S.A.* 104, 18736–18741. doi: 10.1073/pnas.0709419104

Arzate, D. M., Portillo, W., Rodríguez, C., Corona, R., and Paredes, R. G. (2011). Extended paced mating tests induces conditioned place preference without affecting sexual arousal. *Horm. Behav.* 59, 674–680. doi: 10.1016/j.yhbeh.2010.08.016

Azcoitia, I., Sierra, A., Veiga, S., and Garcia-Segura, L. M. (2003). Aromatase expression by reactive astroglia is neuroprotective. *Ann. N. Y. Acad. Sci.* 1007, 298–305. doi: 10.1196/annals.1286.028

Bali, A., and Jaggi, A. S. (2014). Multifunctional aspects of allopregnanolone in stress and related disorders. *Prog. Neuropsychopharmacol. Biol. Psychiatry* 48, 64–78. doi: 10.1016/j.pnpbp.2013.09.005

Barbaccia, M. L., Serra, M., Purdy, R. H., and Biggio, G. (2001). Stress and neuroactive steroids. *Int. Rev. Neurobiol.* 246, 243–272. doi: 10.1016/S0074-7742(01)46065-X

Bauer, B., Hartz, A. M., Fricker, G., and Miller, D.S. (2004). Pregnane X receptor up-regulation of P-glycoprotein expression and transport function at the blood-brain barrier. *Mol. Pharmacol.* 66, 413–419. doi: 10.1124/mol.66.3

Bauer, B., Yang, X., Hartz, A. M., Olson, E. R., Zhao, R., Kalvass, J. C., et al. (2006). *In vivo* activation of human pregnane X receptor tightens the blood-brain barrier to methadone through P-glycoprotein up-regulation. *Mol. Pharmacol.* 70, 1212–1219. doi: 10.1124/mol.106.023796

Billeci, A., Caso, V., Paciaroni, M., Palmerini, F., and Agnelli, G. (2007). Hormone-replacement therapy, dementia and stroke. *Womens Health* 3, 699–710. doi: 10.2217/17455057.3.6.699

Bitran, D., Foley, M., Audette, D., Leslie, N., and Frye, C. A. (2000). Activation of peripheral mitochondrial benzodiazepine receptors in the hippocampus stimulates allopregnanolone synthesis and produces anxiolytic-like effects in the rat. *Psychopharmacology* 151, 64–71. doi: 10.1007/s002130000471

Brinton, R. D. (2013). Neurosteroids as regenerative agents in the brain: therapeutic implications. *Nat. Rev. Endocrinol.* 9, 241–250. doi: 10.1038/nrendo.2013.31

Brunton, P. J., Russell, J. A., and Hirst, J. J. (2014). Allopregnanolone in the brain: Protecting pregnancy and birth outcomes. *Prog. Neurobiol.* 113, 106–136. doi: 10.1016/j.pneurobio.2013.08.005

Camacho, F. J., García-Horsman, P., and Paredes, R. G. (2009). Hormonal and testing conditions for the induction of conditioned place preference by paced mating. *Horm. Behav.* 56, 410–415. doi: 10.1016/j.yhbeh.2009.07.007

Cermenati, G., Abbiati, F., Cermenati, S., Brioschi, E., Volonterio, A., Cavaletti, G., et al. (2012). Diabetes-induced myelin abnormalities are associated with an altered lipid pattern: protective effects of LXR activation. *J. Lipid Res.* 53, 300–310. doi: 10.1194/jlr.M021188

Cermenati, G., Giatti, S., Cavaletti, G., Bianchi, R., Maschi, O., Pesaresi, M., et al. (2010). Activation of the liver X receptor increases neuroactive steroid levels and protects from diabetes-induced peripheral neuropathy. *J. Neurosci.* 30, 11896–11901. doi: 10.1523/JNEUROSCI.1898-10.2010

Chen, J., Chopp, M., and Li, Y. (1999). Neuroprotective effects of progesterone after transient middle cerebral artery occlusion in rat. *J. Neurol. Sci.* 171, 24–30. doi: 10.1016/S0022-510X(99)00247-6

Cheng, Y. J., and Karavolas, H. J. (1975). Subcellular distribution and properties of progesterone (delta4-steroid) 5a-reductase in rat medial basal hypothalamus. *J. Biol. Chem.* 250, 7997–8003.

Dussault, I., and Forman, B. M. (2002). The nuclear receptor PXR: a master regulator of "homeland" defense. *Crit. Rev. Eukaryot. Gene Expr.* 12, 53–64. doi: 10.1615/CritRevEukaryotGeneExpr.v12.i1.30

Edinger, K. L., and Frye, C. A. (2007). Sexual experience of male rats influences anxiety-like behavior and androgen levels. *Physiol. Behav.* 92, 443–453. doi: 10.1016/j.physbeh.2007.04.018

Erskine, M. S. (1985). Effects of paced coital stimulation on estrus duration in intact cycling rats and ovariectomized and ovariectomized-adrenalectomized hormone-primed rats. *Behav. Neurosci.* 99, 151–161. doi: 10.1037/0735-7044.99.1.151

Francis, G. A., Fayard, E., Picard, F., and Auwerx, J. (2002). Nuclear receptors and the control of metabolism. *Annu. Rev. Physiol.* 65, 261–311. doi: 10.1146/annurev.physiol.65.092101.142528

Frye, C. A. (2001a). The role of neurosteroids and nongenomic effects of progestins in the ventral tegmental area in mediating sexual receptivity of rodents. *Horm. Behav.* 40, 226–233. doi: 10.1006/hbeh.2001.1674

Frye, C. A. (2001b). The role of neurosteroids and non-genomic effects of progestins and androgens in mediating sexual receptivity of rodents. *Brain Res. Brain Res. Rev.* 37, 201–222. doi: 10.1016/S0165-0173(01)00119-9

Frye, C. A. (2009). Neurosteroids' effects and mechanisms for social, cognitive, emotional, and physical functions. *Psychoneuroendocrinology* 34, S143–S161. doi: 10.1016/j.psyneuen.2009.07.005

Frye, C. A. (2011). Novel substrates for, and sources of, progestogens for reproduction. *J. Neuroendocrinol.* 23, 961–973. doi: 10.1111/j.1365-2826.2011.02180.x

Frye, C. A., and Bayon, L. E. (1999). Mating stimuli influence endogenous variations in the neurosteroids 3α,5α-THP and 3α-Diol. *J. Neuroendocrinol.* 11, 839–847. doi: 10.1046/j.1365-2826.1999.00379.x

Frye, C. A., Duffy, C. K., and Walf,A. A. (2007). Estrogens and progestins enhance spatial learning of intact and ovariectomized rats in the object placement task. *Neurobiol. Learn. Mem.* 88, 208–216. doi: 10.1016/j.nlm.2007.04.003

Frye, C. A., Koonce, C. J., Edinger, K. L., Osborne, D. M., and Walf, A. A. (2008b). Androgens with activity at estrogen receptor beta have anxiolytic and cognitive-enhancing effects in male rats and mice. *Horm. Behav.* 54, 726–734. doi: 10.1016/j.yhbeh.2008.07.013

Frye, C. A., Koonce, C. J., and Walf, A. A. (2014). Role of pregnane xenobiotic receptor in the midbrain ventral tegmental area for estradiol- and 3α,5α-THP-facilitated lordosis of female rats. *Psychopharmacology.* doi: 10.1007/s00213-013-3406-0. [Epub ahead of print].

Frye, C. A., Koonce, C. J., and Walf, A. A. (in press). Involvement of pregnane xenobiotic receptor in mating-induced allopregnanolone formation in the midbrain and hippocampus and brain-derived neurotrophic factor in the hippocampus among female rats. *Psychopharmacology.* doi: 10.1007/s00213-014-3569-3

Frye, C. A., Koonce, C. J., Walf, A. A., and Rusconi, J. C. (2013). Motivated behaviors and levels of 3α,5α-THP in the midbrain are attenuated by knocking down expression of pregnane xenobiotic receptor in the midbrain ventral tegmental area of proestrous rats. *J. Sex. Med.* 10, 1692–1706. doi: 10.1111/jsm.12173

Frye, C. A., and Paris, J. J. (2011). Progesterone turnover to its 5α-reduced metabolites in the ventral tegmental area of the midbrain is essential for initiating social and affective behavior and progesterone metabolism in female rats. *J. Endocrinol. Invest.* 34, e188–e199. doi: 10.3275/7334

Frye, C. A., Paris, J. J., and Rhodes, M. E. (2008a). Exploratory, anti-anxiety, social, and sexual behaviors of rats in behavioral estrus is attenuated with inhibition of 3α,5α-THP formation in the midbrain ventral tegmental area. *Behav. Brain Res.* 193, 269–276. doi: 10.1016/j.bbr.2008.06.005

Frye, C. A., Paris, J. J., and Rhodes, M. E. (2009). Increasing 3α, 5α-THP following inhibition of neurosteroid biosynthesis in the ventral tegmental area reinstates anti-anxiety, social, and sexual behavior of naturally receptive rats. *Reproduction* 137, 119–128. doi: 10.1530/REP-08-0250

Frye, C. A., Paris, J. J., Walf, A. A., and Rusconi, J. C. (2012). Effects and mechanisms of 3α,5α,-THP on emotion, motivation, and reward functions involving pregnane xenobiotic receptor. *Front. Neurosci.* 195:136. doi: 10.3389/fnins.2011.00136

Frye, C. A., and Rhodes, M. E. (2006). Progestin concentrations are increased following paced mating in midbrain, hippocampus, diencephalon, and cortex of rats in behavioral estrus, but only in midbrain of diestrous rats. *Neuroendocrinology* 83, 336–347. doi: 10.1159/000096051

Frye, C. A., Rhodes, M. E., Petralia, S. M., Walf, A. A., Sumida, K., and Edinger, K. L. (2006). 3alpha-hydroxy-5alpha-pregnan-20-one in the midbrain ventral tegmental area mediates social, sexual, and affective behaviors. *Neuroscience* 138, 1007–1014. doi: 10.1016/j.neuroscience.2005.06.015

Frye, C. A., and Walf, A. A. (2008). Membrane actions of progestins at dopamine type 1-like and GABAA receptors involve downstream signal transduction pathways. *Steroids* 73, 906–913. doi: 10.1016/j.steroids.2008.01.020

Furukawa, A., Miyatake, A., Ohnishi, T., and Ichikawa, Y. (1998). Steroidogenic acute regulatory protein (StAR) transcripts constitutively expressed in the adult rat central nervous system: colocalization of StAR, cytochrome P-450SCC (CYP XIA1), and 3β-hydroxysteroid dehydrogenase in the rat brain. *J. Neurochem.* 71, 2231–2238. doi: 10.1046/j.1471-4159.1998.71062231.x

Geick, A., Eichelbaum, M., and Burk, O. (2001). Nuclear receptor response elements mediate induction of intestinal MDR1 by rifampin. *J. Biol. Chem.* 276, 14581–14587. doi: 10.1074/jbc.M010173200

González-Flores, O., Camacho, F. J., Domínguez-Salazar, E., Ramírez-Orduna, J. M., Beyer, C., and Paredes, R. G. (2004). Progestins and place preference conditioning after paced mating. *Horm. Behav.* 46, 151–157. doi: 10.1016/j.yhbeh.2004.02.006

Harmsen, S., Meijerman, I., Beijnen, J. H., and Schellens, J. H. (2007). The role of nuclear receptors in pharmacokinetic drug-drug interactions in oncology. *Cancer Treat. Rev.* 33, 369–380. doi: 10.1016/j.ctrv.2007.02.003

He, J., Hoffman, S. W., and Stein, D. G. (2004). Allopregnanolone, a progesterone metabolite, enhances behavioral recovery and decreases neuronal loss after traumatic brain injury. *Restor. Neurol. Neurosci.* 22, 19–31.

King, S. R., Manna, P. R., Ishii, T., Syapin, P. J., Ginsberg, S. D., Wilson, K., et al. (2002). An essential component in steroid synthesis, the steroidogenic acute regulatory protein, is expressed in discrete regions of the brain. *J. Neurosci.* 22, 10613–10620.

Kinsley, C. H., and Lambert, K. G. (2008). Reproduction-induced neuroplasticity: natural behavioural and neuronal alterations associated with the production and care of offspring. *J. Neuroendocrinol.* 20, 515–525. doi: 10.1111/j.1365-2826.2008.01667.x

Kliewer, S. A., Goodwin, B., and Willson, T. M. (2002). The nuclear pregnane X receptor: a key regulator of xenobiotic metabolism. *Endocr. Rev.* 23, 687–702. doi: 10.1210/er.2001-0038

Lambert, K. G., Berry, A. E., Griffins, G., Amory-Meyers, E., Madonia-Lomas, L., Love, G., et al. (2005). Pup exposure differentially enhances foraging ability in primiparous and nulliparous rats. *Physiol. Behav.* 84, 799–806. doi: 10.1016/j.physbeh.2005.03.012

Li, X., Bertics, P. J., and Karavolas, H. J. (1997). Regional distribution of cytosolic and particulate 5a-dihydroprogesterone 3a-hydroxysteroid oxidoreductases in female rat brain. *J. Steroid Biochem. Mol. Biol.* 60, 311–318. doi: 10.1016/S0960-0760(96)00195-1

Livak, K. J., and Schmittgen, T. D. (2001). Analysis of relative gene expression data using real-time quantitative PCR and the 2(-Delta Delta C(T)). *Methods* 25, 402–408. doi: 10.1006/meth.2001.1262

Ma, X., Idle, J. R., and Gonzalez, F. J. (2008). The pregnane X receptor: from bench to bedside. *Expert Opin. Drug Metab. Toxicol.* 4, 895–908. doi: 10.1517/17425255.4.7.895

Macbeth, A. H., and Luine, V. N. (2010). Changes in anxiety and cognition due to reproductive experience: a review of data from rodent and human mothers. *Neurosci. Biobehav. Rev.* 34, 452–467. doi: 10.1016/j.neubiorev.2009.08.011

Maki, P. M., and Henderson, V. W. (2012). Hormone therapy, dementia, and cognition: the Women's Health Initiative 10 years on. *Climacteric* 15, 256–262. doi: 10.3109/13697137.2012.660613

Mellon, S. H., and Deschepper, C. F. (1993). Neurosteroid biosynthesis: genes for adrenal steroidogenic enzymes are expressed in the brain. *Brain Res.* 629, 283–292. doi: 10.1016/0006-8993(93)91332-M

Mellon, S. H., Gong, W., and Schonemann, M. D. (2008). Endogenous and synthetic neurosteroids in treatment of Niemann-Pick Type C disease. *Brain Res. Rev.* 57, 410–420. doi: 10.1016/j.brainresrev.2007.05.012

Mitro, N., Cermenati, G., Giatti, S., Abbiati, F., Pesaresi, M., Calabrese, D., et al. (2012). LXR and TSPO as new therapeutic targets to increase the levels of neuroactive steroids in the central nervous system of diabetic animals. *Neurochem. Int.* 60, 616–621. doi: 10.1016/j.neuint.2012.02.025

Murphy, S. J., Littleton-Kearney, M. T., and Hurn, P. D. (2002). Progesterone administration during reperfusion, but not preischemia alone, reduces injury in ovariectomized rats. *J. Cereb. Blood Flow Metab.* 22, 1181–1188. doi: 10.1097/00004647-200210000-00005

Ott, M., Fricker, G., and Bauer, B. (2009). Pregnane X receptor (PXR) regulates P-glycoprotein at the blood-brain barrier: functional similarities between pig and human PXR. *J. Pharmacol. Exp. Ther.* 329, 141–149. doi: 10.1124/jpet.108.149690

Papadopoulos, V., Baraldi, M., Guilarte, T. R., Knudsen, T. B., Lacapère, J. J., Lindemann, P., et al. (2006). Translocator protein (18kDa): new nomenclature for the peripheral-type benzodiazepine receptor based on its structure and molecular function. *Trends Pharmacol. Sci.* 27, 402–409. doi: 10.1016/j.tips.2006.06.005

Paris, J. J., and Frye, C. A. (2008). Estrous cycle, pregnancy, and parity enhance performance of rats in object recognition or object placement tasks. *Reproduction* 136, 105–115. doi: 10.1530/REP-07-0512

Paxinos, G., and Watson, C. (1986). *The Rat Brain.* New York, NY: Academic Press.

Petralia, S. M., and Frye, C. A. (2005). In the ventral tegmental area picrotoxin blocks FGIN 1-27-induced increases in sexual behavior of rats and hamsters. *Psychopharmacology* 178, 174–182. doi: 10.1007/s00213-004-2001-9

Petralia, S. M., Jahagirdar, V., and Frye, C. A. (2005). Inhibiting biosynthesis and/or metabolism of progestins in the ventral tegmental area attenuates lordosis of rats in behavioural oestrus. *J. Neuroendocrinol.* 17, 545–552. doi: 10.1111/j.1365-2826.2005.01342.x

Pinna, G., Agis-Balboa, R. C., Pibiri, F., Nelson, M., Guidotti, A., and Costa, E. (2008). Neurosteroid biosynthesis regulates sexually dimorphic fear and aggressive behavior in mice. *Neurochem. Res.* 33, 1990–2007. doi: 10.1007/s11064-008-9718-5

Pinna, G., and Rasmusson, A. M. (2012). Up-regulation of neurosteroid biosynthesis as a pharmacological strategy to improve behavioural deficits in a putative mouse model of post-traumatic stress disorder. *J. Neuroendocrinol.* 24, 102–116. doi: 10.1111/j.1365-2826.2011.02234.x

Purdy, R. H., Morrow, A. L., Moore, P. H. Jr., and Paul, S. M. (1991). Stress-induced elevations of gamma-aminobutyric acid type A receptor-active steroids in the rat brain. *Proc. Natl. Acad. Sci. U.S.A.* 88, 4553–4557. doi: 10.1073/pnas.88.10.4553

Repa, J. J., Li, H., Frank-Cannon, T. C., Valasek, M. A., Turley, S. D., Tansey, M. G., and Dietschy, J. M. (2007). Liver X receptor activation enhances cholesterol loss from the brain, decreases neuroinflammation, and increases survival of the NPC1 mouse. *J. Neurosci.* 27, 14470–14480. doi: 10.1523/JNEUROSCI.4823-07.2007

Roof, R. L., Duvdevani, R., and Stein, D. G. (1992). Progesterone treatment attenuates brain edema following contusion injury in male and female rats. *Restor. Neurol. Neurosci.* 4, 425–427.

Roof, R. L., Duvdevani, R., and Stein, D.G. (1993). Gender influences outcome of brain injury: progesterone plays a protective role. *Brain Res.* 607, 333–336. doi: 10.1016/0006-8993(93)91526-X

Rossouw, J. E., Anderson, G. L., Prentice, R. L., LaCroix, A. Z., Kooperberg, C., Stefanick, M. L., et al. (2002). Risks and benefits of estrogen plus progestin in healthy postmenopausal women: Principal results from the Women's Health Initiative randomized controlled trial. *JAMA* 288, 321–333. doi: 10.1001/jama.288.3.321

Sandstrom, N. J., and Williams, C. L. (2001). Memory retention is modulated by acute estradiol and progesterone replacement. *Behav. Neurosci.* 115, 384–393. doi: 10.1037/0735-7044.115.2.384

Schmittgen, T. D., and Livak, K. J. (2008). Analyzing real-time PCR data by the comparative C(T) method. *Nat. Protoc.* 3, 1101–1108. doi: 10.1038/nprot.2008.73

Shapiro, S. (2006). Risk of cardiovascular disease in relation to the use of combined postmenopausal hormone therapy: detection bias and resolution of discrepant findings in two Women's Health Initiative studies. *Climacteric* 9, 416–420. doi: 10.1080/13697130601012061

Shumaker, S. A., Legault, C., Rapp, S. R., Thal, L., Wallace, R. B., Ockene, J. K., et al. (2003). Estrogen plus progestin and the incidence of dementia and mild cognitive impairment in postmenopausal women: the Women's Health Initiative Memory Study: a randomized controlled trial. *JAMA* 289, 2651–2662. doi: 10.1001/jama.289.20.2651

Tan, X. J., Dai, Y. B., Wu, W. F., Warner, M., and Gustafsson, J. Å. (2012). Anxiety in liver X receptor β knockout female mice with loss of glutamic acid decarboxylase in ventromedial prefrontal cortex. *Proc. Natl. Acad. Sci. U.S.A.* 109, 7493–7498. doi: 10.1073/pnas.1205189109

Tanabe, F., Miyasaka, N., Kubota, T., and Aso, T. (2004). Estrogen and progesterone improve scopolamine-induced impairment of spatial memory. *J. Med. Dent. Sci.* 51, 89–98.

Tang, W., Ma, Y., Jia, L., Ioannou, Y. A., Davies, J. P., and Yu, L. (2008). Niemann-Pick C1-like 1 is required for an LXR agonist to raise plasma HDL cholesterol in mice. *Arterioscler. Thromb. Vasc. Biol.* 28, 448–454. doi: 10.1161/ATVBAHA.107.160465

Theofilopoulos, S., Wang, Y., Kitambi, S. S., Sacchetti, P., Sousa, K. M., Bodin, K., et al. (2013). Brain endogenous liver X receptor ligands selectively promote midbrain neurogenesis. *Nat. Chem. Biol.* 9, 126–133. doi: 10.1038/nchembio.1156

Toung, T. J., Chen, T. Y., Littleton-Kearney, M. T., Hurn, P. D., and Murphy, S. J. (2004). Effects of combined estrogen and progesterone on brain infarction in reproductively senescent female rats. *J. Cereb. Blood Flow Metab.* 24, 1160–1166. doi: 10.1097/01.WCB.0000135594.13576.D2

Uphouse, L., Adams, S., Miryala, C. S., Hassell, J., and Hiegel, C. (2013). RU486 blocks effects of allopregnanolone on the response to restraint stress. *Pharmacol. Biochem. Behav.* 103, 568–572. doi: 10.1016/j.pbb.2012.09.024

Uphouse, L., Selvamani, A., Lincoln, C., Morales, L., and Comeaux, D. (2005). Mild restraint reduces the time hormonally primed rats spend with sexually active males. *Behav. Brain Res.* 157, 343–350. doi: 10.1016/j.bbr.2004.08.001

Walf, A. A., Rhodes, M. E., and Frye, C. A. (2006). Ovarian steroids enhance object recognition in naturally cycling and ovariectomized, hormone-primed rats. *Neurobiol. Learn. Mem.* 86, 35–46. doi: 10.1016/j.nlm.2006.01.004

Whitney, K. D., Watson, M. A., Collins, J. L., Benson, W. G., Stone, T. M., Numerick, M. J., et al. (2002). Regulation of cholesterol homeostasis by the liver X receptors in the central nervous system. *Mol. Endocrinol.* 16, 1378–1385. doi: 10.1210/mend.16.6.0835

Xu, D. X., Wei, W., Sun, M. F., Wei, L. Z., and Wang, J.P. (2005). Melatonin attenuates lipopolysaccharide-induced down-regulation of pregnane X receptor and its target gene CYP3A in mouse liver. *J. Pineal Res.* 38, 27–34. doi: 10.1111/j.1600-079X.2004.00171.x

Zhang, B., Xie, W., and Krasowski, M.D. (2008). PXR: a xenobiotic receptor of diverse function implicated in pharmacogenetics. *Pharmacogenomics* 9, 1695–1709. doi: 10.2217/14622416.9.11.1695

17

Working memory training improves emotional states of healthy individuals

Hikaru Takeuchi[1]*, Yasuyuki Taki[1,2,3], Rui Nouchi[4], Hiroshi Hashizume[1], Atsushi Sekiguchi[4], Yuka Kotozaki[4], Seishu Nakagawa[5], Carlos Makoto Miyauchi[5], Yuko Sassa[1] and Ryuta Kawashima[1,2,4]

[1] Division of Developmental Cognitive Neuroscience, Institute of Development, Aging and Cancer, Tohoku University, Sendai, Japan
[2] Division of Medical Image Analysis, Department of Community Medical Supports, Tohoku Medical Megabank Organization, Tohoku University, Sendai, Japan
[3] Department of Radiology and Nuclear Medicine, Institute of Development, Aging and Cancer, Tohoku University, Sendai, Japan
[4] Department of Advanced Brain Science, Smart Ageing International Research Center, Institute of Development, Aging and Cancer, Tohoku University, Sendai, Japan
[5] Department of Functional Brain Imaging, Institute of Development, Aging and Cancer, Tohoku University, Sendai, Japan

Edited by:
Manuel Casanova, University of Louisville, USA

Reviewed by:
Hasan Ayaz, Drexel University, USA
Ariana Tart-Zelvin, Idaho State University, USA

***Correspondence:**
Hikaru Takeuchi, Smart Ageing International Research Center, Institute of Development, Aging and Cancer, Tohoku University, 4-1 Seiryo-cho, Aoba-ku, Sendai 980-8575, Japan
e-mail: takehi@idac.tohoku.ac.jp

Working memory (WM) capacity is associated with various emotional aspects, including states of depression and stress, reactions to emotional stimuli, and regulatory behaviors. We have previously investigated the effects of WM training (WMT) on cognitive functions and brain structures. However, the effects of WMT on emotional states and related neural mechanisms among healthy young adults remain unknown. In the present study, we investigated these effects in young adults who underwent WMT or received no intervention for 4 weeks. Before and after the intervention, subjects completed self-report questionnaires related to their emotional states and underwent scanning sessions in which brain activities related to negative emotions were measured. Compared with controls, subjects who underwent WMT showed reduced anger, fatigue, and depression. Furthermore, WMT reduced activity in the left posterior insula during tasks evoking negative emotion, which was related to anger. It also reduced activity in the left frontoparietal area. These findings show that WMT can reduce negative mood and provide new insight into the clinical applications of WMT, at least among subjects with preclinical-level conditions.

Keywords: working memory, training, plasticity, emotion, mood, anger, fMRI

INTRODUCTION

Working memory (WM) is the limited capacity storage system involved in the maintenance and manipulation of information over a short time period (Baddeley, 2003). It is a functionally important system that underlies a wide range of higher-order cognitive activities such as general intelligence, reasoning and problem solving, language comprehension, learning, and response inhibition (Osaka and Nishizaki, 2000; Baddeley, 2003). Reduced WM capacity (WMC) is also associated with a wide variety of emotional aspects, including mood disorders, anxiety, stress, greater emotional responses, and fewer regulatory behaviors (Sorg and Whitney, 1992; Klein and Boals, 2001; Weiland-Fiedler et al., 2004; Schmeichel et al., 2008).

The dorsolateral prefrontal cortex (DLPFC) plays a key role in the central executive system of WM (Baddeley, 2003). The premotor cortex is closely related to DLPFC, both anatomically, and functionally (Fuster, 2006; Takeuchi et al., 2012), and it plays important roles in some executive functions of WM (Wager et al., 2008). Both areas are consistently active during the execution of WM (Reuter-Lorenz et al., 2000). They also play important roles in emotional aspects, and an essential link exists between DLPFC to premotor areas and mood as described below. Functional deficits of DLPFC to dorsal premotor areas are associated with depression (Siegle et al., 2007). DLPFC to premotor areas and other widespread lateral prefrontal and medial prefrontal regions are activated to control negative emotions (Phan et al., 2005; Belden et al., 2014). Rapid-rate transcranial magnetic stimulation (rTMS) over DLPFC as well as premotor areas mitigates depression (Pascual-Leone et al., 1996; Johnson et al., 2013). Activity changes in DLPFC to dorsal premotor areas and the precentral gyrus have been associated with depression (Koenigs and Grafman, 2009; Stuhrmann et al., 2011). DLPFC lesions have been shown to cause apathy and greater vulnerability to fatigue and depression compared with other lesions (Fuster, 2006; Koenigs and Grafman, 2009), and structural abnormalities in DLPFC to premotor areas are associated with fatigue (Chaudhuri and Behan, 2004).

Physical exercise can affect the volume of DLPFC to premotor areas (Colcombe et al., 2004, 2006; Flöel et al., 2010) and improve the cognitive functions that are related to DLPFC to premotor areas (Smith et al., 2010); further, it can robustly improve mood (Arent and Landers, 2000). Other studies have shown that WM training (WMT) can affect the outcomes of psychological measures and neural systems (Uchida and Kawashima, 2008; Klingberg, 2010; Takeuchi et al., 2010b). However, whether WMT can improve cognitive performance is still a matter of debate because several studies have reported different conclusions (Jaeggi et al., 2008; Redick et al., 2013). A recent meta-analysis indicated that WMT has robust effects on WMC and measures of inhibition and attention (Melby-Lervåg and Hulme, 2012). In addition, WMT has been clinically shown to improve fatigue in patients with multiple sclerosis (Takeuchi et al., 2010b) as well as the symptoms of attention deficit hyperactivity disorder (Klingberg et al., 2005), which can affect mood (e.g., impulsivity can lead to a failure in emotional regulation) (Apter et al., 1990). Structural and functional studies that have used magnetic resonance imaging (MRI), positron emission tomography (PET), and near infrared spectroscopy (NIRS), have linked WMT to changes in brain activity during WM and other related tasks, changes in gray and white matter structures, and dopamine D1 receptor density in prefrontal (including DLPFC and premoror) and posterior parietal areas (McNab et al., 2009; Klingberg, 2010; Takeuchi et al., 2010b, 2013b, 2014a; Buschkuehl et al., 2012; McKendrick et al., 2014). In summary, as described, TMS applied to DLPFC to premotor areas improves mood, whereas DLPFC lesions can deteriorate mood. Similarly, deteriorated emotional states have been associated with hypoactivity in DLPFC to premotor areas. Other interventions such as aerobic exercise can improve the structure and functioning of DLPFC to premotor areas and subsequently improve mood (Lawlor and Hopker, 2001). WMT leads to changes in several mechanisms of DLPFC to premotor areas and cognitive functions related to the areas (Takeuchi et al., 2010b, 2013b). Further, emotional states can be changed through a wide range of interventions in both clinical and nonclinical samples (McNair et al., 1992).

These previous findings have led us to question whether WMT can improve emotional states in individuals without apparent cognitive deficits. We investigated this question in the present study in young adults who underwent WMT. The subjects completed self-report questionnaires related to their emotional states before and after WMT and were examined with a functional MRI (fMRI) task to detect negative emotion-related brain activity as they identified faces with negative emotions (angry or afraid) (Hariri et al., 2002). Previously, this task has been used to examine whether individuals at risk for emotional problems (e.g., subjects with a genetic risk for impulsivity and violence) show different activity in emotion-related areas such as the anterior insula (Meyer-Lindenberg et al., 2006). Our primary aim was to investigate the effects of WMT on mood and its underlying neural activity. We believe that there is no evidence that indicates that improvements in emotional states are solely produced by increased emotional regulation. Considering that our emotional states contribute to our everyday well-being, it is important to investigate the extent of their plasticity and develop new methods to improve them, which could lead to the clinical application of WMT. We hypothesized that WMT improves an emotional state and alters neural activity related to negative emotions, particularly in DLPFC to premotor areas and areas related to emotional states. The increase or decrease in task-induced activity after training or interventions depends on many factors. Even when training leads to adaptations in performance or neural mechanisms, a training-related increase in the efficiency of the involved areas (hence, an activity decrease) or a training-related increase in recruitment of the critical areas (hence, an activity increase) may underlie these changes (Erickson et al., 2007). Thus, we did not predict the direction (increase or decrease) of changes.

MATERIALS AND METHODS

SUBJECTS

Subjects characteristics in each group and experiment

We recruited 97 students and graduates to participate in experiments in our laboratory. Of these 97 subjects, 81 were included in the longitudinal intervention experiment, which involved two intervention studies and three groups (a WMT group, another intervention group for another longitudinal study, and a non-intervention control group, **Figure 1**). The remaining

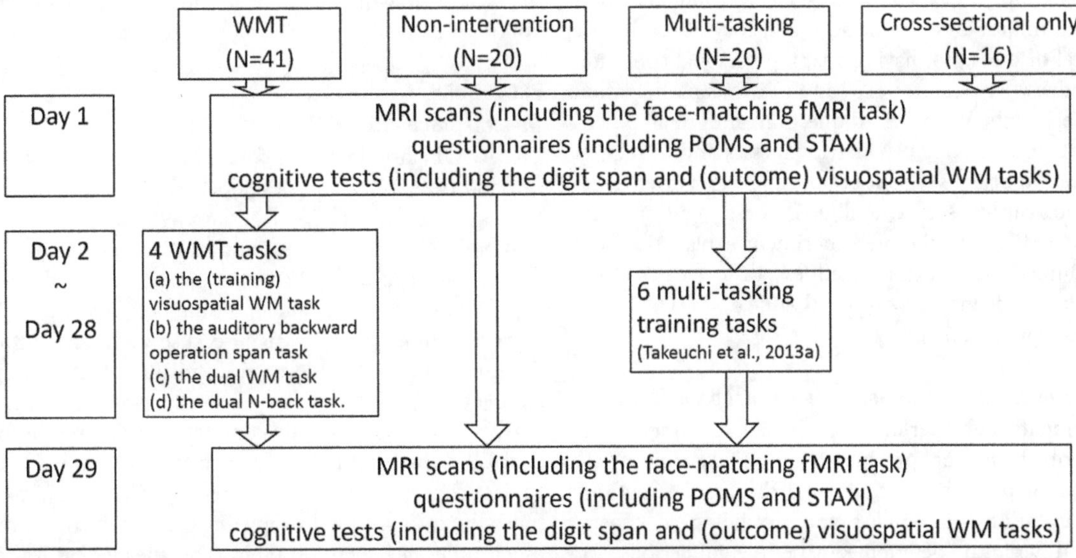

FIGURE 1 | The schema of this study's groups, tasks, and experimental design. A figure illustrating subject flow can be seen in our previous report (Takeuchi et al., 2014b). The measurements for day 1 and day 29 are in no particular order.

16 subjects were included in a cross-sectional experiment that examined brain activity during a face-matching task and completed only all other preintervention procedures [16 women; mean age = 21.6 years; standard deviation (*SD*) = 1.9; age range = 19–27]. Among the 81 subjects included in the longitudinal intervention experiment, 61 were assigned to the WMT or non-intervention control group. The WMT group consisted of 41 subjects (27 men, 14 women) with a mean age of 20.9 years (*SD* = 1.6; age range = 18–24). The non-intervention group consisted of 20 subjects (15 men, 5 women) with a mean age of 21.4 years (*SD* = 2.2; age range = 18–26). Among the 81 subjects included in the longitudinal intervention experiment, the remaining 20 subjects were assigned to a second intervention group (multitasking training group) which is irrelevant to the purpose of this study. Details of this intervention have been described elsewhere (Takeuchi et al., 2014b).

The WMT and control groups were initially similar ($P > 0.1$, two-tailed t-tests) in terms of age, sex, general intelligence scores, WM measures (visuospatial WM and digit span tasks) that were used as outcome measures (Takeuchi et al., 2013b), or mood measures used in this study. Subjects who could not be followed throughout the study because of illness (one subject in the control group) or who failed to submit the required data [one subject in the WMT group did not submit the postintervention Profile of Mood States (POMS) data] were excluded from the relevant analyses. For the description of the subjects flow in the present longitudinal experiment of 81 subjects, please see the figure from our previous report (Takeuchi et al., 2014b).

Subjects' inclusion and exclusion criteria

The study participants were college students at Tohoku University or graduates from the university in the previous year, who were recruited with advertisements posted on bulletin boards or via email, both of which specified the inclusion and exclusion criteria for participation in the study. The exclusion criteria included left-handedness, implanted metal devices, metal around the body, claustrophobia, the use of certain drugs, a history of psychiatric or neurological diseases, not having a laptop personal computer running Windows (Microsoft, USA), and previous participation in related experiments. We provided questionnaires to all potential participants to assess for psychiatric illnesses and to request disclosure of recent drug use. None of the patients reported a history of neurological or psychiatric illness. These questionnaires were administered during the pre-experiment explanation and based on voluntary self-report. Handedness was evaluated using the Edinburgh Handedness Inventory (Oldfield, 1971). All the subjects had normal vision.

Group assignment of participants and experimental periods

Group assignments were performed in a non-arbitrary manner. As described in our previous study (Takeuchi et al., 2013b), groups of participants completed the preintervention- and postinterevention-MRI studies and psychological experiments during different predetermined experimental periods (for example, one group participated in the periods starting 4 weeks from November 4th, another group participated in the periods starting 4 weeks from November 10th, and so on). Participants in one predetermined experimental period were randomly assigned to one of the two groups (e.g., the WMT group or the non-intervention control group). The two groups assigned were different for each predetermined experimental period. This means, for example, that participants in the 4-week periods starting from November 4th and November 25th were assigned to the WMT group or the non-intervention control group, but participants in the 4-week periods starting from November 10th and September 2nd were assigned to the MT training group or the non-intervention control group, yet participants in the 4-week periods starting from November 16th and September 10th were assigned to the WMT group or the MT training group. The participants selected the period they wished to participate in and were not notified that there were two intervention groups before the experiment. Which periods have which two groups are ordered in non-specific manner. Thus, basically, subjects were supposed to be assigned to one of three groups without any bias in a non-arbitrary manner.

The purpose of this study and those of other studies using the data of WMT groups in this study

In this experiment, we aimed to investigate a wide range of distinct research topics, including the effects of polymorphism on cognitive training. We previously investigated the effects of WMT on resting-state FC, regional cerebral blood flow at rest (resting-rCBF), and gray matter structure as well as performance on cognitive tests (Takeuchi et al., 2013b), none of which overlap the measures investigated in the present study. Given these diverse aims and the possible infinite sources of variation, we focused on the effect of WMT on emotional states. More subjects were included in the WMT group to facilitate analysis of polymorphism in WMT, as described above.

Ethical issues

Written informed consent was obtained from each individual for the projects in which they participated. The Ethics Committee of Tohoku University approved all procedures.

PROCEDURE

General procedures of WMT

The WMT task included four computerized tasks that were Borland C++ programs developed in-house. Subjects trained in the task 20–60 min a day for 27 days. We chose a 4-week intervention period because the duration of WMT programs is often 4–5 weeks (Takeuchi et al., 2010b). However, the total training time depended on the level and the time between trials. The length of each training period varied because we did not limit training by time to prevent subjects from finishing the training without completing the tasks properly. Instead, task completion was based on the number of correctly completed trials (in other words, we controlled the length of the tasks based on how many trials each subject completed the tasks correctly). Thus, subjects could not finish the tasks without completing them correctly no matter how much time they spent on them. This means that if the subject's condition was poor, they took longer to complete the training of the day. However, heterogeneity in the amount of overall training among subjects was unlikely because when the subjects recovered the following day they would be able to finish the tasks more quickly (because the level of the tasks would have dropped when the subject's condition was poor). Subjects performed the tasks on their personal computers and were advised to perform the WMT task daily, with two training sessions a week conducted in the laboratory. A log that recorded task performance and the time when subjects completed each trial was used to determine the date and duration of training sessions. Further details can be found in our previous study (Takeuchi et al., 2013b). For the reasons why we used the non-intervention group as a control group, and possible consideration of placebo effects, please see Supplemental Discussion.

Monetary reward

Subjects including those of the control group, received a monetary reward based on the extent to which they participated in the experiments. For training period, to strictly control the amount of training and to motivate subjects to undertake regular training, (a) the subjects received a monetary reward for the training part of the experiment on the basis of the number of sessions they completed; however, (b) they were not given a monetary reward for excessive training (>27 sessions), and (c) the maximum amount of monetary reward was received when one training session was completed each day, even if 27 training sessions were completed. If multiple training sessions were performed in a day, the monetary reward for any second and subsequent training sessions was reduced. For the consideration effects of monetary rewards on moods, see Supplemental Discussion. Basically we failed to find such effects as monetary reward inducement of mood change after the intervention period in this kind of experiment.

TRAINING TASKS

The WMT task is described in our previous report (Takeuchi et al., 2013b). In brief, four WMT tasks were presented during a single training session. In each task, the difficulty (number of items to be remembered) level was modulated on the basis of the subject's performance. Four training tasks were used because increasing the task variability, stimuli, and training situations leads to a more successful transfer (Sweller et al., 1998; Yamnill and McLean, 2001; Green and Bavelier, 2008). The four WMT tasks were as follows: (a) a visuospatial WM task, (b) an auditory backward operation span task, (c) a dual WM task, and (d) a dual N-back task. Additional details are presented in Supplemental Methods. Note that the visuospatial WM task for WMT was different from that used as the outcome measure (Takeuchi et al., 2013b).

We quantified the subjects' performance on all trained WM tasks to analyze their training-related changes in the WM tasks (please see our previous study for details; Takeuchi et al., 2013b). The difference between the composite scores for the first three sessions and the last three sessions was represented as performance changes in the WMT tasks. This method was used in previous studies (Takeuchi et al., 2010a, 2013b, 2014a,b) because it provides a stable performance measure for multiple tasks across three training days.

PSYCHOLOGICAL OUTCOME MEASURES

Neuropsychological tests and questionnaires were administered for preintervention and postintervention evaluation.

POMS

The shortened Japanese version (Yokoyama, 2005) of the POMS (McNair et al., 1992) questionnaire was used to measure a participant's mood on the day of the experiment as well as in the preceding week. The POMS questionnaire consists of six individual subscales: tension/anxiety, depression/dejection, anger/hostility, vigor/activity, fatigue/inertia, and confusion/bewilderment. We used the POMS subscale score for the preceding week to investigate whether WMT improved emotional states. Since its release, POMS has proven to be an excellent measure of fluctuations in affective mood states across a broad population, including psychiatric outpatients, medical patients, and sports subjects (McNair et al., 1992). POMS identifies and assesses transient, fluctuating affective mood states (McNair et al., 1992). It can be administered on a weekly basis, which is a sufficient period for detecting the respondent's mood responses to his or her current life situation but still short enough to assess acute treatment effects (McNair et al., 1992).

State anger scale of the state–trait anger expression inventory

The State Anger scale of the State–Trait Anger Expression Inventory (Spielberger et al., 1999) was used to measure anger. The State Anger scale measures the subjects' mood at the time of the test. These questionnaires can be used to measure the mood of healthy subjects.

Other outcome measures

Several questionnaires designed to assess traits or states related to longer time periods were collected but are not described here. For other performance-type psychological cognitive tests used in this experiment, please see our previous study (Takeuchi et al., 2013b).

FACE-MATCHING TASK (fMRI TASK)

Task procedures

Subjects in the WMT and control groups participated in the fMRI session before and after completing the intervention period. During the fMRI session, subjects performed five blocks of the face-matching task that were alternated with six blocks of a control-matching task involving simple geometric shapes (there was no rest period between blocks). The face-matching task was used to map training-induced changes in negative emotion-related brain activity (Hariri et al., 2002). In each trial, an image of a face portraying anger or fear was presented at the top of a computer screen and was presented at the bottom left and right sides of the screen simultaneously with two additional images of the same face. One of the two bottom images was a face portraying anger, whereas the other face portrayed fear. Subjects were instructed to select one of the faces presented at the bottom of the screen that was identical to the target face (top). Images were presented sequentially per block. Images represented the target affect (angry or fear) and were derived from a standard set of pictures showing facial effects (Kamachi, 2001). In the control-matching task, the faces were replaced with simple geometric shapes, and the subject was instructed to identify the two matching shapes. The subject had to push a button with the first or second finger if he/she selected the bottom left or right shape, respectively.

Four sets of stimuli, each with a duration of 4.0625 s, were presented in a block, with each block lasting 16.25 s Behavioral performance was recorded as the subject's accuracy and reaction time. For a schematic of the task, please refer to the study by Hariri et al. (2002).

Development of stimuli in the previous study

The technical details of how the standard set of pictures of facial effects (Kamachi, 2001) were developed are presented in Kamachi (2001) and Tamamiya and Hiraki (2013). As described in a previous study (Tamamiya and Hiraki, 2013), the database contains 4 females and 6 males and 3 pictures of each model displaying each facial expression. The database also contained the results of a preliminary experiment in which 27 young adults evaluated the intensity of facial expressions and classified the expressions into the following seven categories: happiness, sadness, surprise, anger, disgust, fear, and contempt. The results from that study were used to validate each facial expression.

Rationale for fMRI task paradigm

The behavioral task used in this study has been widely used to detect brain activity related to negative emotions, and it has become the gold standard for tasks that have this purpose. Increased activation in the relevant brain areas when viewing angry or fearful faces indicates the induction of negative emotions during the task (Hariri et al., 2002; Meyer-Lindenberg et al., 2006). These changes simply occurred when subjects viewed the faces without having to identify the emotions they portrayed; thus, this is an implicit task. The emotion face task differs from the present control task in the complexity of the stimuli; however, there are no reasons to assume that such differences contribute to brain activity. The reason for using geometrical shapes in the control task was not provided in its original description. We speculate that the aim of this task is to detect brain activity in emotion-related areas; however, how the activity was induced and what factors induced the activity may not be relevant. The same principle applies to the present study.

Other types of negative emotions include sadness or disgust, and faces showing these emotions could be used as stimuli. We only focused on anger and fear because of time limitations, and we chose to use the same procedures consistently among studies (Hariri et al., 2002; Meyer-Lindenberg et al., 2006). For further explanations of why we used this task and not a task for assessing emotional regulation, please see Supplemental Discussion.

IMAGE ACQUISITION AND ANALYSIS

MRI data acquisition was conducted using a 3-T Philips Achieva scanner. Forty-two transaxial gradient-echo images ($TE = 30$ ms, $FA = 90°$, slice thickness = 3 mm, $FOV = 192$ mm, matrix = 64 × 64) covering the entire brain were acquired at a repetition time of 2.5 s using an echo planar sequence. For the session for negative emotion-related brain activities, 73 functional volumes were obtained. Diffusion-weighted data were acquired using a spin-echo EPI sequence ($TR = 10293$ ms, $TE = 55$ ms, $FOV = 22.4$ cm, $2 \times 2 \times 2\ mm^3$ voxels, 60 slices, SENSE reduction factor = 2, number of acquisitions = 1). The diffusion weighting was isotropically distributed along 32 directions (b-value = 1,000 s/mm^2). Using a spin-echo EPI sequence ($TR = 10293$ ms, $TE = 55$ ms, $FOV = 22.4$ cm, $2 \times 2 \times 2\ mm^3$ voxels, 60 slices), three images with no diffusion weighting (b-value = 0 s/mm^2) ($b = 0$ images) were acquired from 52 subjects and one $b = 0$ image was acquired from nine subjects. From the collected images, FA and ADC maps were calculated (Takeuchi et al., 2011c). These calculated FA and ADC images were used for preprocessing. Other imaging data included scans obtained with fMRI during WM, scans for resting state functional connectivity (FC), arterial spin labeling, and T1-weighted structural images, all of which were used in our previous study of WMT (Takeuchi et al., 2013b).

PREPROCESSING OF FUNCTIONAL ACTIVATION DATA

Preprocessing and analysis of functional activation data were performed using SPM8 implemented in Matlab. Before their analysis, BOLD images from the preintervention and postintervention scans were realigned and resliced to the mean image of the BOLD images from the preintervention scans. For each subject, the skull and skin appearing in the mean BOLD images and $b = 0$ images were removed through intensity thresholding of the spatially smoothed images, as described previously (Takeuchi et al., 2011b). All BOLD images of each subject were coregistered to a skull/skin-stripped $b = 0$ image using the skull/skin-stripped mean BOLD image. Because the $b = 0$ image was aligned with the FA image and ADC map, the BOLD image, $b = 0$ image, FA image, and ADC map were all aligned.

All images were subsequently normalized using a previously validated two-step new segmentation algorithm of diffusion images and the previously validated diffeomorphic anatomical registration through exponentiated lie algebra (DARTEL)-based registration process (Takeuchi et al., 2013a). The voxel size of normalized BOLD images was $3 \times 3 \times 3\ mm^3$.

For additional details on these normalization procedures and their validity, please refer to our previous study (Takeuchi et al., 2013a). In brief, we used these normalization procedures instead of coregistering BOLD and T1-weighted structural images (followed by normalization of the T1-weighted structural image) to ensure precise normalization. Because of the distortion caused by 3-T MRI, the brain's shape in BOLD and T1-weighted structural images can differ, preventing a precise normalization.

INDIVIDUAL-LEVEL STATISTICAL ANALYSIS OF FUNCTIONAL IMAGING DATA

A design matrix was fitted to each participant with one regressor for each of the face-matching task conditions (when compared with controlled task conditions) in the preintervention and postintervention scans using the standard hemodynamic response function (HRF). The design matrix weighted each raw image according to its overall variability to reduce the impact of movement artifacts (Diedrichsen and Shadmehr, 2005). Six parameters obtained by rigid body correction of head motion were regressed out using these variances with the regressor. We removed low-frequency fluctuations with a high-pass filter using a cut-off value of 128 s. The individual-level statistical analyses were performed using a general linear model. After estimation, beta images were smoothed (6-mm full-width half-maximum) and taken to the second level or subjected to random-effect analysis.

In individual analyses, we examined changes in activation related to negative emotion (the face-matching task vs. the control-matching task) before and after a 4-week intervention period. The resulting maps for each participant represented changes in brain activity during the face-matching task condition between the preintervention and postintervention periods as well as the preintervention brain activity during the corresponding condition. The resulting data were forwarded to group analysis.

The present fMRI tasks did not include resting states. Thus, we were not able to determine whether neural activity was affected by interactions among training effects (preintervention, postintervention), task (emotional task, control task), or group (WMT, control group). Even if we included the resting state, fMRI paradigms for comparing individual differences, group differences, and training effects have resting-state differences in neural activity and suffer from the same limitations. Therefore, we used the gold standard procedure for this fMRI task and removed the resting states (Hariri et al., 2002). Furthermore, because repeated exposure to the same tasks alone greatly alters fMRI responses (Luauté et al., 2009), changes in the control group should be considered as a baseline in this type of experiment.

STATISTICAL GROUP-COMPARISON ANALYSIS OF PSYCHOLOGICAL DATA

Behavioral data were analyzed using SPSS 16.0 (SPSS Inc., Chicago, IL). Because training-related improvements were our primary interest and the basis of our hypothesis, we compared test–retest changes in the WMT group with those in the control group using one-tailed One-Way analyses of covariance (ANCOVA), which is the analysis method used in previous studies of WMT (Klingberg et al., 2002, 2005; Takeuchi et al., 2011d, 2013b). The difference between preintervention and postintervention measures was used as the dependent variable, preintervention scores were the independent variable, and group (WMT or control) was the fixed factor ($P < 0.05$). We used ANCOVAs instead of repeated-measure ANOVAs to control for the effects of preintervention test scores. Statistical experts strongly recommend using ANCOVA instead of repeated-measure ANOVA in this type of study design (Dimitrov et al., 2003). With randomized designs, ANCOVA can reduce error variance, whereas with nonrandomized designs (or with analyses involving substantial preexisting group differences), ANCOVA can adjust the postintervention test means for preintervention test differences among groups (Dimitrov et al., 2003). One may recommend using postintervention test scores instead of differences between preintervention test and postintervention test measures. However, when the preintervention test scores are included as covariates, the two analyses return the same statistical value. Using two-tailed tests was not appropriate in this context because statistical tests should be performed against the hypotheses tested. In this study, the hypotheses did not involve a training-related reduction in mood states.

The behavioral data (accuracy and reaction time) recorded in the face-matching and control-matching tasks were analyzed with the same design but with two-tailed analyses because we did not expect changes in these measures (see Results for details).

STATISTICAL GROUP-LEVEL ANALYSIS OF IMAGING DATA

In the group-level imaging analysis, we tested for group-wise differences in functional activity changes across the entire brain during the emotional face-matching task (compared with the control-matching task). We performed voxel-wise ANCOVAs with the difference in each measure between preintervention scans and postintervention scans at each voxel as the dependent variable and the preintervention scan value at each voxel as the independent variable. Biological Parametrical Mapping (BPM) (Casanova et al., 2007) implemented in SPM5 made it possible for us to use these voxel-wise ANCOVAs by including images representing regional values as covariates. We used SPM5 because BPM was not designed and it has not been thoroughly tested against SPM8. Analysis was performed using SPM5 and images representing preintervention to postintervention changes in functional activity during the emotional face-matching task and functional activity during the emotional face-matching task in the preintervention scan. One may think that the difference in the number of subjects in each group may lead to significant differences in measures of preintervention to postintevention activation changes. However, because statistical analyses tested for differences in changes between groups and not within groups (followed by assertions that significant differences were observed in only one group but not in the other group), this was not possible.

Regions with significance were inferred using family-wise error-based cluster-level statistics (Friston et al., 1996). Only clusters with $P < 0.05$ after correction for multiple comparisons at cluster size with a voxel-level cluster-determining threshold of $P < 0.005$ (uncorrected) were considered statistically significant. This voxel-level cluster-determining threshold has been used in previous studies (Takeuchi et al., 2010a, 2011b), and the validation study (Hayasaka and Nichols, 2003) showed that this threshold does not cause anticonservativeness. If anything, it appears to lead to more conservative results compared with more stringent voxel-level cluster-determining thresholds.

We also performed ANCOVA (two-tailed) to compare group differences between the mean beta estimates of preintervention to postintervention changes in functional activity with the mean beta estimates of preintervention functional activity in clusters with significant WMT-related changes in whole brain analysis, preintervention difference of behavioral data (reaction time, accuracy) between the face emotion task and the control-matching task, as well as pre to post changes in difference of behavioral data (reaction time, accuracy) between the face emotion task and the control-matching task.

CORRELATIONS BETWEEN BEHAVIORAL DATA AND FUNCTIONAL ACTIVITY IN SIGNIFICANT CLUSTERS

Furthermore, to reveal the nature of functional activity in areas with significant WMT-related changes, we investigated the association between functional activity and psychological variables using the preintervention data and multiple regression analyses. The dependent variables were the mean beta estimates of functional activity in the clusters with significant WMT-related changes identified in whole brain analysis described above. Independent variables were age, sex, and each psychological variable (scores of measures of emotional states). Data from 95 subjects were included in this analysis. Among the initial 97 subjects considered for the study (see Subjects subsection), data for one subject were not available because of a metal-related problem (Takeuchi et al., 2014b). The data from another subject were removed because the fMRI data were unsuitable. This reduced the number of subjects to 95. We added the data from the additional 16 subjects who only participated in the cross-sectional experiment because they had completed the same protocols for the preintervention period as the subjects in the present study, which included fMRI scans for negative emotion. Excluding these subjects was statistically harmful because it would have reduced the statistical power. For cross-sectional analysis of the brain images, the number of subjects analyzed to determine the effects of WMT (approximately 60 subjects: 41 subjects in the WMT group and 20 subjects in the control group) was quite small; therefore, additional subjects were included in this analysis.

Finally, we investigated whether training-related variables (changes in the composite score of the four WMT tasks), preintervention to postintervention emotional state changes, and preintervention to postintervention functional activity changes in the clusters with significant WMT-related changes identified above were related.

RESULTS

TRAINING DATA

As described in our previous study, to investigate the effect of WMT on resting-state FC, resting-rCBF, and regional gray matter volume using data from the same subjects (Takeuchi et al., 2013b), subjects in the WMT group completed on average 25.87 sessions ($SD = 2.18$) and at least 17 sessions during the 27-day intervention period. The performance on all four trained WM tasks during the last three training sessions was significantly improved compared with that during the first three training sessions (paired t-test, $P < 0.001$). Details of the training data and training-related changes in performance scores on cognitive tests (such as WM tasks) have been described previously (Takeuchi et al., 2013b). WMT task performance significantly improved from the first three training days to the last three training days for all tasks (Takeuchi et al., 2013b). The training-related performance change presented in the previous study is illustrated in Supplemental Table 1. Please note that these behavioral data apply to the training tasks performed during the training period, and no data are available for the control group. Compared with the control group, performance on the untrained verbal and visual WM tasks conducted on the day of the MRI sessions in the WMT significantly improved from preintervention to postintervention, as described previously (Takeuchi et al., 2013b).

THE EFFECT OF WMT ON EMOTIONAL STATES (MAIN PSYCHOLOGICAL ANALYSES OF THIS STUDY)

Compared with the control group, the WMT group showed significantly greater preintervention to postintervention reductions in POMS subscale scores for anger/hostility, depression/dejection, and fatigue/inertia but not for the tension/anxiety, vigor/activity, and confusion/bewilderment subscales. Compared with the control group, the WMT group also showed significantly greater preintervention to postintervention reductions for the STAXI score. The results for the psychological scales are shown in **Table 1**. In these analyses, the statistical values were not corrected for multiple comparisons, which was the case in some previous studies (Klingberg et al., 2002, 2005). Nevertheless, even when these values were corrected using the false discovery rate (Benjamini and Hochberg, 1995), the effects of WMT on the POMS anger/hostility subscale and the STAXI State Anger scale remained significant ($P < 0.05$, corrected). There were also tendencies toward WMT effects ($P < 0.1$) on the

Table 1 | Pretest and posttest scores for psychological measures (mean ± s.e.m.).

	WMT		Control (non-intervention)		Planned contrast	*P*-value[c]
	Pre	Post	Pre	Post		
POMS[a] –tension–anxiety	6.15 ± 4.66	6.55 ± 5.47	6.00 ± 4.03	6.95 ± 3.99	WMT < control	0.322
POMS—depression–dejection	4.50 ± 4.77	3.63 ± 4.39	3.47 ± 3.89	4.95 ± 4.03	WMT < control	0.048*
POMS—anger-hostility	3.73 ± 4.26	3.35 ± 3.85	2.63 ± 2.67	4.79 ± 4.08	WMT < control	0.009**
POMS—vigor–activity	8.28 ± 3.78	7.8 ± 4.54	9.42 ± 3.01	9.11 ± 3.05	WMT > control	0.740
POMS—fatigue–inertia	6.63 ± 4.66	6.18 ± 4.71	7.63 ± 4.34	8.53 ± 4.14	WMT < control	0.050*
POMS—confusion–bewilderment	4.85 ± 3.71	4.93 ± 3.66	4.37 ± 3.52	5.42 ± 3.85	WMT < control	0.219
STAXI[b]—state–anger	11.8 ± 3.7	11.1 ± 3.1	11.3 ± 3.3	12.9 ± 3.2	WMT < control	0.007**

[a] *Profile of Mood States.*

[b] *State–Trait Anger Expression Inventory.*

[c] *One-Way analyses of covariance with test–retest differences in psychological measures as dependent variables and pretest scores of the psychological measures as covariates.*

*$P < 0.05$.

**$P < 0.01$.

POMS depression/dejection and fatigue/inertia subscales, which is congruent with our hypothesis.

Comparisons with a control group are crucial in this type of intervention study. In the present study, average changes in mood scores were observed in the control group. In particular, the score of the POMS anger/hostility subscale significantly increased in the control group ($P = 0.044$, two-tailed paired-t). However, previous studies have shown that mood worsens in the season in which this experiment was performed. Therefore, the changes observed in the control groups may be expected without any intervention or experimental effects. For more details related to this issue, please see Discussion.

THE EFFECT OF WMT ON NEGATIVE EMOTION-RELATED BRAIN ACTIVITIES (MAIN NEUROIMAGING ANALYSES OF THIS STUDY)

We compared changes in negative emotion-related brain activity in the WMT and control groups. This analysis revealed a statistically significant decrease from preintervention measures to postintervention measures in negative emotion-related activities in an anatomical cluster spread around the left posterior insula (**Table 2**; **Figure 2**) and in the anatomical cluster extending from the inferior parietal lobule to the premotor area (**Table 2**; **Figure 3A**). The latter cluster slightly extended into Brodmann's area 8, which includes a small portion of DLPFC. The significance of these results was not affected when any preexisting or postintervention group differences in behavioral performance of fMRI tasks were accounted for.

To determine whether the training-related changes in activity were lateralized to the left hemisphere, we investigated the results using a lenient threshold (uncorrected $P < 0.05$). Please note that we are not making any conclusions about significant results for the right hemisphere using this second threshold; we are merely showing that laterality of the results is unlikely and that no such tendency was observed. This analysis revealed widespread clusters in the frontoparietal area bilaterally and a posterior insula cluster that included the abovementioned significant areas (**Figure 3B**). These three clusters were significant at $P < 0.05$ after correcting for multiple comparisons at the cluster level with a cluster-determining threshold of $P < 0.05$, uncorrected. Thus, the results may not necessarily be lateralized to the left side.

The *P*-values for comparisons between groups with ANCOVA (two-tailed) for the mean beta estimates for changes in functional activity from preintervention to postintervention with the mean beta estimates of preintervention functional activity in the significant clusters presented in **Figures 2, 3A** were 0.0001 and 0.00003, respectively. We next performed ANCOVA (two-tailed) that added the following variables (a–d) as covariates using the mean values of each cluster with significant WMT-related changes: (a) accuracy of preintervention face-matching task—accuracy of preintervention control-matching task; (b) [accuracy of postintervention face-matching task—accuracy of postintervention control-matching task]—[accuracy of preintervention face-matching task—accuracy of preintervention control-matching task]; (c) reaction time of preintervention face-matching task—reaction time of preintervention control-matching task; and (d) [reaction time of postintervention face-matching task—reaction time of postintervention control-matching task]—[reaction time of preintervention face-matching task—reaction time of preintervention control-matching task]. *P*-values from ANCOVAs for the clusters presented in **Figures 2, 3A** were 0.0001 and 0.00002, respectively. These ANCOVA comparisons showed that preexisting group differences in reaction

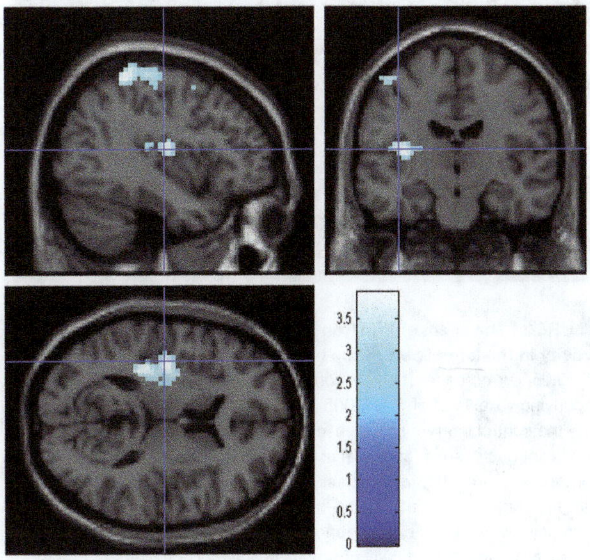

FIGURE 2 | The effect of WMT on negative emotion-related brain activity in the left posterior insula. Results are shown with the threshold of $P < 0.05$, corrected for multiple comparisons at the cluster-level with an underlying voxel-level of $P < 0.005$. Findings were overlaid on a "single-subject T1" SPM5 image. Blue represents the T score. Compared with the control intervention (non-intervention), WMT resulted in a significant decrease in functional activity in a cluster spread around the left posterior insula.

Table 2 | Activity related to WMT and negative emotion decreases compared with the control group.

Area		MNI coordinates of the peak value			T score of the peak value	Corrected *P*-value (cluster)
		x	*y*	*z*		
Posterior insula	L	−39	−15	12	3.91	0.031
Inferior parietal lobule/premotor area/precentral gyrus/postcentral gyrus	L	−39	−42	60	3.79	<0.001

time and accuracy as well as in changes to these behavioral measures did not affect group differences in preintervention to postintervention changes in functional activity for these clusters. We performed these comparisons because covariates (a–d) could not be added to the voxel-by-voxel whole brain analyses because of technical errors in the procedures.

BEHAVIORAL DATA FROM THE fMRI TASKS

The fMRI tasks used in the present study were not cognitively demanding. Therefore, these values were not expected to change, and there is no prior knowledge or theory that suggests individual differences of behavioral performance of this task are even remotely associated with emotion-related cognition. However, preintervetion and postintervention behavioral data for the fMRI tasks are provided in **Table 3**. ANCOVAs with preintervention to postintervention performance changes in each behavioral data set were used as dependent variables that corresponded to the preintervention performance data as covariates. The group difference as a fixed factor revealed no significant WMT-related effects on either accuracy or reaction time during the tasks.

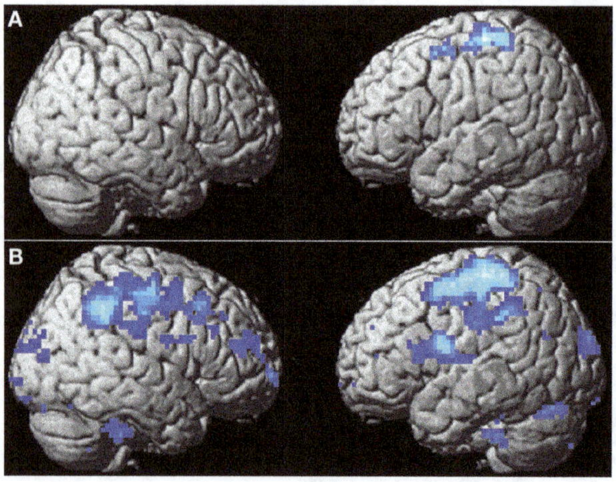

FIGURE 3 | The effect of WMT on negative emotion-related brain activity in the lateral part of the brain. (A) Significant results are $P < 0.05$, corrected for multiple comparisons at the cluster level with an underlying voxel level of $P < 0.005$. Blue represents the T score. Compared with the control intervention (non-intervention), WMT resulted in a significant decrease in functional activity in a cluster spread around the left frontoparietal area. **(B)** Tendencies are $P < 0.05$, uncorrected. Compared with the control intervention (non-intervention), WMT resulted in a tendency toward a decrease in functional activity in a cluster spread bilaterally around the extensive frontoparietal areas. Please note that we are not making any conclusions about significant results in the right hemisphere using this second threshold; we are merely showing that laterality of results is unlikely and that no such tendency was observed.

CORRELATION BETWEEN RELATED PSYCHOLOGICAL VARIABLES AND FUNCTIONAL ACTIVITY IN SIGNIFICANT CLUSTERS BEFORE THE INTERVENTION

To reveal the nature of the functional activity in areas with significant WMT-related changes, we used multiple regression analyses and region of interest (ROI) analysis to investigate the associations between functional activity and psychological variables using data from the preintervention session. In these analyses, the dependent variables were the mean beta estimates of functional activity within the significant clusters presented in **Figures 2, 3A**, while the independent variables were age, sex, and the individual psychological variables. In particular, we tested whether activity in the posterior insula was associated with the state of anger. We examined data from the 95 subjects (see Subjects subsection and correlations between behavioral data and functional activity in significant clusters subsection of Methods).

As expected, activity in the left posterior insula cluster was significantly and positively correlated with the POMS anger/hostility subscale score ($P = 0.019$, $t = 2.38$; effect size $r = 0.228$, **Figure 4**); however, no significant associations were observed with the STAXI State Anger scale score; there was no evidence of outliers in the scatterplot. This correlation remained significant after excluding the 16 abovementioned subjects who only took part in the cross-sectional experiment ($P = 0.039$). The difference could be due to the higher sensitivity for POMS. No other psychological variables, including each POMS subscale score, showed significant correlations with activity. In addition, no significant correlations were observed when the dependent variable was activity in the left frontoparietal cluster.

The present analyses may appear to be slightly circular in nature because the mean values of clusters with significant WMT effects were used (please note that the same problems occur

Table 3 | Preintervention and postintervention behavioral data for the fMRI tasks (mean ± s.e.m.).

	WMT		Control (non-intervention)		Planned contrast	*P*-value[c]
	Pre	Post	Pre	Post		
Control task RT[a] (ms)	7767 ± 1294	7872 ± 1337	8299 ± 884	7905 ± 675	Two-tailed[b]	0.087
Emotional face task RT (ms)	12366 ± 2595	12779 ± 2927	12406 ± 1991	12632 ± 1518	Two-tailed[b]	0.754
Control task accuracy (%)	96.5 ± 3.9	96.8 ± 3.0	98.7 ± 2.0	97.6 ± 3.2	Two-tailed[b]	0.640
Emotional face task accuracy (%)	95.1 ± 6.7	94.3 ± 5.7	96.6 ± 3.7	95.8 ± 5.1	Two-tailed[b]	0.471

[a] *Reaction time.*

[b] *These tasks are not something one has to perform as much as he or she can; therefore, no training-related improvements in these behavioral data have been assumed.*

[c] *One-Way analyses of covariance with test–retest differences in psychological measures as dependent variables and preinterveniton scores of the psychological measures as covariates.*

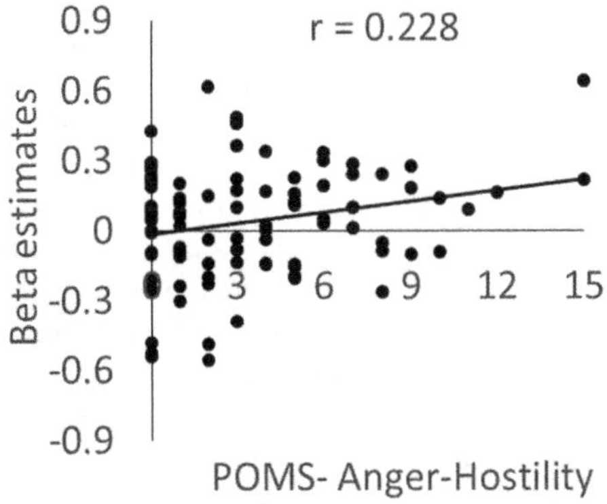

FIGURE 4 | The association between brain activity related to negative emotions and anger mood state. Scatterplot showing the relationship between the POMS Anger–Hostility subscale score and the mean value for brain activity during the preintervention period in a cluster in the left posterior insula in which a significant WMT effect was observed.

even when the peak values of clusters with WMT effects are used). However, even when the effects of group assignments were regressed out of our multiple regression analyses by creating and including a covariate of group assignment (WMT group = −1, control group = +1, other subjects = 0), the significance of the correlation between activity in the cluster in the left posterior insula and the POMS anger/hostility subscale score did not change ($P = 0.030$, $t = 2.20$). This shows that the circular nature of the present analysis does not undermine the finding of an association between anger and brain activity in the anterior insula. These results indicate that the increased activity observed during the face-matching task in fMRI was associated with the state of anger.

CORRELATIONS BETWEEN CHANGES IN RELATED PSYCHOLOGICAL VARIABLES AND CHANGES IN FUNCTIONAL ACTIVITY IN SIGNIFICANT CLUSTERS

Following this, we investigated whether training-related variables (changes in the composite score for the four WMT tasks), emotional state changes, and functional activity changes in two of the significant clusters identified above were related. For this analysis, we performed simple correlational analyses between (a) each functional activity change in the two significant clusters and changes in each score of emotional state measures; (b) each functional activity change in the two significant clusters and changes in the composite score for the WMT tasks; and (c) changes in each score of emotional state measures and changes in the composite score for the WMT tasks among subjects in the WMT group. We found no significant correlations; however, the changes in functional activity in the two significant clusters were highly and positively correlated ($P < 0.001$).

There could be a number of reasons for this lack of correlation. One possible reason is insufficient statistical power because we could only analyze data from subjects in the WMT group in this analysis. On the other hand, large individual differences were observed in the control group for emotional state changes, indicating that much of the variance in emotional state changes in WMT group was also unrelated to WMT. In addition, this experiment was not designed for this type of correlation analysis. Although the amount of training is correlated with training-related changes in neural mechanisms (Takeuchi et al., 2010a), we strictly controlled the amount of training performed by subjects in the WMT group (for the actual SD of the number of training sessions, please see Training data subsection of Results). Therefore, little variance was observed among subjects in this respect. To perform these types of correlation analyses successfully, we should not have controlled the amount of training so strictly. Finally, although WMT is effective in decreasing some negative emotional states, WMT is apparently a cognitively demanding and tiring task. Thus, moderate WMT may be effective for improving mood; however, subjects who exert more effort during training may experience an increase in negative feelings during training and consequently have higher scores for negative moods. This may complicate the association between training and mood changes and negate the correlations among WMT-related changes.

DISCUSSION

In the present study, we investigated whether WMT affected the emotional states and corresponding brain activity in healthy young adults. We observed that individuals who underwent WMT showed decreases in anger, depression, and fatigue as well as decreases in negative emotion-related brain activity in the left posterior insula and in an anatomical cluster near the left frontoparietal area. As discussed below, WMT may reduce anger by increasing the ability to cognitively manage emotional stimuli. WMT may also reduce depressive and fatigue states through previously reported training-induced increases in DLPFC and premotor cortex functioning. These results cannot be entirely explained by preexisting differences between groups because ANCOVA corrected for any preintervention differences. These effects are unlikely to be explained by unknown effects for the non-intervention group, even though the moods in the non-intervention group tended to worsen from the preintervention to postintervention period, as discussed below. The present findings provide new insight into the broader applications of WMT for psychiatric problems, at least among subjects with preclinical-level conditions.

WMT may lead to reduced anger by facilitating cognitive control of situations arousing emotion. Although WMC is not directly related to anger (Hofmann et al., 2008), mental health problems often occur with impaired WMC. For example, substance abuse leads to depression, decreased anger control, suicidal tendencies, and WM deficits (Hoffman et al., 2006). Subjects with a high-functioning WMC are less likely to respond automatically in many situations, including those that provoke emotion (Hofmann et al., 2008). Moreover, they are more likely to correct misapprehensions that lead to anger (Cummins, 2005) and appraise emotional stimuli in an unemotional manner. Thus, they are able to experience and express less emotion in response to such stimuli (Schmeichel et al., 2008). Training-related increases in WMC may lead to decreased anger expression through these mechanisms. Anger and WMC were not correlated despite these previous studies as well as the present study, which may be because anger can lead to arousal and improve performance (Novaco, 1976). Thus, anger and WMC may not reinforce each other through positive feedback.

WMT-related decreases in activity in the frontoparietal region may reflect a decreased cognitive load, which may subsequently allow cognitive management of emotion-inducing stimuli that affect activity in the posterior insula. Numerous studies have shown the posterior insula is associated with pain, anger, and disgust (Calder et al., 2000; Williams et al., 2005; Schultheiss et al., 2008; Paulus et al., 2010). For example, injury to the posterior insula seems to lead to impaired recognition of disgust (Calder et al., 2000). In the present study, subjects performed a face-matching task that involved faces expressing negative emotions, and as they performed the task, activity in the posterior insula was positively correlated with anger/hostility. Thus, the WMT-related decrease in activity in the left posterior insula may reflect a decrease in emotional responses such as anger or other emotions evoked with negative mood-inducing stimuli. On the other hand, the left superior frontal and parietal regions are active during externally directed attention-demanding cognitive tasks (Fox et al., 2005), and this increased activity may generally reflect cognitive load (Takeuchi et al., 2012). Any changes in task-induced activity depends on several factors; and we did not predict the direction of such changes because training-related increases in efficiency (hence an activity decrease) or increase of recruitment of involved areas depend on multiple factors (Erickson et al., 2007). The face-matching task used in the present study appears to have been cognitively demanding because it required additional reaction time. Therefore, the WMT-related decrease in activity in this region may have been related to a decrease in cognitive load during the task. Considering that an increased cognitive capacity allows cognitive management of emotional stimuli, the decreased cognitive load reflected in the frontoparietal area may facilitate cognitive management of emotion-inducing signals that affect posterior insular activity. Alternatively, DLPFC to premotor areas, which are partially included in the frontoparietal area, have been associated with automatic emotion regulation (Mauss et al., 2007). Thus, reduced activity in this area may reflect the load associated with suppression of negative emotion. However, in the present task, the subjects were not required to suppress emotions. Therefore, the nature of task-related activity changes in this area during tasks that induce negative emotion as well as the mechanisms underlying this activity during explicit suppression of emotion remain to be investigated.

It is not clear why after WMT, the frontoparietal area showed activity changes when the extensive DLPFC area that is not overlapped with this area did not. One possibility is a lack of statistical power, considering the right DLPFC showed the same pattern of decreased training-related activity (**Figure 3B**). Further, training-related structural changes of the bilateral DLPFC (Takeuchi et al., 2013b) have been shown, and DLPFC is involved in the voluntary suppression of emotion (Lévesque et al., 2003).

WMT, like other interventions that stimulate DLPFC, may increase the baseline activity of DLPFC to premotor areas and lead to a concomitant reduction in depressive mood. Patients with depression are characterized by hypometabolism in the cortex, particularly in PFC (Fuster, 2006). Loss of initiative and failure to accurately construct thoughts and conversation are characteristics of depression and are underlain by DLPFC dysfunction (Fuster, 2006). TMS applied to DLPFC to premotor areas can decrease depression and increase resting-state activity in DLPFC to premotor areas (Pascual-Leone et al., 1996; Catafau et al., 2001; Knoch et al., 2006; Johnson et al., 2013). Training on complex divided attention speed tasks, which may well recruit DLPFC to premotor areas because divided attention and speed of complex cognitive tasks are both strongly associated with activity of DLPFC to premotor areas (Thomsen et al., 2004; Takeuchi et al., 2012), also prevents depression (Takeuchi and Kawashima, 2012). These findings suggest that strong cortical stimulation, particularly for DLPFC to premotor areas, leads to increased baseline activity in DLPFC to premotor areas and a concomitant reduction in depressive mood, through TMS or cognitive training. However, the possibility of WMT on clinically depressed subjects remains to be clarified. In the case of abovementioned divided attention speed tasks, the training prevents depression, but the effects of the training on subjects who had already developed depression were less clear (Takeuchi and Kawashima, 2012).

WMT may lead to a reduction in fatigue through training-related activity in DLPFC and its related circuits. It was previously shown that WMT can reduce fatigue in patients with multiple sclerosis (Vogt, 2005). Chronic fatigue syndrome is associated with reduced regional gray matter in the bilateral DLPFC (Okada et al., 2004). The fatigue seems to be related to dysfunction in the frontal–subcortical circuits (Okada et al., 2004). Consistent with this notion, lateral PFC lesions lead to apathy (Fuster, 2006). The present results extend the previous finding of WMT-related reductions in fatigue in patients to healthy young adults, and they show that training-related reductions in fatigue can occur without substantial fatigue and cognitive impairments (Takeuchi et al., 2010b). This change may be caused by the previously identified WMT-induced functional and structural changes in DLPFC (Takeuchi et al., 2010b).

Although the mood states in the control group tended to worsen, it is unlikely that the differences between groups in the present study were caused by effects specific to the control group. The group differences in emotional state changes appeared to be mediated by the average aggregation of emotional states in the control group. However, the present experiments were performed in autumn and winter, and a robust increase in negative mood states, as measured by POMS, has been reported during this period (Harris and Dawson-Hughes, 1993). It is also possible that such changes were strengthened because of distressing events at the university that occurred during winter (such as examinations). Even the patterns of mood changes in this study were similar to those observed in the previous study. Although negative moods increased from autumn to winter in both studies, the increases in depression–dejection and anger–hostility were the most robust, and the reduction in positive mood (vigor) was not as clear. Furthermore, we used the non-intervention group as the control, and because of this simple effect of time-related mood changes, this study design was a strength of our study. If certain meaningful active controls were applied, such as videogame playing, we may not have been able to eliminate the possibility of active control group effects on mood states. Because WMT was limited to less than an hour, it is unlikely that reductions in everyday activities replaced by WMT would have strong effects. Thus, based on the use of a control group in intervention studies and the fact that we used a non-intervention control, it is inappropriate to attribute the group differences in mood change to any specific effect associated with the control group.

There are a few potential pitfalls or limitations to this study. While the state of anger reduction was statistically robust and was confirmed by two different measures, the reduction in fatigue and depression was only marginally significant. These WMT-related reductions in mood are congruent with those observed in previous clinical studies examining WMTs or stimulation applied to DLPFC to premotor areas during cognitive training or TMS; however, these findings warrant further replication.

With regard to the negative findings, no significant WMT-related changes in mood were found for anxiety or other POMS subscales. These findings may be attributed to factors such as a lack of statistical power and the inclusion of outliers. However, anxiety differs from apathy and depression (Fuster, 2006). Psychiatric problems such as anxiety and obsessive–compulsive disorder are associated with hyperactivity in the anterior brain regions (Fuster, 2006; Milad and Rauch, 2007), whereas excessive anxiety may be associated with reduced resting-state brain activity (Gur et al., 1987). In the case of anxiety, these anterior regions include parts of the WM network, such as the dorsal part of the anterior cingulate cortex (Milad et al., 2007). Surgical interventions affecting the dorsal part of the anterior cingulate can attenuate these psychiatric problems, including anxiety (Fuster, 2006; Milad et al., 2007). Functional enhancements in certain parts of the WM network, such as the dorsal part of the anterior cingulate cortex, may not reduce anxiety despite other beneficial effects, e.g., an increased cognitive capacity.

ACKNOWLEDGMENTS

We thank Yuki Yamada for operating the MRI scanner, Haruka Nouchi for conducting the psychological tests, the subjects, and all our other colleagues in IDAC, Tohoku University for their support. This study was supported by JST/RISTEX, JST/CREST, a Grant-in-Aid for Young Scientists (B) (KAKENHI 23700306) and a Grant-in-Aid for Young Scientists (A) (KAKENHI 25700012) from the Ministry of Education, Culture, Sports, Science, and Technology. The authors would like to thank Enago (www.enago.jp) for the English language review.

REFERENCES

Apter, A., Van Praag, H., Plutchik, R., Sevy, S., Korn, M., and Brown, S. (1990). Interrelationships among anxiety, aggression, impulsivity, and mood: a serotonergically linked cluster? *Psychiatry Res.* 32, 191–199. doi: 10.1016/0165-1781(90)90086-K

Arent, S., and Landers, M. (2000). The effects of exercise on mood in older adults: a meta-analytic. *J. Ageing Phys. Act.* 8, 407–430.

Bäckman, L., Nyberg, L., Soveri, A., Johansson, J., Andersson, M., Dahlin, E., et al. (2011). Effects of working-memory training on striatal dopamine release. *Science* 333, 718–718. doi: 10.1126/science.1204978

Baddeley, A. (2003). Working memory: looking back and looking forward. *Nat. Rev. Neurosci.* 4, 829–839. doi: 10.1038/nrn1201

Belden, A. C., Luby, J. L., Pagliaccio, D., and Barch, D. M. (2014). Neural activation associated with the cognitive emotion regulation of sadness in healthy children. *Dev. Cogn. Neurosci.* 9, 136–147. doi: 10.1016/j.dcn.2014.02.003

Benjamini, Y., and Hochberg, Y. (1995). Controlling the false discovery rate: a practical and powerful approach to multiple testing. *J. R. Stat. Soc. B (Methodol.)* 57, 289–300.

Brown, A. K., Liu-Ambrose, T., Tate, R., and Lord, S. R. (2009). The effect of group-based exercise on cognitive performance and mood in seniors residing in intermediate care and self-care retirement facilities: a randomised controlled trial. *Br. J. Sports Med.* 43, 608–614. doi: 10.1136/bjsm.2008.049882

Buschkuehl, M., Jaeggi, S. M., and Jonides, J. (2012). Neuronal effects following working memory training. *Dev. Cogn. Neurosci.* 2, S167–S179. doi: 10.1016/j.dcn.2011.10.001

Calder, A. J., Keane, J., Manes, F., Antoun, N., and Young, A. W. (2000). Impaired recognition and experience of disgust following brain injury. *Nat. Neurosci.* 3, 1077–1078. doi: 10.1038/80586

Casanova, R., Srikanth, R., Baer, A., Laurienti, P. J., Burdette, J. H., Hayasaka, S., et al. (2007). Biological parametric mapping: a statistical toolbox for multimodality brain image analysis. *Neuroimage* 34, 137–143. doi: 10.1016/j.neuroimage.2006.09.011

Catafau, A. M., Perez, V., Gironell, A., Martin, J. C., Kulisevsky, J., Estorch, M., et al. (2001). SPECT mapping of cerebral activity changes induced by repetitive transcranial magnetic stimulation in depressed patients. A pilot study. *Psychiatry Res.* 106, 151–160. doi: 10.1016/S0925-4927(01)00079-8

Chaudhuri, A., and Behan, P. O. (2004). Fatigue in neurological disorders. *Lancet* 363, 978–988. doi: 10.1016/S0140-6736(04)15794-2

Clark, F., Azen, S., Zemke, R., Jackson, J., Carlson, M., Mandel, D., et al. (1997). Occupational therapy for independent-living older adults. A randomized controlled trial. *JAMA* 278, 1321–1326. doi: 10.1001/jama.1997.03550160041036

Colcombe, S. J., Erickson, K. I., Scalf, P. E., Kim, J. S., Prakash, R., McAuley, E., et al. (2006). Aerobic exercise training increases brain volume in aging humans. *J. Gerontol. A Biol. Sci. Med. Sci.* 61, 1166–1170. doi: 10.1093/gerona/61.11.1166

Colcombe, S. J., Kramer, A. F., Erickson, K. I., Scalf, P., McAuley, E., Cohen, N. J., et al. (2004). Cardiovascular fitness, cortical plasticity, and aging. *Proc. Natl. Acad. Sci. U.S.A.* 101, 3316–3321. doi: 10.1073/pnas.0400266101

Cummins, P. (2005). "The experience of anger," in *Personal Construct Psychotherapy*, eds D. Winter and L. Viney (London: Whurr), 239–255. doi: 10.1002/9780470713686.ch19

Dahlin, E., Neely, A. S., Larsson, A., Backman, L., and Nyberg, L. (2008). Transfer of learning after updating training mediated by the striatum. *Science* 320, 1510–1512. doi: 10.1126/science.1155466

Dash, D., McNab, F., and Klingberg, T. (2010). "Effect of dual working memory training on a reasoning task- an fMRI study," in *16th Annual Meeting of the Organization for Human Brain Mapping* (Barcelona).

Diedrichsen, J., and Shadmehr, R. (2005). Detecting and adjusting for artifacts in fMRI time series data. *Neuroimage* 27, 624–634. doi: 10.1016/j.neuroimage.2005.04.039

Dimitrov, D. M., Rumrill, J., and Phillip, D. (2003). Pretest-posttest designs and measurement of change. *Work* 20, 159–165.

Erickson, K. I., Colcombe, S. J., Wadhwa, R., Bherer, L., Peterson, M. S., Scalf, P. E., et al. (2007). Training-induced functional activation changes in dual-task processing: an FMRI study. *Cereb. Cortex* 17, 192–204. doi: 10.1093/cercor/bhj137

Flöel, A., Ruscheweyh, R., Krüger, K., Willemer, C., Winter, B., Völker, K., et al. (2010). Physical activity and memory functions: are neurotrophins and cerebral gray matter volume the missing link? *Neuroimage* 49, 2756–2763. doi: 10.1016/j.neuroimage.2009.10.043

Fox, M. D., Snyder, A. Z., Vincent, J. L., Corbetta, M., Van Essen, D. C., and Raichle, M. E. (2005). The human brain is intrinsically organized into dynamic, anticorrelated functional networks. *Proc. Natl. Acad. Sci. U.S.A.* 102, 9673–9678. doi: 10.1073/pnas.0504136102

Friston, K. J., Holmes, A., Poline, J. B., Price, C. J., and Frith, C. D. (1996). Detecting activations in PET and fMRI: levels of inference and power. *Neuroimage* 4, 223–235. doi: 10.1006/nimg.1996.0074

Fuster, J. M. (2006). *The Prefrontal Cortex: Anatomy, Physiology, and Neuropsychology of the Frontal Lobe.* New York, NY: Raven Press.

Green, C. S., and Bavelier, D. (2008). Exercising your brain: a review of human brain plasticity and training-induced learning. *Psychol. Aging* 23, 692–701. doi: 10.1037/a0014345

Gur, R. C., Gur, R. E., Resnick, S. M., Skolnick, B. E., Alavi, A., and Reivich, M. (1987). The effect of anxiety on cortical cerebral blood flow and metabolism. *J. Cereb. Blood Flow Metab.* 7, 173–177. doi: 10.1038/jcbfm.1987.40

Hariri, A. R., Tessitore, A., Mattay, V. S., Fera, F., and Weinberger, D. R. (2002). The amygdala response to emotional stimuli: a comparison of faces and scenes. *Neuroimage* 17, 317–323. doi: 10.1006/nimg.2002.1179

Harris, S., and Dawson-Hughes, B. (1993). Seasonal mood changes in 250 normal women. *Psychiatry Res.* 49, 77–87. doi: 10.1016/0165-1781(93)90031-B

Hayasaka, S., and Nichols, T. E. (2003). Validating cluster size inference: random field and permutation methods. *Neuroimage* 20, 2343–2356. doi: 10.1016/j.neuroimage.2003.08.003

Hoffman, W. F., Moore, M., Templin, R., McFarland, B., Hitzemann, R. J., and Mitchell, S. H. (2006). Neuropsychological function and delay discounting in methamphetamine-dependent individuals. *Psychopharmacology* 188, 162–170. doi: 10.1007/s00213-006-0494-0

Hofmann, W., Gschwendner, T., Friese, M., Wiers, R. W., and Schmitt, M. (2008). Working memory capacity and self-regulatory behavior: toward an individual differences perspective on behavior determination by automatic versus controlled processes. *J. Pers. Soc. Psychol.* 95, 962–977. doi: 10.1037/a0012705

Hróbjartsson, A., and Gøtzsche, P. C. (2001). Is the placebo powerless? An analysis of clinical trials comparing placebo with no treatment. *N. Engl. J. Med.* 344, 1594–1602. doi: 10.1056/NEJM200105243442106

Jaeggi, S. M., Buschkuehl, M., Jonides, J., and Perrig, W. J. (2008). Improving fluid intelligence with training on working memory. *Proc. Natl. Acad. Sci. U.S.A.* 105, 6829–6833. doi: 10.1073/pnas.0801268105

Johnson, K. A., Baig, M., Ramsey, D., Lisanby, S. H., Avery, D., McDonald, W. M., et al. (2013). Prefrontal rTMS for treating depression: location and intensity results from the OPT-TMS multi-site clinical trial. *Brain Stimul.* 6, 108–117. doi: 10.1016/j.brs.2012.02.003

Kamachi, M. (2001). *ATR Facial Affect Database (DB99) Schema. ATR Technical Report.* Kyoto: ATR-Promotions.

Klein, K., and Boals, A. (2001). The relationship of life event stress and working memory capacity. *Appl. Cogn. Psychol.* 15, 565–579. doi: 10.1002/acp.727

Klingberg, T. (2010). Training and plasticity of working memory. *Trends Cogn. Sci.* 14, 317–324. doi: 10.1016/j.tics.2010.05.002

Klingberg, T., Fernell, E., Olesen, P. J., Johnson, M., Gustafsson, P., Dahlström, K., et al. (2005). Computerized training of working memory in children with ADHD-a randomized, controlled trial. *J. Am. Acad. Child Adolesc. Psychiatry* 44, 177–186. doi: 10.1097/00004583-200502000-00010

Klingberg, T., Forssberg, H., and Westerberg, H. (2002). Training of working memory in children with ADHD. *J. Clin. Exp. Neuropsychol.* 24, 781–791. doi: 10.1076/jcen.24.6.781.8395

Knoch, D., Treyer, V., Regard, M., Müri, R., Buck, A., and Weber, B. (2006). Lateralized and frequency-dependent effects of prefrontal rTMS on regional cerebral blood flow. *Neuroimage* 31, 641–648. doi: 10.1016/j.neuroimage.2005.12.025

Koenigs, M., and Grafman, J. (2009). The functional neuroanatomy of depression: distinct roles for ventromedial and dorsolateral prefrontal cortex. *Behav. Brain Res.* 201, 239–243. doi: 10.1016/j.bbr.2009.03.004

Lawlor, D. A., and Hopker, S. W. (2001). The effectiveness of exercise as an intervention in the management of depression: systematic review and meta-regression analysis of randomised controlled trials. *BMJ* 322, 763–767. doi: 10.1136/bmj.322.7289.763

Lévesque, J., Eugène, F., Joanette, Y., Paquette, V., Mensour, B., Beaudoin, G., et al. (2003). Neural circuitry underlying voluntary suppression of sadness. *Biol. Psychiatry* 53, 502–510. doi: 10.1016/S0006-3223(02)01817-6

Luauté, J., Schwartz, S., Rossetti, Y., Spiridon, M., Rode, G., Boisson, D., et al. (2009). Dynamic changes in brain activity during prism adaptation. *J. Neurosci.* 29, 169–178. doi: 10.1523/JNEUROSCI.3054-08.2009

Mahncke, H. W., Connor, B. B., Appelman, J., Ahsanuddin, O. N., Hardy, J. L., Wood, R. A., et al. (2006). Memory enhancement in healthy older adults using a brain plasticity-based training program: a randomized, controlled study. *Proc. Natl. Acad. Sci. U.S.A.* 103, 12523–12528. doi: 10.1073/pnas.0605194103

Mauss, I. B., Bunge, S. A., and Gross, J. J. (2007). Automatic emotion regulation. *Soc. Personal. Psychol. Compass* 1, 146–167. doi: 10.1111/j.1751-9004.2007.00005.x

McKendrick, R., Ayaz, H., Olmstead, R., and Parasuraman, R. (2014). Enhancing dual-task performance with verbal and spatial working memory training: continuous monitoring of cerebral hemodynamics with NIRS. *Neuroimage* 85, 1014–1026. doi: 10.1016/j.neuroimage.2013.05.103

McNab, F., Varrone, A., Farde, L., Jucaite, A., Bystritsky, P., Forssberg, H., et al. (2009). Changes in cortical dopamine D1 receptor binding associated with cognitive training. *Science* 323, 800–802. doi: 10.1126/science.1166102

McNair, D. M., Lorr, M., and Droppleman, L. F. (1992). *Profile of Mood States.* San Diego, CA: Educational and Industrial Testing Service.

Melby-Lervåg, M., and Hulme, C. (2012). Is working memory training effective? A meta-analytic review. *Dev. Psychol.* 49, 270–291. doi: 10.1037/a0028228

Meyer-Lindenberg, A., Buckholtz, J. W., Kolachana, B., Hariri, A. R., Pezawas, L., Blasi, G., et al. (2006). Neural mechanisms of genetic risk for impulsivity and violence in humans. *Proc. Natl. Acad. Sci. U.S.A.* 103, 6269–6274. doi: 10.1073/pnas.0511311103

Milad, M. R., Quirk, G. J., Pitman, R. K., Orr, S. P., Fischl, B., and Rauch, S. L. (2007). A role for the human dorsal anterior cingulate cortex in fear expression. *Biol. Psychiatry* 62, 1191–1194. doi: 10.1016/j.biopsych.2007.04.032

Milad, M. R., and Rauch, S. L. (2007). The role of the orbitofrontal cortex in anxiety disorders. *Ann. N.Y. Acad. Sci.* 1121, 546–561. doi: 10.1196/annals.1401.006

Novaco, R. W. (1976). The functions and regulation of the arousal of anger. *Am. J. Psychiatry* 133, 1124–1128.

Okada, T., Tanaka, M., Kuratsune, H., Watanabe, Y., and Sadato, N. (2004). Mechanisms underlying fatigue: a voxel-based morphometric study of chronic fatigue syndrome. *BMC Neurol.* 4:14. doi: 10.1186/1471-2377-4-14

Oldfield, R. C. (1971). The assessment and analysis of handedness: the Edinburgh inventory. *Neuropsychologia* 9, 97–113. doi: 10.1016/0028-3932(71)90067-4

Olesen, P. J., Westerberg, H., and Klingberg, T. (2004). Increased prefrontal and parietal activity after training of working memory. *Nat. Neurosci.* 7, 75–79. doi: 10.1038/nn1165

Osaka, M., and Nishizaki, Y. (2000). *Brain and Working Memory (in Japanese).* Kyoto: Kyoto University Press.

Pascual-Leone, A., Rubio, B., Pallardó, F., and Catalá, M. D. (1996). Rapid-rate transcranial magnetic stimulation of left dorsolateral prefrontal cortex in drug-resistant depression. *Lancet* 348, 233–237. doi: 10.1016/S0140-6736(96)01219-6

Paulus, M. P., Simmons, A. N., Fitzpatrick, S. N., Potterat, E. G., Van Orden, K. F., Bauman, J., et al. (2010). Differential brain activation to angry faces by elite warfighters: neural processing evidence for enhanced threat detection. *PLoS ONE* 5:e10096. doi: 10.1371/journal.pone.0010096

Phan, K. L., Fitzgerald, D. A., Nathan, P. J., Moore, G. J., Uhde, T. W., and Tancer, M. E. (2005). Neural substrates for voluntary suppression of negative affect: a functional magnetic resonance imaging study. *Biol. Psychiatry* 57, 210–219. doi: 10.1016/j.biopsych.2004.10.030

Price, D., Finniss, D., and Benedetti, F. (2008). A comprehensive review of the placebo effect: recent advances and current thought. *Annu. Rev. Psychol.* 59, 565–590. doi: 10.1146/annurev.psych.59.113006.095941

Redick, T. S., Shipstead, Z., Harrison, T. L., Hicks, K. L., Fried, D. E., Hambrick, D. Z., et al. (2013). No evidence of intelligence improvement after working memory training: a randomized, placebo-controlled study. *J. Exp. Psychol. Gen.* 142, 359–379. doi: 10.1037/a0029082

Reuter-Lorenz, P. A., Jonides, J., Smith, E. E., Hartley, A., Miller, A., Marshuetz, C., et al. (2000). Age differences in the frontal lateralization of verbal and spatial working memory revealed by PET. *J. Cogn. Neurosci.* 12, 174–187. doi: 10.1162/089892900561814

Schmeichel, B. J., Volokhov, R. N., and Demaree, H. A. (2008). Working memory capacity and the self-regulation of emotional expression and experience. *J. Pers. Soc. Psychol.* 95, 1526–1540. doi: 10.1037/a0013345

Schultheiss, O. C., Wirth, M. M., Waugh, C. E., Stanton, S. J., Meier, E. A., and Reuter-Lorenz, P. (2008). Exploring the motivational brain: effects of implicit power motivation on brain activation in response to facial expressions of emotion. *Soc. Cogn. Affect. Neurosci.* 3, 333–343. doi: 10.1093/scan/nsn030

Siegle, G. J., Thompson, W., Carter, C. S., Steinhauer, S. R., and Thase, M. E. (2007). Increased amygdala and decreased dorsolateral prefrontal BOLD responses in unipolar depression: related and independent features. *Biol. Psychiatry* 61, 198–209. doi: 10.1016/j.biopsych.2006.05.048

Smith, P. J., Blumenthal, J. A., Hoffman, B. M., Cooper, H., Strauman, T. A., Welsh-Bohmer, K., et al. (2010). Aerobic exercise and neurocognitive performance: a meta-analytic review of randomized controlled trials. *Psychosom. Med.* 72, 239–252. doi: 10.1097/PSY.0b013e3181d14633

Sorg, B. A., and Whitney, P. (1992). The effect of trait anxiety and situational stress on working memory capacity. *J. Res. Pers.* 26, 235–241. doi: 10.1016/0092-6566(92)90041-2

Spielberger, C. D., Sydeman, S. J., Owen, A. E., and Marsh, B. J. (1999). "Measuring anxiety and anger with the State-Trait Anxiety Inventory (STAI) and the State-Trait Anger Expression Inventory (STAXI)," in *The Use of Psychological Testing for Treatment Planning and Outcomes Assessment, 2nd Edn.*, ed M. Maruish (Mahwah, NJ: Lawrence Erlbaum Associates Publishers), 993–1021.

Stuhrmann, A., Suslow, T., and Dannlowski, U. (2011). Facial emotion processing in major depression: a systematic review of neuroimaging findings. *Biol. Mood Anxiety Disord.* 1, 1–17. doi: 10.1186/2045-5380-1-10

Sweller, J., Van Merrienboer, J. J. G., and Paas, F. (1998). Cognitive architecture and instructional design. *Educ. Psychol. Rev.* 10, 251–296. doi: 10.1023/A:1022193728205

Takeuchi, H., and Kawashima, R. (2012). Effects of processing speed training on cognitive functions and neural systems. *Rev. Neurosci.* 23, 289–301. doi: 10.1515/revneuro-2012-0035

Takeuchi, H., Sekiguchi, A., Taki, Y., Yokoyama, S., Yomogida, Y., Komuro, N., et al. (2010a). Training of working memory impacts structural connectivity. *J. Neurosci.* 30, 3297–3303. doi: 10.1523/JNEUROSCI.4611-09.2010

Takeuchi, H., Sugiura, M., Sassa, Y., Sekiguchi, A., Yomogida, Y., Taki, Y., et al. (2012). Neural correlates of the difference between working memory speed and simple sensorimotor speed: an fMRI study. *PLoS ONE* 7:e30579. doi: 10.1371/journal.pone.0030579

Takeuchi, H., Taki, Y., Hashizume, H., Sassa, Y., Nagase, T., Nouchi, R., et al. (2011a). Effects of training of processing speed on neural systems. *J. Neurosci.* 31, 12139–12148. doi: 10.1523/JNEUROSCI.2948-11.2011

Takeuchi, H., Taki, Y., Hashizume, H., Sassa, Y., Nagase, T., Nouchi, R., et al. (2011b). Failing to deactivate: the association between brain activity during a working memory task and creativity. *Neuroimage* 55, 681–687. doi: 10.1016/j.neuroimage.2010.11.052

Takeuchi, H., Taki, Y., and Kawashima, R. (2010b). Effects of working memory training on cognitive functions and neural systems. *Rev. Neurosci.* 21, 427–450. doi: 10.1515/REVNEURO.2010.21.6.427

Takeuchi, H., Taki, Y., Nouchi, R., Hashizume, H., Sekiguchi, A., Kotozaki, Y., et al. (2013b). Effects of working memory-training on functional connectivity and cerebral blood flow during rest. *Cortex* 49, 2106–2125. doi: 10.1016/j.cortex.2012.09.007

Takeuchi, H., Taki, Y., Nouchi, R., Hashizume, H., Sekiguchi, A., Kotozaki, Y., et al. (2014a). Working memory training impacts the mean diffusivity in the dopaminergic system. *Brain Struct. Funct.* doi: 10.1007/s00429-014-0845-2. [Epub ahead of print].

Takeuchi, H., Taki, Y., Nouchi, R., Hashizume, H., Sekiguchi, A., Kotozaki, Y., et al. (2014b). Effects of multitasking-training on gray matter structure and resting state neural mechanisms. *Hum. Brain Mapp.* 35, 3646–3660. doi: 10.1002/hbm.22427

Takeuchi, H., Taki, Y., Sassa, Y., Hashizume, H., Sekiguchi, A., Fukushima, A., et al. (2011c). Verbal working memory performance correlates with regional white matter structures in the fronto-parietal regions. *Neuropsychologia* 49, 3466–3473 doi: 10.1016/j.neuropsychologia.2011.08.022

Takeuchi, H., Taki, Y., Sassa, Y., Hashizume, H., Sekiguchi, A., Fukushima, A., et al. (2011d). Working memory training using mental calculation impactsregional gray matter of the frontal and parietal regions. *PLoS ONE* 6:e23175. doi: 10.1371/journal.pone.0023175

Takeuchi, H., Taki, Y., Sassa, Y., Hashizume, H., Sekiguchi, A., Nagase, T., et al. (2013a). White matter structures associated with empathizing and systemizing in young adults. *Neuroimage* 77, 222–236. doi: 10.1016/j.neuroimage.2013.04.004

Tamamiya, Y., and Hiraki, K. (2013). Individual differences in the recognition of facial expressions: an event-related potentials study. *PLoS ONE* 8:e57325. doi: 10.1371/journal.pone.0057325

Thomsen, T., Rimol, L. M., Ersland, L., and Hugdahl, K. (2004). Dichotic listening reveals functional specificity in prefrontal cortex: an fMRI study. *Neuroimage* 21, 211–218. doi: 10.1016/j.neuroimage.2003.08.039

Uchida, S., and Kawashima, R. (2008). Reading and solving arithmetic problems improves cognitive functions of normal aged people: a randomized controlled study. *Age* 30, 21–29. doi: 10.1007/s11357-007-9044-x

Vogt, B. A. (2005). Pain and emotion interactions in subregions of the cingulate gyrus. *Nat. Rev. Neurosci.* 6, 533–544. doi: 10.1038/nrn1704

Wager, T. D., Davidson, M. L., Hughes, B. L., Lindquist, M. A., and Ochsner, K. N. (2008). Prefrontal-subcortical pathways mediating successful emotion regulation. *Neuron* 59, 1037–1050. doi: 10.1016/j.neuron.2008.09.006

Weiland-Fiedler, P., Erickson, K., Waldeck, T., Luckenbaugh, D. A., Pike, D., Bonne, O., et al. (2004). Evidence for continuing neuropsychological impairments in depression. *J. Affect. Disord.* 82, 253–258. doi: 10.1016/j.jad.2003.10.009

Westerberg, H., Hirvikoski, T., Forssberg, H., and Klingberg, T. (2004). Visuo-spatial working memory span: a sensitive measure of cognitive deficits in children with ADHD. *Child Neuropsychol.* 10, 155–161. doi: 10.1080/09297040409609806

Williams, L. M., Das, P., Liddell, B., Olivieri, G., Peduto, A., Brammer, M. J., et al. (2005). BOLD, sweat and fears: fMRI and skin conductance distinguish facial fear signals. *Neuroreport* 16, 49–52. doi: 10.1097/00001756-200501190-00012

Yamnill, S., and McLean, G. N. (2001). Theories supporting transfer of training. *Hum. Res. Dev. Q.* 12, 195–208. doi: 10.1002/hrdq.7

Yokoyama, K. (2005). *POMS Shortened Version (in Japanese)*. Tokyo: Kanekoshobo.

18

Time-interval for integration of stabilizing haptic and visual information in subjects balancing under static and dynamic conditions

Jean-Louis Honeine[1] and Marco Schieppati[1,2]*

[1] Department of Public Health, Experimental and Forensic Medicine, University of Pavia, Pavia, Italy
[2] Centro Studi Attività Motorie (CSAM), Fondazione Salvatore Maugeri (IRCSS), Scientific Institute of Pavia, Pavia, Italy

Edited by:
Mikhail Lebedev, Duke University, USA

Reviewed by:
Yoshio Sakurai, Kyoto University, Japan
Robert Peterka, Oregon Health and Science University, USA
David A. E. Bolton, Queen's University Belfast, UK

***Correspondence:**
Marco Schieppati, Centro Studi Attività Motorie (CSAM), Fondazione Salvatore Maugeri (IRCSS), Scientific Institute of Pavia, Via Salvatore Maugeri 4, Pavia 27100, Italy
e-mail: marco.schieppati@unipv.it

Maintaining equilibrium is basically a sensorimotor integration task. The central nervous system (CNS) continually and selectively weights and rapidly integrates sensory inputs from multiple sources, and coordinates multiple outputs. The weighting process is based on the availability and accuracy of afferent signals at a given instant, on the time-period required to process each input, and possibly on the plasticity of the relevant pathways. The likelihood that sensory inflow changes while balancing under static or dynamic conditions is high, because subjects can pass from a dark to a well-lit environment or from a tactile-guided stabilization to loss of haptic inflow. This review article presents recent data on the temporal events accompanying sensory transition, on which basic information is fragmentary. The processing time from sensory shift to reaching a new steady state includes the time to (a) subtract or integrate sensory inputs; (b) move from allocentric to egocentric reference or vice versa; and (c) adjust the calibration of motor activity in time and amplitude to the new sensory set. We present examples of processes of integration of posture-stabilizing information, and of the respective sensorimotor time-intervals while allowing or occluding vision or adding or subtracting tactile information. These intervals are short, in the order of 1–2 s for different postural conditions, modalities and deliberate or passive shift. They are just longer for haptic than visual shift, just shorter on withdrawal than on addition of stabilizing input, and on deliberate than unexpected mode. The delays are the shortest (for haptic shift) in blind subjects. Since automatic balance stabilization may be vulnerable to sensory-integration delays and to interference from concurrent cognitive tasks in patients with sensorimotor problems, insight into the processing time for balance control represents a critical step in the design of new balance- and locomotion training devices.

Keywords: sensory integration, sensory reweighting, haptic, vision, equilibrium, quiet stance, dynamic balance

INTRODUCTION

Maintaining balance involves complex sensorimotor transformations that continually integrate several sensory inputs and coordinate multiple motor outputs to muscles throughout the body (Ting, 2007). The control of quiet-standing posture consists in the maintenance of the center of mass (CoM) of the body within narrow limits. Also under dynamic balance conditions, like riding a platform periodically moving in the antero-posterior direction (Buchanan and Horak, 1999; Corna et al., 1999), the body requires accurate control of the CoM displacement within the range of the platform displacement. In both cases, the spatio-temporal activity of the agonist postural muscles (Schieppati et al., 1994, 1995; Tokuno et al., 2007; Kelly et al., 2012; Wright et al., 2012; Sozzi et al., 2013) is orchestrated by the central nervous system (CNS) based on one or multiple frames of reference (Peterka, 2002; Mergner et al., 2003; Schmid et al., 2007) upon which the body scheme is constructed (Haggard and Wolpert, 2005).

While keeping our body stable during the so-called "quiet stance" condition, feed-forward mechanisms are paramount in modulating the tonic activity in our antigravity extensor muscles and the correcting bursts in the antagonist muscles, which together control the displacement of the center of foot pressure (CoP; Morasso and Schieppati, 1999; Jacono et al., 2004; Bottaro et al., 2005, 2008; Loram et al., 2011; Vieira et al., 2012). In turn, these spatio-temporal patterns of activity rely on the knowledge of our orientation in space and of the relative position of our body segments during stance. This knowledge is built on multiple sensory inputs, which concur in the more or less accurate construction of the "internal model" of our body and of its relationship with the environment (van der Kooij and Peterka, 2011). The accuracy depends on the number and quality of the inflow from the various sensory modalities that have access to the centers integrating and using such information. Feedback obviously contributes to the instant-to-instant control of the stabilizing effort both by engaging reflex responses and by continuously updating the internal model (van Emmerik and van Wegen, 2002). Under steady-state conditions, the feedback contribution may be down-weighted by the brain (Peterka and Loughlin, 2004; Assländer and Peterka, 2014). Under dynamic but stabilized conditions, as when standing on a tilting platform and holding onto a still frame, the proprioceptive feedback from the legs is also down-weighted (Nardone et al., 1990; Schieppati and Nardone, 1991). During locomotion, alteration of the proprioceptive input from the leg muscle produces little effects on gait variables (Courtine et al., 2001). Thus, under predictable, steady-state conditions and tasks, be they static or dynamic, voluntary or produced in response to equilibrium perturbation, the excitability of the circuits ultimately called forth in the control of equilibrium may be tuned down. In general, sensory gating optimizes the execution of ongoing motor tasks (Clarac et al., 1992) by minimizing the effects on the motor command due to the inescapable delay from detection of the relevant information to its transmission to the neural generators of muscle activity (Suzuki et al., 2011). In this context, it is helpful to introduce an operative definition of postural set as it applies to both the control of body orientation in space and to the particular temporary level of excitability of the sensorimotor circuits underpinning the actual state of the body in its environment: "sensorimotor set is a state in which transmission parameters in various sensorimotor pathways have been adjusted to suit a particular task or context" (Prochazka, 1989). As such, the postural set, and in particular the neural circuits' excitability to impending stimuli, is modifiable by the intention to change motor task and by the prediction of a change in the environment.

Stance stability depends on the availability and accuracy of the afferent stimuli that are integrated by the brain. The time-period whereby a sensory input is integrated and incorporated in the control of equilibrium is critical. For example, when the CoM is close to the border of its fixed support base (Schieppati et al., 1994), a handful of milliseconds can be enough to pass this limit and reach a condition that prevents any useful reaction. Any stabilizing information (e.g., vision) must therefore be rapidly integrated and rapidly produce corrective actions. Further, when we maintain the equilibrium during repeated and predictable perturbations of balance, anticipatory postural adjustments occur and in this context changes in visual conditions can quickly lead to appropriate modification in the anticipatory activities with appropriate changes in the balancing strategy (Corna et al., 1999; Schieppati et al., 2002).

The dependence of the control of human stance on sensory information has been the object of a great deal of investigations (Paulus et al., 1984; Day et al., 1993; Bronstein and Buckwell, 1997; Maurer et al., 2006; Guerraz and Bronstein, 2008). Much attention has been devoted to the central integration of afferent input from visual, somatosensory and vestibular receptors (Massion, 1994; Mergner and Rosemeier, 1998; Meyer et al., 2004; Borel et al., 2008). Changes in these sensory inputs lead the CNS to re-evaluate the respective contribution of the different sources of information for regulating posture (Oie et al., 2002; Peterka and Loughlin, 2004).

Ultimately, the more rapid the gain modulation on the insertion (or withdrawal) of a new stabilizing input, the shorter the time-period to reach the new appropriate postural set. Any information from the environment and from the body itself would concur in creating the better condition for the release of the postural muscle bursts apt to brake the displacement of the body's CoM. It would be therefore appropriate if the CNS could integrate the stabilizing information within the shortest possible period of time.

The effects of changing sensory inflow during the performance of a coordinated complex motor task such as maintaining balance under quiet stance or dynamic conditions have received little attention so far (Rabin et al., 2006; Tax et al., 2013). The likelihood that sensory inflow changes during a complex movement is high, not only because of the obvious movement-related changes in proprioceptive input, but also because movement can imply passing from a dark to a lit environment, or from a stationary to a moving visual flow, or from a tactile-guided body displacement to an abrupt loss of such haptic-stabilized condition (Bove et al., 2006). The basic information for addressing these aspects of sensorimotor integration is fragmentary. Hence, the purpose of this review is to discuss sensory reweighting during static or dynamic balancing tasks. Particularly, the review focuses on the time-interval necessary for integration of balance stabilizing haptic or visual inputs, since this topic area is still relatively unexplored with most of the most relevant work having occurred in recent years.

VISUAL INFORMATION AND STANCE STABILIZATION

Vision affects both body sway during quiet stance (Schieppati et al., 1994; Nougier et al., 1998; Slobounov et al., 1998) and postural synergies when balancing on an oscillating platform (Buchanan and Horak, 1999; Corna et al., 1999; De Nunzio et al., 2005; Schmid et al., 2007). In a variety of situations, vision dominates over the proprioceptive input from a great number of postural muscles, the activity of which necessarily accompanies the standing task (Nardone et al., 1990; Bronstein and Buckwell, 1997; Redfern et al., 2001; van Emmerik and van Wegen, 2002; Hagura et al., 2007; Schmid et al., 2008; Carpenter et al., 2010; Murnaghan et al., 2011).

INTERACTION OF VISION AND PROPRIOCEPTION

Regardless of the weight assigned to vision and proprioception by the brain, the interaction between the two sensory inputs may not be based on a simple algebraic sum, not least because of the different time-period necessary for the two inputs to access the brain, as shown by the different latency of their primary components in the cortical evoked potentials (Schieppati and Ducati, 1984; Bodis-Wollner, 1992; Shokur et al., 2013) or to reach consciousness (Barnett-Cowan and Harris, 2009). Further, the ultimate functional effects of either input or of their interaction over time relates to the particular current balance or movement constraints. For example, anticipatory muscle action preceding a predictable perturbation of quiet stance eyes-open is delayed by vibration of leg muscles (Mohapatra et al., 2012). On the other hand, relatively minor effects of muscle vibration are induced on the balancing behavior on a continuously oscillating platform in spite of vision being denied (De Nunzio et al., 2005). These findings open the issue of the effectiveness of leg muscle tendon vibration *per se* in modifying the control of balance, i.e., of a task strongly dependent on proprioception. This is not a matter of interest for this present review. Suffice it to mention here the intriguing finding that tendon vibration operates by triggering a vibration-frequency entrained discharge of the primary afferent fibers from the spindles (Hagbarth et al., 1973; Burke et al., 1976; Roll and Vedel, 1982; Matthews, 1988; Naito, 2002), while quiet stance relies mostly on the inflow of the secondary spindle afferent fibers (Schieppati and Nardone, 1995, 1999; Marque et al., 2001; Nardone and Schieppati, 2004; see also Pettorossi and Schieppati, under review).

Postural control provides an experimental context appropriate to highlight the interaction of multiple sensory inputs originating from different sensory systems (Hatzitaki et al., 2004). Body stability strongly depends on the non-linear aspects of the sensory fusion process and its temporal dynamics (Black and Nashner, 1984; Jeka et al., 2000; Horak and Hlavačka, 2002; Barnett-Cowan and Harris, 2009; Rowland and Stein, 2014). In turn, this depends to a large extent on the nature of the signals involved and their spatiotemporal relationship (Hlavačka et al., 1999). Experiments on the ability of young and elderly subjects to reconfigure their mode of stance control when submitted to successive reduced and augmented visual sensory conditions have shown a deficit in the operation of their central integrative mechanisms responsible for promptly modifying their postural control in the elderly (Teasdale et al., 1991). Young and elderly subjects' body sway increased when occluding vision, while adding vision had a better effect on sway in young than the elderly, suggesting that elderly persons have a deficit in exploiting the stabilizing effect of vision (Jeka et al., 2010).

In a recent study, it was assumed that the sensory organization and the consequent postural set were influenced by the temporal relationship between visual and neck input (Bove et al., 2009), on the premise that re-weighting sensory inputs and re-shaping the postural reference frame must be a time-consuming process. In that paper, the authors investigated whether a given visual condition affects the postural response to neck vibration, and for how long does vision need to be absent prior to perturbation, before its stabilizing contribution be fully abolished. To this aim, the visual condition was time-manipulated to study its effects on the postural response to a balance-perturbing stimulus produced by neck muscle vibration. Notably, neck muscle vibration produces whole-body postural effects under both static and dynamic conditions (Lund, 1980; Roll et al., 1989; Lekhel et al., 1997; Ivanenko et al., 1999, 2000; Kavounoudias et al., 1999; Bove et al., 2001, 2002). The smallest postural response to vibration was observed when the eyes were open with respect to eyes-closed. This shows that vision is sufficient to significantly attenuate sway evoked by neck vibration. Conversely, the postural response to vibration eyes-closed that followed a period during which vision was allowed was significantly smaller than when vision was denied in the foreperiod. This indicated that the postural response to vibration is influenced not only by the visual condition during the administration of the vibratory stimulus, but also by the visual condition immediately preceding the vibration. A second finding was that, in the complete absence of visual references, the amplitude of the postural responses to vibration became progressively larger as a function of the repetition of the stimuli: in spite of the recovery to the initial position after each vibration pulse, the center of pressure moved forward to an increasingly larger extent during the successive neck vibration pulses, as if each vibration pulse found the postural control system progressively more susceptible to the abnormal proprioceptive input, when the absence of vision persisted. In a sense, the repeated proprioceptive perturbation eyes-closed progressively reinstated a heavy dependence of the postural control on proprioception or cancelled any postural reference constructed by visuo-somatosensory integration (Bottini et al., 2001). This sway-increasing phenomenon was not observed under eyes-open/eyes-closed condition, independently of the number of successive vibration pulses in the sequence. Clearly, presence of vision up to the beginning of vibration allows the CNS to define, and retain for a while, a stable postural reference able to cope with the threat represented by the abnormal proprioceptive inflow.

EFFECTS OF VISION ON BALANCING BEHAVIOR DURING A CONTINUOUS PREDICTABLE PERTURBATION OF STANCE

Standing upright quietly can hardly be considered a real balance challenge. Surprisingly, balance control under dynamic conditions (such as standing on a back-and-forth continuously translating platform) is not much more challenging either, at least as based on the observation that neither sensory nor motor impairment represent an unsustainable challenge to the elderly and patients with peripheral neuropathy or movement disorder (Nardone et al., 2000, 2006, 2007, 2008; Nardone and Schieppati, 2005, 2006). Certainly, subjects put in much more cognitive effort to sustain the performance level than under quiet stance (Beckley et al., 1991). Dynamic balancing behavior is an excellent experimental condition for assessing the role of vision in dynamic with respect to static equilibrium. There is indeed a remarkable difference in strategy depending on the availability of vision, whereby the balancing behavior shifts from that of a pendulum to an inverted-pendulum, passing from "head-fixed-in-space" behavior with eyes open to maximal body compliance to the perturbation with eyes closed (Corna et al., 1999). Incidentally, when blind subjects perform the task of balancing while riding a periodically moving platform, their strategy matches that of the sighted subjects performing eyes-closed (Schmid et al., 2007). This shows that long-term absence of visual information cannot be substituted by other sensory inputs (e.g., proprioception) for the selection of the balancing strategy in the control of equilibrium, in spite of the demonstrated cross-modal plasticity in blind subjects (Cohen et al., 1997; Kupers and Ptito, 2014). The findings point to the obligatory (though not unique, e.g., Panichi et al., 2011) role of vision in the processing and integration of other sensory inputs.

Schmid et al. (2008) investigated two competing hypotheses regarding the relationship between visual acuity and balance control strategy. One hypothesis referred to the existence of a threshold value of visual acuity as a turning point between the eyes-open and eyes-closed strategy. The other assumed that the change from eyes-open to eyes-closed balancing behavior is continuous and varies progressively with the worsening of the visual acuity. The findings showed that, in order to stabilize the head in space, visual information of the environment must be distinct. Reducing visual acuity leads to a graded modification of the "head-fixed-in-space" behavior. Thus, the body can produce a continuous mode of balancing patterns as a function of visual acuity. In a sense, this had already been shown by Paulus et al. (1984) for visual control of quiet stance. The findings suggest the notion that the central mechanisms for head and body stabilization operate through linear integration of the visual input with the general somesthetic feedback.

ABRUPT CHANGES IN VISION DURING THE CONTINUOUS PERTURBATION OF BALANCE

The previously mentioned studies have considered balancing behaviors to periodic balance-perturbing stimuli, under stationary sensory conditions (e.g., vision, reduced vision, or no-vision). They ignored relevant aspects of the postural behavior connected to transient sensory events. In subsequent studies, the time interval between the occurrence of a change in the sensory (visual) condition and the corresponding change in the motor behavior was investigated (De Nunzio and Schieppati, 2007). This interval includes the time to (a) integrate subtraction or addition of the sensory inputs; (b) shift from an allocentric reference (vision) to an egocentric reference (no-vision) or vice versa; and (c) adjust the calibration of the motor activity in time and amplitude to reach the best control appropriate to the new sensory set. A related question of adaptation to transient conditions had been previously addressed by Schweigart and Mergner (2008), who described a "sensory reweighting switch", by which subjects change from a control that is referenced to the support to one that is referenced to space. Under optimal visual-acuity levels, on changing visual inflow during the trial (from eyes open to eyes closed or vice versa), the pattern of head and hip movement and of muscle activity turned into that appropriate for the new visual condition in a time-interval broadly ranging from about 1–2.5 s (De Nunzio et al., 2007). On the one hand, the findings indicate that subjects can rapidly adapt their balancing behavior to the new visual condition. On the other hand, the ample range of latencies across trials suggests that subjects refrained from releasing the new behavior when it was inappropriate, but rather released it at an appropriate time in the next platform translation cycle.

ABRUPT CHANGES IN VISION DURING CONTINUOUS PERTURBATION OF BALANCE IN PATIENTS WITH PD

Processing of sensory information and timing operations could be affected in Parkinson's disease (PD) patients, who show abnormal calibration of postural responses (Schieppati and Nardone, 1991) or impaired flexibility of motor strategies (Horak et al., 1992). The capacity and swiftness to pass from a kinesthetic- to a vision-dependent behavior of these patients was investigated during the dynamic balancing task on the same continuously moving platform mentioned above. It turned out that both patients and normal subjects changed kinematics and EMG patterns to those appropriate for the new visual condition. However, PD patients were generally slower in changing their behavior under the eyes-closed to eyes-open condition (De Nunzio et al., 2007). These findings show abnormal temporal features in balancing strategy adaptation when shifting from kinesthetic only to kinesthetic plus visual reference in PD. The delay in the implementation of the vision-dependent behavior was unexpected, given the advantage vision is supposed to confer to motor performance in PD (Cooke et al., 1978). The delay on addition of vision in PD might be connected to an insufficient integration of a new sensory information in their body scheme, or to a delay in the implementation of the change in the appropriate balancing strategy (Bandini et al., 2001; Contreras-Vidal and Buch, 2003). This state might play a role in the instability of patients performing dynamic postural tasks under changing sensory conditions. Although static visual feedback reduces the walking patients' reliance on kinesthetic feedback thereby favoring gait execution (Azulay et al., 1999; Lewis and Byblow, 2002), fast shifting to a new sensory reference may not be adequately exploited in everyday postural tasks. Venkatakrishnan et al. (2011) have suggested that *gradual* shifting of a new afferent input allows PD to better process the sensory input in a pointing movement.

MEASURING THE DELAY BETWEEN VISUAL SHIFT AND IMPLEMENTATION OF THE NEW BALANCING BEHAVIOR IN STATIC CONDITION

The great variability under the dynamic balancing conditions described above (Schieppati et al., 2002) does not allow to adequately address the issue of the sensori-motor processing time during sensory reweighting, owing to the complex motor task at hand. In a much simpler balancing condition, unaffected by the continuously variable kinesthetic inflow and relevant mechanical instability, the onset and time course of postural adjustments may be more clearly detected following abrupt sensory changes (from no-vision to vision or vice versa). Under these conditions, the stabilizing effect of vision is much less conspicuous than under more complex, balance challenging conditions (Buchanan and Horak, 1999; Corna et al., 1999; Ravaioli et al., 2005; Schmid et al., 2007); but it is definitely present (Paulus et al., 1984). The simple question was how long does it take for vision (eyes-closed to eyes-open) to stabilize posture, or how long does it take for the body to become less stable when vision is withdrawn?

The promptness of adaptation of stance control mechanisms was quantified by the latency at which body oscillation and postural muscle activity varied after a shift in visual condition. In a study aimed at estimating the promptness of adaptation to changes in visual conditions (Sozzi et al., 2011), volunteers stood on a force platform with feet parallel or in tandem. Shifts in visual condition were produced by electronic spectacles (LCD goggles that allowed or removed vision on receiving a TTL impulse). On allowing or occluding vision, decrements and increments in the CoP oscillation start occurring within about 2 s. These were preceded by appropriate changes in muscle activity, regardless of the visual-shift direction and the foot position during the standing task (feet parallel or in tandem). After the initial changes, EMG and CoP oscillations slowly reached the steady-state level corresponding to the new sensory condition within about 3 s. These figures were not dependent of the position of the feet, in spite of the overall larger sway under tandem condition, pointing to a constant duration of the sensorimotor integration process, hardly affected by the particular stance conditions at hand.

HAPTIC INFORMATION AND STANCE STABILIZATION

Very much as with vision, contact of the index finger with a stationary surface (Lederman and Klatzky, 2009) attenuates postural sway during quiet stance, even if the applied force itself (1 N) cannot provide mechanical stabilization. It has been proposed that slight changes in contact force at the fingertip give sensory cues about the direction of body sway (Holden et al., 1994; Jeka and Lackner, 1994; Jeka et al., 1997; Rabin et al., 1999, 2006; Krishnamoorthy et al., 2002; Kouzaki and Masani, 2008). Under steady state conditions, the effect of passive tactile cues during standing has been evaluated (Rogers et al., 2001) and the conclusion drawn that, if passive sensory input is available, the postural control process adapts to this input, better so the more cranial the point of application of the stimulus.

Sensory information from light fingertip touch (LFT) on a stationary surface can help in the case of loss of vestibular function (Lackner et al., 1999; Creath et al., 2002; Horak and Hlavačka, 2002). Therefore, LFT is relevant in the control of body orientation in space. Fingertip somatosensory input from an external reference provides spatial cues, which, akin to vision, facilitate the control of body equilibrium (see Wing et al., 2011). LFT has also been shown to suppress the destabilizing effect on posture induced by lower limb muscle vibration (Lackner et al., 2000). Of note, light touch contact between two individuals induced interpersonal stance symmetry (Johannsen et al., 2012). In other terms, the sway of the persons oscillating more would be reduced while the sway of the one oscillating less would be increased.

Stabilizing effects of LFT have been also described in normal subjects after lower-limb muscular fatigue (Vuillerme and Nougier, 2003), in healthy older adults (Tremblay et al., 2004; Baccini et al., 2007), in patients with peripheral neuropathy (Dickstein et al., 2001, 2003) or multiple sclerosis (Kanekar et al., 2013), and in patients with PD (Rabin et al., 2013) or bilateral vestibular loss (Lackner et al., 1999). Interestingly, LFT is able to relieve the perturbing effects of vibration-induced proprioceptive input from the neck, a segment central to postural control and orientation. LFT during neck vibration also attenuates vibration post-effects, further suggesting that its action is not merely mechanical (Bove et al., 2006). All these findings point to a paramount effect of the sensory inflow from light haptic touch on balance control.

HAPTIC EFFECTS ON REFLEX RESPONSES OF POSTURAL MUSCLES

Haptic information from a stable structure not only reduces the sway of the CoP during quiet stance, therefore of the CoM of the body, but also deeply modifies the excitability of the spinal proprioceptive reflexes that normally subserve the reaction to postural perturbations. By using a conditioning-test protocol, major effects of the haptic stabilization on reflex responses to postural perturbations have been observed (Nardone et al., 1990; Schieppati and Nardone, 1991). It was shown that stabilization of stance induced by holding onto a stable frame had a profound depressive action on the size of the medium-latency response to stretch of the postural leg muscles. This phenomenon was attributed to the change in the postural set. Interestingly, the reflex responses began to decrease about 200 ms before subjects touched the frame, but were not fully expressed until well after contact. The initial changes in amplitude of leg muscle responses are therefore not triggered by the go-signal or the contact with the frame itself, suggesting that the modulation is related at least in part to the central command to transition to a new stabilized postural set.

ACTIVE AND PASSIVE INSERTION OR WITHDRAWAL OF HAPTIC INFORMATION DURING STANCE

Thus, touch helps stabilize our standing body very much as vision does, but little is known about the time-interval necessary for the brain to process the haptic inflow (or its removal) and exploit the new information (or counteract its removal). Moreover, under conditions in which haptic information plays a stabilizing role, it would be interesting, on the basis of both basic and applied research data, to assess whether active touch or passive touch are equally effective (Chapman, 1994; Winter et al., 2008; Smith et al., 2009; Sciutti et al., 2010; Waszak et al., 2012), or significant differences exist, since our sensory systems are simultaneously activated as the result of our own actions and of changes in the external word (Von Holst and Mittelstaedt, 1950; Cullen, 2004). Active touch refers to the event where the subject would deliberately touch a surface, while passive touch refers to the event where contact with the surface would be established by external action without movement or anticipation of the stimulus by the subject.

Sozzi et al. (2012) estimated the latency of onset and the time-course of the changes in postural control mode following addition or withdrawal of haptic information produced by touching (eyes-closed) with the tip of the index finger a strain-gauge instrumented touch-pad. Subjects were asked to actively touch the pad, or it was suddenly lowered or raised permitting to study the passive condition. The EMG of postural muscles during tandem stance was also recorded (in order to enhance muscle activity and body sway), to try to get as close as possible to the neural processing of the sensory information by eliminating the effect of the electromechanical delay. It had been shown previously that light touch stabilizes stance under both tandem stance and feet parallel 12 cm apart (Clapp and Wing, 1999). A summary representation of the modification in the medio-lateral and antero-posterior axes occurring around the instant of visual or haptic information shift is reported in **Figure 1**.

Muscle activity and sway adaptively decreased in amplitude on adding stabilizing haptic information. Across the subjects, the time-interval from the sensory shift to decrease in EMG and sway was ~0.5–2 s (Rabin et al., 2006). CoP followed the changes in tibialis anterior muscle EMG by ~0.2 s. Only slightly

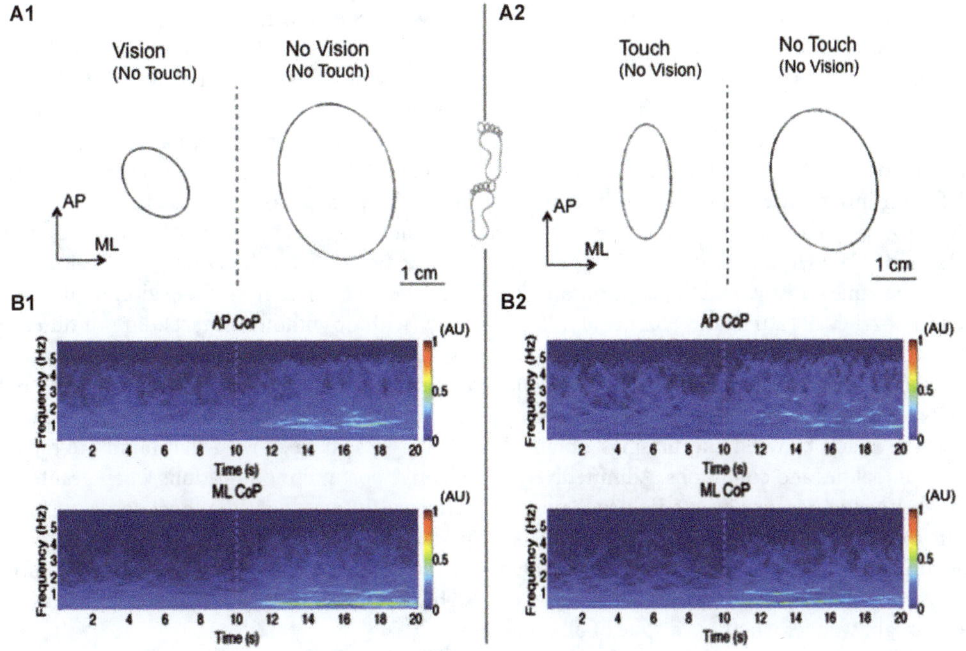

FIGURE 1 | Reweighting of visual or haptic information during tandem stance. This figure shows an elaboration of the results obtained by Sozzi et al. (2011) in one subject standing upright under tandem-stance condition. In this experiment, the subjects' visual sensory information was shifted from vision to no-vision (no touch), while haptic simulation was from touch to no-touch (blindfolded). The sensory shifts occurred at 10 s and were involuntary. The upper panel shows the ellipses of 95% confidence interval of CoP position (mean of 50 trials) during the vision/no-vision shift **(A1)** and touch/no-touch shift **(A2)**. Vision as well as haptic inflow decrease the area of the ellipse. The lower panel shows the "synchro-squeezed" (Daubechies et al., 2011) wavelet transform using a Morlet wavelet of AP CoP (upper traces) and ML CoP (lower traces) between 0.2 and 6 Hz. **(B1)** shows the transform during the vision/no-vision shift, **(B2)** during the touch/no-touch shift. The wavelet transform seen here is the mean of the transforms of 50 trials. The colors in the Figure represent the amplitude of the wavelet coefficient. Dark red represent the highest while dark blue is the lowest wavelets coefficient. Bins of 0.1 s have been chosen in order to better highlight the temporal changes in the coefficients after the sensory shift. Occluding vision or haptic information increases the wavelet coefficients in the frequencies ranging from 0.2 to 3 Hz, which indicates increase in the amplitude of the ML and AP oscillations. Higher frequency components were added up to the spectrum when sensory information was lost. The changes in the wavelets coefficient start increasing after a delay of approx. 1 s, to reach a stationary state in a few more seconds.

shorter intervals were observed following active sensory shifts (Pais-Vieira et al., 2013), in line with the conclusions by Winter et al. (2008) based on a stimulus timing-matching paradigm, who found no advantage on the perceived timing of an active over a passive touch. Latencies of EMG and postural changes were the shortest on removal of haptic information. Following the earliest detectable changes in amplitude, EMG and body sway reached the steady-state corresponding to the new sensory condition within ~1–3 s, under both active and passive tasks. Under control conditions, when subjects were asked to produce deliberate muscle activation in response to the sensory shift in a reaction-time mode, EMG bursts and CoP changes appeared at ~200 ms from the haptic shift, therefore much earlier than the adaptive postural changes seen during stance, signifying the operation of a different order of magnitude of the time scale of these events. Therefore, as much as for the visual information shifts mentioned above, changes in postural behavior require a finite amount of time from haptic shift. In particular, this delay from the sensory shift to the change in postural control mode was significantly longer for haptic than visual cues, the difference being much longer than that between the reaction times to the respective stimuli (Barnett-Cowan and Harris, 2009), indicating a modality-dependence and a heavier computational load for haptic information processing (Vuillerme et al., 2006; Tommerdahl et al., 2010; Bolton et al., 2011a).

The output of the sensory integration process seems to be issued to all relevant muscles. However, the latency of the change was shorter for the tibialis anterior muscle than soleus, likely because the latter rather plays a weight-bearing role (Schmid et al., 2011) while the former, along with peroneus longus, is responsible for providing medial-lateral stability in tandem-stance (Sozzi et al., 2013). Consistent with this role, the cortical projection to the tibialis anterior is stronger than to soleus (Valls-Solé et al., 1994). In this light, the shorter latency of the tibialis anterior changes would be an expression of a prominent supraspinal sensorimotor integration (Bolton et al., 2012) and fast cortical descending control. This finding would be in keeping with the proposals that the cerebral cortex plays a non-negligible role in the control of stance (Tokuno et al., 2009; Pasalar et al., 2010; Murnaghan et al., 2014).

It should be recalled here that the above delays are the result of a statistical estimation. Using statistics to document when a change occurs relies on assumptions and depends on the number of the cases upon which statistics is performed and the data variability, and cannot detect the "true" time at which a change at the CNS level occurs. Rather, the procedure will likely overestimate the true temporal locus of this change at the level of the CNS. Changes at the CNS level in response to visual or tactile inflow certainly occur before a value determined by using statistical tests (Soto-Faraco and Azañón, 2013; Heed and Azañón, 2014; Quinn et al., 2014). However, the same statistics and the same number of cases had been used in Sozzi et al. (2011) and Sozzi et al. (2012) when assessing both addition and withdrawal of information, and when comparing the time-periods to integration of haptic and visual addition (or withdrawal) in body stabilization, allowing a fair comparison to be made between the findings obtained with different sensory modalities and conditions. Admittedly, the "fuzziness" around when actual sensory events influence postural responses requires caution to be exercised to avoid precise claims on absolute times for when sensory signals play their role.

On reflection, one might wonder whether, in spite of all other things being equal, it was legitimate to compare the effect of the haptic sense from a minimal body surface (the tip of the index finger) with the visual information coming from a full binocular visual-field stimulation by the lighted and structured environment. Surprisingly, in spite of these disparities, the duration of the time-periods behind these sensory integrations and the extent of body-sway stabilization was remarkably consistent under both circumstances (Rogers et al., 2001), pointing to a sensory re-weighting phenomenon underpinning a change in reference frame rather than a central detailed analysis of the incoming information. Based on another analytical approach, Riley et al. (1997) had suggested an equivalent time-structure of the haptic and visual effects on the trajectory of the CoP.

HAPTIC INTEGRATION IN BLIND SUBJECTS

Major reorganization of brain areas and reduced cross-modal interaction at the behavioral level follow congenital visual deprivation (Hötting and Röder, 2009; Fiehler and Rösler, 2010; Renier et al., 2014). Vision and touch rapidly lead to postural stabilization in sighted subjects, but is touch-induced stabilization more rapid in blind than in sighted subjects, owing to cross-modal reorganization of function in the blind? In people with impaired visual function, only minor differences in quiet stance control compared to sighted people have been reported (Rougier and Farenc, 2000). Jeka et al. (1996) found no differences between sighted and blind subjects on postural stability while using a cane, a task to which blind people are accustomed. Moreover, when exposed to sudden stance perturbation, the automatic postural responses of the blind are not substantially different from those of sighted persons (Nakata and Yabe, 2001). The same is true also for balancing while riding a periodically moving platform, where the balancing strategy of the blind subjects is similar to that of the sighted subjects performing eyes-closed (Schmid et al., 2007). The sensorimotor integration time of blind subjects should therefore be validly compared to that of sighted people under equal stance conditions. The aim of the Schieppati et al. (2014) study was to assess whether, in spite of known deficits in the processing speed of visual stimuli in the intact visual field of patients with visual system damage (Bola et al., 2013), blind subjects are more prompt than sighted subjects eyes-closed in reducing body sway in response to a haptic cue, based on their past experience and acquired skill in the use of their remaining senses (Pascual-Leone et al., 2005; Cattaneo et al., 2011).

Blind and sighted subjects, standing eyes closed with feet in tandem position, touched a pad with their index finger (LFT) and withdrew the finger from the pad in sequence. Steady-state body sway (with or without contact) did not differ between blind and sighted subjects. On adding the haptic stimulus, postural muscle activity and sway diminished in both groups, but at a significantly shorter latency (by about 0.5 s) in the blind (Schieppati et al., 2014). These data showed that blind are rapid in implementing adaptive postural modifications when granted an external haptic reference. Interestingly, the short delays appeared to be, at least in part, the consequence of a rapid learning process at the beginning of the series of trials, whereby the differences with respect to sighted subjects became obvious after some 10 task repetitions or so.

These findings show that fast processing of the stabilizing haptic spatial-orientation cues may be favored by neural plasticity in the blind, and add new information to the field of sensory-guided dynamic control of equilibrium in man. Under steady-state conditions, the balance control of blind subjects is not superior to that of sighted subjects eyes-closed. However, the former are considerably more rapid than the latter in implementing the appropriate modifications in postural set when confronted with a change in the relationship between body and environment. Coping with the haptic transient (rather than body stabilization *per se* under steady-state condition) seems to be favored by the loss of vision, perhaps through increased reliance on the sense of touch (Wong et al., 2011) and the enhanced functional connectivity between sensory and visual cortex (Ioannides et al., 2013; Ricciardi et al., 2014). The fact that the early-blind subjects showed a more prompt stabilization than late-blind subjects and that the latter were faster than in sighted subjects (Schieppati et al., 2014) suggests a progressive modification over time of the sensorimotor integration processes controlling body orientation in space, as part of their adaptation implying increased attention to non-visual events (Burton et al., 2014). Perhaps, the relatively lesser problems encountered by early-blind subjects in their activities of daily life compared to elderly, low-vision subjects (Chen et al., 2012) may be related to the early onset of plastic changes. In the view of these findings, protocols may be developed for enhancing both postural capacities and tactual object exploration and recognition (Tzovaras et al., 2004).

WHAT DETERMINES THE LENGTH OF THE SENSORIMOTOR PROCESSING TIME?

What mechanisms contribute to the rapid decline in body sway following access to stabilizing haptic or visual sensory inflow? In stance control, under both static and dynamic conditions, we not only track with the CoP the random displacement of the CoM, but we bypass its instantaneous position, in the presumed direction along which it moves, in order to create the torque necessary for braking and reverting its displacement. Indeed, we act on the movement of the CoM, in order to constrain its displacement within a relatively narrow space. In doing so, we rely on the operation of complex processes, whereby ongoing sensory information may be able to inform about future states of instability in a predictive manner (Slobounov et al., 1997, 2009). This may not be dissimilar from the sheepdog task, promptly gathering and fetching moving animals to a pre-defined goal position (Vaughan et al., 1998). The narrower the surface of the ellipse within which the center of feet pressure—the flock—moves, the smaller the energy spent, and the more stable the CoM of the body. In the sheepdog model, the size of the overshoot can be greatly reduced by appropriately tuning the gain parameter—or increasing the dog's anticipatory capacities.

Reducing the overshoot of the CoP with respect to the instantaneous position of the CoM to the extent sufficient for balancing with the minimal possible energy and computation costs would be achieved by increasing the gain of the system controlling the reciprocal positions of the CoM and of CoP, as if the sheepdog became "smarter" in controlling the flock. Changing the gain is likely operating by successive approximations, therefore time consuming, which might explain the relatively long delay of the onset of the changes in postural control mode and the slow time constant of the reduction in sway. Under different conditions (a computer-generated expanding visual field), likely requiring more complex processing than the simple abrupt change in haptic and visual information mentioned above, Jeka et al. (2008) measured the delay necessary for the nervous system to determine the most relevant sensory information for successful control of semi-tandem stance. Seconds from the change were necessary before a steady state was reached. Additionally, their data indicate a low speed for reweighting, when the visual scene motion was reduced, suggesting a temporal asymmetry (a slower process) whenever the change in the information does not threaten balance. Differences in the same sense (longer times to reach steady-state) have been also found on addition compared to withdrawal of stabilizing haptic and visual information, as mentioned above (Sozzi et al., 2012). Notably, under the condition of withdrawal of visual or haptic information, our nervous system could rely on its capacity for sustaining a working memory trace of recent information about the environment for guiding the reaction to postural perturbation (Bove et al., 2009; King et al., 2010; Cheng et al., 2012). Such a memory trace appears to explain our ability to guide targeted compensatory arm responses in the absence of online vision when a postural perturbation occurs (Cheng et al., 2013). However, this mechanism would not justify the *shorter* latencies of sway oscillation changes on withdrawal than addition of visual and haptic information under conditions of maintenance of unperturbed stance.

The timing of sensory modulation may differ when the task demands it and if the threat of an imminent fall increases the rate of gain modulation. For instance, threat of falling (Bolton et al., 2011b) or startling stimuli (Valls-Solé et al., 1999; Alibiglou and MacKinnon, 2012; Stevenson et al., 2014) can drive cortical motor responses faster than expected under normal conditions of voluntary control. Sensorimotor processes could as well be quickened when the task demands it. The slightly shorter latency of postural changes on *withdrawal* than addition of visual and haptic information would be affected by a similar event, since standing in tandem is more demanding in the absence of stabilizing information. Overall, one might note here that, however difficult the task of tandem standing, there is no urgent need to drive a rapid (and possibly metabolically costly) reweighting on the CNS, if a sufficient result can be managed with slower modulation.

CONCLUSIONS AND PERSPECTIVES: BRAIN AUGMENTATION AND NEUROPROSTHESES

The likelihood that the inflow from different senses changes concurrently, or within a short time-interval, is non-negligible. This gives rise to new questions. Do concurrent changes in the "stabilizing" direction (e.g., from no-vision to vision and from no-touch to touch) summate and ultimately assure a "better", more rapid performance? Are there differences when both changes occur in the opposite condition? Each stage of processing sensory information takes a certain amount of time, unique for each sensory modality (Barnett-Cowan and Harris, 2009): do these differences have an impact on the performance? Does the CNS, faced with a movement-balance integration problem, "select" one modality over the other in case of both changing? If so, are there "rules" for this selection? To what extent does the temporal order prevail over the modality? In this context, the expectation that the sensory condition(s) changes during the maintenance of a given (more or less critical) posture or in the preparation of a movement can play a role in the selection of the leading sensory information.

These questions should be taken into account when considering problems of sensorimotor integration in elderly subjects or patients, and when designing simulation models of human balance. In perspective, aged persons (Nardone et al., 1995), Parkinsonian patients, and patients affected by peripheral neuropathies, and blind subjects (Bugnariu and Fung, 2007; Striem-Amit et al., 2012; Maidenbaum et al., 2014) represent examples of different conditions liable to affect the variable at hand, i.e., the sensori-motor processing time, due to progressive losses in function across multiple systems, including sensation, cognition, memory, motor control (Mahncke et al., 2006; De Nunzio et al., 2007; Nardone et al., 2007; Konczak et al., 2008, 2012; Schmid et al., 2008; Aman et al., 2014). A rough attempt at identifying possible steps of the sensorimotor integration process is reported in graphic form in **Figure 2**, where different reweighting coefficients are assumed for different modalities of posture-stabilizing information. Whether the coefficients also affect the delays should be checked by further investigations.

These mechanisms should have an impact on both basic knowledge and applied science: (1) The duration of the process of integration of a change in sensory information is an important variable in the field of sensory-motor coordination. It can be affected by various sensory and motor conditions, and be a marker of a normal state under a given condition. (2) Cognitive processing and integration of sensory inputs for balance require time, and attention influences this processing

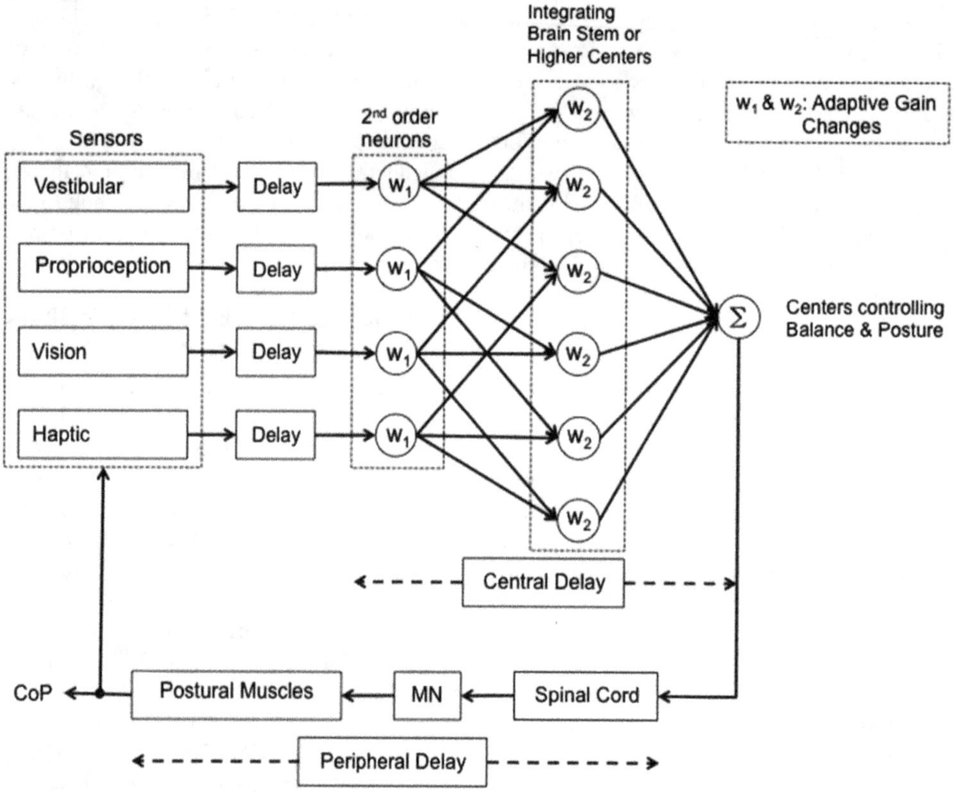

FIGURE 2 | Simplified scheme of the reweighting process during quiet stance. Vestibular, proprioceptive, visual and haptic signals are coded by the peripheral receptors and reach the brain after a corresponding delay. The information is first processed in 2nd order neurons. The afferent information then diverges to higher integrating centers and may be then reweighted according to the availability and accuracy of the other sensory inputs and balance constraints. Then information converges again (Σ) in the centers responsible for the control of balance. Following a short delay the information is transferred to the spinal cord interneuronal circuitry that generates the appropriate spatio-temporal pattern of muscle activity. This implies activation of MN activity and relevant muscle force, the effect of which is measured as displacement of the center of pressure (CoP). Most likely, the main part of the interval between the shift in sensory condition and the change in CoP displacement (approx. 1–2 s) conditional to active or passive addition or withdrawal of sensory information) depends on the operation of the central mechanisms generating the adaptive gain changes.

time, as well as sensory selection by facilitating specific sensory channels. Since performing a concurrent information-processing task may have an effect on the time delay, balance processes in older adults (Papegaaij et al., 2014) or sensory-impaired patients may be vulnerable to sensory-integration delays and to interference from concurrent cognitive tasks (Lacour et al., 2008). (3) Implementation of an appropriate time-lag between changes in a sensory modality, including its effects on balance, seems to represent an important aspect of the design of the control system for humanoid robots (Mahboobin et al., 2008, 2009; Peterka, 2009; Klein et al., 2011; Lebedev et al., 2011; O'Doherty et al., 2011; Rincon-Gonzalez et al., 2011; Demain et al., 2013). Biologically-inspired computational architectures, which are continuous in time and parallel in nature, do not map well onto conventional processors, which are discrete in time and serial in operation (Higgins, 2001). The findings briefly mentioned here would probably foster power- and space-efficient implementation technology. (4) "Rehabilitation robotics" is a new field of investigation between science and technology (Volpe et al., 2003; Casadio et al., 2008). Robots are being used to understand (Mergner, 2007; Mergner et al., 2009) and assist in maintaining balance and equilibrium (Forrester et al., 2014), or in helping movement practice following neurological injury (Krebs and Volpe, 2013), also providing insight into movement recovery. (5) Augmentation protocols of brain function offer enhancements for sensorimotor functions (this issue). For instance, appropriate patterns of vibratory stimulation to the dorsal axial trunk muscles easily reproduce functional mediolateral oscillations of the standing body (De Nunzio et al., 2007) as well as enhance walking cadence and velocity in PD patients (De Nunzio et al., 2010). Moreover, evolved neuroprostheses employing functional neuromuscular stimulation (FNS) can restore basic standing function (Mushahwar et al., 2007; Braz et al., 2009; Capogrosso et al., 2013). Cochlear implants providing vestibular electrodes can enhance the function of the vestibulo-ocular reflex (Perez-Fornos et al., 2014).

Robots can haptically assess sensorimotor performance, administer training, and improve motor recovery. In addition to providing insight into motor control, robotic paradigms and sensory augmentation devices may eventually enhance motor learning and motor recovery beyond the levels possible with conventional training techniques (Steffin, 1997; Bach-y-Rita, 2004; Kärcher et al., 2012; Proulx et al., 2014; Wright, 2014). We hope that defining the sensorimotor processing time for balance can represent a small but critical step in the direction of building new, smarter balance and locomotion training devices.

ACKNOWLEDGMENTS

This study was supported in part by the "Ricerca Finalizzata" grants (GR-2009-1471033 and RF-2011-02352379) from the Italian Ministry of Health and by the "PRIN" grants (2009JMMYFZ and 2010MEFNF7) from the Italian Ministry of University. We would like to sincerely thank the reviewers for their valuable comments and suggestions on our original manuscript.

REFERENCES

Alibiglou, L., and MacKinnon, C. D. (2012). The early release of planned movement by acoustic startle can be delayed by transcranial magnetic stimulation over the motor cortex. *J. Physiol.* 590, 919–936. doi: 10.1113/jphysiol.2011.219592

Aman, J. E., Abosch, A., Bebler, M., Lu, C. H., and Konczak, J. (2014). Subthalamic nucleus deep brain stimulation improves somatosensory function in Parkinson's disease. *Mov. Disord.* 29, 221–228. doi: 10.1002/mds.25731

Assländer, L., and Peterka, R. J. (2014). Sensory reweighting dynamics in human postural control. *J. Neurophysiol.* 111, 1852–1864. doi: 10.1152/jn.00669.2013

Azulay, J. P., Mesure, S., Amblard, B., Blin, O., Sangla, I., and Pouget, J. (1999). Visual control of locomotion in Parkinson's disease. *Brain* 122, 111–120. doi: 10.1093/brain/122.1.111

Baccini, M., Rinaldi, L. A., Federighi, G., Vannucchi, L., Paci, M., and Masotti, G. (2007). Effectiveness of fingertip light contact in reducing postural sway in older people. *Age Ageing* 36, 30–35. doi: 10.1093/ageing/afl072

Bach-y-Rita, P. (2004). Tactile sensory substitution studies. *Ann. N Y Acad. Sci.* 1013, 83–91. doi: 10.1196/annals.1305.006

Bandini, F., Pierantozzi, M., and Bodis-Wollner, I. (2001). Parkinson's disease changes the balance of onset and offset visual responses: an evoked potential study. *Clin. Neurophysiol.* 112, 976–983. doi: 10.1016/s1388-2457(01)00531-4

Barnett-Cowan, M., and Harris, L. R. (2009). Perceived timing of vestibular stimulation relative to touch, light and sound. *Exp. Brain Res.* 198, 221–231. doi: 10.1007/s00221-009-1779-4

Beckley, D. J., Bloem, B. R., Remler, M. P., Roos, R. A., and Van Dijk, J. G. (1991). Long latency postural responses are functionally modified by cognitive set. *Electroencephalogr. Clin. Neurophysiol.* 81, 353–358. doi: 10.1016/0168-5597(91)90024-r

Black, F. O., and Nashner, L. M. (1984). Vestibulo-spinal control differs in patients with reduced versus distorted vestibular function. *Acta Otolaryngol. Suppl.* 406, 110–114. doi: 10.3109/00016488309123015

Bodis-Wollner, I. (1992). Sensory evoked potentials: PERG, VEP and SEP. *Curr. Opin. Neurol. Neurosurg.* 5, 716–726.

Bola, M., Gall, C., and Sabel, B. A. (2013). The second face of blindness: processing speed deficits in the intact visual field after pre- and post-chiasmatic lesions. *PLoS One* 8:e63700. doi: 10.1371/journal.pone.0063700

Bolton, D. A., Brown, K. E., McIlroy, W. E., and Staines, W. R. (2012). Transient inhibition of the dorsolateral prefrontal cortex disrupts somatosensory modulation during standing balance as measured by electroencephalography. *Neuroreport* 23, 369–372. doi: 10.1097/WNR.0b013e328352027c

Bolton, D. A., McIlroy, W. E., and Staines, W. R. (2011a). The impact of light fingertip touch on haptic cortical processing during a standing balance task. *Exp. Brain Res.* 212, 279–291. doi: 10.1007/s00221-011-2728-6

Bolton, D. A. E., Patel, R., Staines, W. R., and McIlroy, W. E. (2011b). Transient inhibition of primary motor cortex suppresses hand muscle responses during a reactive reach to grasp. *Neurosci. Lett.* 504, 83–87. doi: 10.1016/j.neulet.2011.09.001

Borel, L., Lopez, C., Péruch, P., and Lacour, M. (2008). Vestibular syndrome: a change in internal spatial representation. *Neurophysiol. Clin.* 38, 375–389. doi: 10.1016/j.neucli.2008.09.002

Bottaro, A., Casadio, M., Morasso, P. G., and Sanguineti, V. (2005). Body sway during quiet standing: is it the residual chattering of an intermittent stabilization process? *Hum. Mov. Sci.* 24, 588–615. doi: 10.1016/j.humov.2005.07.006

Bottaro, A., Yasutake, Y., Nomura, T., Casadio, M., and Morasso, P. (2008). Bounded stability of the quiet standing posture: an intermittent control model. *Hum. Mov. Sci.* 27, 473–495. doi: 10.1016/j.humov.2007.11.005

Bottini, G., Karnath, H. O., Vallar, G., Sterzi, R., Frith, C. D., Frackowiak, R. S., et al. (2001). Cerebral representations for egocentric space: functional-anatomical evidence from caloric vestibular stimulation and neck vibration. *Brain* 124, 1182–1196. doi: 10.1093/brain/124.6.1182

Bove, M., Bonzano, L., Trompetto, C., Abbruzzese, G., and Schieppati, M. (2006). The postural disorientation induced by neck muscle vibration subsides on lightly touching a stationary surface or aiming at it. *Neuroscience* 143, 1095–1103. doi: 10.1016/j.neuroscience.2006.08.038

Bove, M., Courtine, G., and Schieppati, M. (2002). Neck muscle vibration and spatial orientation during stepping in place in humans. *J. Neurophysiol.* 88, 2232–2241. doi: 10.1152/jn.00198.2002

Bove, M., Diverio, M., Pozzo, T., and Schieppati, M. (2001). Neck muscle vibration disrupts steering of locomotion. *J. Appl. Physiol. (1985)* 91, 581–588.

Bove, M., Fenoggio, C., Tacchino, A., Pelosin, E., and Schieppati, M. (2009). Interaction between vision and neck proprioception in the control of stance. *Neuroscience* 164, 1601–1608. doi: 10.1016/j.neuroscience.2009.09.053

Braz, G. P., Russold, M., Smith, R. M., and Davis, G. M. (2009). Efficacy and stability performance of traditional versus motion sensor-assisted strategies for FES standing. *J. Biomech.* 42, 1332–1338. doi: 10.1016/j.jbiomech.2009.03.003

Bronstein, A. M., and Buckwell, D. (1997). Automatic control of postural sway by visual motion parallax. *Exp. Brain Res.* 113, 243–248. doi: 10.1007/bf02450322

Buchanan, J. J., and Horak, F. B. (1999). Emergence of postural patterns as a function of vision and translation frequency. *J. Neurophysiol.* 81, 2325–2339.

Bugnariu, N., and Fung, J. (2007). Aging and selective sensorimotor strategies in the regulation of upright balance. *J. Neuroeng. Rehabil.* 20, 4–19. doi: 10.1186/1743-0003-4-19

Burke, R. E., Rudomin, P., and Zajac, F. E. 3rd. (1976). The effect of activation history on tension production by individual muscle units. *Brain Res.* 109, 515–529. doi: 10.1016/0006-8993(76)90031-7

Burton, H., Snyder, A. Z., and Raichle, M. E. (2014). Resting state functional connectivity in early blind humans. *Front. Syst. Neurosci.* 8:51. doi: 10.3389/fnsys.2014.00051

Capogrosso, M., Wenger, N., Raspopovic, S., Musienko, P., Beauparlant, J., Bassi Luciani, L., et al. (2013). A computational model for epidural electrical stimulation of spinal sensorimotor circuits. *J. Neurosci.* 33, 19326–19340. doi: 10.1523/JNEUROSCI.1688-13.2013

Carpenter, M. G., Murnaghan, C. D., and Inglis, J. T. (2010). Shifting the balance: evidence of an exploratory role for postural sway. *Neuroscience* 171, 196–204. doi: 10.1016/j.neuroscience.2010.08.030

Casadio, M., Sanguineti, V., Morasso, P., and Solaro, C. (2008). Abnormal sensorimotor control, but intact force field adaptation, in multiple sclerosis subjects with no clinical disability. *Mult. Scler.* 14, 330–342. doi: 10.1177/1352458507085068

Cattaneo, Z., Fantino, M., Tinti, C., Pascual-Leone, A., Silvanto, J., and Vecchi, T. (2011). Spatial biases in peripersonal space in sighted and blind individuals revealed by a haptic line bisection paradigm. *J. Exp. Psychol. Hum. Percept. Perform.* 37, 1110–1121. doi: 10.1037/a0023511

Chapman, C. E. (1994). Active versus passive touch: factors influencing the transmission of somatosensory signals to primary somatosensory cortex. *Can. J. Physiol. Pharmacol.* 72, 558–570. doi: 10.1139/y94-080

Chen, N., Huang, T. L., Tsai, R. K., and Sheu, M. M. (2012). Prevalence and causes of visual impairment in elderly Amis aborigines in Eastern Taiwan (the Amis Eye Study). *Jpn. J. Ophthalmol.* 56, 624–630. doi: 10.1007/s10384-012-0178-8

Cheng, K. C., McKay, S. M., King, E. C., and Maki, B. E. (2012). Reaching to recover balance inunpredictable circumstances: is online visual control of the reach-to-grasp reaction necessary or sufficient? *Exp. Brain Res.* 218, 589–599. doi: 10.1007/s00221-012-3051-6

Cheng, K. C., Pratt, J., and Maki, B. E. (2013). Effects of spatial-memory decay and dual-task interference on perturbation-evoked reach-to-grasp reactions in the absence of online visual feedback. *Hum. Mov. Sci.* 32, 328–342. doi: 10.1016/j.humov.2012.11.001

Clapp, S., and Wing, A. M. (1999). Light touch contribution to balance in normal bipedal stance. *Exp. Brain Res.* 125, 521–524. doi: 10.1007/s002210050711

Clarac, F., el Manira, A., and Cattaert, D. (1992). Presynaptic control as a mechanism of sensory-motor integration. *Curr. Opin. Neurobiol.* 2, 764–769. doi: 10.1016/0960-9822(92)90095-r

Cohen, L. G., Celnik, P., Pascual-Leone, A., Corwell, B., Falz, L., Dambrosia, J., et al. (1997). Functional relevance of cross-modal plasticity in blind humans. *Nature* 389, 180–183. doi: 10.1038/38278

Contreras-Vidal, J. L., and Buch, E. R. (2003). Effects of Parkinson's disease on visuomotor adaptation. *Exp. Brain Res.* 150, 25–32. doi: 10.1007/s00221-003-1403-y

Cooke, J. D., Brown, J. D., and Brooks, V. B. (1978). Increased dependence on visual information for movement control in patients with Parkinson's disease. *Can. J. Neurol. Sci.* 5, 413–415.

Corna, S., Tarantola, J., Nardone, A., Giordano, A., and Schieppati, M. (1999). Standing on a continuously moving platform: is body inertia counteracted or exploited? *Exp. Brain Res.* 124, 331–341. doi: 10.1007/s002210050630

Courtine, G., Pozzo, T., Lucas, B., and Schieppati, M. (2001). Continuous, bilateral Achilles' tendon vibration is not detrimental to human walk. *Brain Res. Bull.* 55, 107–115. doi: 10.1016/s0361-9230(01)00504-4

Creath, R., Kiemel, T., Horak, F., and Jeka, J. J. (2002). Limited control strategies with the loss of vestibular function. *Exp. Brain Res.* 145, 323–333. doi: 10.1007/s00221-002-1110-0

Cullen, K. E. (2004). Sensory signals during active versus passive movement. *Curr. Opin. Neurobiol.* 14, 698–706. doi: 10.1016/j.conb.2004.10.002

Daubechies, I., Jianfeng, L., and Hau-Tiemg, W. (2011). Synchrosqueezed wavelet transforms: an empirical mode decomposition-like tool. *Appl. Comput. Harmon. Anal.* 30, 243–261. doi: 10.1016/j.acha.2010.08.002

Day, B. L., Steiger, M. J., Thompson, P. D., and Marsden, C. D. (1993). Effect of vision and stance width on human body motion when standing: implications for afferent control of lateral sway. *J. Physiol.* 469, 479–499.

Demain, S., Metcalf, C. D., Merrett, G. V., Zheng, D., and Cunningham, S. A. (2013). Narrative review on haptic devices: relating the physiology and psychophysical properties of the hand to devices for rehabilitation in central nervous system disorders. *Disabil. Rehabil. Assist. Technol.* 8, 181–189. doi: 10.3109/17483107.2012.697532

De Nunzio, A. M., Grasso, M., Nardone, A., Godi, M., and Schieppati, M. (2010). Alternate rhythmic vibratory stimulation of trunk muscles affects walking cadence and velocity in Parkinson's disease. *Clin. Neurophysiol.* 121, 240–247. doi: 10.1016/j.clinph.2009.10.018

De Nunzio, A. M., Nardone, A., and Schieppati, M. (2005). Head stabilization on a continuously oscillating platform: the effect of a proprioceptive disturbance on the balancing strategy. *Exp. Brain Res.* 165, 261–272. doi: 10.1007/s00221-005-2297-7

De Nunzio, A. M., Nardone, A., and Schieppati, M. (2007). The control of equilibrium in Parkinson's disease patients: delayed adaptation of balancing strategy to shifts in sensory set during a dynamic task. *Brain Res. Bull.* 74, 258–270. doi: 10.1016/j.brainresbull.2007.06.020

De Nunzio, A. M., and Schieppati, M. (2007). Time to reconfigure balancing behaviour in man: changing visual condition while riding a continuously moving platform. *Exp. Brain Res.* 178, 18–36. doi: 10.1007/s00221-006-0708-z

Dickstein, R., Peterka, R. J., and Horak, F. B. (2003). Effects of light fingertip touch on postural responses in subjects with diabetic neuropathy. *J. Neurol. Neurosurg. Psychiatry* 74, 620–626. doi: 10.1136/jnnp.74.5.620

Dickstein, R., Shupert, C. L., and Horak, F. B. (2001). Fingertip touch improves postural stability in patients with peripheral neuropathy. *Gait Posture* 14, 238–247. doi: 10.1016/s0966-6362(01)00161-8

Fiehler, K., and Rösler, F. (2010). Plasticity of multisensory dorsal stream functions: evidence from congenitally blind and sighted adults. *Restor. Neurol. Neurosci.* 28, 193–205. doi: 10.3233/RNN-2010-0500

Forrester, L. W., Roy, A., Krywonis, A., Kehs, G., Krebs, H. I., and Macko, R. F. (2014). Modular ankle robotics training in early subacute stroke: a randomized controlled pilot study. *Neurorehabil. Neural Repair* 28, 678–687. doi: 10.1177/1545968314521004

Guerraz, M., and Bronstein, A. M. (2008). Ocular versus extraocular control of posture and equilibrium. *Neurophysiol. Clin.* 38, 391–398. doi: 10.1016/j.neucli.2008.09.007

Hagbarth, K. E., Wallin, G., and Löfstedt, L. (1973). Muscle spindle responses to stretch in normal and spastic subjects. *Scand. J. Rehabil. Med.* 5, 156–159.

Haggard, P. D., and Wolpert (2005). "Disorders of body schema," in *High-Order Motor Disorders: From Neuroanatomy and Neurobiology to Clinical Neurology*, eds J. Freund, M. Jeannerod, M. Hallett and R. Leiguarda (Oxford: Oxford University Press), 261–271.

Hagura, N., Takei, T., Hirose, S., Aramaki, Y., Matsumura, M., Sadato, N., et al. (2007). Activity in the posterior parietal cortex mediates visual dominance over kinesthesia. *J. Neurosci.* 27, 7047–7053. doi: 10.1523/jneurosci.0970-07.2007

Hatzitaki, V., Pavlou, M., and Bronstein, A. M. (2004). The integration of multiple proprioceptive information: effect of ankle tendon vibration on postural responses to platform tilt. *Exp. Brain Res.* 154, 345–354. doi: 10.1007/s00221-003-1661-8

Heed, T., and Azañón, E. (2014). Using time to investigate space: a review of tactile temporal order judgments as a window onto spatial processing in touch. *Front. Psychol.* 5:76. doi: 10.3389/fpsyg.2014.00076

Higgins, C. M. (2001). Sensory architectures for biologically inspired autonomous robotics. *Biol. Bull.* 200, 235–242. doi: 10.2307/1543322

Hlavačka, F., Shupert, C. L., and Horak, F. B. (1999). The timing of galvanic vestibular stimulation affects responses to platform translation. *Brain Res.* 821, 8–16. doi: 10.1016/s0006-8993(98)01356-0

Holden, M., Ventura, J., and Lackner, J. R. (1994). Stabilization of posture by precision contact of the index finger. *J. Vestib. Res.* 4, 285–301.

Horak, F. B., and Hlavačka, F. (2002). Vestibular stimulation affects medium latency postural muscle responses. *Exp. Brain Res.* 144, 95–102. doi: 10.1007/s00221-002-1041-9

Horak, F. B., Nutt, J. G., and Nashner, L. M. (1992). Postural inflexibility in PD subjects. *J. Neurol. Sci.* 111, 46–58. doi: 10.1016/0022-510x(92)90111-w

Hötting, K., and Röder, B. (2009). Auditory and auditory-tactile processing in congenitally blind humans. *Hear. Res.* 258, 165–174. doi: 10.1016/j.heares.2009.07.012

Ioannides, A. A., Liu, L., Poghosyan, V., Saridis, G. A., Gjedde, A., Ptito, M., et al. (2013). MEG reveals a fast pathway from somatosensory cortex to occipital areas via posterior parietal cortex in a blind subject. *Front. Hum. Neurosci.* 7:429. doi: 10.3389/fnhum.2013.00429

Ivanenko, Y. P., Grasso, R., and Lacquaniti, F. (2000). Neck muscle vibration makes walking humans accelerate in the direction of gaze. *J. Physiol.* 525, 803–814. doi: 10.1111/j.1469-7793.2000.t01-1-00803.x

Ivanenko, Y. P., Talis, V. L., and Kazennikov, O. V. (1999). Support stability influences postural responses to muscle vibration in humans. *Eur. J. Neurosci.* 11, 647–654. doi: 10.1046/j.1460-9568.1999.00471.x

Jacono, M., Casadio, M., Morasso, P. G., and Sanguineti, V. (2004). The sway-density curve and the underlying postural stabilization process. *Motor Control* 8, 292–311.

Jeka, J. J., Allison, L. K., and Kiemel, T. (2010). The dynamics of visual reweighting in healthy and fall-prone older adults. *J. Mot. Behav.* 42, 197–208. doi: 10.1080/00222895.2010.481693

Jeka, J. J., Easton, R. D., Bentzen, B. L., and Lackner, J. R. (1996). Haptic cues for orientation and postural control in sighted and blind individuals. *Percept. Psychophys.* 58, 409–423. doi: 10.3758/bf03206817

Jeka, J. J., and Lackner, J. R. (1994). Fingertip contact influences human postural control. *Exp. Brain Res.* 100, 495–502. doi: 10.1007/bf00229188

Jeka, J., Oie, K. S., and Kiemel, T. (2000). Multisensory information for human postural control: integrating touch and vision. *Exp. Brain Res.* 134, 107–125. doi: 10.1007/s002210000412

Jeka, J. J., Oie, K. S., and Kiemel, T. (2008). Asymmetric adaptation with functional advantage in human sensorimotor control. *Exp. Brain Res.* 191, 453–463. doi: 10.1007/s00221-008-1539-x

Jeka, J. J., Schöner, G., Dijkstra, T., Ribeiro, P., and Lackner, J. R. (1997). Coupling of fingertip somatosensory information to head and body sway. *Exp. Brain Res.* 113, 475–483. doi: 10.1007/pl00005600

Johannsen, L., Wing, A. M., and Hatzitaki, V. (2012). Contrasting effects of finger and shoulder interpersonal light touch on standing balance. *J. Neurophysiol.* 107, 216–225. doi: 10.1152/jn.00149.2011

Kanekar, N., Lee, Y. J., and Aruin, A. S. (2013). Effect of light finger touch in balance control of individuals with multiple sclerosis. *Gait Posture* 38, 643–647. doi: 10.1016/j.gaitpost.2013.02.017

Kärcher, S. M., Fenzlaff, S., Hartmann, D., Nagel, S. K., and König, P. (2012). Sensory augmentation for the blind. *Front. Hum. Neurosci.* 6:37. doi: 10.3389/fnhum.2012.00037

Kavounoudias, A., Gilhodes, J. C., Roll, R., and Roll, J. P. (1999). From balance regulation to body orientation: two goals for muscle proprioceptive information processing? *Exp. Brain Res.* 124, 80–88. doi: 10.1007/s002210050602

Kelly, L. A., Kuitunen, S., Racinais, S., and Cresswell, A. G. (2012). Recruitment of the plantar intrinsic foot muscles with increasing postural demand. *Clin. Biomech. (Bristol, Avon)* 27, 46–51. doi: 10.1016/j.clinbiomech.2011.07.013

King, E. C., McKay, S. M., Cheng, K. C., and Maki, B. E. (2010). The use of peripheral vision to guide perturbation-evoked reach-to-grasp balance-recovery reactions. *Exp. Brain Res.* 207, 105–118. doi: 10.1007/s00221-010-2434-9

Klein, A., Jeka, J., Kiemel, T., and Lewis, M. A. (2011). Navigating sensory conflict in dynamic environments using adaptive state estimation. *Biol. Cybern.* 105, 291–304. doi: 10.1007/s00422-011-0466-2

Konczak, J., Li, K. Y., Tuite, P. J., and Poizner, H. (2008). Haptic perception of object curvature in Parkinson's disease. *PLoS One* 3:e2625. doi: 10.1371/journal.pone.0002625

Konczak, J., Sciutti, A., Avanzino, L., Squeri, V., Gori, M., Masia, L., et al. (2012). Parkinson's disease accelerates age-related decline in haptic perception by altering somatosensory integration. *Brain* 135, 3371–3379. doi: 10.1093/brain/aws265

Kouzaki, M., and Masani, K. (2008). Reduced postural sway during quiet standing by light touch is due to finger tactile feedback but not mechanical support. *Exp. Brain Res.* 188, 153–158. doi: 10.1007/s00221-008-1426-5

Krebs, H. I., and Volpe, B. T. (2013). Rehabilitation robotics. *Handb. Clin. Neurol.* 110, 283–294. doi: 10.1016/B978-0-444-52901-5.00023-X

Krishnamoorthy, V., Slijper, H., and Latash, M. L. (2002). Effects of different types of light touch on postural sway. *Exp. Brain Res.* 147, 71–79. doi: 10.1007/s00221-002-1206-6

Kupers, R., and Ptito, M. (2014). Compensatory plasticity and cross-modal reorganization following early visual deprivation. *Neurosci. Biobehav. Rev.* 41, 36–52. doi: 10.1016/j.neubiorev.2013.08.001

Lackner, J. R., DiZio, P., Jeka, J., Horak, F., Krebs, D., and Rabin, E. (1999). Precision contact of the fingertip reduces postural sway of individuals with bilateral vestibular loss. *Exp. Brain Res.* 126, 459–466. doi: 10.1007/s002210050753

Lackner, J. R., Rabin, E., and DiZio, P. (2000). Fingertip contact suppresses the destabilizing influence of leg muscle vibration. *J. Neurophysiol.* 84, 2217–2224.

Lacour, M., Bernard-Demanze, L., and Dumitrescu, M. (2008). Posture control, aging and attention resources: models and posture-analysis methods. *Neurophysiol. Clin.* 38, 411–421. doi: 10.1016/j.neucli.2008.09.005

Lebedev, M. A., Tate, A. J., Hanson, T. L., Li, Z., O'Doherty, J. E., Winans, J. A., et al. (2011). Future developments in brain-machine interface research. *Clinics (Sao Paulo)* 66, 25–32. doi: 10.1590/s1807-59322011001300004

Lederman, S. J., and Klatzky, R. L. (2009). Haptic perception: a tutorial. *Atten. Percept. Psychophys.* 71, 1439–1459. doi: 10.3758/app.71.7.1439

Lekhel, H., Popov, K., Anastasopoulos, D., Bronstein, A., Bhatia, K., Marsden, C. D., et al. (1997). Postural responses to vibration of neck muscles in patients with idiopathic torticollis. *Brain* 120, 583–591. doi: 10.1093/brain/120.4.583

Lewis, G. N., and Byblow, W. D. (2002). Altered sensorimotor integration in Parkinson's disease. *Brain* 125, 2089–2099. doi: 10.1093/brain/awf200

Loram, I. D., Gollee, H., Lakie, M., and Gawthrop, P. J. (2011). Human control of an inverted pendulum: is continuous control necessary? Is intermittent control effective? Is intermittent control physiological? *J. Physiol.* 589, 307–324. doi: 10.1113/jphysiol.2010.194712

Lund, S. (1980). Postural effects of neck muscle vibration in man. *Experientia* 36:1398. doi: 10.1007/bf01960120

Mahboobin, A., Loughlin, P., Atkeson, C. G., and Redfern, M. (2009). A mechanism for sensory re-weighting in postural control. *Med. Biol. Eng. Comput.* 47, 921–929. doi: 10.1007/s11517-009-0477-5

Mahboobin, A., Loughlin, P. J., Redfern, M. S., Anderson, S. O., Atkeson, C. G., and Hodgins, J. K. (2008). Sensory adaptation in human balance control: lessons for biomimetic robotic bipeds. *Neural Netw.* 21, 621–627. doi: 10.1016/j.neunet.2008.03.013

Mahncke, H. W., Bronstone, A., and Merzenich, M. M. (2006). Brain plasticity and functional losses in the aged: scientific bases for a novel intervention. *Prog. Brain Res.* 157, 81–109. doi: 10.1016/s0079-6123(06)57006-2

Maidenbaum, S., Abboud, S., and Amedi, A. (2014). Sensory substitution: closing the gap between basic research and widespread practical visual rehabilitation. *Neurosci. Biobehav. Rev.* 41, 3–15. doi: 10.1016/j.neubiorev.2013.11.007

Marque, P., Nicolas, G., Marchand-Pauvert, V., Gautier, J., Simonetta-Moreau, M., and Pierrot-Deseilligny, E. (2001). Group I projections from intrinsic foot muscles to motoneurones of leg and thigh muscles in humans. *J. Physiol.* 536, 313–327. doi: 10.1111/j.1469-7793.2001.t01-1-00313.x

Massion, J. (1994). Postural control system. *Curr. Opin. Neurobiol.* 4, 877–887. doi: 10.1016/0959-4388(94)90137-6

Matthews, P. B. (1988). Proprioceptors and their contribution to somatosensory mapping: complex messages require complex processing. *Can. J. Physiol. Pharmacol.* 66, 430–438. doi: 10.1139/y88-073

Maurer, C., Mergner, T., and Peterka, R. J. (2006). Multisensory control of human upright stance. *Exp. Brain Res.* 171, 231–250. doi: 10.1007/s00221-005-0256-y

Mergner, T. (2007). Modeling sensorimotor control of human upright stance. *Prog. Brain Res.* 165, 283–297. doi: 10.1016/s0079-6123(06)65018-8

Mergner, T., Maurer, C., and Peterka, R. J. (2003). A multisensory posture control model of human upright stance. *Prog. Brain Res.* 142, 189–201. doi: 10.1016/s0079-6123(03)42014-1

Mergner, T., and Rosemeier, T. (1998). Interaction of vestibular, somatosensory and visual signals for postural control and motion perception under terrestrial and microgravity conditions—a conceptual model. *Brain Res. Brain Res. Rev.* 28, 118–135. doi: 10.1016/s0165-0173(98)00032-0

Mergner, T., Schweigart, G., and Fennell, L. (2009). Vestibular humanoid postural control. *J. Physiol. Paris* 103, 178–194. doi: 10.1016/j.jphysparis.2009.08.002

Meyer, P. F., Oddsson, L. I., and De Luca, C. J. (2004). The role of plantar cutaneous sensation in unperturbed stance. *Exp. Brain Res.* 156, 505–512. doi: 10.1007/s00221-003-1804-y

Mohapatra, S., Krishnan, V., and Aruin, A. S. (2012). Postural control in response to an external perturbation: effect of altered proprioceptive information. *Exp. Brain Res.* 217, 197–208. doi: 10.1007/s00221-011-2986-3

Morasso, P. G., and Schieppati, M. (1999). Can muscle stiffness alone stabilize upright standing? *J. Neurophysiol.* 82, 1622–1626.

Murnaghan, C. D., Horslen, B. C., Inglis, J. T., and Carpenter, M. G. (2011). Exploratory behavior during stance persists with visual feedback. *Neuroscience* 195, 54–59. doi: 10.1016/j.neuroscience.2011.08.020

Murnaghan, C. D., Squair, J. W., Chua, R., Inglis, J. T., and Carpenter, M. G. (2014). Cortical contributions to control of posture during unrestricted and restricted stance. *J. Neurophysiol.* 111, 1920–1926. doi: 10.1152/jn.00853.2012

Mushahwar, V. K., Jacobs, P. L., Normann, R. A., Triolo, R. J., and Kleitman, N. (2007). New functional electrical stimulation approaches to standing and walking. *J. Neural Eng.* 4, S181–S197. doi: 10.1088/1741-2560/4/3/s05

Naito, E. (2002). Perceptual distortion of intrapersonal and near-personal space sensed by proprioception. *Percept. Mot. Skills* 94, 499–505. doi: 10.2466/pms.2002.94.2.499

Nakata, H., and Yabe, K. (2001). Automatic postural response systems in individuals with congenital total blindness. *Gait Posture* 14, 36–43. doi: 10.1016/s0966-6362(00)00100-4

Nardone, A., Galante, M., Grasso, M., and Schieppati, M. (2008). Stance ataxia and delayed leg muscle responses to postural perturbations in cervical spondylotic myelopathy. *J. Rehabil. Med.* 40, 539–547. doi: 10.2340/16501977-0214

Nardone, A., Galante, M., Pareyson, D., and Schieppati, M. (2007). Balance control in sensory neuron disease. *Clin. Neurophysiol.* 118, 538–550. doi: 10.1016/j.clinph.2006.11.012

Nardone, A., Giordano, A., Corrà, T., and Schieppati, M. (1990). Responses of leg muscles in humans displaced while standing. Effects of types of perturbation and of postural set. *Brain* 113, 65–84. doi: 10.1093/brain/113.1.65

Nardone, A., Grasso, M., and Schieppati, M. (2006). Balance control in peripheral neuropathy: are patients equally unstable under static and dynamic conditions? *Gait Posture* 23, 364–373. doi: 10.1016/j.gaitpost.2005.04.002

Nardone, A., Grasso, M., Tarantola, J., Corna, S., and Schieppati, M. (2000). Postural coordination in elderly subjects standing on a periodically moving platform. *Arch. Phys. Med. Rehabil.* 81, 1217–1223. doi: 10.1053/apmr.2000.6286

Nardone, A., and Schieppati, M. (2004). Group II spindle fibres and afferent control of stance. Clues from diabetic neuropathy. *Clin. Neurophysiol.* 115, 779–789. doi: 10.1016/j.clinph.2003.11.007

Nardone, A., and Schieppati, M. (2005). Reflex contribution of spindle group Ia and II afferent input to leg muscle spasticity as revealed by tendon vibration in hemiparesis. *Clin. Neurophysiol.* 116, 1370–1381. doi: 10.1016/j.clinph.2005.01.015

Nardone, A., and Schieppati, M. (2006). Balance in Parkinson's disease under static and dynamic conditions. *Mov. Disord.* 21, 1515–1520. doi: 10.1002/mds.21015

Nardone, A., Siliotto, R., Grasso, M., and Schieppati, M. (1995). Influence of aging on leg muscle reflex responses to stance perturbation. *Arch. Phys. Med. Rehabil.* 76, 158–165. doi: 10.1016/s0003-9993(95)80025-5

Nougier, V., Bard, C., Fleury, M., and Teasdale, N. (1998). Contribution of central and peripheral vision to the regulation of stance: developmental aspects. *J. Exp. Child Psychol.* 68, 202–215. doi: 10.1006/jecp.1997.2427

O'Doherty, J. E., Lebedev, M. A., Ifft, P. J., Zhuang, K. Z., Shokur, S., Bleuler, H., et al. (2011). Active tactile exploration using a brain-machine-brain interface. *Nature* 479, 228–231. doi: 10.1038/nature10489

Oie, K. S., Kiemel, T., and Jeka, J. J. (2002). Multisensory fusion: simultaneous re-weighting of vision and touch for the control of human posture. *Brain Res. Cogn. Brain Res.* 14, 164–176. doi: 10.1016/s0926-6410(02)00071-x

Pais-Vieira, M., Lebedev, M. A., Wiest, M. C., and Nicolelis, M. A. (2013). Simultaneous top-down modulation of the primary somatosensory cortex and thalamic nuclei during active tactile discrimination. *J. Neurosci.* 33, 4076–4093. doi: 10.1523/JNEUROSCI.1659-12.2013

Panichi, R., Botti, F. M., Ferraresi, A., Faralli, M., Kyriakareli, A., Schieppati, M., et al. (2011). Self-motion perception and vestibulo-ocular reflex during whole body yaw rotation in standing subjects: the role of head position and neck proprioception. *Hum. Mov. Sci.* 30, 314–332. doi: 10.1016/j.humov.2010.10.005

Papegaaij, S., Taube, W., Baudry, S., Otten, E., and Hortobágyi, T. (2014). Aging causes a reorganization of cortical and spinal control of posture. *Front. Aging Neurosci.* 6:28. doi: 10.3389/fnagi.2014.00028

Pasalar, S., Ro, T., and Beauchamp, M. S. (2010). TMS of posterior parietal cortex disrupts visual tactile multisensory integration. *Eur. J. Neurosci.* 31, 1783–1790. doi: 10.1111/j.1460-9568.2010.07193.x

Pascual-Leone, A., Amedi, A., Fregni, F., and Merabet, L. B. (2005). The plastic human brain cortex. *Annu. Rev. Neurosci.* 28, 377–401. Review. doi: 10.1146/annurev.neuro.27.070203.144216

Paulus, W. M., Straube, A., and Brandt, T. (1984). Visual stabilization of posture. Physiological stimulus characteristics and clinical aspects. *Brain* 107, 1143–1163. doi: 10.1093/brain/107.4.1143

Perez-Fornos, A., Guinand, N., van de Berg, R., Stokroos, R., Micera, S., Kingma, H., et al. (2014). Artificial balance: restoration of the vestibulo-ocular reflex in humans with a prototype vestibular neuroprosthesis. *Front. Neurol.* 5:66. doi: 10.3389/fneur.2014.00066

Peterka, R. J. (2002). Sensorimotor integration in human postural control. *J. Neurophysiol.* 88, 1097–1118. doi: 10.1152/jn.00605.2001

Peterka, R. J. (2009). Comparison of human and humanoid robot control of upright stance. *J. Physiol.* 103, 149–158. doi: 10.1016/j.jphysparis.2009.08.001

Peterka, R. J., and Loughlin, P. J. (2004). Dynamic regulation of sensorimotor integration in human postural control. *J. Neurophysiol.* 91, 410–423. doi: 10.1152/jn.00516.2003

Prochazka, A. (1989). Sensorimotor gain control: a basic strategy of motor systems? *Prog. Neurobiol.* 33, 281–307. doi: 10.1016/0301-0082(89)90004-x

Proulx, M. J., Brown, D. J., Pasqualotto, A., and Meijer, P. (2014). Multisensory perceptual learning and sensory substitution. *Neurosci. Biobehav. Rev.* 41, 16–25. doi: 10.1016/j.neubiorev.2012.11.017

Quinn, B. T., Carlson, C., Doyle, W., Cash, S. S., Devinsky, O., Spence, C., et al. (2014). Intracranial cortical responses during visual-tactile integration in humans. *J. Neurosci.* 34, 171–181. doi: 10.1523/JNEUROSCI.0532-13.2014

Rabin, E., Bortolami, S. B., DiZio, P., and Lackner, J. R. (1999). Haptic stabilization of posture: changes in arm proprioception and cutaneous feedback for different arm orientations. *J. Neurophysiol.* 82, 3541–3549.

Rabin, E., Chen, J., Muratori, L., Di Francisco-Donoghue, J., and Werner, W. G. (2013). Haptic feedback from manual contact improves balance control in people with Parkinson's disease. *Gait Posture* 38, 373–379. doi: 10.1016/j.gaitpost.2012.12.008

Rabin, E., DiZio, P., and Lackner, J. R. (2006). Time course of haptic stabilization of posture. *Exp. Brain Res.* 170, 122–126. doi: 10.1007/s00221-006-0348-3

Ravaioli, E., Oie, K. S., Kiemel, T., Chiari, L., and Jeka, J. J. (2005). Nonlinear postural control in response to visual translation. *Exp. Brain Res.* 160, 450–459. doi: 10.1007/s00221-004-2030-y

Redfern, M. S., Yardley, L., and Bronstein, A. M. (2001). Visual influences on balance. *J. Anxiety Disord.* 15, 81–94. Review. doi: 10.1016/s0887-6185(00)00043-8

Renier, L., De Volder, A. G., and Rauschecker, J. P. (2014). Cortical plasticity and preserved function in early blindness. *Neurosci. Biobehav. Rev.* 41, 53–63. doi: 10.1016/j.neubiorev.2013.01.025

Ricciardi, E., Bonino, D., Pellegrini, S., and Pietrini, P. (2014). Mind the blind brain to understand the sighted one! Is there a supramodal cortical functional architecture? *Neurosci. Biobehav. Rev.* 41, 64–77. doi: 10.1016/j.neubiorev.2013.10.006

Riley, M. A., Wong, S., Mitra, S., and Turvey, M. T. (1997). Common effects of touch and vision on postural parameters. *Exp. Brain Res.* 117, 165–170. doi: 10.1007/s002210050211

Rincon-Gonzalez, L., Warren, J. P., Meller, D. M., and Tillery, S. H. (2011). Haptic interaction of touch and proprioception: implications for neuroprosthetics. *IEEE Trans. Neural Syst. Rehabil. Eng.* 19, 490–500. doi: 10.1109/tnsre.2011.2166808

Rogers, M. W., Wardman, D. L., Lord, S. R., and Fitzaptrick, R. C. (2001). Passive tactile sensory input improves stability during standing. *Exp. Brain Res.* 136, 514–522. doi: 10.1007/s002210000615

Roll, J. P., and Vedel, J. P. (1982). Kinaesthetic role of muscle afferents in man, studied by tendon vibration and microneurography. *Exp. Brain Res.* 47, 177–190. doi: 10.1007/bf00239377

Roll, J. P., Vedel, J. P., and Ribot, E. (1989). Alteration of proprioceptive messages induced by tendon vibration in man: a microneurographic study. *Exp. Brain Res.* 76, 213–222. doi: 10.1007/bf00253639

Rougier, P., and Farenc, I. (2000). Adaptative effects of loss of vision on upright undisturbed stance. *Brain Res.* 871, 165–174. doi: 10.1016/s0006-8993(00)02357-x

Rowland, B. A., and Stein, B. E. (2014). A model of the temporal dynamics of multisensory enhancement. *Neurosci. Biobehav. Rev.* 41, 78–84. doi: 10.1016/j.neubiorev.2013.12.003

Schieppati, M., and Ducati, A. (1984). Short-latency cortical potentials evoked by tactile air-jet stimulation of body and face in man. *Electroencephalogr. Clin. Neurophysiol.* 58, 418–425. doi: 10.1016/0013-4694(84)90138-x

Schieppati, M., and Nardone, A. (1991). Free and supported stance in Parkinson's disease. The effect of posture and postural set on leg muscle responses to perturbation and its relation to the severity of the disease. *Brain* 114, 1227–1244. doi: 10.1093/brain/114.3.1227

Schieppati, M., and Nardone, A. (1995). Time course of 'set'-related changes in muscle responses to stance perturbation in humans. *J. Physiol.* 487, 787–796.

Schieppati, M., and Nardone, A. (1999). Group II spindle afferent fibers in humans: their possible role in the reflex control of stance. *Prog. Brain Res.* 123, 461–472. doi: 10.1016/s0079-6123(08)62882-4

Schieppati, M., Giordano, A., and Nardone, A. (2002). Variability in a dynamic postural task attests ample flexibility in balance control mechanisms. *Exp. Brain Res.* 144, 200–210. doi: 10.1007/s00221-002-1028-6

Schieppati, M., Hugon, M., Grasso, M., Nardone, A., and Galante, M. (1994). The limits of equilibrium in young and elderly normal subjects and in parkinsonians. *Electroencephalogr. Clin. Neurophysiol.* 93, 286–298. doi: 10.1016/0168-5597(94)90031-0

Schieppati, M., Nardone, A., Siliotto, R., and Grasso, M. (1995). Early and late stretch responses of human foot muscles induced by perturbation of stance. *Exp. Brain Res.* 105, 411–422. doi: 10.1007/bf00233041

Schieppati, M., Schmid, M., and Sozzi, S. (2014). Rapid processing of haptic cues for postural control in blind subjects. *Clin. Neurophysiol.* 125, 1427–1439. doi: 10.1016/j.clinph.2013.11.011

Schmid, M., Bottaro, A., Sozzi, S., and Schieppati, M. (2011). Adaptation to continuous perturbation of balance: progressive reduction of postural muscle activity with invariant or increasing oscillations of the center of mass depending on perturbation frequency and vision conditions. *Hum. Mov. Sci.* 30, 262–278. doi: 10.1016/j.humov.2011.02.002

Schmid, M., Casabianca, L., Bottaro, A., and Schieppati, M. (2008). Graded changes in balancing behavior as a function of visual acuity. *Neuroscience* 153, 1079–1091. doi: 10.1016/j.neuroscience.2008.03.024

Schmid, M., Nardone, A., De Nunzio, A. M., Schmid, M., and Schieppati, M. (2007). Equilibrium during static and dynamic tasks in blind subjects: no evidence of cross-modal plasticity. *Brain* 130, 2097–2107. doi: 10.1093/brain/awm157

Schweigart, G., and Mergner, T. (2008). Human stance control beyond steady state response and inverted pendulum simplification. *Exp. Brain Res.* 185, 635–653. doi: 10.1007/s00221-007-1189-4

Sciutti, A., Squeri, V., Gori, M., Masia, L., Sandini, G., and Konczak, J. (2010). Predicted sensory feedback derived from motor commands does not improve haptic sensitivity. *Exp. Brain Res.* 200, 259–267. doi: 10.1007/s00221-009-1996-x

Shokur, S., O'Doherty, J. E., Winans, J. A., Bleuler, H., Lebedev, M. A., and Nicolelis, M. A. (2013). Expanding the primate body schema in sensorimotor cortex by virtual touches of an avatar. *Proc. Natl. Acad. Sci. U S A* 110, 15121–15126. doi: 10.1073/pnas.1308459110

Slobounov, S., Cao, C., Jaiswal, N., and Newell, K. M. (2009). Neural basis of postural instability identified by VTC and EEG. *Exp. Brain Res.* 199, 1–16. doi: 10.1007/s00221-009-1956-5

Slobounov, S. M., Moss, S. A., Slobounova, E. S., and Newell, K. M. (1998). Aging and time to instability in posture. *J. Gerontol. A Biol. Sci. Med. Sci.* 53, B71–B78. doi: 10.1093/gerona/53a.1.b71

Slobounov, S. M., Slobounova, E. S., and Newell, K. M. (1997). Virtual time-to-collision and human postural control. *J. Mot. Behav.* 29, 263–281. doi: 10.1080/00222899709600841

Smith, A. M., Chapman, C. E., Donati, F., Fortier-Poisson, P., and Hayward, V. (2009). Perception of simulated local shapes using active and passive touch. *J. Neurophysiol.* 102, 3519–3529. doi: 10.1152/jn.00043.2009

Soto-Faraco, S., and Azañón, E. (2013). Electrophysiological correlates of tactile remapping. *Neuropsychologia* 51, 1584–1594. doi: 10.1016/j.neuropsychologia.2013.04.012

Sozzi, S., Do, M. C., Monti, A., and Schieppati, M. (2012). Sensorimotor integration during stance: processing time of active or passive addition or withdrawal of visual or haptic information. *Neuroscience* 212, 59–76. doi: 10.1016/j.neuroscience.2012.03.044

Sozzi, S., Honeine, J. L., Do, M. C., and Schieppati, M. (2013). Leg muscle activity during tandem stance and the control of body balance in the frontal plane. *Clin. Neurophysiol.* 124, 1175–1186. doi: 10.1016/j.clinph.2012.12.001

Sozzi, S., Monti, A., De Nunzio, A. M., Do, M. C., and Schieppati, M. (2011). Sensori-motor integration during stance: time adaptation of control mechanisms on adding or removing vision. *Hum. Mov. Sci.* 30, 172–189. doi: 10.1016/j.humov.2010.06.002

Steffin, M. (1997). Virtual reality therapy of multiple sclerosis and spinal cord injury: design consideration for a haptic-visual interface. *Stud. Health Technol. Inform.* 44, 185–208.

Stevenson, A. J., Chiu, C., Maslovat, D., Chua, R., Gick, B., Blouin, J. S., et al. (2014). Cortical involvement in the StartReact effect. *Neuroscience* 269, 21–34. doi: 10.1016/j.neuroscience.2014.03.041

Striem-Amit, E., Cohen, L., Dehaene, S., and Amedi, A. (2012). Reading with sounds: sensory substitution selectively activates the visual word form area in the blind. *Neuron* 76, 640–652. doi: 10.1016/j.neuron.2012.08.026

Suzuki, Y., Nomura, T., and Morasso, P. (2011). Stability of a double inverted pendulum model during human quiet stance with continuous delay feedback control. *Conf. Proc. IEEE Eng. Med. Biol. Soc.* 2011, 7450–7453. doi: 10.1109/iembs.2011.6091747

Tax, C. M., Bom, A. P., Taylor, R. L., Todd, N., Cho, K. K., Fitzpatrick, R. C., et al. (2013). The galvanic whole-body sway response in health and disease. *Clin. Neurophysiol.* 124, 2036–2045. doi: 10.1016/j.clinph.2012.12.041

Teasdale, N., Stelmach, G. E., Breunig, A., and Meeuwsen, H. J. (1991). Age differences in visual sensory integration. *Exp. Brain Res.* 85, 691–696. doi: 10.1007/bf00231755

Ting, L. H. (2007). Dimensional reduction in sensorimotor systems: a framework for understanding muscle coordination of posture. *Prog. Brain Res.* 165, 299–321. doi: 10.1016/s0079-6123(06)65019-x

Tokuno, C. D., Carpenter, M. G., Thorstensson, A., Garland, S. J., and Cresswell, A. G. (2007). Control of the triceps surae during the postural sway of quiet standing. *Acta Physiol. (Oxf.)* 191, 229–236. doi: 10.1111/j.1748-1716.2007.01727.x

Tokuno, C. D., Taube, W., and Cresswell, A. G. (2009). An enhanced level of motor cortical excitability during the control of human standing. *Acta Physiol. (Oxf)* 195, 385–395. doi: 10.1111/j.1748-1716.2008.01898.x

Tommerdahl, M., Favorov, O. V., and Whitsel, B. L. (2010). Dynamic representations of the somatosensory cortex. *Neurosci. Biobehav. Rev.* 34, 160–170. doi: 10.1016/j.neubiorev.2009.08.009

Tremblay, F., Mireault, A. C., Dessureault, L., Manning, H., and Sveistrup, H. (2004). Postural stabilization from fingertip contact: I. Variations in sway attenuation, perceived stability and contact forces with aging. *Exp. Brain Res.* 157, 275–285. doi: 10.1007/s00221-004-1830-4

Tzovaras, D., Nikolakis, G., Fergadis, G., Malasiotis, S., and Stavrakis, M. (2004). Design and implementation of haptic virtual environments for the training of the visually impaired. *IEEE Trans. Neural Syst. Rehabil. Eng.* 12, 266–278. doi: 10.1109/tnsre.2004.828756

Valls-Solé, J., Alvarez, R., and Tolosa, E. S. (1994). Responses of the soleus muscle to transcranial magnetic stimulation. *Electroencephalogr. Clin. Neurophysiol.* 93, 421–427. doi: 10.1016/0168-5597(94)90148-1

Valls-Solé, J., Rothwell, J. C., Goulart, F. R., Cossu, G., and Muñoz, E. (1999). Patterned ballistic movements triggered by a startle in healthy humans. *J. Physiol.* 516, 931–938. doi: 10.1111/j.1469-7793.1999.0931u.x

van der Kooij, H., and Peterka, R. J. (2011). Non-linear stimulus-response behavior of the human stance control system is predicted by optimization of a system with sensory and motor noise. *J. Comput. Neurosci.* 30, 759–778. doi: 10.1007/s10827-010-0291-y

van Emmerik, R. E., and van Wegen, E. E. (2002). On the functional aspects of variability in postural control. *Exerc. Sport Sci. Rev.* 30, 177–183. doi: 10.1097/00003677-200210000-00007

Vaughan, R., Sumpter, N., Frost, A., and Cameron, S. (1998). "Robot sheepdog project achieves automatic flock control," in *Proceedings of the Fifth International Conference on Simulation of Adaptive Behavior on From Animals to Animats 5* (Cambridge, MA: MIT Press), 489–493.

Venkatakrishnan, A., Banquet, J. P., Burnod, Y., and Contreras-Vidal, J. L. (2011). Parkinson's disease differentially affects adaptation to gradual as compared to sudden visuomotor distortions. *Hum. Mov. Sci.* 30, 760–769. doi: 10.1016/j.humov.2010.08.020

Vieira, T. M., Loram, I. D., Muceli, S., Merletti, R., and Farina, D. (2012). Recruitment of motor units in the medial gastrocnemius muscle during human quiet standing: is recruitment intermittent? What triggers recruitment? *J. Neurophysiol.* 107, 666–676. doi: 10.1152/jn.00659.2011

Volpe, B. T., Krebs, H. I., and Hogan, N. (2003). Robot-aided sensorimotor training in stroke rehabilitation. *Adv. Neurol.* 92, 429–433.

Von Holst, E., and Mittelstaedt, H. (1950). Das Reafferezprinzip. Wechselwirkungen zwischen Zentralnerven-System und Peripherie. *Naturwiss.* 37, 467–476. doi: 10.1007/BF00622503

Vuillerme, N., Isableu, B., and Nougier, V. (2006). Attentional demands associated with the use of a light fingertip touch for postural control during quiet standing. *Exp. Brain Res.* 169, 232–236. doi: 10.1007/s00221-005-0142-7

Vuillerme, N., and Nougier, V. (2003). Effect of light finger touch on postural sway after lower-limb muscular fatigue. *Arch. Phys. Med. Rehabil.* 84, 1560–1563. doi: 10.1016/s0003-9993(03)00235-1

Waszak, F., Cardoso-Leite, P., and Hughes, G. (2012). Action effect anticipation: neurophysiological basis and functional consequences. *Neurosci. Biobehav. Rev.* 36, 943–959. doi: 10.1016/j.neubiorev.2011.11.004

Wing, A. M., Johannsen, L., and Endo, S. (2011). Light touch for balance: influence of a time-varying external driving signal. *Philos. Trans. R. Soc. Lond. B Biol. Sci.* 366, 3133–3141. doi: 10.1098/rstb.2011.0169

Winter, R., Harrar, V., Gozdzik, M., and Harris, L. R. (2008). The relative timing of active and passive touch. *Brain Res.* 1242, 54–58. doi: 10.1016/j.brainres.2008.06.090

Performance enhancement at the cost of potential brain plasticity: neural ramifications of nootropic drugs in the healthy developing brain

Kimberly R. Urban*[1] *and Wen-Jun Gao*[2]

[1] *Department of Psychology, University of Delaware, Newark, DE, USA*
[2] *Department of Neurobiology and Anatomy, Drexel University College of Medicine, Philadelphia, PA, USA*

Edited by:
Mikhail Lebedev, Duke University, USA

Reviewed by:
Kimberly Simpson, University of Mississippi Medical Center, USA
Christopher R. Madan, University of Alberta, Canada

****Correspondence:***
Wen-Jun Gao, Department of Neurobiology and Anatomy, Drexel University College of Medicine, 2900 Queen Lane, Philadelphia, PA 19129, USA
e-mail: wgao@drexelmed.edu

Cognitive enhancement is perhaps one of the most intriguing and controversial topics in neuroscience today. Currently, the main classes of drugs used as potential cognitive enhancers include psychostimulants (methylphenidate (MPH), amphetamine), but wakefulness-promoting agents (modafinil) and glutamate activators (ampakine) are also frequently used. Pharmacologically, substances that enhance the components of the memory/learning circuits—dopamine, glutamate (neuronal excitation), and/or norepinephrine—stand to improve brain function in healthy individuals beyond their baseline functioning. In particular, non-medical use of prescription stimulants such as MPH and illicit use of psychostimulants for cognitive enhancement have seen a recent rise among teens and young adults in schools and college campuses. However, this enhancement likely comes with a neuronal, as well as ethical, cost. Altering glutamate function via the use of psychostimulants may impair behavioral flexibility, leading to the development and/or potentiation of addictive behaviors. Furthermore, dopamine and norepinephrine do not display linear effects; instead, their modulation of cognitive and neuronal function maps on an inverted-U curve. Healthy individuals run the risk of pushing themselves beyond optimal levels into hyperdopaminergic and hypernoradrenergic states, thus vitiating the very behaviors they are striving to improve. Finally, recent studies have begun to highlight potential damaging effects of stimulant exposure in healthy juveniles. This review explains how the main classes of cognitive enhancing drugs affect the learning and memory circuits, and highlights the potential risks and concerns in healthy individuals, particularly juveniles and adolescents. We emphasize the performance enhancement at the potential cost of brain plasticity that is associated with the neural ramifications of nootropic drugs in the healthy developing brain.

Keywords: methylphenidate, modafinil, ampakine, cognitive enhancement, synaptic plasticity, brain development

INTRODUCTION

Cognitive enhancement, and the ethical considerations that go along with it, is one of the hottest current topics in the neuroscience community. Humans have sought substances to improve our cognitive function for centuries, from ancient civilizations using hallucinogens in an attempt to raise their consciousness to commune with their gods, to the rise of coffee, to the more recent development of drugs such as stimulants and glutamate activators. Some might argue, therefore, that seeking to improve ourselves is a human trait, and therefore cognitive enhancement is nothing more than our application of new scientific approaches to meet our age-old desire for self-improvement and development. However, others argue that artificially enhancing one's cognitive abilities is unfair and gives an unbeatable advantage to the richer populations who will have more ready access to the drugs (Butcher, 2003; Cakic, 2009). The issue of cognitive enhancement has even been likened to the steroid debate in sports (Cakic, 2009).

There are many comprehensive reviews and articles published on the ethical concerns of cognitive enhancement; however, literature on the safety of consuming these drugs in youth is starkly lacking despite the significant increase in teen misuse and abuse of stimulants reported in a recent national study (Goldberg, 2013). Therefore, for the purpose of this review, we will concentrate on examining potential neurobiological ramifications of the popular cognitive enhancers, and highlight recent data on these drugs' actions in developing brains. It is likely that a large proportion of the population is exposed to cognitive enhancing drugs and pressure to take them may be especially high among college and high school students; these individuals are facing more stringent college and graduate school acceptance criteria, limited job pools and an ever-increasing pressure to perform better and better if they hope to succeed (Goodman, 2010; Franke et al., 2011; Lynch et al., 2011). However, individuals in this population may be the ones most likely at risk for potential neurological consequences,

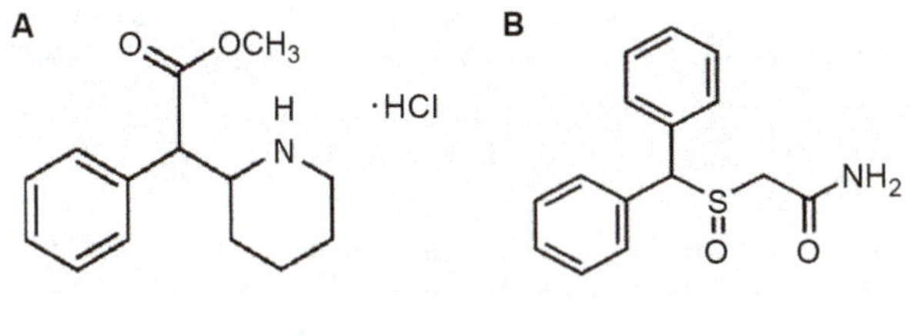

FIGURE 1 | (A) Chemical structure of methylphenidate (Ritalin©). **(B)** Chemical structure of modafinil (Provigil©). The drug bears a striking resemblance to methylphenidate and other stimulants.

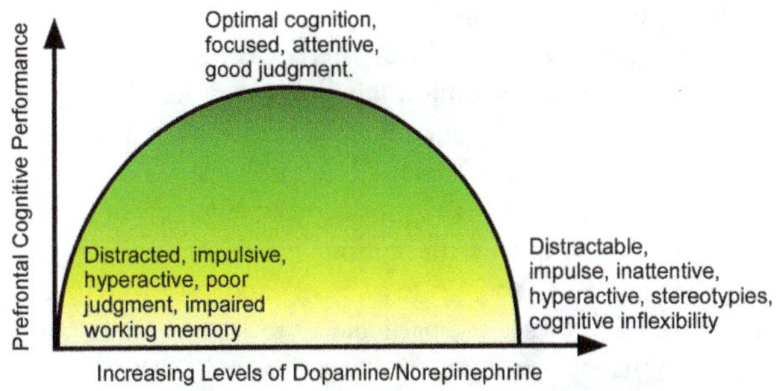

FIGURE 2 | Relationship of dopamine/norepinephrine to prefrontal function. At lower than optimal levels, the PFC is underactive, and the individual suffers from symptoms of ADHD (impulsivity, poor judgment, inattentiveness, motor hyperactivity). As levels rise, the function improves, until cognition and executive function reaches peak performance at optimal levels of dopamine/norepinephrine. As levels of the neurotransmitters continue to rise past the optimal point, cognition again becomes impaired, with the individual showing distractability, impulsivity, stereotypical behaviors and cognitive inflexibility.

due to their still-developing brains. We express regret that we are not able to cite many other good articles due to the topic specificity and sparsity of existing research; however, interesting information on cognitive enhancers that was outside the scope of this review can be found in these additional references (Dresler et al., 2013; Pang and Hannan, 2013; Ragan et al., 2013; Madan, 2014).

METHYLPHENIDATE AND THE DEVELOPING BRAIN

One of the most popular drugs under consideration for cognitive enhancement was originally developed to treat attention deficit-hyperactivity disorder (ADHD). Methylphenidate (Ritalin©; MPH; **Figure 1A**) is currently the most commonly prescribed medications for the treatment of ADHD (Challman and Lipsky, 2000; Spiller et al., 2013). MPH is a psychostimulant, related to amphetamine and cocaine and exerts its effects by blocking the transporters that reuptake dopamine and norepinephrine into the presynaptic neuron following their release; thus, it increases the levels or prolongs the availability of these neurotransmitters in the synapses to exert effects on postsynaptic neurons (Kuczenski and Segal, 2005).

However, a large proportion of literature on the safety and efficacy of MPH comes from studies performed on normal, healthy adult animals, as there is currently no sufficiently reliable animal model for ADHD. Several decades ago, studies began emerging that suggested that reduced hyperactivity and impulsivity in stimulant-treated ADHD patients were not "paradoxical" effects, but in fact also occurred in healthy individuals given the same doses (Rapoport et al., 1978, 1980). More recent MPH studies in both humans and rats have found that low doses of MPH that correspond to those given to ADHD patients in the clinic appear to enhance prefrontal-dependent functions and cognition in much the same way in healthy humans and rats as they do in ADHD patients and disease model rat strains (Mehta et al., 2001; Askenasy et al., 2007; Dow-Edwards et al., 2008; Agay et al., 2010; Linssen et al., 2012). These facts led to not only the acceptance of MPH study in normal subjects, but also the consideration of the medication as a cognitive enhancer.

The vast majority of studies on the cognitive enhancing effects of MPH and its effects on the normal brain have been performed in adult animals or humans. Higher doses (doses greater than those given to treat ADHD; 5–10 mg/kg intraperitoneal in rats) increase locomotor activity and impair attention and performance on prefrontal cortex-dependent cognitive tasks; however, lower doses (doses equivalent to the range given to ADHD patients; 0.5–2 mg/kg intraperitoneal in rats) improve cognitive performance and reduce locomotor activity in healthy individuals (Mehta et al., 2001). Likewise, lower doses of MPH (0.25–1 mg/kg, intraperitoneal, i.p.) in normal adult rats resulted in increased performance on attention tasks along with no effect on locomotor activity, while higher doses impaired performance and caused hyperactivity; doses beyond 10 mg/kg resulted in "stereotypes" (repetitive, fine motor movements similar to the tics seen in disorders like Tourette's syndrome) (Mehta et al., 2001). The low doses of MPH result in slight increases in dopamine and norepinephrine selectively in the prefrontal cortex, while not affecting other brain regions (Berridge et al., 2006). This allows for improvements in executive control and working memory (WM) without inducing locomotor activity or stereotypes.

However, the dangers of cognitive enhancement with stimulants like MPH lie in their potential effects on the regulation of dopamine and norepinephrine (**Figure 2**). At optimal doses, dopamine binds to higher-affinity D1-like receptors, and norepinephrine binds to $\alpha 2$ receptors, leading to an increase in prefrontal cortical signal-to-noise ratio and enhancing the flow of information and strengthening neuronal communication (Arnsten and Li, 2005). When the levels of dopamine and norepinephrine rise beyond the optimal levels, they begin to activate dopamine D2-class receptors and noradrenergic $\alpha 1$ and β receptors, which leads to weakening of the signal-to-noise ratio via activation of neurons that may not be involved in the current task (Arnsten and Li, 2005; Arnsten, 2009b). This nonspecific activation impairs attentional selectivity and results in a manifestation of locomotor hyperactivity, distractability and poor impulse control.

Levels of dopamine and norepinephrine in a normal, healthy brain are not universal and they may vary slightly over time within the same individual based on season, time of day, or activity (Otter and Nurmand, 1980; Petrović et al., 1980). Currently, there is no reliable method for determining optimal levels of these neurotransmitters in living human brains; thus, predicting how a certain dose of MPH will affect a particular person is largely an educated approximation. It is also possible that, although many studies found no overt cognitive differences between the effects of low-dose MPH on normal individuals and ADHD patients, molecular or cellular differences may exist that await detection by the development of more advanced technology. Thus, one must examine the research on MPH as a cognitive enhancer and studies using normal individuals with caution.

MPH is currently most often abused and sold on the black market among adolescents, particularly in high schools and on college campuses (Goodman, 2010; Franke et al., 2011). Students look for the medication when they have exams, or need to stay awake for long hours, in order to boost their energy and memory. This rather commonplace usage among adolescents is particularly frightening in light of the developmental timeline of the prefrontal cortex. This brain region, the center of control of judgment, behavioral inhibition and emotion, WM, logical thinking and decision making, does not finish developing until young adulthood; in humans this falls around the end of the second decade or the beginning of the third decade of life (Casey et al., 2008). During adolescent development, the levels of norepinephrine and dopamine surge and wane to allow for maturation of the executive control and reward pathways (Kanitz et al., 2011). Introducing a substance that alters dopamine and norepinephrine levels, such as MPH, might disrupt the maturation of the prefrontal cortex and have lasting behavioral consequences.

Indeed, research has recently begun to shift toward understanding MPH's actions in a juvenile brain. These pioneering studies have yielded striking results, indicating that early life treatment with MPH may alter circadian rhythms, induce anxiety that persists into adulthood, and even impair object-recognition memory (Lee et al., 2009; Algahim et al., 2010). However, many of the studies have not been particularly stringent in their dosing regimens, and the reader must examine the amount of drug used in each study very carefully. In adult rats, a therapeutic, clinically-relevant dose of MPH is one that produces blood plasma levels of 8–40 ng/dL; this appears to be in the range of 0.25–1 mg/kg given in an intraperitoneal injection (i.p.) (Berridge et al., 2006). We have recently completed several studies examining the effects of a low therapeutic dose (1 mg/kg, i.p.) on juvenile rats. We reported that a single dose of MPH resulted in significant depression of neuronal excitability and synaptic transmission in the prefrontal cortex; treatment with a chronic regimen of 3 weeks resulted in even further depression (Urban et al., 2012). In adult rats, however, the same low dosage increased neuronal activity (Urban et al., 2012). These results suggest that there is an age-dependent difference in MPH's actions, and that in healthy juveniles and adolescents, the doses previously thought to be therapeutic and cognitively enhancing may in fact be inducing excessive levels of dopamine and norepinephrine and in fact impairing certain aspects of cognition. Further supporting this theory, we discovered that the depression of neuronal activity was due, at least in part, to activation of a channel known as the hyperpolarization-activated non-specific cation channel (HCN; Urban et al., 2012). The HCN channel allows for flow of positively-charged ions, particularly potassium, out of the neuron, lowering its voltage potential and making it harder for the neuron to fire action potentials. The HCN channel is also known to be activated by a hyperdopaminergic state; thus, its role in juvenile treatment with MPH suggests that the dosage is inducing excessive dopamine, and possibly norepinephrine as well (Arnsten, 2009a).

One important unique property of the prefrontal cortex is its high level of plasticity, allowing for executive functions like WM and active decision-making; this plasticity may be a product of the slow maturation of this region (Jernigan et al., 1991; Kuboshima-Amemori and Sawaguchi, 2007; Spencer-Smith and Anderson, 2009; Newman and McGaughy, 2011; Teffer and Semendeferi, 2012; Selemon, 2013). Plasticity is controlled by levels of α-amino-3-hydroxy-5-methyl-4-isoxazolepropionic acid (AMPA) receptors and n-methyl-d-aspartate (NMDA) receptors. NMDA receptors contain two NR1 subunits with a combination of either NR2A or NR2B; NR2B conveys slower kinetics to the channel, allowing it to remain partially open during multiple stimulations (Cull-Candy et al., 2001). This property results in summation of responses and the continuation of the neural activity briefly after input has stopped, which is thought to be the neuronal correlate of WM (Wang et al., 2008, 2013). In most cortical brain regions, the ratio of NR2B/NR2A is high at birth, and declines over development; however, in prefrontal cortex it remains high (Wang et al., 2008). This allows for retention of plasticity throughout life, allowing the prefrontal cortex to continually adapt to incoming information and adjust behavioral output. We recently discovered that low dose (1 mg/kg, i.p.) treatment of juvenile rats with MPH induced a selective decrease in the levels of NR2B without affecting NR2A subunits (Urban et al., 2013). This finding supports our theory that the juvenile brain may be hypersensitive to dopamine levels; excessive levels of dopamine induce internalization of NR2B receptors via activation of glycogen synthase kinase (GSK)-3β, which causes phosphorylation of β-catenin, disrupting the β-catenin-NR2B interaction that stabilizes the NR2B subunit (Li et al., 2009). With β-catenin unbound, the NR2B subunits become targeted for internalization.

What do our findings mean for the healthy adolescent taking MPH? The prefrontal cortex's uniquely high levels of NR2B subunits throughout life impart the ability of the neurons to summate responses to incoming stimuli, resulting in the short-term potentiation of neural activity necessary for WM; thus, decreasing the levels of NR2B in prefrontal cortex leads to a reduction in the summation, which should impair WM (Wang et al., 2008, 2013; Urban et al., 2013). However, long-term potentiation (LTP) was found to be enhanced following juvenile treatment with MPH (Urban et al., 2013). The exact roles of NR2A versus NR2B receptor subunits in LTP regulation in the prefrontal cortex are not well understood, but it is currently believed that the direction of plasticity in prefrontal cortex (potentiation or depression) is dependent on the ratio of NR2A/NR2B, rather than exact levels of each subunit (Massey et al., 2004; Xu et al., 2009; Foster et al., 2010). Thus, reducing NR2B levels without altering NR2A levels, as was seen following juvenile MPH treatment, was enough to alter the direction of PFC long-term plasticity (Urban et al., 2013). The behavioral ramifications of altering LTP and long-term depression (LTD) in the prefrontal cortex are unclear, as it is not known exactly what LTP is representing in this region. However, it has been hypothesized that, if short-term potentiation is a cellular constituent of WM, then LTP might be a marker of sustained attention and long-term memory consolidation. Thus, perhaps treatment of the healthy juvenile brain with these low doses of MPH results in impaired WM and behavioral flexibility, but enhanced sustained attention and long-term memory? If this is the case, it could indicate that MPH-treated children who do not in fact have ADHD would appear successfully treated in a classroom setting—these children would be paying attention to the teacher, less hyperactive and learning might improve. However, stringent testing of their behavioral flexibility and WM might reveal subtle deficits that may affect their lives. For example, behavioral flexibility is needed for driving an automobile—the driver must be able to quickly shift attention from the road, to road signs, other approaching vehicles, back to the road and so on. Rigid attention and lack of flexibility could potentially result in inattentive or distracted driving. Behavioral flexibility is also a critical component of interpersonal skills; one must be able to adapt to different individuals and, in a work setting, shift plans and roles within the group in order to achieve the goal. Again, behavioral and cognitive inflexibility could impair the individual's function at their job and lead to reduced pay, unemployment or disciplinary action. Finally, behavioral flexibility is a critical component of resisting and recovering from drug abuse. Kalivas and Volkow identified alterations in glutamatergic signaling that result in an inability to alter one's behavior in cocaine addicts (Kalivas and Volkow, 2005, 2011; Kalivas et al., 2005). MPH has been shown to reduce the likelihood of later drug abuse in individuals diagnosed with ADHD, but, as the drug appears to affect glutamatergic signaling, it could potentially result in similar behavioral rigidity and lead to an increased likelihood for obsessive-compulsive or addictive behaviors (Newman and McGaughy, 2011).

MODAFINIL—POTENTIAL FOR STIMULANT-LIKE EFFECTS?

MPH's effects on brain development are surely interesting and potentially frightening; however, it is not the only cognitive enhancing medication that alters dopamine and glutamate transmission. Another cognitive enhancer that has begun to receive attention in the scientific community is modafinil (Provigil©), which bears a striking structural resemblance to methylphenidate (MPH) and other stimulants (**Figure 1B**). Originally developed in France in the 1970s, modafinil elevates hypothalamic histamine levels, but also appears to have a striking affinity for cell surface dopamine transporters (Engber et al., 1998; Ishizuka et al., 2008; Zolkowska et al., 2009). Its exact mechanism of action remains under debate, although arguments have been made both for its performing more as a wakefulness-promoting reagent via the hypocretin/orexin system of the hypothalamus, and as a classical psychostimulant via its blockade of the dopamine reuptake inhibitor (Ishizuka et al., 2003; Zolkowska et al., 2009). However, modafinil still promotes wakefulness in orexin knockout mice, so it appears that the orexin system is not required for therapeutic benefits (Willie et al., 2005). Whatever the mechanism, or mechanisms, of action may turn out to be, modafinil is currently a heavily studied drug with multiple uses. It is currently approved by the US Food and Drug Administration (FDA) for the treatment of narcolepsy, shift-work disorder and obstructive sleep apnea (Erman and Rosenberg, 2007; Cephalon, 2013). It has been shown to reduce jet lag and improve mood among shift workers, who often struggle with depression and chronic fatigue, forgetfulness and general cognitive impairments brought on by their work hours not allowing for a steady sleep-wake cycle (O'Connor, 2004; Hart et al., 2006). Modafinil has also been studied as an alternative to amphetamines for military usage—the military provides stimulants to soldiers in sleep-deprivation or high stress situations that require extreme alertness for long stretches of time. It is currently approved for Air Force missions in the US, and is also used in the UK and India (Taylor and Keys, 2003; Wheeler, 2006; Sharma, 2011).

Although modafinil is considered a first-line therapy for excessive daytime sleepiness (EDS) associated with narcolepsy in adults; it is also widely used in the treatment of EDS in children (Ivanenko et al., 2003; Sullivan, 2012). Caution is again the rule, especially at younger ages, due to reports of serious adverse events (such as tachycardia, insomnia, agitation, dizziness and anxiety) in elevated modafinil doses (Spiller et al., 2009), and in fact, the manufacturer recommends against use of modafinil in younger children. Despite these reports, modafinil is FDA-approved for use in children over age 16 years (Sullivan, 2012).

The usefulness of modafinil in improving alertness and wakefulness in non-sleep-deprived, healthy individuals, and its military involvement, has led to the consideration of the drug as a cognitive enhancer (Turner et al., 2003; Baranski et al., 2004; Randall et al., 2005b). Most studies agree that modafinil induces improvements in pattern recognition memory, digit span recall and mental digit manipulation (performing addition/subtraction/multiplication in one's mind), but the effects on spatial memory, attention and other aspects of executive function are more ambiguous, and appear to depend on the baseline performance of the individual in question (Turner et al., 2003; Baranski et al., 2004; Müller et al., 2004; Randall et al., 2005b). In a study of healthy student volunteers, modafinil improved target sensitivity in a rapid visual information processing (RVIP) task, and speed of color naming and drawing, but only in individuals with a "low" (mean 106 + 6) IQ; it had no significant effect on individuals with "higher" (mean 115 + 5) IQs (Randall et al., 2005a). In rats, these results are replicated, with low responding rats showing improvement on stop-signal reaction time tests after modafinil; higher performing rats showed no improvement (Eagle et al., 2007). Interestingly, MPH also shows sensitivity to baseline performance; many studies have indicated that MPH induces greater improvement in low-performing individuals than in higher performing individuals, and in some cases may actually cause deficits in higher performers (Eagle et al., 2007; Finke et al., 2010).

A recent study conducted in healthy human subjects reported that modafinil differs from other arousal-enhancing agents in chemical structure, neurochemical profile, and behavioral effects (Rasetti et al., 2010). Unlike most functional neuroimaging studies that focused on the effect of modafinil only on information processing underlying executive cognition, this study examined the effect of modafinil on neural circuits underlying affective processing and cognitive functions. They underwent blood-oxygen-level dependent (BOLD) functional magnetic resonance imaging (MRI, or functional MRI, fMRI) while performing an emotion information-processing task that activates the amygdala and two prefrontally dependent cognitive tasks—a WM task and a variable attentional control (VAC) task. BOLD fMRI revealed significantly decreased amygdala reactivity to fearful stimuli on modafinil compared with the placebo condition. During executive cognition tasks, a WM task and a VAC task, modafinil reduced BOLD signal in the prefrontal cortex and anterior cingulate. This study suggested that modafinil in low doses has a unique physiological profile compared with stimulant drugs: it enhances the efficiency of prefrontal cortical cognitive information processing, while dampening reactivity to threatening stimuli in the amygdala, a brain region implicated in anxiety (Rasetti et al., 2010).

The baseline performance sensitivity, and dopamine reuptake transporter affinity, indicates that modafinil could induce similar effects on the brain as psychostimulants like MPH. If this is the case, cause for concern arises when modafinil is considered as a cognitive enhancer in adolescents and young adults. To enlist in the Air Force, where modafinil is currently in use for pilots, one must be between 17–27 years of age (U. S. Air Force, 2013). The prefrontal cortex, under tight regulation by levels of dopamine and norepinephrine, and the brain's main center of attention and executive processing, does not finish development until the late 20's to early 30's for humans; thus, young pilots may be at risk for modafinil inducing excessive levels of dopamine in this brain region (Casey et al., 2008). One can expect that the potential ramifications of modafinil use in healthy young adults and teenagers would be similar to those seen in juvenile/adolescent use of MPH (Urban et al., 2012, 2013). Thus, modafinil could induce changes in plasticity or behavioral rigidity, and potentially damage WM, logical thinking and decision making. It has been reported that prolonged wakefulness induces experience-dependent synaptic plasticity in mouse hypocretin/orexin neurons (Rao et al., 2007). Specifically, acute and chronic prolonged wakefulness in mice induced by modafinil treatment produced LTP of glutamatergic synapses on hypocretin/orexin neurons in the lateral hypothalamus, a well-established arousal/wake-promoting center. A similar potentiation of synaptic strength at glutamatergic synapses on hypocretin/orexin neurons was also seen when mice were sleep deprived for 4 h. These results indicate that synaptic plasticity due to prolonged wakefulness occurs in circuits responsible for arousal and may contribute to changes in the brain of animals experiencing sleep loss. It is therefore likely that misuse and abuse of modafinil in the teens will eventually result in brain plasticity, especially brain regions related to sleep and motivation such as hypothalamus and dopamine-rich prefrontal cortex, hippocampus and nucleus accumbens. Future studies will need to address these shortcomings in order to determine the safety and efficacy of modafinil as a true cognitive enhancer. Recent reviews proposed some interesting mechanisms that may explain the likelihood of cognitive enhancement (Lynch et al., 2011; Roesler and Schröder, 2011; Lynch and Gall, 2013) but experiments are warranted for further exploration. The current research is contradictory in that some studies have noted clear improvements in sustained attention in humans, while others have failed to find any effect of the drug (Turner et al., 2003; Randall et al., 2005b). Similar discrepancies can be found in rodent studies; however, more recent studies are pointing to the possibility that modafinil selectively enhances WM without affecting consolidation of memories into long-term storage (Béracochéa et al., 2002; Turner et al., 2003; Müller et al., 2004; Randall et al., 2005b; Minzenberg and Carter, 2008). These studies are interesting, and suggest striking utility of modafinil as a cognitive enhancer; however, they have been performed on adult humans and rodents. MPH has also been shown in studies of healthy adults and children with ADHD to apparently enhance WM (Mehta et al., 2004; Pietrzak et al., 2006; Kobel et al., 2009; Marquand et al., 2011), yet recent juvenile rat studies suggest that in a healthy, developing brain, the drug might actually impair WM at low doses thought to be clinically relevant, i.e., doses that produce blood plasma levels of 8–40 ng/dL (Urban et al., 2013). Modafinil's profile by showing improvements in WM in healthy adults and sleep-deprived individuals (the population the drug was originally developed for) is analogous to MPH promoting improvements for healthy adults and children with ADHD; since both drugs appear to affect dopamine levels through blockade of the reuptake transporters, and alter glutamate signaling, it stands to reason that they could result in similar effects on WM in healthy, juvenile brains. Thus, modafinil at certain doses might cause a reduction in NMDA receptor levels, impairments in short-term plasticity and alterations in long-term plasticity much as MPH does (Urban et al., 2013). Future studies of modafinil as a cognitive enhancer should examine this possibility, and establish whether the drug shows an age- and dose-dependent profile of effects like the classic psychostimulants.

AMPAKINES—DRUGS FOR TREATMENT OF ALZHEIMER'S DISEASE—TURNED COGNITIVE ENHANCERS

The final classes of medications we will discuss in this review are the ampakines, which also have potential for significant effects on the developing glutamatergic system. Ampakines are a class of drugs that bind to the glutamatergic AMPA receptor, enhancing its activity by slowing deactivation and attenuating desensitization of AMPA receptor currents, increasing synaptic responses and enhancing LTP (Arai and Kessler, 2007). AMPA receptors are critically involved in regulating cortical plasticity; trafficking of AMPA receptors to the synapse is crucial for maintenance of excitability that leads to LTP (Malinow and Malenka, 2002; Huganir and Nicoll, 2013). However, there is more to the story of how AMPA regulates excitability; it does not function alone in the process. A second class of ionotropic glutamate receptors, NMDA receptors, actually trigger the induction of LTP; however, these receptors are normally blocked by magnesium at resting membrane potentials (Dingledine et al., 1999; Cull-Candy et al., 2001; Paoletti et al., 2013). Activation of AMPA receptors induces EPSCs, which depolarize the neuron and remove the magnesium block of NMDA, allowing for the induction of LTP. Then, NMDA receptors increase trafficking of more AMPA receptors to the synapse, maintaining the LTP (Lu et al., 2001; Paoletti et al., 2013). No ampakines are currently FDA approved, but they are being investigated as treatments for Alzheimer's senility, Parkinson's disease, ADHD, Rhett syndrome, schizophrenia, depression, autism, and Angelman syndrome (AS; Goff et al., 2001; Arai and Kessler, 2007; Ogier et al., 2007; Wezenberg et al., 2007; Simmons et al., 2009; Baudry et al., 2012; Silverman et al., 2013). However, they've also shown effectiveness at improving memory and cognition in healthy adult volunteers and rats (Ingvar et al., 1997; Hampson et al., 1998; Lynch and Gall, 2006; Wezenberg et al., 2007). Ampakines are also being studied by the US military for use as cognitive enhancers and alertness promoters for soldiers in high-stress extended combat situations; the lack of central nervous stimulation (such as would occur with modafinil, amphetamines or MPH make the ampakines very attractive (Saletan, 2008). Although ampakines have few adverse effects at therapeutically relevant concentrations and protect neurons against neurotoxic insults in adults (Arai and Kessler, 2007), the ampakine faramptor can cause headache, somnolence and nausea (Wezenberg et al., 2007).

While the ampakines represent perhaps the most promising group of pharmaceuticals for low-risk cognitive enhancement, as well as a potential relief for sufferers of psychiatric illnesses, they are likely not without danger to teens, adolescents, and young adults. First, very little is known about these drugs; the only example to reach human clinical trials is Cortex Pharmaceuticals' CX-717, which was evaluated in Phase I for the treatment of Alzheimer's disease; histological damage was seen in animal studies but Cortex claimed this was an artifact of tissue fixation (Stoll and Griesel, 2007). The FDA denied the application, and CX-717 approval halted. None of the other ampakines is known to currently be in human trials, so little can be proven about their efficacy or safety in healthy individuals. However, we can speculate based on knowledge of plasticity and the glutamate system.

The first concern when stimulating glutamate transmission in the brain is the potential for excitotoxicity. Glutamate toxicity generally occurs when excess glutamate storms the AMPA and NMDA receptors, causing a mass influx of calcium. This excess calcium in the cells activates a number of enzymes like proteases and phospholipases, which induce damage to organelles, the cell membrane, and DNA (Manev et al., 1989; Ankarcrona et al., 1995). However, activating AMPA receptors directly would cause a similar mass influx of cations and could also induce excitotoxicity. A recent study reported that ampakines promote spine actin polymerization, LTP, and learning in a mouse model of AS (Baudry et al., 2012). AS is a neurodevelopmental disorder largely due to abnormal maternal expression of the UBE3A gene leading to the deletion of E6-associated protein. AS subjects have severe cognitive impairments for which there are no therapeutic interventions. Mouse models (knockouts of the maternal UBE3A gene: "AS mice") of the disorder have substantial deficits in LTP and learning. Baudry et al reported that ampakine CX929 significantly enhanced LTP and notably, reduced dendritic spine abnormality and learning impairments (Baudry et al., 2012). This minimally invasive drug treatment is certainly promising for AS, and probably other neurodevelopmental disorders such as fragile X syndrome and autism (Rueda et al., 2009; Silverman et al., 2013) as well. However, such a magnitude of effects on synaptic plasticity and dendritic spine integrity also raises serious concern for immature brains of young children using ampakines as cognitive enhancers. It is not difficult to imagine that ampakines would have similar effects on the synaptic transmission and neuronal communication in the normal brain, eventually eliciting brain plasticity in the regions that are associated with emotional and affective functions. This could potentially lead to poor emotional regulation and impaired behavioral inhibition if plasticity is excessive and unregulated. Indeed, one of the important mechanisms by which the brain connections are maintained and tuned is through synaptic pruning, whereby highly active synapses are strengthened and less active synapses are removed through axon retraction (Luo and O'Leary, 2005; Gazzaniga and Mangum, 2009; Kolb et al., 2012). At first thought, heightened plasticity might seem to be a benefit—translating to faster learning and improved cognitive function; however, the excessive plasticity could also lead to high activity in all synapses and therefore reduce synaptic pruning. Impairments in synaptic pruning have in fact been associated with autistic spectrum disorders (Belmonte et al., 2004). The excessive connectivity leads to a heightened overall brain activation but the reduction in selectivity of activation is such that the signal-to-noise ratio is greatly lowered (Belmonte, 2000; Belmonte and Yurgelun-Todd, 2003). Thus, one can clearly see the potential dangers associated with unregulated plasticity, and how ampakines (which strengthen synapses and heighten plasticity by promoting dendritic spine growth) might lead to autism-like syndromes.

Although no studies have yet noted this in humans, doses of ampakines given to humans thus far have been tightly controlled. If the drug became available as a cognitive enhancer, or reached the black market, individuals could easily exceed safe doses and suffer neuronal damage from glutamate toxicity. Furthermore, the main purported therapeutic action of the ampakines is an alteration of plasticity; they are known to lower the threshold for induction of LTP and also increase the magnitude of LTP achieved (Lynch and Gall, 2006). While this alteration of plasticity may improve many aspects of learning and cognition, such as alertness, enhancement of LTP will likely come with a concomitant decrease in the opposite direction of plasticity, i.e., LTD. LTD is crucial for formation of spatial maps, and might play a role in cerebellar motor learning as well (although studies of motor performance after LTD impairment have been somewhat contradictory) (Aiba et al., 1994; Manahan-Vaughan, 2005; Kemp and Manahan-Vaughan, 2007). Thus, shifting plasticity in favor of LTP could lead to impairments in spatial memory and perhaps motor function. Careful determination of a dose-response curve, excitotoxic effects and species differences in metabolism/reaction to ampakines will need to be completed in the future in order to determine their true utility as cognitive enhancers.

CONCLUSION AND FUTURE PERSPECTIVE

In this review, we have examined three major pharmaceuticals under consideration as cognitive enhancers—MPH, modafinil and the ampakines. We have reported striking and deeply concerning effects of clinically relevant doses of MPH on the juvenile prefrontal cortex function and plasticity, compared them to the potential ramifications of modafinil treatment, and suggested several potential risks of ampakine exposure in healthy individuals. It is clear from the current lack of research in the field that much work needs to be done in order to determine the safety of cognitive enhancers, particularly among adolescents, the population most likely to take advantage of these drugs should they become available. There is already a high demand on college campuses and in high schools for MPH; thus, many healthy adolescents and young adults are already being exposed to unregulated doses of this substance. Understanding the behavioral and functional ramifications in cellular and molecular changes in the yet immature brains is paramount to mitigating risks for potential brain plasticity and consequent emotional and behavioral changes (Urban and Gao, 2012, 2013).

It is currently unclear if the dose range of stimulants that translates to effective ADHD symptom alleviation and cognitive enhancement in the healthy adult will translate to the same behavioral effects in juveniles; however, our recent studies suggest that the juvenile brain is hypersensitive to the effects of MPH (Urban et al., 2012). Thus, even a low, purportedly clinically relevant dose is likely to cause excessive levels of dopamine and norepinephrine, and impair executive functions and WM. This excessive dopamine/norepinephrine is likely also a potential risk of juvenile treatment with modafinil. It is far less clear how the ampakines might affect juvenile brain function, but their effects on plasticity through the glutamatergic system warrants further exploration. The desire for development of cognitive enhancing substances is unlikely to diminish with time; it may represent the next stage in evolution—man's desire for self-improvement driving artificial enhancement of innate abilities. It is therefore the responsibility of scientists and the medical community to stringently evaluate and research each new candidate substance, furthering our understanding of the brain in the process. Perhaps most importantly, the role of age and developmental stage in individual responses to cognitive enhancing substances needs to be thoroughly examined. Juvenile metabolic rates compared to adult are not clear in humans or rodent models; the dose-response curve for juveniles compared to adults for MPH, modafinil and the ampakines, as well as many other psychoactive medications, has not been examined. Finally, a potential long-term ramification of early life exposure of the healthy juvenile brain to these substances is only a very recent emerging topic of research, and much care needs to be taken to answer the questions expediently. Cognitive enhancement is no longer a scientific fiction; we must consider the unique dynamics of the developing brain and proceed cautiously until thorough safety and efficacy parameters have been established.

ACKNOWLEDGMENTS

This study was supported by grant R01MH085666 to Wen-Jun Gao from the National Institutes of Health, USA.

REFERENCES

Agay, N., Yechiam, E., Carmel, Z., and Levkovitz, Y. (2010). Non-specific effects of methylphenidate (Ritalin) on cognitive ability and decision-making of ADHD and healthy adults. *Psychopharmacology (Berl)* 210, 511–519. doi: 10.1007/s00213-010-1853-4

Aiba, A., Kano, M., Chen, C., Stanton, M. E., Fox, G. D., Herrup, K., et al. (1994). Deficient cerebellar long-term depression and impaired motor learning in mGluR1 mutant mice. *Cell* 79, 377–388. doi: 10.1016/0092-8674(94)90205-4

Algahim, M. F., Yang, P. B., Burau, K. D., Swann, A. C., and Dafny, N. (2010). Repetitive ritalin treatment modulates the diurnal activity pattern of young SD male rats. *Cent. Nerv. Syst. Agents Med. Chem.* 10, 247–257. doi: 10.2174/1871524911006030247

Ankarcrona, M., Dypbukt, J. M., Bonfoco, E., Zhivotovsky, B., Orrenius, S., Lipton, S. A., et al. (1995). Glutamate-induced neuronal death: a succession of necrosis or apoptosis depending on mitochondrial function. *Neuron* 15, 961–973. doi: 10.1016/0896-6273(95)90186-8

Arai, A. C., and Kessler, M. (2007). Pharmacology of ampakine modulators: from AMPA receptors to synapses and behavior. *Curr. Drug Targets* 8, 583–602. doi: 10.2174/138945007780618490

Arnsten, A. F. (2009a). Stress signalling pathways that impair prefrontal cortex structure and function. *Nat. Rev. Neurosci.* 10, 410–422. doi: 10.1038/nrn2648

Arnsten, A. F. (2009b). Toward a new understanding of attention-deficit hyperactivity disorder pathophysiology: an important role for prefrontal cortex dysfunction. *CNS Drugs* 1(Suppl. 1), 33–41. doi: 10.2165/00023210-200923000-00005

Arnsten, A. F., and Li, B. M. (2005). Neurobiology of executive functions: catecholamine influences on prefrontal cortical functions. *Biol. Psychiatry* 57, 1377–1384. doi: 10.1016/j.biopsych.2004.08.019

Askenasy, E. P., Taber, K. H., Yang, P. B., and Dafny, N. (2007). Methylphenidate (Ritalin): behavioral studies in the rat. *Int. J. Neurosci.* 117, 757–794. doi: 10.1080/00207450600910176

Baranski, J. V., Pigeau, R., Dinich, P., and Jacobs, I. (2004). Effects of modafinil on cognitive and meta-cognitive performance. *Hum. Psychopharmacol.* 19, 323–332. doi: 10.1002/hup.596

Baudry, M., Kramar, E., Xu, X., Zadran, H., Moreno, S., Lynch, G., et al. (2012). Ampakines promote spine actin polymerization, long-term potentiation and learning in a mouse model of Angelman syndrome. *Neurobiol. Dis.* 47, 210–215. doi: 10.1016/j.nbd.2012.04.002

Belmonte, M. (2000). Abnormal attention in autism shown by steady-state visual evoked potentials. *Autism* 4, 269–285. doi: 10.1177/1362361300004003004

Belmonte, M. K., Allen, G., Bekel-Mitchener, A., Boulanger, L. M., Carper, R. A., and Webb, S. J. (2004). Autism and abnormal development of brain connectivity. *J. Neurosci.* 24, 9228–9231. doi: 10.1523/jneurosci.3340-04.2004

Belmonte, M. K., and Yurgelun-Todd, D. A. (2003). Functional anatomy of impaired selective attention and compensatory processing in autism. *Brain Res. Cogn. Brain Res.* 17, 651–664. doi: 10.1016/s0926-6410(03)00189-7

Béracochéa, D., Celerier, A., Borde, N., Valleau, M., Peres, M., and Pierard, C. (2002). Improvement of learning processes following chronic systemic administration of modafinil in mice. *Pharmacol. Biochem. Behav.* 73, 723–728. doi: 10.1016/s0091-3057(02)00877-8

Berridge, C. W. D., Devilbiss, D. M., Andrzejewski, M. E., Arnsten, A. F., Kelley, A. E., Schmeichel, B., et al. (2006). Methylphenidate preferentially increases catecholamine neurotransmission within the prefrontal cortex at low doses that enhance cognitive function. *Biol. Psychiatry* 60, 1111–1120. doi: 10.1016/j.biopsych.2006.04.022

Butcher, J. (2003). Cognitive enhancement raises ethical concerns. Academics urge pre-emptive debate on neurotechnologies. *Lancet* 362, 132–133. doi: 10.1016/s0140-6736(03)13897-4

Cakic, V. (2009). Smart drugs for cognitive enhancement: ethical and pragmatic considerations in the era of cosmetic neurology. *J. Med. Ethics* 35, 611–615. doi: 10.1136/jme.2009.030882

Casey, B. J., Jones, R. M., and Hare, T. A. (2008). The adolescent brain. *Ann. N Y Acad. Sci.* 1124, 111–126. doi: 10.1196/annals.1440.010

Cephalon, I. (2013). Provigil(R)-modafinil. As accessed 10-22-2013. www.provigil.com

Challman, T. D., and Lipsky, J. J. (2000). Methylphenidate: its pharmacology and uses. *Mayo Clin. Proc.* 75, 711–721. doi: 10.4065/75.7.711

Cull-Candy, S., Brickley, S., and Farrant, M. (2001). NMDA receptor subunits: diversity, development and disease. *Curr. Opin. Neurobiol.* 11, 327–335. doi: 10.1016/s0959-4388(00)00215-4

Dingledine, R., Borges, K., Bowie, D., and Traynelis, S. F. (1999). The glutamate receptor ion channels. *Pharmacol. Rev.* 51, 7–61.

Dow-Edwards, D. L., Weedon, J. C., and Hellmann, E. (2008). Methylphenidate improves performance on the radial arm maze in periadolescent rats. *Neurotoxicol. Teratol.* 30, 419–427. doi: 10.1016/j.ntt.2008.04.001

Dresler, M., Sandberg, A., Ohla, K., Bublitz, C., Trenado, C., Mroczko-Wasowicz, A., et al. (2013). Non-pharmacological cognitive enhancement. *Neuropharmacology* 64, 529–543. doi: 10.1016/j.neuropharm.2012.07.002

Eagle, D. M., Tufft, M. R., Goodchild, H. L., and Robbins, T. W. (2007). Differential effects of modafinil and methylphenidate on stop-signal reaction time task performance in the rat and interactions with the dopamine receptor antagonist cis-flupenthixol. *Psychopharmacology (Berl)* 192, 193–206. doi: 10.1007/s00213-007-0701-7

Engber, T. M., Koury, E. J., Dennis, S. A., Miller, M. S., Contreras, P. C., and Bhat, R. V. (1998). Differential patterns of regional c-Fos induction in the rat brain by amphetamine and the novel wakefulness-promoting agent modafinil. *Neurosci. Lett.* 241, 95–98. doi: 10.1016/s0304-3940(97)00962-2

Erman, M. K., and Rosenberg, R., Modafinil Shift Work Sleep Disorder Study Group. (2007). Modafinil for excessive sleepiness associated with chronic shift work sleep disorder: effects on patient functioning and health-related quality of life. *Prim. Care Companion J. Clin. Psychiatry* 9, 188–194. doi: 10.4088/pcc.v09n0304

Finke, K., Dodds, C. M., Bublak, P., Regenthal, R., Baumann, F., Manly, T., et al. (2010). Effects of modafinil and methylphenidate on visual attention capacity: a TVA-based study. *Psychopharmacology (Berl)* 210, 317–329. doi: 10.1007/s00213-010-1823-x

Foster, K. A., McLaughlin, N., Edbauer, D., Phillips, M., Bolton, A., Constantine-Paton, M., et al. (2010). Distinct roles of NR2A and NR2B cytoplasmic tails in long-term potentiation. *J. Neurosci.* 30, 2676–2685. doi: 10.1523/jneurosci.4022-09.2010

Franke, A. G., Bonertz, C., Christmann, M., Huss, M., Fellgiebel, A., Hildt, E., et al. (2011). Non-medical use of prescription stimulants and illicit use of stimulants for cognitive enhancement in pupils and students in Germany. *Pharmacopsychiatry* 44, 60–66. doi: 10.1055/s-0030-1268417

Gazzaniga, M. S., and Mangum, G. R. (2009). *Cognitive Neuroscience: The Biology of the Mind.* New York, NY: W. W. Norton and Company.

Goff, D. C., Leahy, L., Berman, I., Posever, T., Herz, L., Leon, A. C., et al. (2001). A placebo-controlled pilot study of the ampakine CX516 added to clozapine in schizophrenia. *J. Clin. Psychopharmacol.* 21, 484–487. doi: 10.1097/00004714-200110000-00005

Goldberg, C. (2013). National study: teen misuse and abuse of prescription drugs up 33 percent since 2008 stimulants contributing to sustained Rx epidemic. Newsroom, The Partnership at DrugFree.org. Accessed 11-1-2013. http://www.drugfree.org/newsroom

Goodman, R. (2010). Cognitive enhancement, cheating, and accomplishment. *Kennedy Inst. Ethics J.* 20, 145–160. doi: 10.1353/ken.0.0309

Hampson, R. E., Rogers, G., Lynch, G., and Deadwyler, S. A. (1998). Facilitative effects of the ampakine CX516 on short-term memory in rats: enhancement of delayed-nonmatch-to-sample performance. *J. Neurosci.* 18, 2740–2747.

Hart, C. L., Haney, M., Vosburg, S. K., Comer, S. D., Gunderson, E., and Foltin, R. W. (2006). Modafinil attenuates disruptions in cognitive performance during simulated night-shift work. *Neuropsychopharmacology* 31, 1526–1536. doi: 10.1038/sj.npp.1300991

Huganir, R. L., and Nicoll, R. A. (2013). AMPARs and synaptic plasticity: the last 25 years. *Neuron* 80, 704–717. doi: 10.1016/j.neuron.2013.10.025

Ingvar, M., Ambros-Ingerson, J., Davis, M., Granger, R., Kessler, M., Rogers, G. A., et al. (1997). Enhancement by an ampakine of memory encoding in humans. *Exp. Neurol.* 146, 553–559. doi: 10.1006/exnr.1997.6581

Ishizuka, T., Murakami, M., and Yamatodani, A. (2008). Involvement of central histaminergic systems in modafinil-induced but not methylphenidate-induced increases in locomotor activity in rats. *Eur. J. Pharmacol.* 578, 209–215. doi: 10.1016/j.ejphar.2007.09.009

Ishizuka, T., Sakamoto, Y., Sakurai, T., and Yamatodani, A. (2003). Modafinil increases histamine release in the anterior hypothalamus of rats. *Neurosci. Lett.* 339, 143–146. doi: 10.1016/s0304-3940(03)00006-5

Ivanenko, A., Tauman, R., and Gozal, D. (2003). Modafinil in the treatment of excessive daytime sleepiness in children. *Sleep Med.* 4, 579–582. doi: 10.1016/s1389-9457(03)00162-x

Jernigan, T. L., Trauner, D. A., Hesselink, J. R., and Tallal, P. A. (1991). Maturation of human cerebrum observed in vivo during adolescence. *Brain* 114(Pt. 5), 2037–2049. doi: 10.1093/brain/114.5.2037

Kalivas, P. W., and Volkow, N. D. (2005). The neural basis of addiction: a pathology of motivation and choice. *Am. J. Psychiatry* 162, 1403–1413. doi: 10.1176/appi.ajp.162.8.1403

Kalivas, P. W., and Volkow, N. D. (2011). New medications for drug addiction hiding in glutamatergic neuroplasticity. *Mol. Psychiatry* 16, 974–986. doi: 10.1038/mp.2011.46

Kanitz, E., Otten, W., Hameister, T., Tuchscherer, M., Puppe, B., and Tuchscherer, A. (2011). Age-related changes in corticosteroid receptor expression and monoamine neurotransmitter concentrations in various brain regions of post-natal pigs. *J. Neurosci. Res.* 89, 1134–1141. doi: 10.1002/jnr.22621

Kalivas, P. W., Volkow, N., and Seamans, J. (2005). Unmanageable motivation in addiction: a pathology in prefrontal-accumbens glutamate transmission. *Neuron* 45, 647–650. doi: 10.1016/j.neuron.2005.02.005

Kemp, A., and Manahan-Vaughan, D. (2007). Hippocampal long-term depression: master or minion in declarative memory processes? *Trends Neurosci.* 30, 111–118. doi: 10.1016/j.tins.2007.01.002

Kobel, M., Bechtel, N., Weber, P., Specht, K., Klarhofer, M., Scheffler, K., et al. (2009). Effects of methylphenidate on working memory functioning in children with attention deficit/hyperactivity disorder. *Eur. J. Paediatr. Neurol.* 13, 516–523. doi: 10.1016/j.ejpn.2008.10.008

Kolb, B., Mychasiuk, R., Muhammad, A., Li, Y., Frost, D. O., and Gibb, R. (2012). Experience and the developing prefrontal cortex. *Proc. Natl. Acad. Sci. U S A* 109, 17186–17193. doi: 10.1073/pnas.1121251109

Kuboshima-Amemori, S., and Sawaguchi, T. (2007). Plasticity of the primate prefrontal cortex. *Neuroscientist* 13, 229–240. doi: 10.1177/1073858406298554

Kuczenski, R., and Segal, D. S. (2005). Stimulant actions in rodents: implications for attention-deficit/hyperactivity disorder treatment and potential substance abuse. *Biol. Psychiatry* 57, 1391–1396. doi: 10.1016/j.biopsych.2004.12.036

Lee, M. J., Yang, P. B., Wilcox, V. T., Burau, K. D., Swann, A. C., and Dafny, N. (2009). Does repetitive Ritalin injection produce long-term effects on SD female adolescent rats? *Neuropharmacology* 57, 201–207. doi: 10.1016/j.neuropharm.2009.06.008

Li, Y. C., Xi, D., Roman, J., Huang, Y. Q., and Gao, W. J. (2009). Activation of glycogen synthase kinase-3 beta is required for hyperdopamine and D2 receptor-mediated inhibition of synaptic NMDA receptor function in the rat prefrontal cortex. *J. Neurosci.* 29, 15551–15563. doi: 10.1523/JNEUROSCI.3336-09.2009

Linssen, A. M., Vuurman, E. F., Sambeth, A., and Riedel, W. J. (2012). Methylphenidate produces selective enhancement of declarative memory consolidation in healthy volunteers. *Psychopharmacology (Berl)* 221, 611–619. doi: 10.1007/s00213-011-2605-9

Lu, W., Man, H., Ju, W., Trimble, W. S., MacDonald, J. F., and Wang, Y. T. (2001). Activation of synaptic NMDA receptors induces membrane insertion of new AMPA receptors and LTP in cultured hippocampal neurons. *Neuron* 29, 243–254. doi: 10.1016/s0896-6273(01)00194-5

Luo, L., and O'Leary, D. D. (2005). Axon retraction and degeneration in development and disease. *Annu. Rev. Neurosci.* 28, 127–156. doi: 10.1146/annurev.neuro.28.061604.135632

Lynch, G., and Gall, C. M. (2006). Ampakines and the threefold path to cognitive enhancement. *Trends Neurosci.* 29, 554–562. doi: 10.1016/j.tins.2006.07.007

Lynch, G., and Gall, C. M. (2013). Mechanism based approaches for rescuing and enhancing cognition. *Front. Neurosci.* 7:143. doi: 10.3389/fnins.2013.00143

Lynch, G., Palmer, L. C., and Gall, C. M. (2011). The likelihood of cognitive enhancement. *Pharmacol. Biochem. Behav.* 99, 116–129. doi: 10.1016/j.pbb.2010.12.024

Madan, C. R. (2014). Augmented memory: a survey of the approaches to remembering more. *Front. Syst. Neurosci.* 8:30. doi: 10.3389/fnsys.2014.00030

Malinow, R., and Malenka, R. C. (2002). AMPA receptor trafficking and synaptic plasticity. *Annu. Rev. Neurosci.* 25, 103–126. doi: 10.1146/annurev.neuro.25.112701.142758

Manahan-Vaughan, D. (2005). "Hippocampal long-term depression as a declarative memory mechanism. in: H.E.S.," in *Synaptic Plasticity and Transsynaptic Signaling Scharfman*, eds P. K. Scharfman and C. Bramham (Springer: Berlin), 305–319.

Manev, H., Favaron, M., Guidotti, A., and Costa, E. (1989). Delayed increase of Ca2+ influx elicited by glutamate: role in neuronal death. *Mol. Pharmacol.* 36, 106–112.

Marquand, A. F., De Simoni, S., O'Daly, O. G., Williams, S. C., Mourao-Miranda, J., and Mehta, M. A. (2011). Pattern classification of working memory networks reveals differential effects of methylphenidate, atomoxetine and placebo in healthy volunteers. *Neuropsychopharmacology* 36, 1237–1247. doi: 10.1038/npp.2011.9

Massey, P. V. J., Johnson, B. E., Moult, P. R., Auberson, Y. P., Brown, M. W., Molnar, E., et al. (2004). Differential roles of NR2A and NR2B-containing NMDA receptors in cortical long-term potentiation and long-term depression. *J. Neurosci.* 24, 7821–7828. doi: 10.1523/jneurosci.1697-04.2004

Mehta, M. A., Goodyer, I. M., and Sahakian, B. J. (2004). Methylphenidate improves working memory and set-shifting in AD/HD: relationships to baseline memory capacity. *J. Child Psychol. Psychiatry* 45, 293–305. doi: 10.1111/j.1469-7610.2004.00221.x

Mehta, M. A., Sahakian, B. J., Mavaddat, N., Pickard, J. D., and Robbins, T. W. (2001). "Comparative psychopharmacology of methylpyhenidate and related drugs in human volunteers, patients with ADHD and experimental animals," in *Stimulant Drugs and ADHD: Basic and Clinical Neuroscience.*, eds M. V. A. Solanto, A. F. T. Arnsten and F. X. Castellanos (New York: Oxford University Press), 303–331.

Minzenberg, M. J., and Carter, C. S. (2008). Modafinil: a review of neurochemical actions and effects on cognition. *Neuropsychopharmacology* 33, 1477–1502. doi: 10.1038/sj.npp.1301534

Müller, U., Steffenhagen, N., Regenthal, R., and Bublak, P. (2004). Effects of modafinil on working memory processes in humans. *Psychopharmacology (Berl)* 177, 161–169. doi: 10.1007/s00213-004-1926-3

Newman, L. A., and McGaughy, J. (2011). Adolescent rats show cognitive rigidity in a test of attentional set shifting. *Dev. Psychobiol.* 53, 391–401. doi: 10.1002/dev.20537

O'Connor, A. (2004). *Wakefulness Finds a Powerful Ally.* New York: The New York Times.

Ogier, M., Wang, H., Hong, E., Wang, Q., Greenberg, M. E., and Katz, D. M. (2007). Brain-derived neurotrophic factor expression and respiratory function improve after ampakine treatment in a mouse model of Rett syndrome. *J. Neurosci.* 27, 10912–10917. doi: 10.1523/jneurosci.1869-07.2007

Otter, M., and Nurmand, L. B. (1980). Seasonal fluctuations in the catecholamine content in the brain of white rats. *Biull. Eksp. Biol. Med.* 89, 215–217.

Pang, T. Y. C., and Hannan, A. J. (2013). Enhancement of cognitive function in models of brain disease through environmental enrichment and physical activity. *Neuropharmacology* 64, 515–528. doi: 10.1016/j.neuropharm.2012.06.029

Paoletti, P., Bellone, C., and Zhou, Q. (2013). NMDA receptor subunit diversity: impact on receptor properties, synaptic plasticity and disease. *Nat. Rev. Neurosci.* 14, 383–400. doi: 10.1038/nrn3504

Petrović, V. M., Maksimović, K., and Davidović, V. (1980). Chemical sympathectomy and diurnal fluctuations of noradrenaline calorigenic action in the rat. *Arch. Int. Physiol. Biochim.* 88, 273–276. doi: 10.3109/13813458009104866

Pietrzak, R. H., Mollica, C. M., Maruff, P., and Snyder, P. J. (2006). Cognitive effects of immediate-release methylphenidate in children with attention-deficit/hyperactivity disorder. *Neurosci. Biobehav. Rev.* 30, 1225–1245. doi: 10.1016/j.neubiorev.2006.10.002

Ragan, C. I., Bard, I., and Singh, I. (2013). What should we do about student use of cognitive enhancers? An analysis of current evidence. *Neuropharmacology* 64, 588–595. doi: 10.1016/j.neuropharm.2012.06.016

Randall, D. C., Shneerson, J. M., and File, S. E. (2005a). Cognitive effects of modafinil in student volunteers may depend on IQ. *Pharmacol. Biochem. Behav.* 82, 133–139. doi: 10.1016/j.pbb.2005.07.019

Randall, D. C., Viswanath, A., Bharania, P., Elsabagh, S. M., Hartley, D. E., Shneerson, J. M., et al. (2005b). Does modafinil enhance cognitive performance in young volunteers who are not sleep-deprived? *J. Clin. Psychopharmacol.* 25, 175–179. doi: 10.1097/01.jcp.0000155816.21467.25

Rao, Y., Liu, Z. W., Borok, E., Rabenstein, R. L., Shanabrough, M., Lu, M., et al. (2007). Prolonged wakefulness induces experience-dependent synaptic plasticity in mouse hypocretin/orexin neurons. *J. Clin. Invest.* 117, 4022–4033. doi: 10.1172/jci32829

Rapoport, J. L., Buchsbaum, M. S., Zahn, T. P., Weingartner, H., Ludlow, C., and Mikkelsen, E. J. (1978). Dextroamphetamine: cognitive and behavioral effects in normal prepubertal boys. *Science* 199, 560–563. doi: 10.1126/science.341313

Rapoport, J. L. B., Buchsbaum, M. S., Weingartner, H., Zahn, T. P., Ludlow, C., and Mikkelsen, E. J. (1980). Dextroamphetamine- its cognitive and behavioral effects in normal and hyperactive boys and normal men. *Arch. Gen. Psychiatry* 37, 933–943. doi: 10.1001/archpsyc.1980.01780210091010

Rasetti, R., Mattay, V. S., Stankevich, B., Skjei, K., Blasi, G., Sambataro, F., et al. (2010). Modulatory effects of modafinil on neural circuits regulating emotion and cognition. *Neuropsychopharmacology* 35, 2101–2109. doi: 10.1038/npp.2010.83

Roesler, R., and Schröder, N. (2011). Cognitive enhancers: focus on modulatory signaling influencing memory consolidation. *Pharmacol. Biochem. Behav.* 99, 155–163. doi: 10.1016/j.pbb.2010.12.028

Rueda, J. R., Ballesteros, J., and Tejada, M. I. (2009). Systematic review of pharmacological treatments in fragile X syndrome. *BMC Neurol.* 9:53. doi: 10.1186/1471-2377-9-53

Saletan, W. (2008). Night of the living meds: the US military's sleep-reduction program, slate magazine. *The Slate Group.* Accessed 11-1-2013. http://www.slate.com/articles/health_and_science/human_nature/2008/07/night_of_the_living_meds.html

Selemon, L. D. (2013). A role for synaptic plasticity in the adolescent development of executive function. *Transl. Psychiatry* 3:e238. doi: 10.1038/tp.2013.7

Sharma, V. (2011). Pilot pill project, pruneMirror.in. Accessed 10-22-2013. http://www.punemirror.in/article/2/20110216201102160633164458771 4a65/Pilot-pill-project.html

Silverman, J. L., Oliver, C. F., Karras, M. N., Gastrell, P. T., and Crawley, J. N. (2013). AMPAKINE enhancement of social interaction in the BTBR mouse model of autism. *Neuropharmacology* 64, 268–282. doi: 10.1016/j.neuropharm.2012.07.013

Simmons, D. A., Rex, C. S., Palmer, L., Pandyarajan, V., Fedulov, V., Gall, C. M., et al. (2009). Up-regulating BDNF with an ampakine rescues synaptic plasticity and memory in Huntington's disease knockin mice. *Proc. Natl. Acad. Sci. U S A* 106, 4906–4911. doi: 10.1073/pnas.0811228106

Spencer-Smith, M., and Anderson, V. (2009). Healthy and abnormal development of the prefrontal cortex. *Dev. Neurorehabil.* 12, 279–297. doi: 10.3109/17518420903090701

Spiller, H. A., Borys, D., Griffith, J. R., Klein-Schwartz, W., Aleguas, A., Sollee, D., et al. (2009). Toxicity from modafinil ingestion. *Clin. Toxicol. (Phila)* 47, 153–156. doi: 10.1080/15563650802175595

Spiller, H. A., Hays, H. L., and Aleguas, A. Jr. (2013). Overdose of drugs for attention-deficit hyperactivity disorder: clinical presentation, mechanisms of toxicity and management. *CNS Drugs* 27, 531–543. doi: 10.1007/s40263-013-0084-8

Stoll, R. G. M. E., and Griesel, D. (2007). Cortex's AMPAKINE CX717 toxicoloy data package submitted to the FDA, cortex pharmaceuticals.

Sullivan, S. S. (2012). Current treatment of selected pediatric sleep disorders. *Neurotherapeutics* 9, 791–800. doi: 10.1007/s13311-012-0149-2

Taylor, G. P. Jr., and Keys, R. E. (2003). *Modafinil and Management of Aircrew Fatigue.* Washington, DC: United States Department of the Air Force.

Teffer, K., and Semendeferi, K. (2012). Human prefrontal cortex: evolution, development, and pathology. *Prog. Brain Res.* 195, 191–218. doi: 10.1016/B978-0-444-53860-4.00009-X

Turner, D. C., Robbins, T. W., Clark, L., Aron, A. R., Dowson, J., and Sahakian, B. J. (2003). Cognitive enhancing effects of modafinil in healthy volunteers. *Psychopharmacology (Berl)* 165, 260–269. doi: 10.1007/s00213-002-1250-8

Urban, K. R., and Gao, W. J. (2012). Evolution of the study of methylphenidate and its actions on the adult versus juvenile brain. *J. Atten. Disord.* 24, 65–74. doi: 10.1177/1087054712455504

Urban, K. R., and Gao, W.-J. (2013). Methylphenidate and the juvenile brain: enhancement of attention at the expense of cortical plasticity? *Med. Hypotheses* 81, 988–994. doi: 10.1016/j.mehy.2013.09.009

Urban, K. R., Li, Y. C., and Gao, W. J. (2013). Treatment with a clinically-relevant dose of methylphenidate alters NMDA receptor composition and synaptic plasticity in the juvenile rat prefrontal cortex. *Neurobiol. Learn. Mem.* 101, 65–74. doi: 10.1016/j.nlm.2013.01.004

Urban, K. R., Waterhouse, B. D., and Gao, W. J. (2012). Distinct age-dependent effects of methylphenidate on developing and adult prefrontal neurons. *Biol. Psychiatry* 72, 880–888. doi: 10.1016/j.biopsych.2012.04.018

U. S. Air Force. (2013). Joining the air force-enlisted overview. Accessed 10-22-2013. http://www.airforce.com/joining-the-air-force/enlisted-overview/

Wang, H., Stradtman, G. G. 3rd., Wang, X. J., and Gao, W. J. (2008). A specialized NMDA receptor function in layer 5 recurrent microcircuitry of the adult rat prefrontal cortex. *Proc. Natl. Acad. Sci. U S A* 105, 16791–16796. doi: 10.1073/pnas.0804318105

Wang, M., Yang, Y., Wang, C.-J., Gamo, N. J., Jin, L. E., Mazer, J. A., et al. (2013). NMDA receptors subserve persistent neuronal firing during working memory in dorsolateral prefrontal cortex. *Neuron* 77, 736–749. doi: 10.1016/j.neuron.2012.12.032

Wezenberg, E., Verkes, R. J., Ruigt, G. S., Hulstijn, W., and Sabbe, B. G. (2007). Acute effects of the ampakine farampator on memory and information processing in healthy elderly volunteers. *Neuropsychopharmacology* 32, 1272–1283. doi: 10.1038/sj.npp.1301257

Wheeler, B. (2006). *UK Army Tested "Stay Awake" Pills.* London: BBC News.

Willie, J. T., Renthal, W., Chemelli, R. M., Miller, M. S., Scammell, T. E., Yanagisawa, M., et al. (2005). Modafinil more effectively induces wakefulness in orexin-null mice than in wild-type littermates. *Neuroscience* 130, 983–995. doi: 10.1016/j.neuroscience.2004.10.005

Xu, Z., Chen, R. Q., Gu, Q. H., Yan, J. Z., Wang, S. H., Liu, S. Y., et al. (2009). Metaplastic regulation of long-term potentiation/long-term depression threshold by activity-dependent changes of NR2A/NR2B ratio. *J. Neurosci.* 29, 8764–8773. doi: 10.1523/jneurosci.1014-09.2009

Zolkowska, D., Jain, R., Rothman, R. B., Partilla, J. S., Roth, B. L., Setola, V., et al. (2009). Evidence for the involvement of dopamine transporters in behavioral stimulant effects of modafinil. *J. Pharmacol. Exp. Ther.* 329, 738–746. doi: 10.1124/jpet.108.146142

20

A little elastic for a better performance: kinesiotaping of the motor effector modulates neural mechanisms for rhythmic movements

Riccardo Bravi[1], Eros Quarta[1], Erez J. Cohen[1], Anna Gottard[2] and Diego Minciacchi[1]*

[1] Department of Experimental and Clinical Medicine, University of Florence, Florence, Italy
[2] Department of Statistics, Informatics, Applications, University of Florence, Florence, Italy

Edited by:
Mikhail Lebedev, Duke University, USA

Reviewed by:
Peter Praamstra, Radboud University Nijmegen, Netherlands
Yuri P. Ivanenko, IRCCS Fondazione Santa Lucia, Italy

***Correspondence:**
Diego Minciacchi, Department of Experimental and Clinical Medicine, University of Florence, Viale Morgagni 63, Florence I-50134, Italy
e-mail: diego@unifi.it

A rhythmic motor performance is brought about by an integration of timing information with movements. Investigations on the millisecond time scale distinguish two forms of time control, event-based timing and emergent timing. While event-based timing asserts the existence of a central internal timekeeper for the control of repetitive movements, the emergent timing perspective claims that timing emerges from dynamic control of nontemporal movements parameters. We have recently demonstrated that the precision of an isochronous performance, defined as performance of repeated movements having a uniform duration, was insensible to auditory stimuli of various characteristics (Bravi et al., 2014). Such finding has led us to investigate whether the application of an elastic therapeutic tape (Kinesio® Tex taping; KTT) used for treating athletic injuries and a variety of physical disorders, is able to reduce the timing variability of repetitive rhythmic movement. Young healthy subjects, tested with and without KTT, have participated in sessions in which sets of repeated isochronous wrist's flexion-extensions (IWFEs) were performed under various auditory conditions and during their recall. Kinematics was recorded and temporal parameters were extracted and analyzed. Our results show that the application of KTT decreases the variability of rhythmic movements by a 2-fold effect: on the one hand KTT provides extra proprioceptive information activating cutaneous mechanoreceptors, on the other KTT biases toward the emergent timing thus modulating the processes for rhythmic movements. Therefore, KTT appears able to render movements less audio dependent by relieving, at least partially, the central structures from time control and making available more resources for an augmented performance.

Keywords: sensory-motor integration, timing, isochronous movements, auditory imagery, music

INTRODUCTION

Considerable evidence suggest that the study of human motor rhythmic performance synchronized to auditory stimuli is useful in unraveling neural aspects of action timing. The effects of different types of audio information (i.e., metronome or music) on motor performance have been extensively investigated in studies of finger tapping (Repp, 1999a,b; del Olmo and Cudeiro, 2005) and of gait (see Wittwer et al., 2013). The interest for the effects of paced auditory stimuli on rhythmic activities stems from the proven notion that this design of sensorimotor integration is shown to be an effective tool for gross motor rehabilitation in neurological diseases by improving spatial-temporal parameters and decreasing temporal variability (Thaut et al., 1996; McIntosh et al., 1997; del Olmo and Cudeiro, 2005; del Olmo et al., 2006; Hausdorff et al., 2007; Arias and Cudeiro, 2008; de Dreu et al., 2012).

In a recent study we showed how do auditory stimuli with distinct characteristics, streams of clicks or excerpts of music, influence the precision of repeated isochronous wrist's flexion-extensions (IWFEs), performed with no direct surface opposition and minimizing visual information (Bravi et al., 2014). Some reports have described a reduction of temporal variability for rhythmic movements in the presence of paced auditory stimuli. Our data, however, displayed clearly that when both tactile and visual information are minimized, the listening alone to paced auditory stimuli does not improve the precision of an isochronous performance. Also, in a previous study on timing of rhythmic movements a lack of reduction in temporal variability was observed during paced tapping when compared to unpaced tapping (Schlerf et al., 2007). These findings have prompted us to investigate other tools that might augment the precision of rhythmic movement.

In addition, investigations on the millisecond time scale distinguish two forms of time control, explicit timing and implicit

Abbreviations: bpm, beats per minute; Cl, while listening to a stream of clicks; Cl2, after 2 min from the end of the Cl condition; CVs, coefficients of variation; Fr, free, in absence of auditory information; IWFEs, isochronous wrist's flexion-extensions; KTT, Kinesio® Tex taping; Mu, while listening to an excerpt of music; Mu2, after 2 min from the end of the Mu condition; N/KTT, no KTT; w$\gamma(1)$, windowed lag-one autocorrelations.

timing, later renamed as event-based timing and emergent timing, respectively, (Spencer and Ivry, 2005). Event-based timing has evolved from the information processing approach, asserting the existence of internal timekeepers for motor control, and is well represented by the two-level model proposed by Wing and Kristofferson (1973a,b). According to the Wing and Kristofferson model, temporal precision in a self-paced tapping is limited by variability in the central timekeeper and by variability arising from the peripheral motor system (Semjen et al., 2000). The emergent timing perspective is derived from the dynamic systems theory, claiming that there are no representational clocks (Kugler et al., 1980; Kelso, 1995) and that timing emerges from dynamic control of nontemporal movements parameters (Schoner, 2002; Huys et al., 2008) such as stiffness which is playing a major role for determining movement frequency (Turvey, 1977; Delignières et al., 2004). For the study of timing, the task most widely employed was the performance of repeated movements. Among the rhythmic motor tasks, tapping is thought to be under the control of the event-based timing while circle drawing is thought to be under the control of the emergent timing (Zelaznik et al., 2002). Air tapping, a motor task performed in the air with no surface contact, represents a more recent approach for the study of timing. This motor task possesses specific characteristics of both the event-based and emergently motor rhythmic tasks due to the presence of salient motor events and smooth effector trajectories (Delignières and Torre, 2011).

The participation of the cerebellum in timing was once a controversial issue (Leiner et al., 1993; Rao et al., 2001). To date, the cerebellar timing hypothesis, first formulated by Keele and Ivry (1990), is widely accepted. According to this hypothesis, the cerebellum functions as an internal timing device in the milliseconds range for both motor and non-motor processes (Ivry and Spencer, 2004). In particular, the involvement of the inferior olive and the climbing fiber system in timing was shown to take part in encoding temporal information independent of motor behavior (Xu et al., 2006). Investigations using rhythmic tapping tasks have provided evidences to support this hypothesis. In a study on individuals with unilateral cerebellar lesions, participants were asked to perform timed tapping, intermittent circle drawing, and continuous circle drawing tasks. Performances were impaired only when tasks were executed with the ipsilesional hand and involved movements theorized to require event-based but not emergent timing (Spencer et al., 2003).

The timing mode of rhythmic movements can change over time within a single task (Studenka and Zelaznik, 2008; Zelaznik and Rosenbaum, 2010; Delignières and Torre, 2011). The discrete or continuous character of movements performed in the rhythmic tasks is considered to be a key factor for the involvement of the event-based or the emergent timing mode (Robertson et al., 1999; Huys et al., 2008). In addition, neurophysiological and neuroanatomical studies provided bases to suggest that neural circuits are not completely independent of the timing functions. For discrete movements, it is proposed that explicit processes for timing arise as coordinated activity in the core striatal and olivo-cerebellar networks that are interconnected, with each other and with the cerebral cortex, through multiple synaptic pathways (Spencer et al., 2007; Teki et al., 2012). Conversely continuous movements, by nature, lack an event structure. For these movements timing may be achieved through the control of a secondary variable, such as angular velocity, which does not involve the cerebellum.

Kinesio® Tex Tape is an elastic cotton strip with an acrylic adhesive developed by Japanese chiropractor, Dr. Kenso Kase, in the 1970's (Kase et al., 2013). Kinesio® Tex taping (KTT) is a kinesthetic method commonly used in clinical practice for treating athletic injuries and a variety of physical disorders, with the purpose of mimicking the thickness and flexibility of the skin (Morris et al., 2013). It is claimed that the application of KTT causes micro convolutions, or folds, in the skin; it brings about a lifting of the skin away from the tissue beneath, favoring the release of pressure from tender tissues underneath and providing space for lymphatic fluid movement (Morris et al., 2013).

It was proposed that KTT is able to enhance somatosensory inputs and influence proprioception through stimulation of cutaneous mechanoreceptors (Callaghan et al., 2002; Kneeshaw, 2002; Halseth et al., 2004). We have, therefore, chosen KTT as a tool for possibly augmenting the precision of rhythmic movements. While little is known about the potential proprioceptive effect of KTT, the stimulation of cutaneous mechanoreceptors is believed to be induced by the pressure and stretching effect provoked by KTT application on the skin (Grigg, 1994).

In the current study we investigate whether the application of KTT on skin is able to reduce the timing variability of repetitive rhythmic movements. We also attempt to understand whether a causal relationship subsists between such reduction and functional augmentation of central structures involved, brought about by relieving, at least partially, these structures from time control.

We thus performed an experiment in which subjects, tested with and without KTT, participated in sessions in which sets of repeated IWFEs were performed under different conditions (i.e., without audio information, with paced audio in the form of clicks or music, and in the recall conditions; see Bravi et al., 2014). Our IWFEs performed with no direct surface opposition and while minimizing visual information, could potentially employ, as air finger tapping movements, both event-based and emergent timing processes. Participants were not instructed about the way to perform the IWFEs since it was showed that in the absence of specific instructions, the production of movements with no contact surface elicits alternatively different timing modes (Delignières and Torre, 2011).

We hypothesize that KTT, due to its aforementioned characteristics, is able to cause an improvement of the wrist joint proprioception due to augmented afferent input via the stimulation of cutaneous mechanoreceptors (Riemann and Lephart, 2002). The improvement in wrist joint proprioception would stabilize the motor effector during the performance, causing the IWFEs to be less discrete and thus smoother. Consequently this would entail the shifting from an event-based to emergent process to control the production of the IWFEs (Spencer et al., 2007; Huys et al., 2008). Therefore, by relieving, at least partially, the central structures from timing control, KTT would release resources and allow for a net augmentation of the central efficiency and, consequently, reduce the timing variability of IWFEs.

MATERIALS AND METHODS

PARTICIPANTS

A group of 25 right-handed volunteers (21 males, ages 20–27, mean 24.1 ± 2.4 years; 4 females, ages 18–27, mean 23.0 ± 2.7 years) took part in the recording sessions. All participants were naive to the purpose of the study; they were neither musically trained nor listeners of a classical music repertoire, and reported no auditory, motor, or other neurological impairments. The experimental protocol conformed to the requirements of the Federal Policy for the Protection of Human Subjects (U.S. Office of Science and Technology Policy) and of the Declaration of Helsinki, and has been approved by the Research Ethics Board of our Institution (Local Ethics Committee, Azienda Ospedaliero Universitaria Careggi, Florence, Italy). All participants provided an informed consent in written form.

SET UP

Each subject was tested individually, sitting upright on a chair with the legs comfortably positioned on leg-rest (**Figure 1A**). The participant's right forearm was placed on the armrest, in a relaxed horizontal position. The wrist and hand of the subject were free to move in mid-air with no direct opposition, thus minimizing tactile information. In order to reduce possible interference of visual information, the subject was requested to wear a blindfold. Environmental noise was reduced by the use of headphones (K 240 Studio, AKG Acoustics GmbH, Wien, AT), which were also used for the clean delivery of audio information. This setup was designed to minimize all information that is known to influence motor strategies (i.e., visual, tactile, and environmental noise) and that may result in a different motor performance (Bove et al., 2009; Saijo and Gomi, 2010). A triaxial accelerometer (ADXL330, Analog Devices Inc., Norwood, MA 02062) was placed on the dorsal aspect of the hand, over the proximal part of the 2nd–3rd metacarpal bones. The sensor, placed in a small pocket, was kept in position by an elastic band and secured by a Velcro strap. Sensor output was acquired and digitized at 200 Hz through PCI-6071E (12-Bit E Series Multifunction DAQ, National Instruments, Austin, TX, USA).

STIMULI

Audio stimuli were paced streams of clicks and excerpts of music. Music excerpts of 60 s duration were extracted from original professional productions. Selected fragments had a simple and explicit rhythmic structure and a tempo that remained constant throughout time. Music fragments were taken from musical styles popular among young people: rock, techno, dance, trance, hard rock, and film music. Three musical experts (professionals with musical experience) were asked to verify independently the tempo of the excerpts in order to be as accurate and sure as possible in the choice of unambiguous paced excerpts. It is known that the determination of perceptual musical tempo can be ambiguous (McKinney and Moelants, 2007) and that algorithms for music tempo extraction have several limitations (McKinney et al., 2007), although recent effort has been put into methods to possibly improve the evaluation metrics used for automatic tempo estimation (Levy, 2011). Only fragments for which the experts collectively agreed of having a single musical tempo were selected.

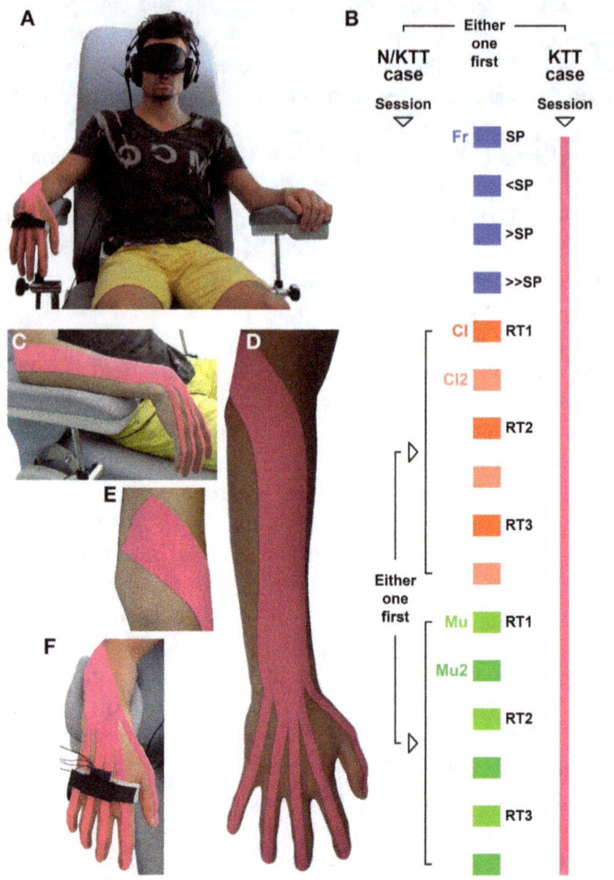

FIGURE 1 | (A) The subject is seated on a chair with armrests, wearing an eye-mask and headphones. The triaxial accelerometer is placed over the 2nd–3rd metacarpal bones. Subject is asked to perform sets of IWFEs. **(B)** The two sessions, one with N/KTT and one with KTT (color-coded in pink) are designed to record first IWFEs in condition free from auditory information (in the absence of auditory information, free = Fr, self-paced = SP; slower than SP = <SP; faster than SP = >SP; faster than >SP = >>SP) and then in conditions related to clicks (during the listening of clicks = Cl; recall after 2 min from the end of the Cl condition = Cl2; one block consisting of three pairs of Cl and Cl2 sets performed at three different reference tempi: RT1, RT2, and RT3) followed by those related to music (during the listening of music = Mu; recall after 2 min from the end of the Mu condition = Mu2; one block consisting of three pairs Mu and Mu2 sets performed at three different reference tempi: RT1, RT2, and RT3), or vice versa. In this and in the following figures the conditions and associated results are color-coded. **(C)** KTT was placed between the lateral epicondyle of the humerus and phalanges, at the position of maximum flexion. **(D)** KTT was applied over the extensor carpi ulnaris, extensor carpi radialis longus and brevis, extensor digitorum, extensor indicis, extensor digiti minimi, and extensor pollicis longus. **(E)** Proximally, KTT was placed from 5 cm proximal to muscles insertion. **(F)** Each branch of tape was applied down on the back of phalanx until the nail. As in the N/KTT set up, the accelerometer was placed on the dorsal aspect of the hand, over the proximal part of the 2nd–3rd metacarpal bones, into a pocket kept in position by an elastic band and secured by a Velcro strap.

All chosen fragments had small tempo variations due to live performance. Therefore, the tempo for each fragment was analyzed, beat-mapped, and set to fixed beats per minute (bpm, used as a measure of tempo in music) using the softwares Jackson (http://vanaeken.com/; accuracy is within a 0.001 bpm margin) and Audacity (GNU/GPL, http://audacity.sourceforge.net/). Our time manipulations were all well below 5% deviation of the mean music tempo (professional performances have minimal deviations from mean tempo; Dannenberg and Mohan, 2011) and thus below the detection threshold for temporal changes in music (Ellis, 1991; Madison and Paulin, 2010). We didn't use fragments likely to be familiar to the listeners since it has been shown that high familiarity with a song installs an accurate long-term memory of its tempo (Levitin and Cook, 1996; Quinn and Watt, 2006). Streams of clicks of 60 s duration were produced using the audio editor Audacity, via the Generate Click Track function. The duration of an individual click was set to 10 ms and the click sound was set to white noise. The music and clicks stimuli were set to eight reference tempi ranging from 64 to 176 bpm (937.21 to 340.95 ms, **Table 1**). The same eight tempi were chosen for both streams of clicks and excerpts of music. Audio files were all normalized to −0.3 dB as the highest peak and stored as waveform (waveform audio file; 44.1 kHz; 16-bit depth) using Audacity. Fade in and fade out (10 ms) were placed at the beginning and end of each file. Audio stimuli were presented binaurally to the subjects through headphones (**Figure 1A**).

DATA FORMAT

Subjects were asked to perform sets of IWFEs and kinematic parameters were evaluated. Data from the sensor were stored and an off-line analysis of raw data from the triaxial accelerometer was implemented. The signal extracted from the accelerometer presented a minimum when the wrist reached the maximum flexion and a maximum when it reached the maximum extension. The duration of a single wrist's flexion-extension (i.e., IWFE duration) was calculated as the difference between two consecutive flexion-extension minima (custom software developed in Matlab®). To avoid initial and final transients, the first and last 5 s of each recording were excluded from analysis (Repp, 2005, 2011). Considering that tempi of the recorded IWFEs sets were remarkably variable, giving rise to a quantitative redundancy of tempi obtained in overall, we have decided to rank them as ranges (**Table 1**). IWFEs sets were then assigned to a defined range according to their tempo.

SESSION

Each subject had participated in two sessions, one with no KTT (N/KTT) and one with KTT (**Figure 1B**), that were performed at a week's distance. The order in which subjects performed the N/KTT or KTT sessions were set to obtain equivalent number of subjects that played first one or the other. The KTT session started approximately 10 min after mounting the tape since this interval is needed to overcome perception of tape on the skin (Kase et al., 2013). In each session the subject performed 16 sets of repeated IWFEs under various conditions. A single session was comprised of a baseline recording (4 sets) and 2 blocks (12 sets). In a single session the performance of the IWFEs sets was executed under five conditions: in absence of auditory information (free, Fr), while listening to a stream of clicks (Cl), after 2 min from the end of the Cl condition (Cl2), while listening to an excerpt of music (Mu), after 2 min from the end of the Mu condition (Mu2). Sets of IWFEs were recorded in all conditions. For each block IWFEs sets were performed using one type of auditory stimulus (Cl or Mu). One block consisted of three pairs of Cl and Cl2 sets, or Mu and Mu2 sets, performed at three different reference tempi, for the auditory Cl or Mu sets; the same tempi were then used for the auditory sets of the second block (**Figure 1B**). The order in which the clicks or music stimuli were presented was set to obtain equivalent number of subjects that received first one or the other.

The subject was instructed to restrain from listening to music during the day of the session. Each session began with instructions on how the sets of wrist's flexion-extensions were to be performed, followed by a short practice test. During the practice test, IWFEs were recorded and evaluated to assess whether the instructions were understood; after the practice test, the subject was asked if he/she felt comfortable with the task. Recordings from the practice test were not used for further analyses. The session started with recording in the Fr condition, which consisted of four IWFEs sets. In the first set, the subject was asked to perform IWFEs in a self-paced manner. In the second set, the subject was asked to perform IWFEs slower than those of the first set. In the third and fourth sets, the subject was asked to perform IWFEs faster than first recording and then faster than the third recording. The subject was then instructed to perform a set of repetitive IWFEs while listening to clicks or music at a similar pace concurrently with the tempo of the delivered audio

Table 1 | Musical names, ranking, and tempo equivalences between ranges of movement durations in Hertz and milliseconds.

Musical names	Rank	Tempo equivalences					
		Ranges (Hz)			Ranges (ms)		
		Reference	From	To	Reference	From	To
Adagio	1	1.067	1.017	1.133	937.21	983.28	882.61
Andante	2	1.333	1.283	1.400	750.19	779.42	714.29
	3	1.600	1.550	1.667	625.00	645.16	599.88
Moderato	4	1.867	1.817	1.933	535.62	550.36	517.33
	5	2.133	2.083	2.200	468.82	480.08	454.55
Allegro	6	2.400	2.350	2.467	416.67	425.53	405.35
	7	2.700	2.617	2.800	370.37	382.12	357.14
Presto	8	2.933	2.817	3.000	340.95	354.99	333.33

(i.e., maintaining an in-phase 1:1 relationship between repeated wrist's flexion-extensions and the tempo of the audio, conditions Cl or Mu). Then, instructions to subject for IWFEs performances in recalls were of the kind: "now, try to hear in your head the auditory stimulus just heard" (immediately after the end of the stimulus, see Zatorre and Halpern, 2005). After a 2 min break, the subject was asked to perform IWFEs as accurately as possible at the tempo of the auditory stimulus just heard while concurrently hearing mentally the stimulus itself (conditions Cl2 or Mu2). The session continued with the recordings of IWFEs in a reversed order (i.e., with the Mu conditions if Cl was recorded first, or vice versa). In order to obtain a balanced number of performances for the eight chosen reference tempi, the three tempi that were selected for the blocks were randomized for each single session.

KINESIO® TEX TAPE APPLICATION

The Kinesio® Tex Tape is comprised of a polymer elastic strand wrapped by 100% cotton fibers. It allow for a longitudinal stretch of 55–60% of its resting length. The Kinesio® Tex Tape is applied to the paper substrate with 25% of tension; the adhesive is 100% acrylic (Kase et al., 2013). For the KTT (Kinesio® Tex Gold™ FP—2″ Red) application the subject, already seated on the chair with own right forearm rested on the armrest, was asked to keep the wrist in a position of maximum flexion, and the distance between the lateral epicondyle of the humerus and the distal end of the third phalanx of the middle finger was measured. The purpose was to apply the tape over the open kinetic chain including wrist, metacarpal, and finger joints. During the application of KTT, between the lateral epicondyle of the humerus and phalanges, the wrist and forearm were maintained in full flexion and full pronation, respectively (**Figure 1C**). After manually assessing the origin and insertion of muscles, KTT was applied over the extensor carpi ulnaris, extensor carpi radialis longus and brevis, extensor digitorum, extensor indicis, extensor digiti minimi, and extensor pollicis longus (**Figures 1D–F**). The strip of Kinesio® Tex was cut 5 cm longer than the maximum length of the kinetic chain measured with the wrist in maximum flexion (Kase et al., 2013). The course of the tendons of the extensor muscles (for each finger) was then identified on the back of subject's hand and distances were measured between the distal end of each phalanx and the wrist. Measurements were used to cut the distal side of the elastic band into five branches to be placed over the metacarpal area and fingers following the course of the tendons. KTT was then applied from 5 cm proximal to muscles insertion to facilitate muscle function; the application tension was light, about 25%. From the lateral humeral epicondyle, KTT was applied—in a wave-like pattern—to wrap the wrist's extensors until reaching the wrist. Each branch was then applied down on the back of phalanx until the nail.

STATISTICAL ANALYSIS

To model directly the observed IWFEs durations we adopted random effect ANOVA models for repeated measurements (Pinheiro and Bates, 2000; Diggle et al., 2002). Separate models were adopted for different kinds of conditions and also the response variable was chosen differently according to the presence of audio. In particular, the differences between observed and the expected IWFEs durations were considered as response variable for performances under audio (Cl and Mu) and recall (Cl2 and Mu2) conditions. This response variable measures the error observed in the IWFEs durations, the observed IWFEs duration was instead considered as the response variable for performances in the Fr condition. As the response variables have been recorded several times for each performance and for each individual, a random effect part had to be included to take into account the lack of independence among the observations. Typically, in the random effect ANOVA models adopted for the analyses, the main effects concern the effect of the overall mean of the absence/presence of KTT (N/KTT vs. KTT) and of the tempo (fast if <517.33 ms, slow otherwise). The random effect part of the ANOVA models was specified in order to separately measure the variability within individuals and within performances. Moreover, the residual variance among observations, once taken into account for the main fixed and the random effects, was further modeled to take into account possible residual heteroscedasticity.

Moreover, in order to evaluate the precision of IWFEs, we used coefficients of variation (CVs = standard deviation/mean × 100). CVs of IWFEs durations were used to investigate whether the KTT influences the precision of IWFEs performances under different conditions and, if not indicated otherwise, are to be considered as the condition's and the range's means.

Lag-one autocorrelation analysis is used as statistical signature to investigate the processes for temporal regulation. It is assumed (see Wing and Kristofferson, 1973a,b) that series of produced time intervals regulated by the event-based process should have negative lag-one autocorrelation values (between -0.5 and 0). Conversely, emergent timing is characterized by positive lag-one autocorrelation values (between 0 and 0.5). To study the influence of KTT in the Cl and Cl2 conditions we computed series of windowed lag-one autocorrelations $w\gamma(1)$ (Delignières and Torre, 2011) for each set of IWFEs. Each windowed autocorrelation coefficient was computed as the mean of a set of 30 autocorrelations. Moving the set along the sequence, a series of windowed autocorrelation coefficients was computed for each performance, measuring autoregressive linear dependency within the IWFEs. Then, we calculated the mean of the obtained windowed lag series for each performance. We considered the mean $w\gamma(1)$ as an estimator of overall dependence in the performance. Furthermore, we calculated the percentage of positive and negative windowed $w\gamma(1)$ values for each performance. If not indicated otherwise, the mean of $w\gamma(1)$ and the percentage of positive and negative $w\gamma(1)$ are to be considered as the condition's and the range's means. To analyze the observed $w\gamma(1)$ we adopted random effects ANOVA model for repeated measurements. In order to allow an appropriate use of parametric statistical tests, the Fisher's Z-transformation was used to normalize the distribution of autocorrelation coefficients (Nolte et al., 2004; Freyer et al., 2012).

RESULTS

TIMING VARIABILITY

Examples of our datasets are illustrated in **Figure 2** as parallel box plots, for the Mu and Mu2 conditions. It is interesting to note that pairs of N/KTT—KTT plots are relatively analogous when compared for slow ($\geq$517.33 ms) or fast ($<$517.33 ms) movements durations. Also, it is easily appreciable that while median, upper and lower hinges and whiskers are visibly similar for pairs of N/KTT—KTT parallel box plots in the slow and fast collections of movements durations, the position and especially number of outside values is reduced when KTT is applied, with the lonely exception of a single far out value in the condition Mu2 for slow movements with KTT.

We estimated separate random effect ANOVA models for the different conditions: without audio information (Fr), with clicks (Cl), or music (Mu), and in the recall conditions (Cl2 and Mu2). The estimates for the main effects for the models in the two audio conditions Cl and Mu are reported in **Table 2**, together with their *p*-values and confidence intervals. As aforementioned, for these models the response variable is the difference between the observed and the expected IWFEs durations. As can be seen in **Table 2**, the overall mean is negative and significant in both models. This implies that, under a slow stimulus, observed IWFEs durations are, on mean, shorter than expected. The effect of tempo (movement duration) is significant in both Cl and Mu conditions, correcting the mean error toward zero. Conversely, KTT has no significant effect on the mean error.

The parameters concerning the random effects are also of interest. These parameters specifically shape the variability of the response variable. All the parameters for the random effects reported in **Table 2** are significant according to the appropriate likelihood ratio test. Remarkably, the most relevant result concerns the fact that the residual variability resulted heterogeneous between N/KTT or KTT cases. The KTT-specific residual variances (usually called factor-specific residual variances, see Muthén, 1989; for details on random effects model for heterogeneous population) result significantly different (**Table 3**). **Table 3** reports the estimate of the ratio between the residual variance for N/KTT and KTT cases. Both in the case of Mu and of Cl stimuli, this ratio is significantly less than one, assessing that the presence of the tape significantly help to decrease the variability of the errors in IWFEs durations. In particular, residual variance for KTT cases is about 14% less of the variance for N/KTT cases in Cl and 8% less in Mu.

A similar model was adopted for the recalls Cl2 and Mu2, recorded 2 min after the audio stimuli (**Table 4**). In this second model, the main effects are the overall mean, the condition and the movement duration, and the absence or presence of KTT. None of the estimates are significant, suggesting that, on mean, there is no evidence of a systematic error in IWFEs durations when movements are performed during recalls of music or clicks, recalls of fast or slow audio stimuli, and recalls with N/KTT or KTT. Interestingly, the presence of KTT still helps to significantly reduce the residual variance of about 6% (**Table 3**). The

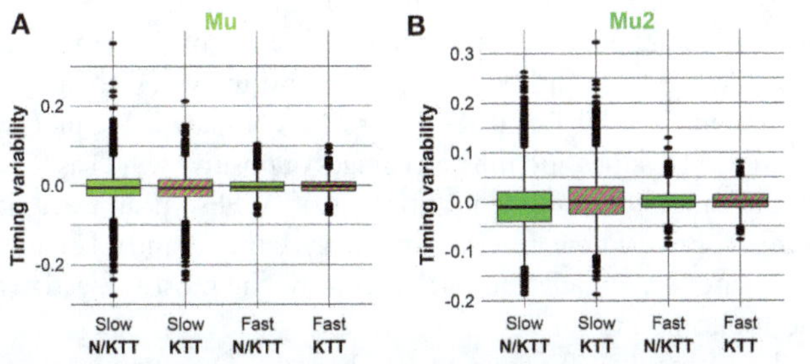

FIGURE 2 | (A,B) Box plots of the response variable, i.e., the difference between the observed and the expected interval durations, for datasets in the conditions Mu and Mu2, respectively. Pairs of N/KTT—KTT box plots are noticeably similar when compared for slow (≥517.33 ms) vs. fast (<517.33 ms) IWFEs durations. Also, easily appreciable is that the median, the upper and lower hinges and the whiskers are very similar for pairs of N/KTT—KTT parallel box plots in slow and fast collections of IWFEs durations. Conversely, the queues of the distributions are reduced when KTT is applied (the only exception is a single far out value in the condition Mu2 for slow IWFEs with KTT). KTT reduces the variability of IWFEs durations.

Table 3 | Factor specific residual variances (σ^2) for N/KTT vs. KTT movements.

Condition	N/KTT (σ^2)	KTT (σ^2)	N/KTT vs. KTT (*p*-value)
Cl	0.00076729	0.0006625549	< 0.0001
Mu	0.000772	0.000714	< 0.0001
Recalls (Cl2 and Mu2)	0.00085849	0.0008080108	< 0.0001
Fr	0.00082369	0.0007996383	0.005

Table 2 | Estimate, *p*-values (in parenthesis) and confidence intervals for model parameters in random effects ANOVA models for the Cl and Mu conditions.

	Cl		Mu	
Main fixed effects	**Estimate (*p*-value)**	**95% confidence interval**	**Estimate (*p*-value)**	**95% confidence interval**
Overall mean	−0.0063 (0.0000)	−0.0086; −0.0039	−0.0056 (0.0100)	−0.0099; −0.0013
Movement duration	0.0021 (0.0283)	0.0002; 0.0040	0.0042 (0.0401)	0.0002; 0.0083
N/KTT vs. KTT	−0.0009 (0.3349)	−0.0009; 0.0026	−0.0020 (0.3004)	−0.0058; 0.0018
Random effects	**Estimate**	**95% confidence interval**	**Estimate**	**95% confidence interval**
Within-individual SD	0.0045	0.0032; 0.0064	0.0066	0.0042; 0.0101
Within-set SD	0.0049	0.0042; 0.0057	0.0115	0.0101; 0.131
KTT residual variance ratio	0.8635	0.8440; 0.8835	0.9242	0.9036; 0.9452

Table 4 | Estimate, *p*-values (in parenthesis) and confidence intervals for model parameters in random effects ANOVA models for the Recalls and Fr conditions.

	Recalls (Cl2 and Mu2)		Fr	
Main fixed effects	**Estimate (*p*-value)**	**95% confidence interval**	**Estimate (*p*-value)**	**95% confidence interval**
Overall mean	−0.0014 (0.7492)	−0.0071; −0.0099	0.7218 (0.0000)	0.6865; 0.7571
Movement duration	−0.0034 (0.4347)	−0.0121; 0.0052	−0.3147 (0.0000)	−0.3571; −0.2723
N/KTT vs. KTT	0.0031 (0.4836)	−0.0055; 0.0117	0.0114 (0.5934)	−0.0306; 0.0533
Random effects	**Estimate**	**95% confidence interval**	**Estimate**	**95% confidence interval**
Within-individual SD	0.0031	1e-04; 0.0993	0.0127	1e-04; 1.2508
Within-set SD	0.0377	0.0347; 0.0410	0.1452	0.1306; 0.1614
KTT residual variance ratio	0.9412	0.9252; 0.9575	0.9708	0.9511; 0.9908

KTT residual variance ratio is estimated 0.9412 (95% confidence interval: 0.9252; 0.9575).

For the condition without audio stimulus (Fr), the model considers as the response variable directly the observed duration (**Table 4**). Consequently, the overall mean simply measures the mean movement duration chosen for performances of slow movements with N/KTT, while the main effect of movement duration measures the increment in bpm implied by a faster tempo. The overall mean and the main effect of tempo are then obviously significant by construction. The main effect of KTT is not significant. For this particular model, this result implies that individuals choose the tempo of the performance independently of the presence of the tape on their arm. Regarding the random part of the model, again it is worth to notice that the effect of the KTT in reducing the residual variability is still significant (**Table 3**). The residual variance, small but still present, is about the 3% less in KTT cases (estimate: 0.9708; 95% confidence interval: 0.9511; 0.9908).

The CV of IWFEs is used to normalize measures of temporal variability. We plotted the CVs of IWFEs as a function of the ranges of movement duration to visualize the rate dependent changes of the precision of isochronous performances and the interactions between these changes and the different experimental cases (N/KTT or KTT). The CVs of IWFEs, ranked per within-ranges of IWFEs durations, are illustrated in **Figure 3** for all conditions (**Figures 3A–E**). CVs values appear to change with movement duration. In particular, CVs of IWFEs become smaller as IWFEs become faster and, within the same condition and for the same range of movement duration, CVs values are very often smaller in KTT than in N/KTT cases. In **Figure 3F** the five within-condition CVs of IWFEs durations are compared for N/KTT and KTT cases. The CVs values of IWFEs are below 5% in all conditions and for both N/KTT and KTT cases. It is also noticeable that the within-condition CVs values are always smaller in KTT, when values for the same condition are compared, and that the difference is maximal for the condition Cl. Also, in **Figure 3G** are shown the percent reductions for the within-condition CVs in the case of KTT application. The percent reduction for the within-condition CVs values is maximal when IWFEs are performed while listening to an audio stimulus such as clicks (10.33%, for Cl). Impressively, a percent reduction for within-condition CVs values in KTT is visible in all other conditions (5.47%, for Mu; 4.03%, for Cl2; 5.96%, for Mu2; and 3.50%, for Fr; see **Figure 3G**).

THE PROCESSES FOR TEMPORAL REGULATION

To explore whether, and to what extent, the processes for temporal regulation are influenced by the application of KTT, the mean wγ(1) values and the percentages of positive wγ(1) of IWFEs computed in N/KTT and KTT cases are compared. We plot the mean wγ(1) values and the percentages of positive wγ(1) as function of ranges of movement durations of IWFEs. As an exemplar comparison, we here describe and analyze the Cl and Cl2 conditions since we already showed them to be the most subjective to the application of KTT.

The mean wγ(1) values of IWFEs ranked per within-ranges of movement durations are displayed in **Figure 4** for the N/KTT and KTT cases of the Cl and Cl2 conditions. In all cases mean wγ(1) values appear to change with movement durations. In the N/KTT case of the Cl condition (**Figure 4A**) mean wγ(1) values are almost all negative with only one exception in range 5 (for this and the following references to ranges of movement durations see **Table 1**) whereas in the KTT case of the Cl condition (**Figure 4A**) mean wγ(1) values are negative for only the half of eight ranges of movement durations. The highest peaks of mean wγ(1) values are expressed within the moderato, allegro and presto tempi in the last four ranges of interval durations (Cl of N/KTT) and in the last five ranges of movement durations (Cl of KTT).

In the N/KTT case of the Cl2 condition (**Figure 4B**) mean wγ(1) values are all negative with only one exception in range 6 whereas in the KTT case of the Cl2 condition (**Figure 4B**) mean wγ(1) values are positive for more than half of ranges of movement durations. The highest peaks of mean wγ(1) values for the Cl2 condition are expressed within the moderato, allegro and presto tempi in the last five ranges of movement durations in both N/KTT and KTT cases.

The percentages of positive and negative wγ(1) values ranked per within-ranges of movement durations are displayed in **Figure 5** as radar charts for the N/KTT and KTT cases of the Cl and Cl2 conditions. Here also, it appears evident that the percentage of positive wγ(1) values is sensitive to movement durations.

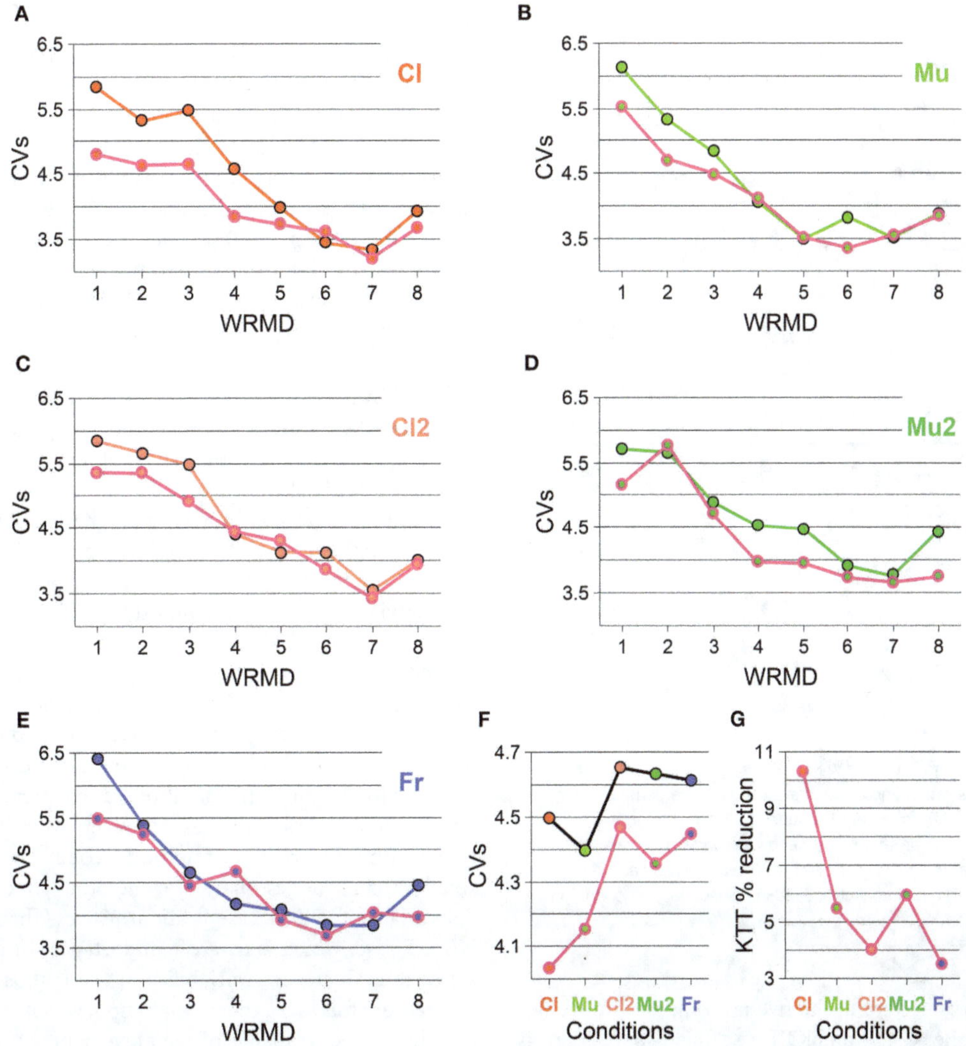

FIGURE 3 | (A–E) For each condition the CVs of IWFEs durations, ranked per within-ranges of durations, are illustrated. **(F)** The five within-condition CVs of IWFEs durations are compared for N/KTT and KTT. **(G)** The percent reduction of the within-condition CVs values when KTT is applied. The reduction is more than 3% in all conditions; the most evident reduction, more than 10%, is for the Cl condition. Values are plotted as black (N/KTT) and pink (KTT) outlined circles, filled-in color-coded per condition. Color-coded connecting lines are shown to ease reading. CVs = within-range or, in **(F)**, within-condition CVs values. WRMD, within-ranges movements durations.

The values of wγ(1) of IWFEs in the Cl condition are mostly negative for the N/KTT case (75.27% of negative values and 24.73% of positive values). In the KTT case, although the amount of positive values increases, negative wγ(1) values continue to outnumber positive ones (61.43% of negative values and 38.57% of positive values). In the N/KTT case of the Cl condition (**Figure 5A**), percentages of positive wγ(1) values are extremely low in the first four ranges of movement durations. The highest peaks for percentages of positive wγ(1) are evident in the last four ranges of movement durations. The highest peaks for percentages of positive wγ(1) values are always less than 50%, with only one exception (range 6, 53.23%). In the KTT case of the Cl condition (**Figure 5C**), percentages of positive wγ(1) values are extremely low only in the first two ranges of movement durations. However, the percentages of positive wγ(1) values in the two successive ranges (3 and 4) increase from the 2.19 and 12.38% in the N/KTT case to the 34.38 and 49.93% in the KTT case, respectively. Also, in the last four ranges of movement durations of KTT case, the percentages of positive wγ(1) values are similar to those in N/KTT case.

The values of wγ(1) of IWFEs in the Cl2 condition are somewhat negative for the N/KTT case (61.09% of negative values and 38.91% of positive values) while in the KTT case negative wγ(1) values slightly outnumber positive ones (54.74% of negative values and 45.26% of positive values). In the N/KTT case of the Cl2 condition (**Figure 5B**), percentages of positive wγ(1) reach lowest values in the first and third ranges of movement durations. In the KTT case of the Cl2 condition (**Figure 5D**), percentages of positive wγ(1) reach extremely low values only in the first three ranges of movement durations. The highest peaks for percentages

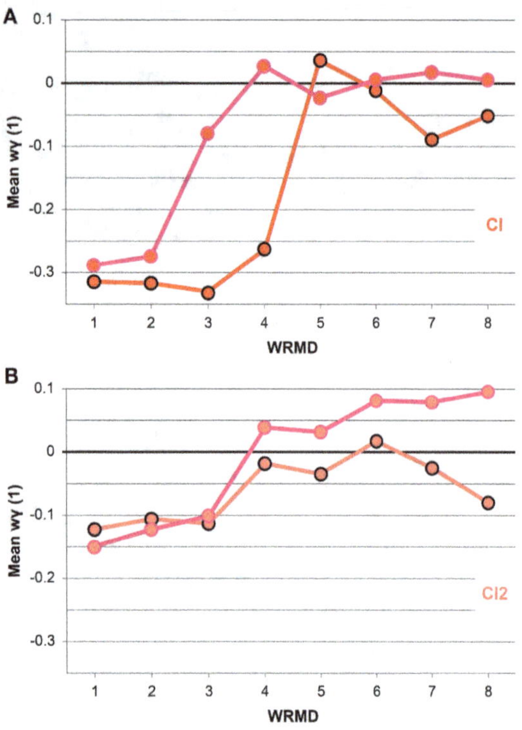

FIGURE 4 | (A,B) Mean windowed wγ(1) values, ranked per within-ranges of durations, are illustrated. The conditions Cl and Cl2 are compared for N/KTT and KTT. Note that mean wγ(1) values appear to change with movement durations and are, for both Cl and Cl2 conditions, biased toward more positive values when KTT is applied. Values are plotted as black (N/KTT) and pink (KTT) outlined circles, filled-in color-coded per condition. WRMD, within-ranges movements durations.

of positive wγ(1) values are in the five last ranges of movement durations both in the N/KTT and KTT case. It is also well perceivable that while in the N/KTT case only one of the within-range percentage of positive wγ(1) values is above the 50%, in the KTT case five of the eight within-range percentages of positive wγ(1) values are above the 50%.

In **Figures 5E,F** the percentages of positive wγ(1) values of N/KTT vs. KTT cases are compared separately for the Cl and the Cl2 conditions. As illustrated, the area generated by eight ranges percentages of positive wγ(1) values is wider in the KTT than in the N/KTT case, both for the Cl and the Cl2 conditions. For the Cl condition, the differential percent of positive wγ(1) values is of 13.84% (calculated as difference between the percentages of positive wγ(1) of 38.57% in KTT case and that of 24.73% in N/KTT case). This differential percent is equivalent to an increase of 55.96% of positive wγ(1) values in the KTT case (**Figure 5G**). Similarly, for the Cl2 condition, the differential percent of positive wγ(1) values is of 6.34% (calculated as difference between the percentages of positive wγ(1) of 45.26% in the KTT case and that of 38.91% in the N/KTT case). In the Cl2 condition, the differential percent is equivalent to an increase of 16.30% of positive wγ(1) values in the KTT case.

Finally, random effect ANOVA model for repeated measurements is performed for the wγ(1) values in Cl and Cl2 conditions, respectively. The model for Cl reveals a highly significant effect for the presence of KTT [$F_{(1, 98)} = 15.126, p < 0.001$] and tempo [$F_{(1, 98)} = 59.62, p < 0.001$]. The interaction between the presence of KTT and tempo shows also a significant effect [$F_{(1, 98)} = 5.05, p < 0.05$]. The model for Cl2 fails to reveal a significant effect of presence of KTT, [$F_{(1, 101)} = 0.34, p > 0.05$] and tempo, [$F_{(1, 101)} = 3.69, p > 0.05$]. Conversely, the interaction between the presence of KTT and tempo shows a significant effect [$F_{(1, 101)} = 5.05, p < 0.05$]. It should be remembered here that in the Cl2 condition mean within-range wγ(1) values become more positive in KTT than in N/KTT only for fast tempi (see **Figure 4B**).

DISCUSSION

In this study, we examined whether the application of KTT on skin is able to reduce the timing variability of repetitive rhythmic movements in healthy subjects.

Overall, our results indicate that the temporal variability of IWFEs is influenced by the application of KTT. Using a task of auditory-motor integration recently developed in our laboratory (see Bravi et al., 2014) we demonstrate that the timing variability is reduced in the KTT case, independently of the type of sensorimotor integration required from the participant to accomplish the motor performance (i.e., without audio information, with paced audio in the form of clicks or music, and in the recall conditions). Quantitatively, the reduction in the timing variability is different for the different conditions, and is greatest for the Cl and smallest for the Fr conditions. However, even though the reduction in timing variability for the Fr condition is quantitatively smaller than those estimated for the other conditions, the residual variance for KTT case is about 3% less than the variance of N/KTT case, which is of great importance. In fact, the residual variance evaluates the variability in the IWFEs durations when subjects are following their own tempo, which is mostly linked to the physical performance of the movement, without the effort of following or recalling a tempo proposed by others. Also, our analysis of the CVs of IWFEs show that, in general, when IWFEs are performed in presence of KTT the within-condition CVs values are smaller than those obtained in the N/KTT case. Here, again, the reduction in the CVs value is maximal when IWFEs are performed while listening to an audio stimulus such as clicks and minimal when performed in the Fr condition.

Our first experimental hypothesis is that KTT brings about an improvement of wrist joint proprioception due to augmented afferent input via the stimulation of cutaneous mechanoreceptors. This effect would, in turn, augment the coordination of the wrist joint during the rhythmic motor performance and consequently contribute to the reduction in timing variability of the IWFEs. The type of KTT application that we used allowed us to speculate about this possible effect provided by KTT: indeed, since the elastic band, placed between the lateral epicondyle of the humerus and the phalanges, is applied with the wrist positioned in maximum flexion, it cannot provide a facilitation of the ascent phase of the movement by means of elastic return to the starting position. This consents us to discard the possibility that the reduction of timing variability in the KTT condition is due to the dampening of gravity, but leads us toward an explanation

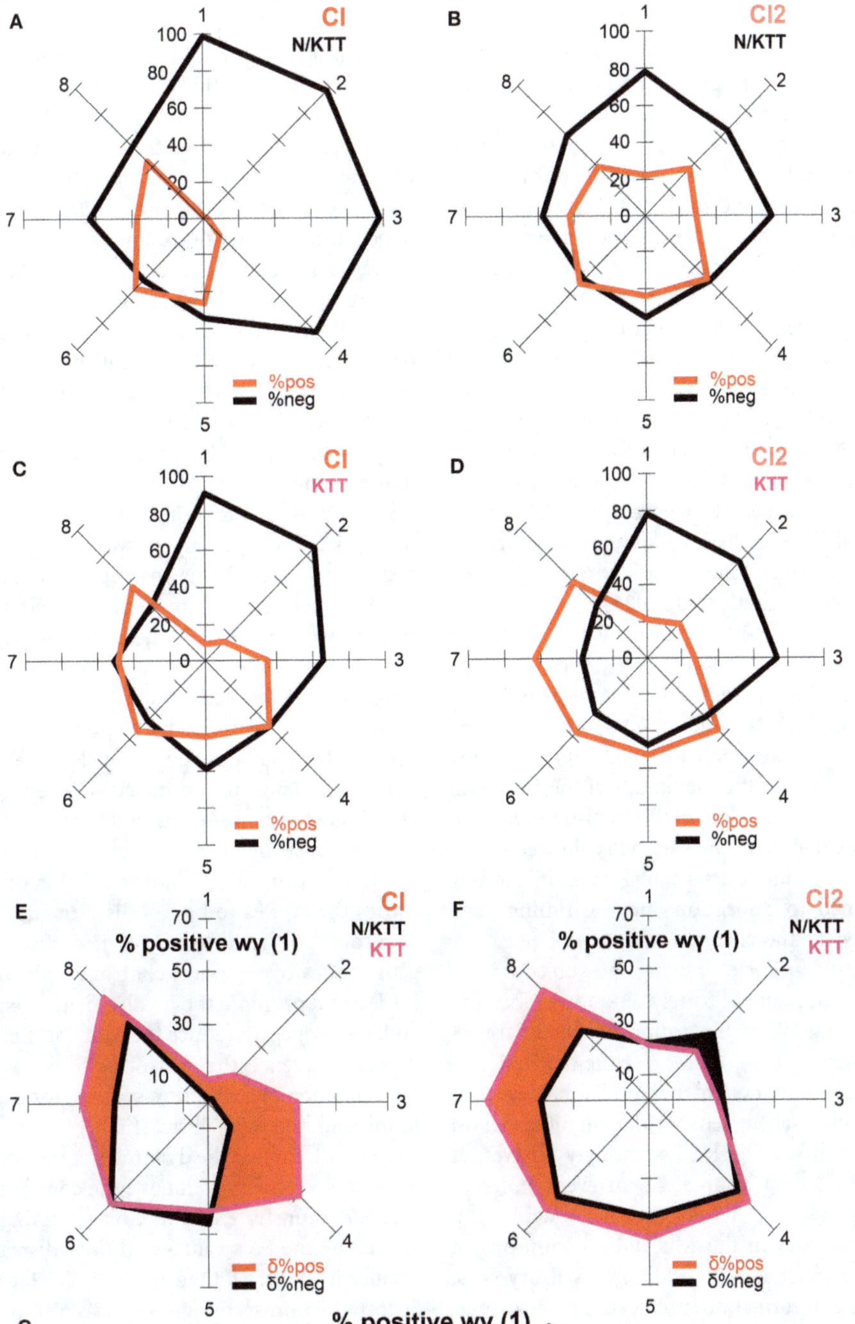

G % positive wγ (1)

CI

N/KTT	KTT	KTT δ%pos
24.73	38.57	55.96

CI2

N/KTT	KTT	KTT δ%pos
38.91	45.26	16.30

FIGURE 5 | (A–D) On the radar charts are illustrated, for the N/KTT and KTT cases of CI and CI2 conditions, the percentages of positive and negative wγ(1) values ranked per within-ranges of durations. Note that the areas generated by the eight within-range percentages of positive wγ(1) values are wider in the KTT than in N/KTT cases for both CI and CI2 conditions. **(E,F)** The percentages of N/KTT vs. KTT positive wγ(1) values are compared for the CI and the CI2 conditions, respectively. The red area indicates for each of the eight within-ranges of durations the differential percent of positive wγ(1) values. This area is wider in the KTT than in the N/KTT case, both for the CI and the CI2 conditions. Compound shapes are obtained by combination of areas of positive wγ(1) values in the N/KTT and KTT cases for both the CI and CI2 conditions. The overlapping area was excluded, turning the filled region into a hole. **(G)** The increase of positive wγ(1) values in the KTT case is comprehensively indicated as differential percent equivalent both for the CI and CI2 conditions (see text for more explanations). %pos (red) = percentages of positive wγ(1) values. %neg (black) = percentages of negative wγ(1) values. δ%pos (red) = differential percent equivalent for percentages of positive wγ(1) values. δ%neg (black) = differential percent equivalent for percentages of negative wγ(1) values.

that KTT might enhance proprioceptive information provided by activating cutaneous receptors.

Proprioception consists of a combination of joint position sense, i.e., the ability to sense the position and movement of a limb in space (Aydin et al., 2001), and the sense of muscular effort and tension (Proske and Gandevia, 2009). The joint position sense is a very important contributor to joint coordination, maintenance of muscle stiffness, and to the production of natural movements for appropriate task performance (Han and Lee, 2014). It was demonstrated that the principal muscle receptor in joint position sense is the muscle spindle; however, also cutaneous receptors have become recognized as playing an important role (Proske and Gandevia, 2009). The cutaneous receptors, subserving a sense of position and movement, respond to the stretching of skin (Proske and Gandevia, 2009). As proposed by Grigg (1994), it is plausible that the application of KTT induces, during the joint movement, a pressure and a stretching/deformation of the skin, thus activating cutaneous mechanoreceptors. Therefore, the mechanical effects of KTT applied to skin, augmenting skin receptor output, might enhance kinesthetic and joint position sense (Simoneau et al., 1997; Halseth et al., 2004).

Zelaznik and Rosenbaum (2010) performed an analysis in which timing precision was measured at different locations during both the performance of tapping and circle drawing tasks. Evidences showed that the highest values of CVs during the performance of the tapping task were at a location opposite to the specified timing location, that is, the maximum of the extension point. Earlier, Semjen and Garcia-Colera (1986) also noted that, in a tapping motor performance, timing variability showed smallest values at the instructed timing location. Hence, in tapping tasks the subject is timed to a location and the timing variability is best controlled at the corresponding event (e.g., the contact with the tap key); in circle drawing the subject is not timed to a place (i.e., is not required to rely on a target location or event) but is controlling evenly the entire movement trajectory (Spencer and Zelaznik, 2003). Our experimental design is not based on a tapping task, although the IWFEs, having clear turning points that provide salient sensory information (Elliott et al., 2009), are fairly similar. The KTT seemingly relieves, at least in part, from the need of a target or an event inherent with the kinematics of IWFEs. This is particularly evident in the Cl (see **Figure 3**) but also in the Mu audio conditions in which movements are performed with additional sensory cues. The extra proprioceptive information provided by KTT, augmenting the stability of wrist joint during the performance, could very well account for the reduction in IWFEs temporal variability that we observed as being more pronounced in our cued conditions.

In addition, we explore the possible influences of our KTT on the neural processes governing the temporal regulation for production of rhythmic movements. The mean wγ(1) values and the percentages of positive wγ(1) of IWFEs, calculated in N/KTT and KTT cases, and compared for the exemplar Cl and Cl2 conditions, show that the processes for temporal regulation can be influenced by the application of KTT. We demonstrate that the mean wγ(1) and percentages of positive wγ(1) are in fact biased toward values congruent with the emergent mode for control of timing.

Overall, these results have important implications for the event-emergent timing distinction. Heretofore, it was suggested that a task is controlled via event timing or via emergent timing depending on the kinematic of the performed movement (Zelaznik and Rosenbaum, 2010). Huys et al. (2008) using a rhythmic motor task, such as tapping, have demonstrated that discrete and continuous movements are two classes of movements topologically distinct. Indeed, it was shown that when finger flexion-extensions are performed as slow and discrete movements, the engagement of an explicit timing (event-based) process is required; whereas when the tapping is performed as rapid and smooth movements, the employment of a self-organized limit-cycle (emergent) process is necessary. The clarity with which such events are delineated in a particular experimental situation is considered to be the factor determining the weight of the event-based timing component. The continuity of the movement largely determines the strength of emergent timing component (Repp and Steinman, 2010). In addition, in a timing study on air finger tapping, participants performed discrete movements, being instructed to pause before each flexion cycle, and continuous movements, being instructed to move as smoothly as possible without pausing (Spencer et al., 2007). Despite the subtle difference between these discrete and continuous movements, activation in the cerebellum was greater when participants were instructed to perform discrete movements, suggesting that the engagement of the cerebellum may depend on how movements are produced or, even better, on how they are represented (Spencer et al., 2007).

Our experimental hypothesis is that the application of KTT, by stabilization of the motor effector during the performance, causes the IWFEs to be less discrete and thus more continuous. According to the dichotomic view of the event-based vs. emergent modes of temporal control (Delignières and Torre, 2011), KTT could promote the involvement of emergent timing control and, consequently, reduce the contribution of event-based timing. As a consequence, the control for timing would no longer need to refer to a nervous structure such as, for example, the cerebellum, in the building of an abstract representation of the time intervals to produce. Rather, the dynamics of the system could be sufficient *per se* to keep the movement cycle constant.

We demonstrate a reduction in timing variability with KTT, as seen by the CVs values and their dispersion, being very often smaller in the KTT than in the N/KTT cases (see **Figures 2, 3**). Such reduction seemingly suggests a transition toward an emergent timing control. This emergence of the emergent timing strategy (see **Figures 4, 5E–G**) appears to be by virtue of the KTT's to render movements less audio sensitive or dependent (compare, in **Figures 5A–C** vs. **B–D**). This mechanism ultimately results in a reduced variability and thus, in a better—more homogenous—performance. The same concept is analogous to a computer that allocates memory for a better performance; so do the cortical and subcortical circuits, which are usually required to bear the load of motor control and of other cognitive activities. Being less dependent on external/discrete events, central structures are partially relieved from timing control, thus freeing resources and allowing for a net augmentation of the central efficiency for motor control and cognition.

In conclusion, KTT was used in this study as a tool to possibly augment the precision of rhythmic movements. Our results show that KTT does, in fact, reduce the timing variability of rhythmic movements performed with no direct surface opposition and minimizing visual information. In particular, our results suggest that KTT—on the one hand by providing extra proprioceptive information, and on the other hand by relieving, at least partially, the central structures from time control—allows for a net augmentation of the central efficiency for motor control.

AUTHOR CONTRIBUTIONS

Riccardo Bravi: Substantial contributions to the conception of the work, the data acquisition, analysis, and the interpretation of data; Substantial contribution in drafting the work and revising it critically for important intellectual content; final approval of the version to be published; agreement to be accountable for accuracy and integrity of any part of the work. Eros Quarta: Substantial contributions to the design of the work and data acquisition; Substantial contribution in drafting the work; final approval of the version to be published; agreement to be accountable for accuracy and integrity of any part of the work. Erez J. Cohen: Substantial contributions to the design and the data acquisition of the work; Substantial contribution in drafting the work; final approval of the version to be published; agreement to be accountable for accuracy and integrity of any part of the work. Anna Gottard: Substantial contributions to the analysis and interpretation of data for the work; Substantial contribution in drafting the work; final approval of the version to be published; agreement to be accountable for accuracy and integrity of any part of the work. Diego Minciacchi: Substantial contributions to the conception of the work, analysis, and interpretation of data for the work; Substantial contribution in revising the work critically for important intellectual content; final approval of the version to be published; agreement to be accountable for accuracy and integrity of any part of the work.

ACKNOWLEDGMENTS

We are grateful for the seminal contribution of Dr. Giacomo Margiacchi, for the valuable contribution of Dr. Claudia del Tongo and Dr. Stefano Marletta during the setup of the experimental design and to the first experiments. We are also indebted with Mr. Filippo Cocchetti who kindly helped for the realization of the methodological Figure.

REFERENCES

Arias, P., and Cudeiro, J. (2008). Effects of rhythmic sensory stimulation (auditory, visual) on gait in Parkinson's disease patients. *Exp. Brain Res.* 186, 589–601. doi: 10.1007/s00221-007-1263-y

Aydin, T., Yildiz, Y., Yanmis, I., Yildiz, C., and Kalyon, T. A. (2001). Shoulder proprioception: a comparison between the shoulder joint in healthy and surgically repaired shoulders. *Arch. Orthop. Trauma Surg.* 121, 422–425. doi: 10.1007/s004020000245

Bove, M., Tacchino, A., Pelosin, E., Moisello, C., Abbruzzese, G., and Ghilardi, M. F. (2009). Spontaneous movement tempo is influenced by observation of rhythmical actions. *Brain Res. Bull.* 80, 122–127. doi: 10.1016/j.brainresbull.2009.04.008

Bravi, R., Del Tongo, C., Cohen, E. J., Dalle Mura, G., Tognetti, A., and Minciacchi, D. (2014). Modulation of isochronous movements in a flexible environment: links between motion and auditory experience. *Exp. Brain Res.* 232, 1663–1675. doi: 10.1007/s00221-014-3845-9

Callaghan, M. J., Selfe, J., Bagley, P. J., and Oldham, J. A. (2002). The effects of patellar taping on knee joint proprioception. *J. Athl. Train.* 37, 19–24. doi: 10.1016/S0031-9406(05)61377-6

Dannenberg, R. B., and Mohan, S. (2011). *Characterizing Tempo Change in Musical Performances.* Ann Arbor, MI: ICMC Proc.

de Dreu, M. J., van der Wilk, A. S. D., Poppe, E., Kwakkel, G., and van Wegen, E. E. H. (2012). Rehabilitation, exercise therapy and music in patients with Parkinson's disease: a meta-analysis of the effects of music-based movement therapy on walking ability, balance and quality of life. *Parkinsonism Relat. Disord.* 18(Suppl. 1), S114–S119. doi: 10.1016/S1353-8020(11)70036-0

Delignières, D., Lemoine, L., and Torre, K. (2004). Time intervals production in tapping and oscillatory motion. *Hum. Mov. Sci.* 23, 87–103. doi: 10.1016/j.humov.2004.07.001

Delignières, D., and Torre, K. (2011). Event-based and emergent timing: dichotomy or continuum? A reply to Repp and Steinman (2010). *J. Mot. Behav.* 43, 311–318. doi: 10.1080/00222895.2011.588274

del Olmo, M. F., Arias, P., Furio, M. C., Pozo, M. A., and Cudeiro, J. (2006). Evaluation of the effect of training using auditory stimulation on rhythmic movement in Parkinsonian patients–a combined motor and [18F]-FDG PET study. *Parkinsonism Relat. Disord.* 12, 155–164. doi: 10.1016/j.parkreldis.2005.11.002

del Olmo, M. F., and Cudeiro, J. (2005). Temporal variability of gait in Parkinson disease: effects of a rehabilitation programme based on rhythmic sound cues. *Parkinsonism Relat. Disord.* 11, 25–33. doi: 10.1016/j.parkreldis.2004.09.002

Diggle, P., Heagerty, P., Liang, K. Y., and Zeger, S. (2002). *Analysis of Longitudinal Data.* New York, NY: Oxford University Press.

Elliott, M. T., Welchman, A. E., and Wing, A. M. (2009). Being discrete helps keep to the beat. *Exp. Brain Res.* 192, 731–737. doi: 10.1007/s00221-008-1646-8

Ellis, M. (1991). Thresholds for detecting tempo change. *Psychol. Music* 19, 164–169. doi: 10.1177/0305735691192007

Freyer, F., Reinacher, M., Nolte, G., Dinse, H. R., and Ritter, P. (2012). Repetitive tactile stimulation changes resting-state functional connectivity-implications for treatment of sensorimotor decline. *Front. Hum. Neurosci.* 6:144. doi: 10.3389/fnhum.2012.00144

Grigg, P. (1994). Peripheral neural mechanisms in proprioception. *J. Sport Rehabil.* 3, 2–17.

Halseth, T., McChesney, J. W., Debeliso, M., Vaughn, R., and Lien, J. (2004). The effects of kinesio™ taping on proprioception at the ankle. *J. Sports Sci. Med.* 3, 1–7.

Han, J. T., and Lee, J. H. (2014). Effects of kinesiology taping on repositioning error of the knee joint after quadriceps muscle fatigue. *J. Phys. Ther. Sci.* 26, 921–923. doi: 10.1589/jpts.26.921

Hausdorff, J. M., Lowenthal, J., Herman, T., Gruendlinger, L., Peretz, C., and Giladi, N. (2007). Rhythmic auditory stimulation modulates gait variability in Parkinson's disease. *Eur. J. Neurosci.* 26, 2369–2375. doi: 10.1111/j.1460-9568.2007.05810.x

Huys, R., Studenka, B. E., Rheaume, N. R., Zelaznik, H. N., and Jirsa, V. K. (2008). Distinct timing mechanisms produce discrete and continuous movements. *PLoS Comput. Biol.* 4:e1000061. doi: 10.1371/journal.pcbi.1000061

Ivry, R. B., and Spencer, R. (2004). The neural representation of time. *Curr. Opin. Neurobiol.* 14, 225–232. doi: 10.1016/j.conb.2004.03.013

Kase, K., Wallis, J., and Kase, T. (2013). *Clinical Therapeutic Applications of the Kinesio Taping Method*, 3rd Edn. New Mexico: Kinesio Taping Ass.

Keele, S. W., and Ivry, R. (1990). Does the cerebellum provide a common computation for diverse tasks? A timing hypothesis. *Ann. N.Y. Acad. Sci.* 608, 179–207. doi: 10.1111/j.1749-6632.1990.tb48897.x

Kelso, J. A. S. (1995). *Dynamic Patterns.* Cambridge, MA: MIT Press.

Kneeshaw, D. (2002). Shoulder taping in the clinical setting. *J. Body Mov. Ther.* 6, 2–8. doi: 10.1054/jbmt.2001.0233

Kugler, P. N., Kelso, J. A. S., and Turvey, M. T. (1980). "On the concept of coordinative structures as dissipative structures I. Theoretical lines of convergence" in *Tutorials in Motor Behavior*, eds G. E. Stelmach and J. Requin (Amsterdam: North Holland), 3–47.

Leiner, H. C., Leiner, A. L., and Dow, R. S. (1993). Cognitive and language functions of the human cerebellum. *Trends Neurosci.* 16, 444–447. doi: 10.1016/0166-2236(93)90072-T

Levitin, D. J., and Cook, P. R. (1996). Memory for musical tempo: additional evidence that auditory memory is absolute. *Percept. Psychophys.* 58, 927–935. doi: 10.3758/BF03205494

Levy, M. (2011). "Improving perceptual tempo estimation with crowd-sourced annotations," in *12th International Society for Music Information Retrieval Conference (ISMIR 2011)* (Miami, FL), 317–322.

Madison, G., and Paulin, J. (2010). Ratings of speed in real music as a function of both original and manipulated beat tempo. *J. Acoust. Soc. Am.* 128, 3032–3040. doi: 10.1121/1.3493462

McIntosh, G. C., Brown, S. H., Rice, R. R., and Thaut, M. H. (1997). Rhythmic auditory-motor facilitation of gait patterns in patients with Parkinson's disease. *J. Neurol. Neurosurg. Psychiatry* 62, 22–26. doi: 10.1136/jnnp.62.1.22

McKinney, M. F., and Moelants, D. (2007). Ambiguity in tempo perception: what draws listeners to different metric levels? *Music Percept.* 24, 155–165. doi: 10.1525/mp.2006.24.2.155

McKinney, M. F., Moelants, D., Davies, E. P., and Klapuri, A. (2007). Evaluation of audio beat tracking and music tempo extraction algorithms. *J. New Music Res.* 36, 1–16. doi: 10.1080/09298210701653252

Morris, D., Jones, D., Ryan, H., and Ryan, C. G. (2013). The clinical effects of Kinesio® Tex taping: a systematic review. *Physiother. Theory Pract.* 29, 259–270. doi: 10.3109/09593985.2012.731675

Muthén, B. O. (1989). Latent variable modeling in heterogeneous populations. *Psychometrika* 54, 557–585. doi: 10.1007/BF02296397

Nolte, G., Bai, O., Wheaton, L., Mari, Z., Vorbach, S., and Hallett, M. (2004). Identifying true brain interaction from EEG data using the imaginary part of coherency. *Clin. Neurophysiol.* 115, 2292–2307. doi: 10.1016/j.clinph.2004.04.029

Pinheiro, J. C., and Bates, D. M. (2000). *Mixed Effects Models in S and S-PLUS*. New York, NY: Springer-Verlag.

Proske, U., and Gandevia, S. C. (2009). The kinaesthetic senses. *J. Physiol. (Lond.)* 587, 4139–4146. doi: 10.1113/jphysiol.2009.175372

Quinn, S., and Watt, R. (2006). The perception of tempo in music. *Perception* 35, 267–280. doi: 10.1068/p5353

Rao, S. M., Mayer, A. R., and Harrington, D. L. (2001). The evolution of brain activation during temporal processing. *Nat. Neurosci.* 4, 317–323. doi: 10.1038/85191

Repp, B. H. (1999a). Detecting deviations from metronomic timing in music: effects of perceptual structure on mental timekeeper. *Percept. Psychophys.* 61, 529–548. doi: 10.3758/BF03211971

Repp, B. H. (1999b). Control of expressive and metronomic timing in pianists. *J. Motor Behav.* 31, 145–164. doi: 10.1080/00222899909600985

Repp, B. H. (2005). Sensorimotor synchronization: a review of the tapping literature. *Psychon. Bull. Rev.* 12, 969–992. doi: 10.3758/BF03206433

Repp, B. H. (2011). Temporal evolution of the phase correction response in synchronization of taps with perturbed two-interval rhythms. *Exp. Brain Res.* 208, 89–101. doi: 10.1007/s00221-010-2462-5

Repp, B. H., and Steinman, S. R. (2010). Simultaneous event-based and emergent timing: synchronization, continuation, and phase correction. *J. Mot. Behav.* 42, 111–126. doi: 10.1080/00222890903566418

Riemann, B., and Lephart, S. (2002). The sensorimotor system, Part II: the role of proprioception in motor control and functional joint stability. *J. Athl. Train.* 37, 80–84.

Robertson, S. D., Zelaznik, H. N., Lantero, D. A., Bojczyk, K. G., Spencer, R. M., Doffin, J. G., et al. (1999). Correlations for timing consistency among tapping and drawing tasks: evidence against a single timing process for motor control. *J. Exp. Psychol. Hum. Percept. Perform.* 25, 1316–1330. doi: 10.1037/0096-1523.25.5.1316

Saijo, N., and Gomi, H. (2010). Multiple motor learning strategies in visuomotor rotation. *PLoS ONE* 5:e9399. doi: 10.1371/journal.pone.0009399

Schlerf, J. E., Spencer, R. M., Zelaznik, H. N., and Ivry, R. B. (2007). Timing of rhythmic movements in patients with cerebellar degeneration. *Cerebellum* 6, 221–231. doi: 10.1080/14734220701370643

Schoner, G. (2002). Timing, clocks, and dynamical systems. *Brain Cogn.* 48, 31–51. doi: 10.1006/brcg.2001.1302

Semjen, A., and Garcia-Colera, A. (1986). Planning and timing of finger- tapping sequences with a stressed element. *J. Mot. Behav.* 18, 287–322. doi: 10.1080/00222895.1986.10735383

Semjen, A., Schulze, H. H., and Vorberg, D. (2000). Timing precision in continuation and synchronization tapping. *Psychol. Res.* 63, 137–147. doi: 10.1007/PL00008172

Simoneau, G. G., Degner, R. M., Kramper, C. A., and Kittleson, K. H. (1997). Changes in ankle joint proprioception resulting from strips of athletic tape applied over the skin. *J. Athl. Train.* 32, 141–147.

Spencer, R. M. C., and Ivry, R. B. (2005). Comparison of patients with Parkinson's disease or cerebellar lesions in the production of periodic movements involving event-based or emergent timing. *Brain Cogn.* 58, 84–93. doi: 10.1016/j.bandc.2004.09.010

Spencer, R. M. C., Verstynen, T., Brett, M., and Ivry, R. (2007). Cerebellar activation during discrete and not continuous timed movements: an fMRI study. *Neuroimage* 36, 378–387. doi: 10.1016/j.neuroimage.2007.03.009

Spencer, R. M. C., and Zelaznik, H. N. (2003). Weber (slope) analyses of timing variability in tapping and drawing tasks. *J. Mot. Behav.* 35, 371–382. doi: 10.1080/00222890309603157

Spencer, R. M. C., Zelaznik, H. N., Diedrichsen, J., and Ivry, R. B. (2003). Disrupted timing of discontinuous but not continuous movements by cerebellar lesions. *Science* 300, 1437–1439. doi: 10.1126/science.1083661

Studenka, B. E., and Zelaznik, H. N. (2008). The influence of dominant versus non-dominant hand on event and emergent motor timing. *Hum. Mov. Sci.* 27, 29–52. doi: 10.1016/j.humov.2007.08.004

Teki, S., Grube, M., and Griffiths, T. D. (2012). A unified model of time perception accounts for duration-based and beat-based timing mechanisms. *Front. Integr. Neurosci.* 5:90. doi: 10.3389/fnint.2011.00090

Thaut, M. H., McIntosh, G. C., Rice, R. R., Miller, R. A., Rathbun, J., and Brault, J. M. (1996). Rhythmic auditory stimulation in gait training for Parkinson's disease patients. *Mov. Disord.* 11, 193–200. doi: 10.1002/mds.870110213

Turvey, M. T. (1977). "Preliminaries to a theory of action with reference to vision," in *Perceiving, Acting and Knowing: Toward an Ecological Psychology*, eds R. Shaw and J. Bransford (Hillsdale, NJ: Erlbaum), 211–265.

Wing, A. M., and Kristofferson, A. B. (1973a). The timing of inter-response intervals. *Percept. Psychophys.* 13, 455–460. doi: 10.3758/BF03205802

Wing, A. M., and Kristofferson, A. B. (1973b). Response delays and timing of discrete motor responses. *Percept. Psychophys.* 14, 5–12. doi: 10.3758/BF03198607

Wittwer, J. E., Webster, K. E., and Hill, K. (2013). Music and metronome cues produce different effects on gait spatiotemporal measures but not gait variability in healthy older adults. *Gait Posture* 37, 219–222. doi: 10.1016/j.gaitpost.2012.07.006

Xu, D., Liu, T., Ashe, J., and Bushara, K. O. (2006). Role of the olivo-cerebellar system in timing. *J. Neurosci.* 26, 5990–5995. doi: 10.1523/JNEUROSCI.0038-06.2006

Zatorre, R. J., and Halpern, A. R. (2005). Mental concerts: musical imagery and auditory cortex. *Neuron* 47, 9–12. doi: 10.1016/j.neuron.2005.06.013

Zelaznik, H. N., and Rosenbaum, D. A. (2010). Timing processes are correlated when tasks share a salient event. *J. Exp. Psychol. Hum. Percept. Perform.* 36, 1565–1575. doi: 10.1037/a0020380

Zelaznik, H. N., Spencer, R. M. C., and Ivry, R. B. (2002). Dissociation of explicit and implicit timing in repetitive tapping and drawing movements. *J. Exp. Psychol. Hum. Percept. Perform.* 28, 575–588. doi: 10.1037/0096-1523.28.3.575

21

Multifaceted effects of noisy galvanic vestibular stimulation on manual tracking behavior in Parkinson's disease

Soojin Lee[1], Diana J. Kim[1], Daniel Svenkeson[2], Gabriel Parras[2], Meeko Mitsuko K. Oishi[2] and Martin J. McKeown[1]*

[1] *Pacific Parkinson's Research Centre, Department of Medicine, University of British Columbia, Vancouver, BC, Canada*
[2] *Department of Electrical and Computer Engineering, University of New Mexico, Albuquerque, NM, USA*

Edited by:
Ioan Opris, Wake Forest University, USA

Reviewed by:
Michael Noll-Hussong, University of Ulm, Germany
Filip Bergquist, University of Gothenburg, Sweden

***Correspondence:**
Martin J. McKeown, Pacific Parkinson's Research Centre, Department of Medicine, University of British Columbia, M31, Purdy Pavilion, 2221 Wesbrook Mall, Vancouver, BC V6T 2B5, Canada
e-mail: martin.mckeown@ubc.ca

Parkinson's disease (PD) is a neurodegenerative movement disorder that is characterized clinically by slowness of movement, rigidity, tremor, postural instability, and often cognitive impairments. Recent studies have demonstrated altered cortico-basal ganglia rhythms in PD, which raises the possibility of a role for non-invasive stimulation therapies such as noisy galvanic vestibular stimulation (GVS). We applied noisy GVS to 12 mild-moderately affected PD subjects (Hoehn and Yahr 1.5–2.5) off medication while they performed a sinusoidal visuomotor joystick tracking task, which alternated between 2 task conditions depending on whether the displayed cursor position underestimated the actual error by 30% ('Better') or overestimated by 200% ('Worse'). Either sham or subthreshold, noisy GVS (0.1–10 Hz, 1/f-type power spectrum) was applied in pseudorandom order. We used exploratory (linear discriminant analysis with bootstrapping) and confirmatory (robust multivariate linear regression) methods to determine if the presence of GVS significantly affected our ability to predict cursor position based on target variables. Variables related to displayed error were robustly seen to discriminate GVS in all subjects particularly in the Worse condition. If we considered higher frequency components of the cursor trajectory as "noise," the signal-to-noise ratio of cursor trajectory was significantly increased during the GVS stimulation. The results suggest that noisy GVS influenced motor performance of the PD subjects, and we speculate that they were elicited through a combination of mechanisms: enhanced cingulate activity resulting in modulation of frontal midline theta rhythms, improved signal processing in neuromotor system via stochastic facilitation and/or enhanced "vigor" known to be deficient in PD subjects. Further work is required to determine if GVS has a selective effect on corrective submovements that could not be detected by the current analyses.

Keywords: Parkinson's disease, vestibular system, GVS, manual tracking, discriminant analysis

INTRODUCTION

Motor symptoms in Parkinson's disease (PD) characteristically manifest themselves as tremor, rigidity, akinesia/bradykinesia and postural instability. While levodopa is the gold standard treatment for PD, chronic use eventually leads to the long-term development of side effects, such as motor fluctuations, dyskinesias, and psychiatric disorders (Pontone et al., 2006; Weintraub et al., 2006). Surgical treatments, including deep brain stimulation targeted to subcortical nuclei, have provided effective therapeutic benefits, but are complex and invasive (Okun, 2012). With recent technological advances, numerous novel stimulatory techniques for PD treatment are presently being explored (Fuentes et al., 2009; Thevathasan et al., 2010; Samoudi et al., 2012; Faught and Tatum, 2013). Non-invasive brain stimulation techniques are currently a growing avenue of interest for PD and other neurological disorders due to their safety, tolerability and minimally invasive nature (Fregni and Pascual-Leone, 2007). Additionally, these methods, such as transcranial current brain stimulation (tCS), arguably influence solely the targeted site of stimulation, but also exert effects on associated brain connectivity patterns (Luft et al., 2014). Since PD is characterized by abnormally exaggerated beta synchronization throughout a basal ganglia (BG)-cortical network (Eusebio et al., 2009), non-invasive stimulatory approaches could potentially be used to modulate aberrant network dynamics (Fregni and Pascual-Leone, 2007).

A few studies have suggested that non-invasive stimulation of vestibular nerves via noisy galvanic vestibular stimulation (GVS) may improve motor deficits in PD (Yamamoto et al., 2005; Pan et al., 2008; Pal et al., 2009; Samoudi et al., 2012). Noisy GVS delivers currents with randomly varying amplitudes in time to vestibular afferents and subsequently influences resting state cortical electroencephalography (EEG) activity, suggesting that cortical-subcortical connections are also modulated by GVS (Kim et al., 2013). Akin to how tCS strengthens connectivity patterns in premotor, motor, and sensorimotor areas while subjects are engaged in a finger tapping task (Polanía et al., 2011), noisy GVS hypothetically is also able to influence functional BG-cortical motor networks depending on the brain state during stimulation. It is not fully established, however, whether noisy GVS improves motor performance. Yamamoto et al. (2005) measured trunk dynamics as well as reaction time in a Go/NoGo paradigm whereas Pan et al. (2008) measured wrist activity in akinetic PD patients. Effects of noisy GVS on postural and balance responses have also been measured in both humans and rat models (Pal et al., 2009; Samoudi et al., 2012), although none of these studies have directly investigated the effects of GVS on bradykinesia with respect to motor coordination and sensorimotor processing.

One potential way to rigorously assess the motoric effect of GVS is to utilize a visuomotor task, which is useful for understanding mechanisms that contribute to motor coordination with accuracy and stability (Ryu and Buchanan, 2012). Corrective movements and behavior are required in response to varying visual error feedback, which are important for maintaining effective perception-action or sensorimotor processing (Ryu and Buchanan, 2012). With respect to clinical significance, the ability to continually adapt one's behavior to changing environmental or sensory stimuli is particularly relevant in PD as these patients demonstrate impaired switching between motor paradigms (Engel and Fries, 2010).

In the present study, we implemented a visuomotor tracking task and investigated the effect of noisy GVS on motor performance. Our visuomotor task required subjects to respond to visual error feedback that was, unbeknownst to the subjects, either minimized to 30% of the actual error, or amplified by 200% to create the appearance of 'Better' or 'Worse' motor performance, respectively. We used linear discriminant analysis (LDA; Duda et al., 2012) to identify parameters significantly influenced by GVS and to investigate if the effects of GVS are dependent on the task conditions. We then analyzed our data using a robust multivariate linear regression method (Filzmoser and Todorov, 2011) to test if tracking movement was affected by GVS. We show that subthreshold GVS resulted in robust changes in tracking, mostly related to increased sensitivity to perceived error.

MATERIALS AND METHODS

SUBJECTS

Twelve PD subjects (10 males, 2 females; mean age 61.4 ± 6.5 years; 11 right-handed, 1 left-handed) participated in the study. None of the participants had any reported vestibular or auditory disorders. All PD subjects were recruited from the Pacific Parkinson's Research Centre (Vancouver, BC, Canada). PD subjects had mild to moderate disease severity (Hoehn and Yahr stages 1.5–2.5) with UPDRS (Unified Parkinson's Disease Rating Scale) Part III motor scores at a mean of 22.3 ± 7.8 (**Table 1**). All PD subjects were tested in the off-medicated state after a 12-h overnight withdrawal from L-dopa medication. Other medications that some subjects were on included: amantadine, ramipril, and atorvastatin.

ETHICS STATEMENT

The study was approved by the University of British Columbia Clinical Research Ethics Board. All subjects gave written, informed consent prior to participation. Research was conducted according to the principles expressed in the Declaration of Helsinki.

VISUOMOTOR TRACKING TASK

Subjects were comfortably seated 80 cm in front of a screen and performed a manual tracking task. On the screen, a target (blue) and cursor (yellow) connected by a black horizontal rod were displayed (**Figure 1**). The target box oscillated vertically up and down with the summation of two frequencies (0.06 and 0.1 Hz). Subjects controlled the cursor using a joystick with the objective of matching the horizontal position of the cursor to the target – i.e., to keep the horizontal black rod straight. The tracking error (Δ, difference between the actual positions of the target and cursor) was scaled by a factor (α) to determine the displayed position of the cursor: $\Delta \times \alpha =$ displayed visual error feedback. In the 'Better' (B) task condition, α was set to 0.3, and in the 'Worse' (W)

Table 1 | PD subjects' characteristics for behavior task.

Patient number	Age (yr)	Sex	Duration since diagnosis (yr)	UPDRS motor score	Hoehn and Yahr stage	Handedness
1	58	M	4	18	2	R
2	64	F	4	12	1.5	R
3	67	M	4	16	2	R
4	56	M	2.5	21	2	L
5	53	M	3	32	2.5	R
6	49	M	7.5	35	2	R
7	65	F	5	32	2	R
8	68	M	1.5	22	2	R
9	66	M	1	24	2	R
10	70	M	1	21	2	R
11	59	M	1.5	10	2	R
12	62	M	3.5	24	2	R

UPDRS, unified Parkinson's disease rating scale.

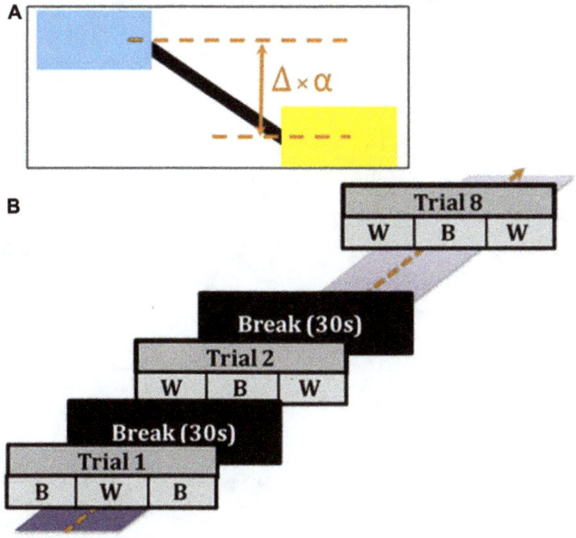

FIGURE 1 | Behavior task. (A) Subjects faced a screen with a target (blue) that moved vertically up and down, and controlled a cursor (yellow) using a joystick. The error difference (Δ) between the actual positions of the target and cursor was amplified by a scaling factor (α): Δ × α = displayed visual error feedback. In the 'Better' (B) condition, α was set to 0.3, and in the 'Worse' (W) condition, α was set to 2, such that it appeared that subjects performed better or worse respectively based on their visual error feedback. **(B)** Trials (90 s) alternated between B and W conditions (each condition 30 s). Each trial was followed by a break of 30 s until a culmination of eight trials total were completed for the experiment.

task condition, α was set to 2, such that it artificially appeared to subjects that they performed better or worse, respectively, based on their scaled error feedback.

During the experiment, subjects performed a total of eight trials. Each trial (90 s) was comprised of three alternating blocks (30 s each) of B and W conditions – with Trial 1 ordered as B-W-B and Trial 2 ordered as W-B-W (**Figure 1**). During each trial, either a subthreshold *verum* current (90% of cutaneous sensory threshold) or *sham* current stimulation was delivered. Four trials contained *verum* GVS delivery whereas the other four trials contained *sham* stimulation. Subjects were unaware of either *verum* or *sham* stimulation since the order in which stimuli were delivered was pseudorandom, and the *verum* stimulation was imperceptible to the subject. Each trial was followed by a break (30 s) to preclude a hysteretic effect carrying over to the next trial. Before starting the experiment, subjects were allowed to practice tracking the target and using the joystick as needed in at least one practice trial. Practice trials were differently structured from the eight experiment trials described above. Due to technical details of the data capture system, the cursor position was irregularly sampled at ~55 Hz. We then resampled the data at exactly 50 Hz using linear interpolation before further analyses.

STIMULUS

Galvanic vestibular stimulation was delivered to subjects through carbon rubber electrodes (17 cm^2) in a bilateral, bipolar fashion. For bilateral stimulation, an electrode was placed over the mastoid process behind each ear, and coated with Tac gel (Pharmaceutical Innovations, NJ, USA) to optimize conductivity and adhesiveness. The average impedance of the subjects was measured around 1 kΩ. Digital signals were generated on a computer using MATLAB and converted to analog signals via a NI USB-6221 BNC digital acquisition module (National Instruments, TX, USA). The analog command voltage signals were subsequently passed to a constant current stimulator (Model DS5, Digitimer, Hertfordshire, UK), which was connected to the stimulating electrodes.

Bipolar stimulation signals were zero-mean, linearly detrended, noisy currents with a 1/f-type power spectrum (pink noise) as previously applied to PD and healthy subjects (Soma et al., 2003; Yamamoto et al., 2005; Pan et al., 2008). The stimulation signal was generated between 0.1 and 10 Hz with a Gaussian probability density, with the command signal delivered to the constant-current amplifier at 60 Hz (**Figure 2**). The stimulus was applied at an

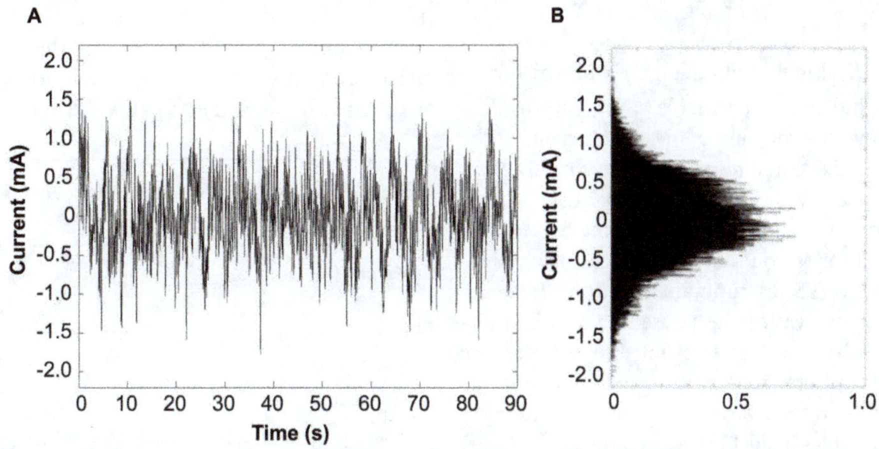

FIGURE 2 | Characteristics of the stimulus. (A) Typical recording from a subject receiving a noisy stimulus applied for 90 s duration. The stimulus presented is at the highest current intensity (current level 6), which is set to 90% of the subject's individual sensory threshold (RMS current value of 266 μA). **(B)** Probability density function of the stimulus current follows a Gaussian distribution.

imperceptible level to avoid effects by general arousal and/or voluntary selective attention, with the current level individually determined according to each subject's cutaneous sensory threshold.

Since perception of GVS is inherently subjective, we utilized systematic procedures that have been previously used in determining subliminal current levels for both GVS and transcranial stimuli (Hummel et al., 2005; Utz et al., 2011; Wilkinson et al., 2012). Starting from a basal current level of 20 μA, noisy test stimuli were delivered for 20 s periods with gradual stepwise increases (20 μA) in current intensity until subjects perceived a mild, local tingling in the area of the stimulating electrodes. As performed previously, a threshold value was defined once subjects reported a tingling sensation (Utz et al., 2011; Wilkinson et al., 2012), which lasted for the duration of the test stimulus. The current level was then decreased each time by one level until sensation was no longer reported during delivery of test stimulus pulses, and increased by one step in current intensity to confirm threshold. Each delivery of a test stimulus was followed by a period of no stimulation for at least 30 s to preclude a hysteretic effect carrying over to the next test stimulus. Subjects were blind to the onset and duration of test stimuli, as well as the threshold-testing scheme. After completing the threshold test and throughout the experiment, stimuli were delivered at subthreshold intensity (190–900 μA), which is achieved at 90% of the determined cutaneous sensory threshold value.

BEHAVIORAL DATA ANALYSIS

We employed both exploratory and hypothesis-driven analysis methods to analyze the behavioral data. We initially analyzed the data on a subject-by-subject basis as we were unclear whether or not there would be substantial intersubject variability to GVS response. LDA was first used to see if tracking behavior could be reliably discriminated depending upon whether GVS was applied or not. We derived a GVS linear discrimination function, g(X), to create maximum separation between means of the projected classes with minimum variance within each projected class:

$$g(\mathbf{X}) = w_1 \mathbf{X}_1 + w_2 \mathbf{X}_2 + \cdots + w_{21} \mathbf{X}_{21} + \omega_0 = \mathbf{w}^t \mathbf{X}^t + \omega_0 \quad (1)$$

where $\mathbf{X} = [\mathbf{X}_1\ \mathbf{X}_2\ \ldots\ \mathbf{X}_{21}]$ is a input data matrix in which each column represents an independent variable, $\mathbf{w} = [w_1, w_2, \ldots, w_{21}] \in \mathbb{R}^{21}$ the weight vector containing linear coefficients of the variables in the data matrix **X**, and ω_0 the bias-weight. LDA was applied to the "Better" and "Worse" conditions separately.

For this exploratory part of the analysis, we included linear (first-order) and non-linear (second- and third-order) combinations of variables in the GVS discriminant function (**Table 2**). During the experiment, we varied the phase of the initial target trajectory not only between subjects but also between the trials to prevent the subjects from easily predicting upcoming target movement. Therefore, variables from X_1 to X_9 were included as nuisance variables in the LDA to account for the target differences.

To test for significance of the LDA results, we employed bootstrapping techniques. We permuted the GVS labels (on/off) and then re-computed the LDA function with the permuted data.

Table 2 | Variables in linear discriminant analysis (LDA) model.

Notation	Variables
X_1, X_2, X_3	$T(t), T(t)^2, T(t)^3$
X_4, X_5, X_6	$V_T(t), V_T(t)^2, V_T(t)^3$
X_7, X_8, X_9	$A_T(t), A_T(t)^2, A_T(t)^3$
X_{10}, X_{11}, X_{12}	$D(t) - T(t), \{D(t) - T(t)\}^2, \{D(t) - T(t)\}^3$
X_{13}, X_{14}, X_{15}	$V_D(t) - V_T(t), \{V_D(t) - V_T(t)\}^2, \{V_D(t) - V_T(t)\}^3$
X_{16}, X_{17}, X_{18}	$D(t+\Delta t) - D(t), \{D(t+\Delta t) - D(t)\}^2, \{D(t+\Delta t) - D(t)\}^3$
X_{19}, X_{20}, X_{21}	$V_D(t+\Delta t) - V_D(t), \{V_D(t+\Delta t) - V_D(t)\}^2, \{V_D(t+\Delta t) - V_D(t)\}^3$

T, target position; V_T, target velocity; A_T, target acceleration; D, displayed cursor position; V_D, displayed cursor velocity; t, time index, and Δt, reaction delay of 0.5 s (Jordan et al., 1992).

This was repeated 1000 times. Any weight value from the original LDA function g(X) whose absolute value was greater than all the weights computed from the permuted data was considered to be significantly influenced by GVS.

In addition, a multivariate linear regression model was used to test the hypothesis that GVS had a significant effect on cursor position during tracking. As the traditional least squares regression may be sensitive to noisy and gross errors (Akkaya and Tiku, 2008), we chose a robust regression method to analyze our data ("robustfit" function in MATLAB). This method is known to be robust to outliers utilizing an iteratively reweighted scheme to deweight the influences of outliers. With cursor position as a response variable (Y_i), the following regression model was proposed:

$$Y_i = \boldsymbol{A}_i \boldsymbol{\beta} + \boldsymbol{\varepsilon}_i \quad (2)$$

where for each data point i we have the vector of independent variables $\boldsymbol{A}_i = [A_{i1}, \cdots, A_{i5}]$, the vector of regression coefficients solved by a bisquare weighting function $\boldsymbol{\beta}$, and the residual $\boldsymbol{\varepsilon}_i$ (assumed to be independent and identically distributed Gaussian). The selected independent variables are summarized in **Table 3** (note that A_1, A_2 and A_3 are same as the variables X_1, X_4 and X_{10} in eq.1, respectively). The categorical variable of GVS was denoted with either 0 (GVSoff) or 1 (GVSon). We tested for significance

Table 3 | Estimated coefficients in the robust regression model (eq.2) and the *p*-values.

Variables (*A*)	Coefficient estimates (*β*)	*p*-value
Target position (A_1)	1.00	0.0000
Target velocity (A_2)	−7.79e-02	0.0000
Displayed cursor position – target position (A_3)	5.01e-01	0.0000
Cursor velocity – target velocity (A_4)	−1.60e-02	0.0002
GVS (A_5)	3.99e-05	0.0410

R^2 = 0.8811.

of the coefficients under the null hypothesis that the coefficient estimates were equal to zero.

For a signal-to-noise ratio (SNR) analysis, we utilized "snr" function in MATLAB to calculate SNR of cursor trajectories. This examines the fundamental frequencies of the tracking trajectory plus the next six harmonics, and assumes that any power in the spectrum than these peaks are "noise."

RESULTS

RESULTS OF LDA IN WORSE CONDITION

Coefficients of GVS discriminant function (eq.1) were calculated for each subject and are plotted as black lines in **Figure 3**. For clarity, nuisance variables related to absolute target position (i.e., X_1–X_9) are not shown. The 1000 sets of linear coefficients generated from the bootstrapping are depicted as blue lines. In most subjects, the coefficients w_{10}, w_{11}, and w_{12} of g(X; representing linear and higher powers of the perceived error between the target and the displayed cursor position) were robustly modulated by GVS. In addition, displayed cursor velocity (w_{16} or w_{17}) and acceleration (w_{19}, w_{20}, or w_{21}) were also found to be significantly affected by GVS across subjects.

RESULTS OF LDA IN BETTER CONDITION

Figure 4 shows the LDA results in the better condition. As before, coefficients w_{10}, w_{11}, and w_{12} were significant among all the subjects. In addition, 10 out of 12 subjects showed significant w_{18} weightings. Other coefficients were not robustly seen in all subjects. For example, unlike the LDA results of the Worse condition, displayed cursor acceleration (w_{19}, w_{20}, or w_{21}) was no longer significantly influenced by GVS in the Better condition.

RESULTS OF ROBUST REGRESSION MODEL

Table 3 is the coefficient estimates of the variables of the multivariate regression model (eq.2) and their p-values. The computed R^2 of the regression model was 0.8811. GVS was significantly associated with cursor position across all subjects ($p < 0.05$).

EFFECT OF GVS ON CURSOR OVERSHOOTING

In order to get an intuitive interpretation of GVS effects, we calculated the GVS discriminant function values (eq.1) for each subject. We used data from trials 1 and 7 for the calculation as these two trials had identical phases of the trajectories, with a difference in whether or not GVS was delivered (GVSon for trial 1). Then, Δg was computed by subtracting the function values of trial 7 from trial 1. By plotting Δg, we could not only locate GVS effects on the cursor trajectory but also directly make visual comparison of the cursor movement in the identified location. **Figure 5** shows target trajectory, cursor trajectory and Δg for each subject.

The effect of GVS was greatest near sinusoidal peaks. This trend was found in most of the subjects regardless of how well the subjects tracked the target. For instance, subject 5 tracked the target relatively better compared to the other subjects, and Δg was significant around at 5, 20, 65, and 80 s. Subjects 11 and 12 performed the tracking task poorly, but the GVS effects still appeared near sinusoidal peaks.

One of the noticeable features on the peaks is a degree of overshooting of cursor trajectories. To assess a possible relationship to GVS stimulation, we compared the difference between the cursor position and the target on the peaks. **Figure 6** shows a representative example of cursor overshooting near sinusoidal peaks in target. The peaks in cursor appeared with some lagged

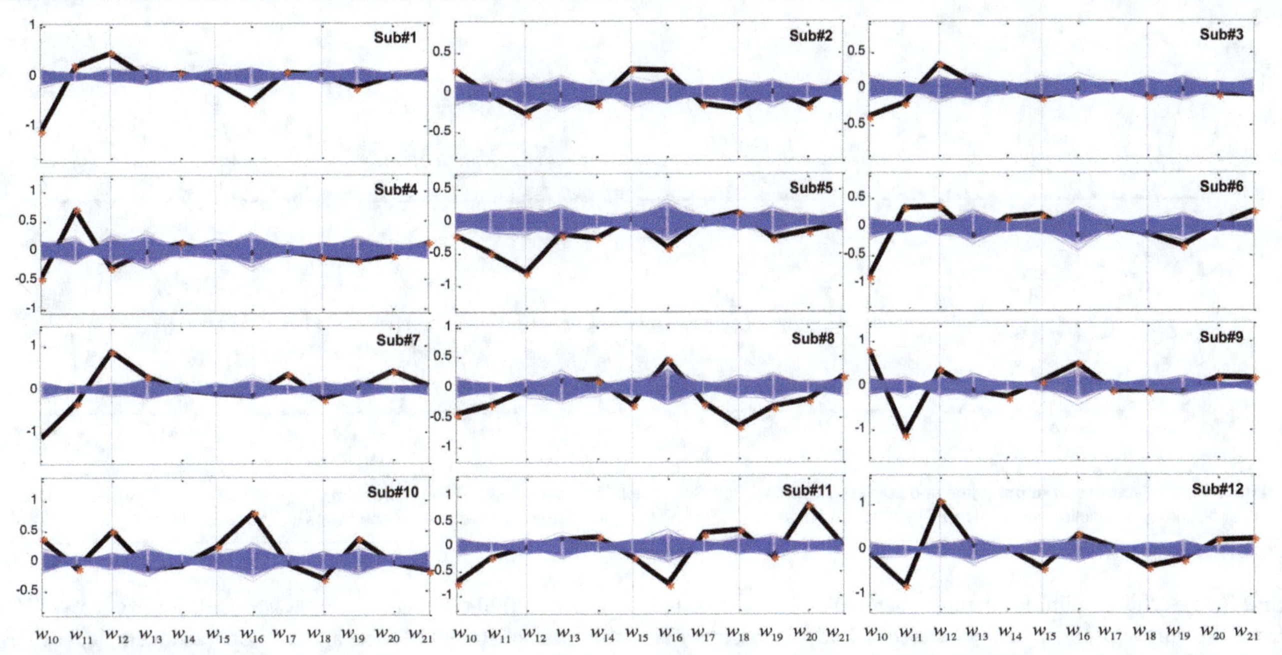

FIGURE 3 | Coefficients of the variables of the linear discriminant function in the Worse condition. The x-axis represents variables from X_{10} to X_{21} in **Table 2** while the y-axis represents weight (w) value. The computed coefficients are depicted as black for the GVS discriminant function and blue for bootstrapping. Red asterisks denote coefficients that are outside the 95% confidence interval of bootstrapping.

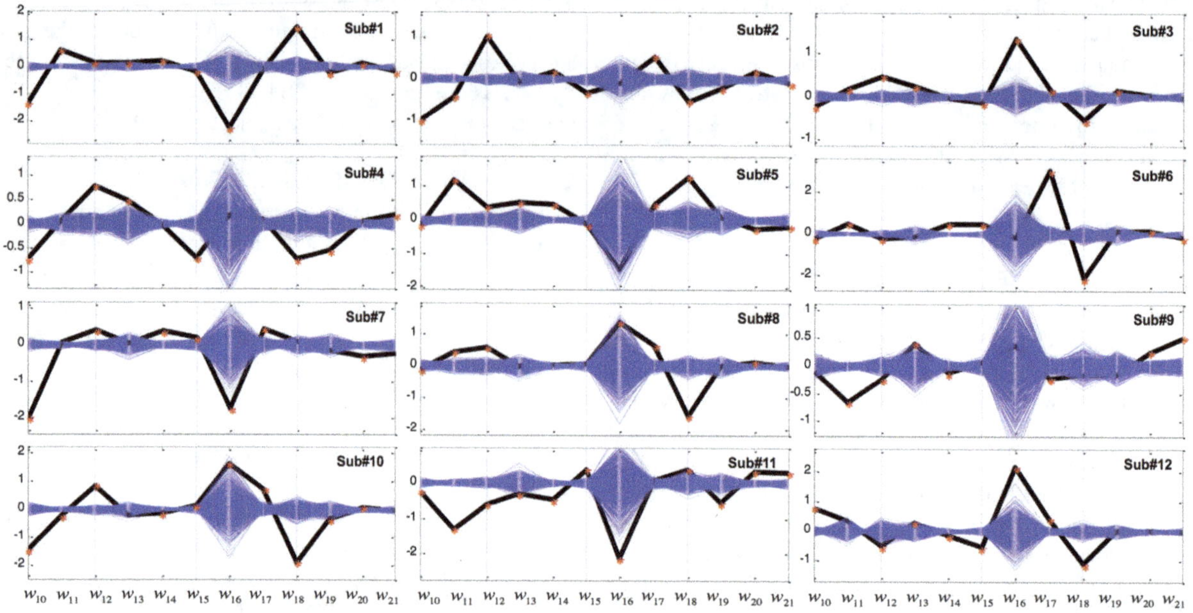

FIGURE 4 | Coefficients of the variables of the linear discriminant function in the Better condition. The *x*-axis represents variables from X_{10} to X_{21} in **Table 2** while the *y*-axis represents weight (*w*) value. The computed coefficients are depicted as black for the GVS discriminant function and blue for bootstrapping. Red asterisks denote coefficients that are outside the 95% confidence interval of bootstrapping.

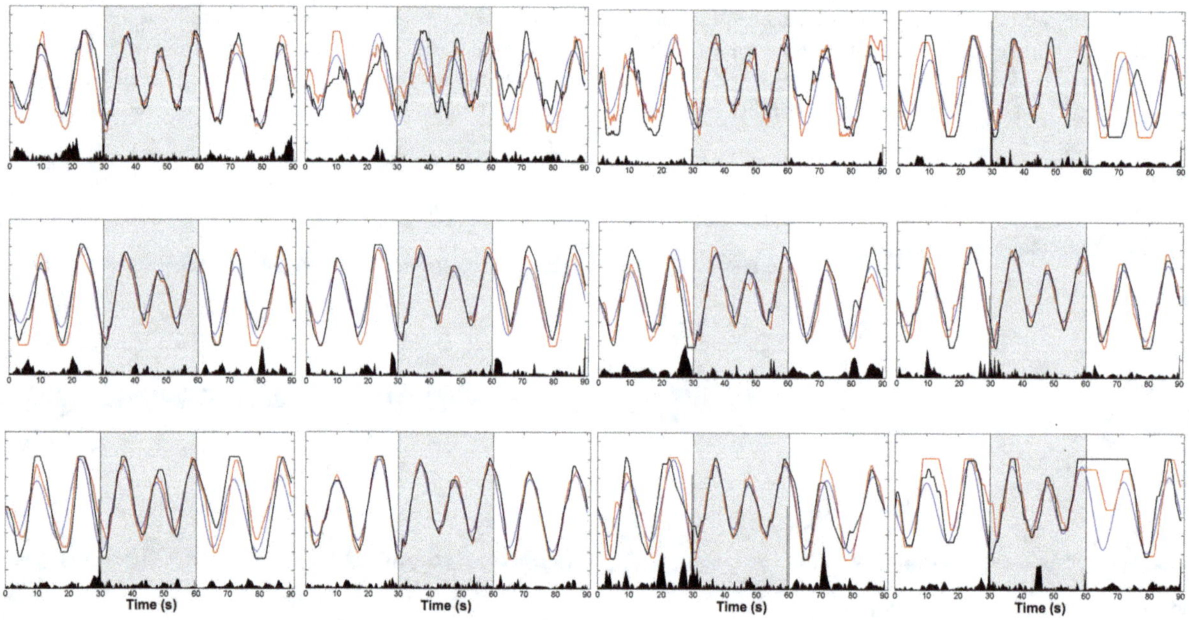

FIGURE 5 | Trajectories of target (blue) and cursor (GVSon: red, GVSoff: black) and Δg (black bar in the bottom). Δg was computed by subtracting the linear discriminant function values of trial 7 (GVSoff) from trial 1 (GVSon). The trials alternated between W-B-W conditions (each condition 30 s).

time (Δt). The amplitude of the target peaks was subtracted from the cursor peaks, and the difference (Δd) was defined as cursor overshooting. Cursor peak was defined when the cursor position was at its max/min point. Cursor overshooting was calculated for all trials and subjects, then averaged depending on the task conditions and presence of GVS stimulation as shown in **Table 4**. The *p*-value was calculated from ANOVA of the means between GVSon and GVSoff (i.e., a single, two-level factor).

In Worse condition, the subjects tended to overshoot significantly less on the lower peaks while stimulated by GVS. On the upper peaks, the mean overshooting of GVSon was also smaller

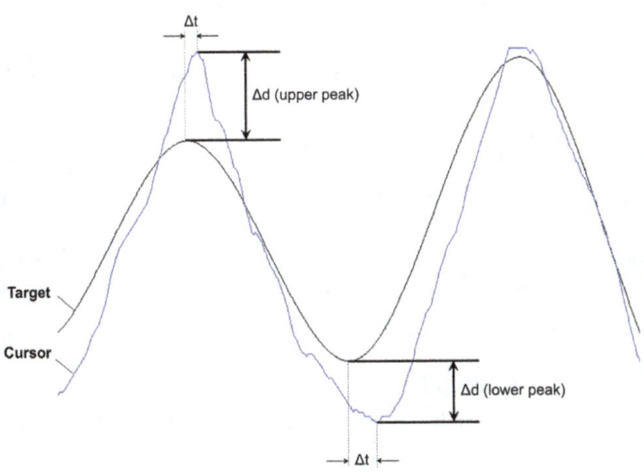

FIGURE 6 | Representative example of cursor overshooting on upper and lower peaks from Subject 1 Cursor overshooting (Δd) was calculated as cursor position – target position. Δt represents time difference between peaks in cursor and target trajectories.

Table 4 | Means of cursor overshooting on sinusoidal peaks and ANOVA results.

	Lower peak			Upper peak		
	GVSon	GVSoff	*p*-value	GVSon	GVSoff	*p*-value
Worse	−0.0517	−0.0714	0.0036	0.0695	0.0784	0.22
Better	−0.0946	−0.0451	0.0038	0.0890	0.0690	0.14

than GVSoff, but the difference was not significant. In Better condition, however, there was an increasing tendency for cursor overshooting with stimulation.

EFFECT OF GVS ON SNR OF CURSOR TRAJECTORY

Movement variability is another important feature to characterize the tracking performance. Particularly, in goal-directed behavior, the variability originates from collateral movement to the main goal of a task. In this sense, the cursor trajectories in our tracking test can be seen to a combination of two components. One is the primary movement whose form is similar to the target trajectory, and the other is submovement that may appear as noise superimposed on the primary movement. In order to investigate if GVS had affected movement variability of the subjects, we calculated SNR of cursor trajectories and compared differences in between GVSon and GVSoff conditions. As shown in **Figure 7**, the mean SNR of 12 PD subjects was 27.6 when GVS was applied, which was significantly greater than 21.3 in GVSoff condition ($p < 0.05$).

DISCUSSION

Our results demonstrate that noisy GVS robustly influences motor tracking performance in PD patients off dopaminergic medication. Motor improvements are consistent with results previously reported in hemiparkinsonian rats (Samoudi et al., 2012) whereby

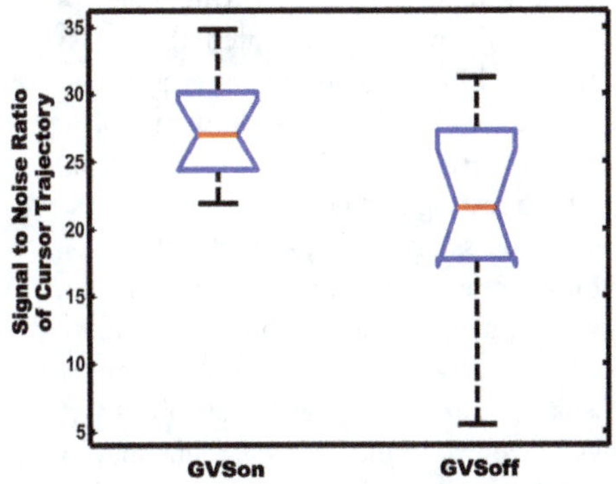

FIGURE 7 | Comparison of SNR of cursor trajectories between GVSon and GVSoff conditions.

GVS with a 1/f power density improved rod performance. Previously, we demonstrated that noisy GVS has the ability to modulate synchronization of broadband EEG oscillations in healthy subjects (Kim et al., 2013). Our recordings of EEG rhythms were observed at resting-state, suggesting that noisy GVS was able to modulate cortical activity and presumably connected subcortical-cortical projections. In this study, we observed a functional effect of GVS on sensorimotor processing and motor performance in a visuomotor task, suggesting that noisy vestibular stimulation modulates motor networks in PD subjects.

Our results seem to indicate that noisy GVS affects the sensitivity of motor responses (in this case, joystick-controlled cursor position) to visualized error (displayed cursor position – target position). We do not believe that our observed results are the consequence of an attentional or general arousal effect, such as through activation of the reticular activating system. The imperceptible nature of our stimulus, which subjects were not aware of throughout the experiment trials, precludes this issue which is present with other forms of minimally invasive stimulation methods (Fuentes et al., 2009).

Depending on the stimulus parameters (i.e., current intensity, frequency, signal shape), GVS is known to induce a broad range of effects, including eye movements, postural control and movements (Fitzpatrick and Day, 2004). Therefore, one interpretation of our results may include the confounding effects of nystagmus and/or ocular torsion through activation of the vestibulo-ocular reflex (VOR; Zink et al., 1998). Since subjects rely on visual error feedback, ocular torsion would potentially hamper the perceived error feedback through a subjective tilt in the visual perceptual field (Zink et al., 1998). However, we note that our stimulus levels were weak, subthreshold currents with the highest current delivered at around 140 ± 113 μA, whereas the preferred GVS current intensities for inducing ocular torsion and subsequent perceptual tilts through GVS are much higher at around 1–3 mA (Zink et al., 1998). Therefore, we presume that our subthreshold stimulus was not strong enough to notably induce confounding visual effects and corollary perceptual changes in our experiment.

Noisy GVS is known to modulate EEG spectral power. Wilkinson et al. (2012) have demonstrated that noisy GVS is able to modulate the EEG spectral power during a face processing task. Our previous study has demonstrated that noisy GVS is able to modulate the EEG synchrony patterns in healthy subjects (Kim et al., 2013). Altogether, these findings combined with our present results suggest that noisy GVS is able to modulate oscillatory activity in resting and task-related networks, which involve sensorimotor processing in our particular study.

The motoric effects of GVS may be related to modulation of oscillations related to integration of information and error-processing. Since perceived error (i.e., the error between the target and the displayed cursor position) was robustly detected by the LDA analysis, fronto–midline (FM) theta may be a candidate oscillation to be modulated by GVS in PD subjects. FM-theta shows an increased amplitude during tasks requiring concentration (Mitchell et al., 2008), which is related to error-related negativity (ERN), an event-related potential seen after errors are made. FM-theta may represent a universal mechanism for action monitoring with the midcingulate cortex acting as hub for the integration of information (Cavanagh et al., 2012). Thus, our results suggest that GVS may regulate FM-theta activity in PD subjects.

The increased SNR shown in **Figure 7** suggests that application of noisy GVS may have increased synchronization in neuromotor system via stochastic facilitation. Stochastic facilitation is a term to describe phenomena where stochastic biological noise elicits functional benefits in a non-linear system such as the nervous system (McDonnell and Ward, 2011). Several studies have reported that a presence of additive noise allows a weak input signal to be better detected, resulting in an increase in SNR in EEG (Galambos and Makeig, 1992; Srebro and Malladi, 1999; Elias et al., 2003; Kitajo et al., 2007; Keita et al., 2008; Ward et al., 2010; Doren et al., 2014) and sensorimotor performance (Ignacio et al., 2012). These findings suggest that noisy GVS input may also be able to modulate detection and transmission of the sensorimotor system via stochastic facilitation, resulting in an increase in synchronization of the neuromotor system. However, a further investigation is required to elucidate whether the synchronization is limited to cortical areas or if it could give rise to corticomuscular synchronization (Ignacio et al., 2012).

We further speculate that our results may be at least partly explained by modulation of cortico-BG rhythms involved in sensorimotor processing. Growing observations suggest a concept that the BG regulates action motivation or response 'vigor' (Niv et al., 2007; Salamone et al., 2009) as well as the speed and size of movement (Spraker et al., 2007; Thobois et al., 2007). Deficient scaling of the initial burst of earliest agonist muscle activity (EMG) to meet the demands of a motor task is frequently observed in clinical disorders of the BG, such as PD. The link between motivation and movement gain may be universally weakened in Parkinsonian subjects (Ballanger et al., 2006; Thobois et al., 2007). We thus speculate that GVS may also correct deficient vigor caused by BG dysfunction through modulation of pathological brain rhythms.

We note that we used a single noisy stimulus for all subjects. However, the results shown in **Figure 3** also emphasize the importance of looking at patient-specific stimuli. For instance, the coefficients regarding the difference between cursor and target velocities (w_{13}, w_{14}, and w_{15}) were found to be significant in some subjects, but were indistinguishable from bootstrapping for the rest subjects.

Finally, we note that GVS had fewer effects in the Better condition compared to the Worse condition. Presumably, subjects would have made fewer corrective movements in the former condition. This raises the possibility that GVS may also depend upon the number and form of corrective submovements. As submovements were not captured by the global LDA and multivariate regression methods used here, this warrants further investigation.

ACKNOWLEDGMENT

This work was partly funded by PPRI/UBC chair in Parkinson's Disease (Martin J. McKeown). This material is based upon work supported by the National Science Foundation under Grant Number CMMI-1254990 (Meeko Mitsuko K. Oishi CAREER Award). Any opinions, findings, and conclusions or recommendations expressed in this material are those of the authors and do not necessarily reflect the views of the National Science Foundation.

REFERENCES

Akkaya, A. D., and Tiku, M. L. (2008). Robust estimation in multiple linear regression model with non-Gaussian noise. *Automatica* 44, 407–417. doi: 10.1016/j.automatica.2007.06.029

Ballanger, B., Thobois, S., Baraduc, P., Turner, R. S., Broussolle, E., and Desmurget, M. (2006). "Paradoxical kinesis" is not a hallmark of Parkinson's disease but a general property of the motor system. *Mov. Disord.* 21, 1490–1495. doi: 10.1002/mds.20987

Cavanagh, J. F., Zambrano-Vazquez, L., and Allen, J. J. B. (2012). Theta lingua franca: a common mid-frontal substrate for action monitoring processes. *Psychophysiology* 49, 220–238. doi: 10.1111/j.1469-8986.2011.01293.x

Doren, J. V., Langguth, B., and Schecklmann, M. (2014). Electroencephalographic effects of transcranial random noise stimulation in the auditory cortex. *Brain Stimul.* 7, 807–812. doi: 10.1016/j.brs.2014.08.007

Duda, R. O., Hart, P. E., and Stork, D. G. (2012). *Pattern Classification.* New York: John Wiley & Sons.

Elias, M., Gerardo, R., Ignacio, M., and Amira, F. (2003). Stochastic resonance within the somatosensory system: effects of noise on evoked field potentials elicited by tactile stimuli. *J. Neurosci.* 23, 1997–2001.

Engel, A. K., and Fries, P. (2010). Beta-band oscillations — signalling the status quo? *Curr. Opin. Neurobiol.* 20, 156–165. doi: 10.1016/j.conb.2010.02.015

Eusebio, A., Pogosyan, A., Wang, S., Averbeck, B., Gaynor, L. D., Cantiniaux, S., et al. (2009). Resonance in subthalamo-cortical circuits in Parkinson's disease. *Brain* 132, 2139–2150. doi: 10.1093/brain/awp079

Faught, E., and Tatum, W. (2013). Trigeminal stimulation: a superhighway to the brain? *Neurology* 80, 780–781. doi: 10.1212/WNL.0b013e318285c17d

Filzmoser, P., and Todorov, V. (2011). Review of rubust multivariate statistical methods in high dimension. *Anal. Chim. Acta* 705, 2–14. doi: 10.1016/j.aca.2011.03.055

Fitzpatrick, R. C., and Day, B. L. (2004). Probing the human vestibular system with galvanic stimulation. *J. Appl. Physiol.* 96, 2301–2316. doi: 10.1152/japplphysiol.00008.2004

Fregni, F., and Pascual-Leone, A. (2007). Technology insight: noninvasive brain stimulation in neurology-perspectives on the therapeutic potential of rTMS and tDCS. *Nat. Clin. Pract. Neurol.* 3, 383–393. doi: 10.1038/ncpneuro0530

Fuentes, R., Petersson, P., Siesser, W. B., Caron, M. G., and Nicolelis, M. A. L. (2009). Spinal cord stimulation restores locomotion in animal models of Parkinson's disease. *Science* 323, 1578–1582. doi: 10.1126/science.1164901

Galambos, R., and Makeig, S. (1992). Physiological studies of central masking in man. I: the effects of noise on the 40-Hz steady-state response. *J. Acoust. Soc. Am.* 92, 2683–2690. doi: 10.1121/1.404383

Hummel, F., Celnik, P., Giraux, P., Floel, A., Wu, W.-H., Gerloff, C., et al. (2005). Effects of non-invasive cortical stimulation on skilled motor function in chronic stroke. *Brain* 128, 490–499. doi: 10.1093/brain/awh369

Ignacio, M., Elias, M., Jürgen, S., Frank, H., Jesus, A. T., Marie-Claude, H., et al. (2012). Improved sensorimotor performance via stochastic resonance. *J. Neurosci.* 32, 12612–12618. doi: 10.1523/JNEUROSCI.0680-12.2012

Jordan, N., Sagar, H. J., and Cooper, J. A. (1992). Cognitive components of reaction time in Parkinson's disease. *J. Neurol. Neurosurg. Psychiatry* 55, 658–664. doi: 10.1136/jnnp.55.8.658

Keita, T., Kawakatsu, M., and Nemoto, I. (2008). Stochastic resonance in auditory steady-state responses in a magnetoencephalogram. *Clin. Neurophysiol.* 119, 2104–2110. doi: 10.1016/j.clinph.2008.05.007

Kim, D. J., Yogendrakumar, V., Chiang, J., Ty, E., Wang, Z. J., and Mckeown, M. J. (2013). Noisy galvanic vestibular stimulation modulates the amplitude of EEG synchrony patterns. *PLoS ONE* 8:e69055. doi: 10.1371/journal.pone.0069055

Kitajo, K., Doesburg, S. M., Yamanaka, K., Nozaki, D., Ward, L. M., and Yamamoto, Y. (2007). Noise-induced large-scale phase synchronization of human-brain activity associated with behavioural stochastic resonance. *Europhys. Lett.* 80:40009. doi: 10.1209/0295-5075/80/40009

Luft, C. D. B., Pereda, E., Banissy, M., and Bhattacharya, J. (2014). Best of both worlds: promise of combining brain stimulation and brain connectome. *Front. Syst. Neurosci.* 8:132. doi: 10.3389/fnsys.2014.00132

McDonnell, M. D., and Ward, L. M. (2011). The benefits of noise in neural systems: bridging theory and experiment. *Nat. Rev. Neurosci.* 12, 415–426. doi: 10.1038/nrn3061

Mitchell, D. J., Mcnaughton, N., Flanagan, D., and Kirk, I. J. (2008). Frontal-midline theta from the perspective of hippocampal "theta." *Prog. Neurobiol.* 86, 156–185. doi: 10.1016/j.pneurobio.2008.09.005

Niv, Y., Daw, N. D., Joel, D., and Dayan, P. (2007). Tonic dopamine: opportunity costs and the control of response vigor. *Psychopharmacology* 191, 507–520. doi: 10.1007/s00213-006-0502-4.

Okun, M. S. (2012). Deep-brain stimulation for Parkinson's disease. *N. Eng. J. Med.* 367, 1529–1538. doi: 10.1056/NEJMct1208070

Pal, S., Rosengren, S. M., and Colebatch, J. G. (2009). Stochastic galvanic vestibular stimulation produces a small reduction in sway in Parkinson's disease. *J. Vestib. Res.* 19, 137–142. doi: 10.3233/VES-2009-0360

Pan, W., Soma, R., Kwak, S., and Yamamoto, Y. (2008). Improvement of motor functions by noisy vestibular stimulation in central neurodegenerative disorders. *J. Neurol.* 255, 1657–1661. doi: 10.1007/s00415-008-0950-3.

Polanía, R., Nitsche, M. A., and Paulus, W. (2011). Modulating functional connectivity patterns and topological functional organization of the human brain with transcranial direct current stimulation. *Hum. Brain Mapp.* 32, 1236–1249. doi: 10.1002/hbm.21104

Pontone, G., Williams, J. R., Bassett, S. S., and Marsh, L. (2006). Clinical features associated with impluse control disorders in Parkinson disease. *Neurology* 67, 1258–1261. doi: 10.1212/01.wnl.0000238401.76928.45

Ryu, Y. U., and Buchanan, J. J. (2012). Accuracy, Stability, and Corrective Behavior in a Visuomotor Tracking Task: a Preliminary Study. *PLoS ONE* 7:e38537. doi: 10.1371/journal.pone.0038537

Salamone, J. D., Correa, M., Farrar, A. M., Nunes, E. J., and Pardo, M. (2009). Dopamine, behavioral economics, and effort. *Front. Behav. Neurosci.* 3:13. doi: 10.3389/neuro.08.013.2009

Samoudi, G., Nissbrandt, H., Dutia, M. B., and Bergquist, F. (2012). Noisy galvanic vestibular stimulation promotes GABA release in the substantia nigra and improves locomotion in hemiparkinsonian rats. *PLoS ONE* 7:e29308. doi: 10.1371/journal.pone.0029308

Soma, R., Kwak, S., and Yamanoto, Y. (2003). "Functional stochastic resonance in human baroreflex induced by 1/f-type noisy galvanic vestibular stimulation," in *Proceeding of SPIE 5110 – the International Society for Optical Engineering, Fluctuations and Noise in Biological, Biophysical, and Biomedical Systems*, Tokyo, 69. doi: 10.1117/12.500315

Spraker, M. B., Yu, H., Corcos, D. M., and Vaillancourt, D. E. (2007). Role of individual basal ganglia nuclei in force amplitude generation. *J. Neurophysiol.* 98, 821–834. doi: 10.1152/jn.00239.2007

Srebro, R., and Malladi, P. (1999). Stochastic Resonance of the Visually Evoked Potential. *Phys. Rev. E* 59, 2566–2570. doi: 10.1103/PhysRevE.59.2566

Thevathasan, W., Mazzone, P., Jha, A., Djamshidian, A., Dileone, M., Di Lazzaro, V., et al. (2010). Spinal cord stimulation failed to relieve akinesia or restore locomotion in Parkinson disease. *Neurology* 74, 1325–1327. doi: 10.1212/WNL.0b013e3181d9ed58

Thobois, S., Ballanger, B., Baraduc, P., Le Bars, D., Lavenne, F., Broussolle, E., et al. (2007). Functional anatomy of motor urgency. *Neuroimage* 37, 243–252. doi: 10.1016/j.neuroimage.2007.04.049

Utz, K. S., Korluss, K., Schmidt, L., Rosenthal, A., Oppenländer, K., Keller, I., et al. (2011). Minor adverse effects of galvanic vestibular stimulation in persons with stroke and healthy individuals. *Brain Inj.* 25, 1058–1069. doi: 10.3109/02699052.2011.607789

Ward, L. M., MacLean, S. E., and Kirschner, A. (2010). Stochastic resonance modulates neural synchronization within and between cortical sources. *PLoS ONE* 5:e14371. doi: 10.1371/journal.pone.0014371

Weintraub, D., Siderowf, A. D., Potenza, M. N., Goveas, J., Morales, K. H., Duda, J. E., et al. (2006). Dopamine agonist use is associated with impulse control disorders in Parkinson's disease. *Arch. Neurol.* 63, 969–973. doi: 10.1001/archneur.63.7.969

Wilkinson, D., Ferguson, H. J., and Worley, A. (2012). Galvanic vestibular stimulation modulates the electrophysiological response during face processing. *Vis. Neurosci.* 29, 255–262. doi: 10.1017/S0952523812000235

Yamamoto, Y., Struzik, Z. R., Soma, R., Ohashi, K., and Kwak, S. (2005). Noisy vestibular stimulation improves autonomic and motor responsiveness in central neurodegenerative disorders. *Ann. Neurol.* 58, 175–181. doi: 10.1002/ana.20574

Zink, R., Bucher, S. F., Weiss, A., Brandt, T., and Dieterich, M. (1998). Effects of galvanic vestibular stimulation on otolithic and semicircular canal eye movements and perceived vertical. *Electroencephalogr. Clin. Neurophysiol.* 107, 200–205. doi: 10.1016/S0013-4694(98)00056-X

22

Control of humanoid robot via motion-onset visual evoked potentials

***Wei Li*[1,2]*, *Mengfan Li*[2] and *Jing Zhao*[2]**

[1] *Department of Computer and Electrical Engineering and Computer Science, California State University, Bakersfield, CA, USA*
[2] *School of Electrical Engineering and Automation, Tianjin University, Tianjin, China*

Edited by:
Mikhail Lebedev, Duke University, USA

Reviewed by:
Ana-Maria Cebolla, Université Libre de Bruxelles, Belgium
Emmanuele Tidoni, Fondazione Santa Lucia, Italy
Arzu Güneysu, Bogaziçi University, Turkey

***Correspondence:**
Wei Li, Department of Computer and Electrical Engineering and Computer Science, California State University, 9001 Stockdale Highway, Bakersfield, CA 93311, USA
e-mail: wli@csub.edu

This paper investigates controlling humanoid robot behavior via motion-onset specific N200 potentials. In this study, N200 potentials are induced by moving a blue bar through robot images intuitively representing robot behaviors to be controlled with mind. We present the individual impact of each subject on N200 potentials and discuss how to deal with individuality to obtain a high accuracy. The study results document the off-line average accuracy of 93% for hitting targets across over five subjects, so we use this major component of the motion-onset visual evoked potential (mVEP) to code people's mental activities and to perform two types of on-line operation tasks: navigating a humanoid robot in an office environment with an obstacle and picking-up an object. We discuss the factors that affect the on-line control success rate and the total time for completing an on-line operation task.

Keywords: brain robot interaction, mind-controlled humanoid robot, N200 potentials, humanoid robot behavior, visual feedback

INTRODUCTION

Event related potentials (ERPs) are able to set up a communication between external stimuli and people's cognitive tasks. Assigning specific meanings to visual stimuli allows to "read" people's mind by identifying a target stimulus related with their attention (Lebedev and Nicolelis, 2006). A P300 model based on visual attention mechanism (Jin et al., 2012) is commonly used in the ERP-based brain-computer-interfaces (BCIs). When we evaluated the P300 model on Cerebot—a mind-controlled humanoid robot (Li et al., 2011, 2012), we noted some issues of this model (Li et al., 2013a,b). First, this model needs to flash a visual stimulus by growing its visual contrast, which easily causes people's visual fatigue (Hong et al., 2009). Second, the P300 potential is correlated with both the people's attention allocation (Farwell and Donchin, 1988) and the biological determinants of cognitive operation (Polich and Kok, 1995), so the people's states and experimental environments significantly affect the P300 signal quality. Considering the problems above, we investigate a N200 potential-based robot brain interaction (BRI) model.

The stimulus appearing in moving a bar through images instead of flashing the images (Heinrich, 2007) induces a N200 potential with a negative deflection occurring at 180–325 ms post-stimulus (Patel and Azzam, 2005). The N200 potential is an involuntary component that less depends on people's attention, and even people's fixation can induce this kind of potential (Frensel and Neubert, 2010). N200 potentials may promise a useful BCI model for controlling external devices due to the interface's low requirements of luminance and contrast, the large amplitude of the induced brain signal, and the low individual difference of mVEP (Schaeff et al., 2012). A N200-speller based Internet browser (Liu et al., 2010) reports that the N200 stimulus interface causes less visual discomfort and the induced N200 potential is more stable and less affected by the adaption effect. A BCI system is presented by combining mVEP and P300 potentials (Jin et al., 2012).

Comparing with manipulators and mobile robots, humanoid robots are more advanced as they are created to imitate some of the same physical and mental tasks that humans undergo daily (Hirai et al., 1998), but control of humanoid robots is much more complex. Humanoid robots are being developed to perform a wide range of complex tasks like personal assistance, where they should be able to assist the sick and elderly, and dirty or dangerous jobs. Recently, controlling a humanoid robot via brainwaves becomes more attractive. Bell et al. (2008) and Choi et al. (Choi and Jo, 2013) used ERPs to select an object as a target that a humanoid robot should reach, while our study focuses on telepresence control of humanoid robot behavior via the N200 potentials, including walking in an environment with obstacles and picking-up an object. The challenge to develop an ERP-based model is to make a trade-off between improving the classification accuracy and shortening the intervals between commands in controlling the humanoid robot in real time under the limited information transfer rate (ITR) (Wolpaw et al., 2000).

When investigating the P300-based BRI models (Li et al., 2013a,b), we noticed that the N200 components in brainwaves acquired from our experiments were stable and their amplitudes were relative high. The prominent shape of ERP is very helpful to build feature vectors for improving the classification accuracy. In this article, we propose a BRI model based on the N200 potentials. In order to acquire N200 potentials with high quality, we design an interface by replacing characters in a regular speller with robot images representing robot behaviors to be controlled with mind.

We evaluate this N200-based model by telepresence controlling a humanoid robot with live video feedback. We analyze the N200 potentials induced by the experiment procedure to suggest how to improve the proposed model.

The paper is organized as follows. In Section Materials and Methods, we present the materials and methods for this study, including our mind-controlled humanoid robot system-Cerebot, the detailed experiment procedure, and the method for analyzing and recognizing the N200 potentials. In section Results, we off-line analyze the N200 potentials elicited by the experiment procedure and present the model performance regarding the accuracy, the ITR and the practical bit rate (PBR) (Jin et al., 2012). In this section, we apply the N200-based model to telepresence control a humanoid robot to accomplish two types of tasks. In section Discussion, we discuss the factors that affect the performance of the on-line control operation tasks and draw some conclusions.

MATERIALS AND METHODS

CEREBOT

Cerebot is a mind-controlled humanoid robot platform (Li et al., 2011, 2012). Cerebus™ is the neural signal acquisition system in this platform. It is able to record both invasive and noninvasive neural signals and its processor can deal with on-line signal pre-processing, such as filtering and line noise removing. The platform uses two kinds of humanoid robots. The first one is a NAO humanoid robot made by Aldebaran in France [http://www.aldebaran.com/en]. The other one is a KT-X PC humanoid robot made by Kumotek in USA [http://kumotek.com]. Both of the humanoid robots with high degree of freedoms (DOFs) are equipped with microphones, a camera, a sonar rangefinder, etc., to provide environment information. The Cerebot platform can be used: first, to challenge brainwave-based methods since control of a humanoid robot with full body movements is difficult; second, to evaluate different methods for controlling a humanoid robot under a uniform platform; third, to testify neuroscience assumptions; fourth, to investigate the effect of telepresence control on the subject's mental activities. In this study, we implement the N200 model on Cerebot to on-line navigate a NAO humanoid robot in an office environment and to pick-up an object based on live videos sent back by the camera embedded in the robot.

The control architecture of Cerebot is developed under the OpenViBE-based programming environment. OpenViBE is a free and open-source software platform for designing, testing, and using brain-computer interfaces. It consists of a set of modules devoted to the acquisition, pre-processing, processing, and visualization of cerebral data, as well as to the interaction with Virtual Reality (VR) (Renard et al., 2010). It offers a powerful interface named "Virtual-Reality Peripheral Network (VRPN)" to communicate with other scripts programmed in Matlab or Python. In the Cerebot system (Zhao et al., 2013), OpenViBE integrates the signal acquisition section, the signal processing section, and the control section, as shown in **Figure 1**. In order to control the NAO robot via N200 potentials, an OpenViBE module generates a serial of visual stimuli in a random order to a subject who focuses on a target stimulus (a robot image) that codes the subject's mental activity. Cerebus™ records brainwaves and sends them to the signal processing section to pre-process them, to extract their features of N200 potentials, and to classify them according to the codes of the subject mental activities. Once the subject mental activity is identified, its corresponding control command is sent to the control section to activate the robot behavior.

N200 MODEL

Flow diagram

We implemented the N200 model on Cerebot under the OpenViBE programming environment. **Figure 2** shows the model flow diagram. The white boxes in the diagram are the toolboxes provided by the OpenViBE packages, while the colored boxes are modules developed in C++ or Matlab. The arrows in the diagram

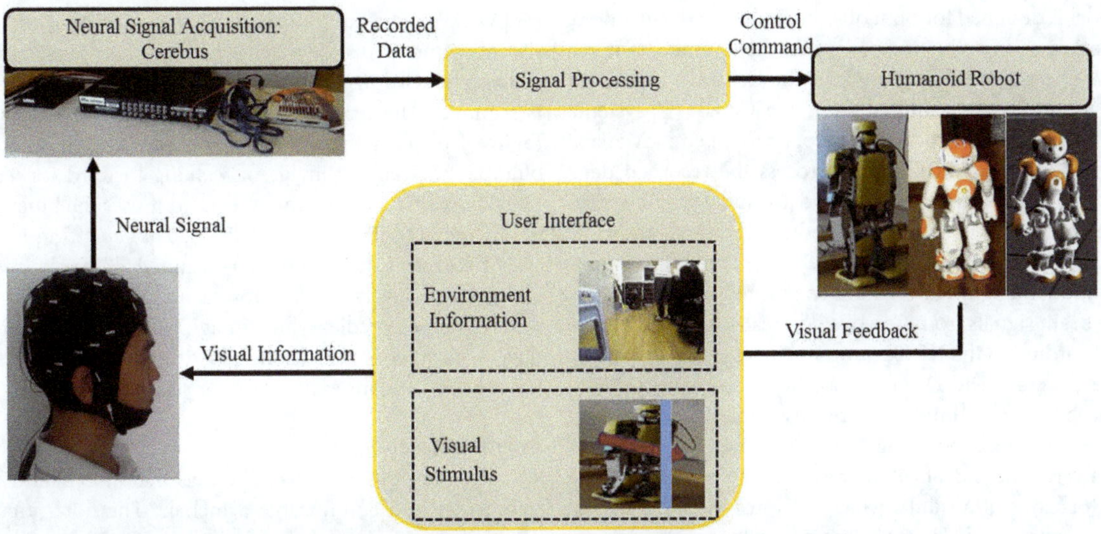

FIGURE 1 | A N200 model based mind-controlled humanoid robot.

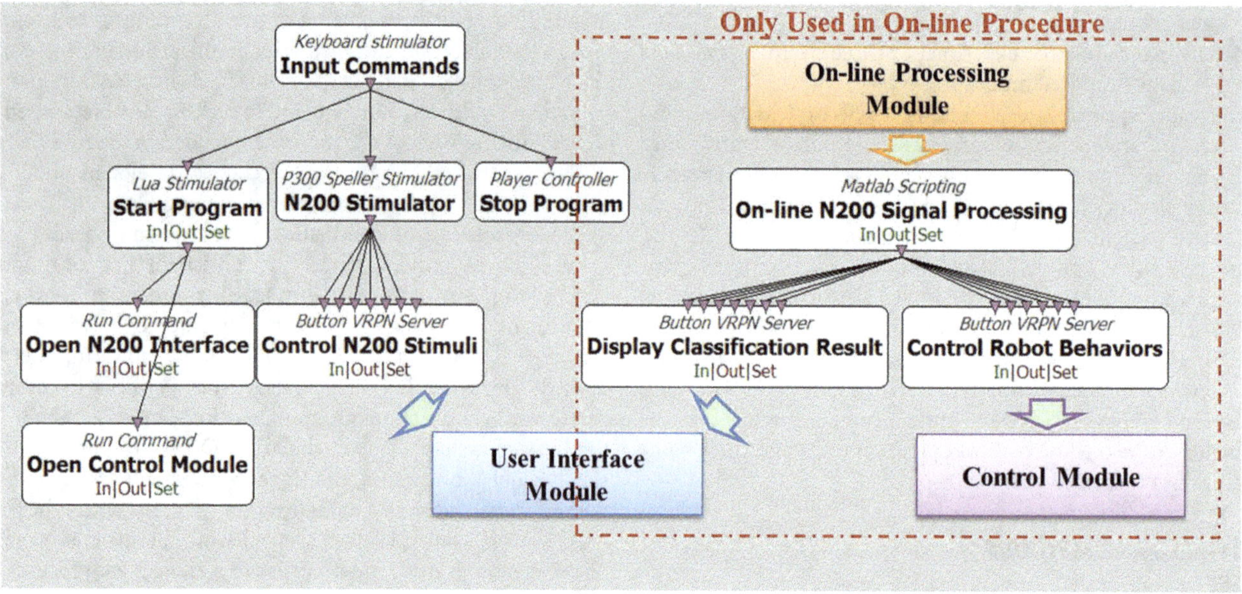

FIGURE 2 | Diagram of N200 model under the OpenViBE programming environment. The white boxes are functions provided by the OpenViBE software package, and the colored boxes are the modules for the N200 model. The boxes enclosed in the red dashed rectangle are only for the on-line control procedure.

indicate data flow paths. The N200 model uses the Start Program toolbox and the Open N200 Interface toolbox in **Figure 2** to start up the User Interface module programmed in C++. To start an experiment, the N200 model uses the N200 Stimulator toolbox provided by OpenViBE to determine the settings, e.g., the stimulating timeline of the visual stimuli, for the User Interface module. The communication from the N200 Stimulator toolbox to the User Interface module is established via VRPN. The User Interface module activates six robot images in random order as the visual stimuli to evoke N200 potentials and sends their event markers to Cerebus™ via serial port to lock the time point at which the relevant image is activated.

The model is designed for both off-line analyzing the acquired N200 potentials and on-line controlling the humanoid robot via brainwaves. The off-line procedure uses the Central software to record the brain signals acquired from the Cerebus™ system. The off-line N200 signal processing scripts developed in Matlab, which are not displayed in **Figure 2**, process the recorded data to analyze the brain signal features and to investigate classification algorithms. In the on-line procedure, the On-line N200 Signal Processing toolbox starts up the On-line Processing module via the Matlab engine to load the configured parameters, to acquire the brain signals from Cerebus™ in real-time and to classify them according to the N200 feature vectors generated during the off-line process. The Display Classification Result toolbox displays the hit visual stimulus on the user interface by framing the corresponding robot image. The Control Robot Behavior toolbox converts the classification result to its corresponding command for Control Module, which activates the behavior to be controlled with mind. **Figure 2** shows how the toolboxes and modules exchange data with each other under the OpenViBE environment.

Interface and protocol for acquiring N200 potentials

Figure 3A shows the user interface with a 2 × 3 matrix of images. These images taken from the real represent six robot behaviors: walking forward, walking backward, shifting left, shifting right, turning left and turning right. We attached red arrows on the images to make the meanings of the images more impressive. In order to induce N200 potentials, a blue bar scans an image from right to left. **Figure 3B** shows that the blue bar is moving on the image to activate the visual stimulus of robot working forward.

We applied the Single Character (SC) method (Guger et al., 2009) to randomly activate the images one by one with the probability of 1/6. The duration of the stimulus onset asynchrony (SOA) (Wei and Luo, 2010) is 220 ms consisting of 150 ms for scanning and 70 ms for a break between two consecutive activations. A repetition is defined as a process in which each image is scanned. The repetition duration is 220 ms × 6 = 1320 ms. **Figure 4** displays the entire process of a repetition. It uses the blue bar to scan the image of walking forward for 150 ms and takes a break for 70 ms, and afterward it uses the blue bar to scan the image of turning left, and so on. The repetition is completed after 1320 ms as the blue bar has scanned all the six images. Each image is randomly selected for scanning in a repetition, so the subject cannot predict which image will be the next visual stimulus. A number of repetitions constitute a trial in which the blue bar repeatedly scans each image for several times.

Experiment procedure

We conducted experiments in a quiet environment and asked subjects to sit in a comfortable armchair. The horizontal distance between the armchair and a monitor was 70 cm. The monitor was a 22-inch LCD one with a resolution of 1280×1024 pixels. The electroencephalogram (EEG) signals were recorded at

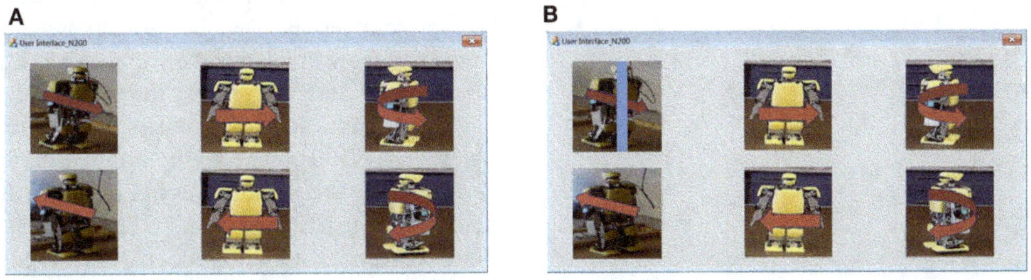

FIGURE 3 | (A) User interface of visual stimuli is a 2 × 3 matrix of six robot images depicting six humanoid robot behaviors. **(B)** The visual stimulus for walking forward is activated by using a blue bar to scan the robot walking forward image from left to right.

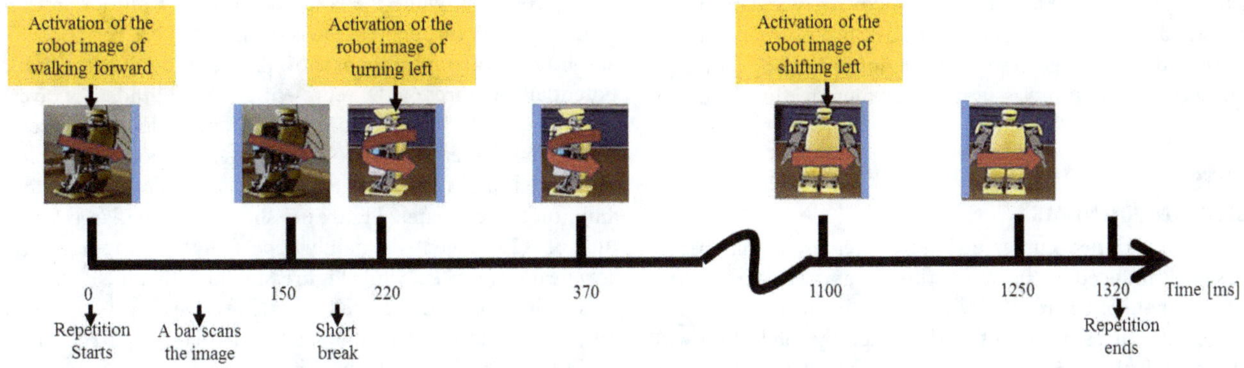

FIGURE 4 | Protocol of inducing N200 potentials activates the six visual stimuli one by one in a random order.

1000 Hz from 32 surface channels using an EEG cap according to the "International 10-20 system." The linked mastoids were reference channels and the channel AFz was the ground channel.

Five subjects (one female, four males, aged 26–28) signed a written informed consent to participate in experiments. Tianjin medical university general hospital ethics committee gives the oral approval of the consent form and experimental procedure before any subjects participated. All of their visual acuities were normal or corrected to normal. Three of them had no prior experience on the experiments. Each subject conducted 360 repetitions, i.e., 36 trials. In each trial, the subject selected a robot image as a target stimulus according to his/her mental activity. During a trial, the subject needed to focus on the target stimulus, tried his/her best to ignore the non-target stimuli, and had to avoid making any movements. Cerebus™ received the visual stimuli and simultaneously recorded the evoked potentials.

SIGNAL ANALYSIS AND FEATURE EXTRACTION

Signal analysis

We analyzed the recorded brain signals to extract their features. First, the brain signals were cut into epochs that were simultaneously with the visual stimuli. The length of each epoch was from post-stimulus 0 ms to post-stimulus 800 ms to cover the potentials. Because the delta (0.5–4 Hz) and theta (4–7.5 Hz) oscillation contribute to the N200 potentials (Karakas et al., 2000a) and the drift mainly appears in a low band, a digital band-pass filter with 1–10 Hz was chosen to process the epochs. Second, we removed the signal drift by the method of common average reference (CAR). Finally, the epochs were divided into two groups: the epochs induced by the target stimulus and the ones induced by the non-target stimulus, and then both the groups of the epochs were averaged, respectively.

Feature extraction and classification

Being able to represent the feature of brain signals in low dimension space can reduce the amount of computation (Bian and Zhang, 2000). According to Shannon's theorem, we were able to reduce the dimension of the feature vectors by down-sampling the data epochs from 1000 to 20 Hz (Krusienski et al., 2008). We used the N200 signal processing scripts to remove noises from the epoch from post-stimulus 100–500 ms and to average the epochs induced by the same visual stimulus in a trial. The brain signals from a single channel yielded an 8-dimension [(500-100)/1000 × 20] feature vector. If n channels were used to extract the features, the total dimension of a vector was $8 \times n$. The selected channel number depended on the characteristics of individual subject's brain signals.

We adopted the Fisher's linear discriminant analysis (FLDA) as a two-class classifier to discover which visual stimulus was the target one by checking each feature vector. The idea of this algorithm is to find the optimal direction of projections that groups the vectors with the same features into a class (Mika et al., 1999) as bellow:

$$\mathbf{w} = \mathbf{S}_w^{-1} (\mathbf{M}_1 - \mathbf{M}_2)$$

$$\mathbf{S}_w = \mathbf{S}_1 + \mathbf{S}_2$$

$$\mathbf{S}_i = \sum_{\mathbf{x}_k \in \mathbf{X}_i} (\mathbf{x}_k - \mathbf{M}_i)(\mathbf{x}_k - \mathbf{M}_i)^T, i = 1, 2$$

$$\mathbf{M}_i = \frac{1}{n_i} \sum_{\mathbf{x}_k \in \mathbf{X}_i} \mathbf{x}_k, i = 1, 2$$

where $\mathbf{x}_k$ is the feature vector, X_i represents the class set and n_i is the number of feature vectors in the ith class.

We trained the FLDA classifier using the feature vectors and tested it by the brain signals recorded in a trial that established six feature vectors according to the six visual stimuli. The trained classifier processed each feature vector successively and outputted the classified value. The classifier outputted no control command if it classified the six features vectors as non-targets or outputted a control command if it classified one or more feature vectors as targets.

RESULTS

INDUCED N200 POTENTIALS

The solid and dotted curves in **Figure 5** represent the average brain signals induced by the target stimulus and non-target stimulus from channel P3, respectively. The brain signal induced by the target stimulus appears with a sharp negative deflection with amplitude of 5 uV at 258 ms and a positive deflection with amplitude of 3.5 uV at 358 ms. The negative deflection is known as the N200 potential that is the response to scanning over the target image by the blue bar. The positive deflection resembles the P300 potential. The brain signals induced by the non-target stimuli do not appear with obvious deflection. The results demonstrate that the designed interface can induce N200 potentials by scanning over a target image with the blue bar. The negative deflection provides a recognizable feature of the N200 potential for us to classify the brain signals.

We plot the average brain signals acquired from each subject through channels P3 and CP3 to discuss their individual difference, as shown in **Figures 6A,B**. The black thick curve is the average N200 potentials across the five subjects, while the other thin color curves are the N200 potentials from the individual subject. The N200 potential amplitudes acquired from the subj5, represented by the green curves in **Figures 6A,B**, are smaller than the others. The latencies of the N200 potentials acquired by the subj4, represented by the pink curves in **Figures 6A,B**, is 20 ms shorter than the average latency. The N200 potentials induced from the subjects show different amplitude distributions over channels P3 and CP3. For example, the N200 potential amplitude acquired from the subj2 through channel P3 is larger than the one through channel CP3, represented by the blue curves in **Figures 6A,B**, while the N200 potentials amplitudes acquired from the subj5 through channels P3 and CP3 are very close. The amplitude topographic maps show the distribution of the induced potentials. **Figures 6C,D** represent the amplitudes of average brain signals at 258 ms and 358 ms after the visual stimuli, respectively. The darker the red color indicates the positive amplitude the greater, and the darker the blue color indicates the negative amplitude the greater. **Figure 6C** shows that the largest amplitude of N200 potentials mainly appears in the temporal-parietal area near channel P3, while **Figure 6D** shows that the P300 potentials mainly distribute in the parietal area. We draw two following remarks. First, although the N200 potentials acquired from the subjects are slightly different, they exhibit the N200 potentials' features that are important to control the robot behavior. Second, the N200 and P300 potentials mainly appear in the parietal and temporal areas in a window of post-stimulus 100–500 ms and the channels from which the recognizable N200 potentials are acquired vary due to the individuality, so we determine time windows and select the best channels for the individual subject for processing N200 potentials to control the humanoid robot.

The electrical potentials caused by eye movement and blinking can be much larger than the ERPs (Joyce et al., 2004) and

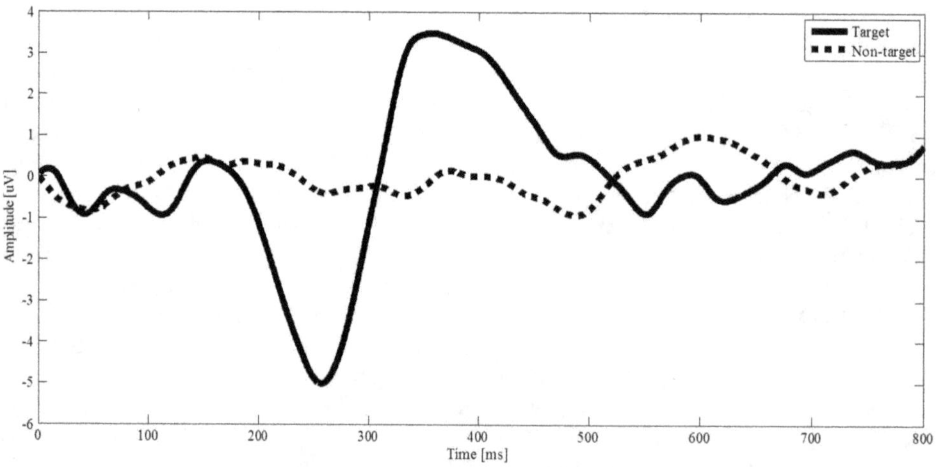

FIGURE 5 | Evoked potentials from channel P3 are averaged. The solid curve is the brainwave of a target stimulus, and the dotted curve is the brainwave of a non-target stimulus.

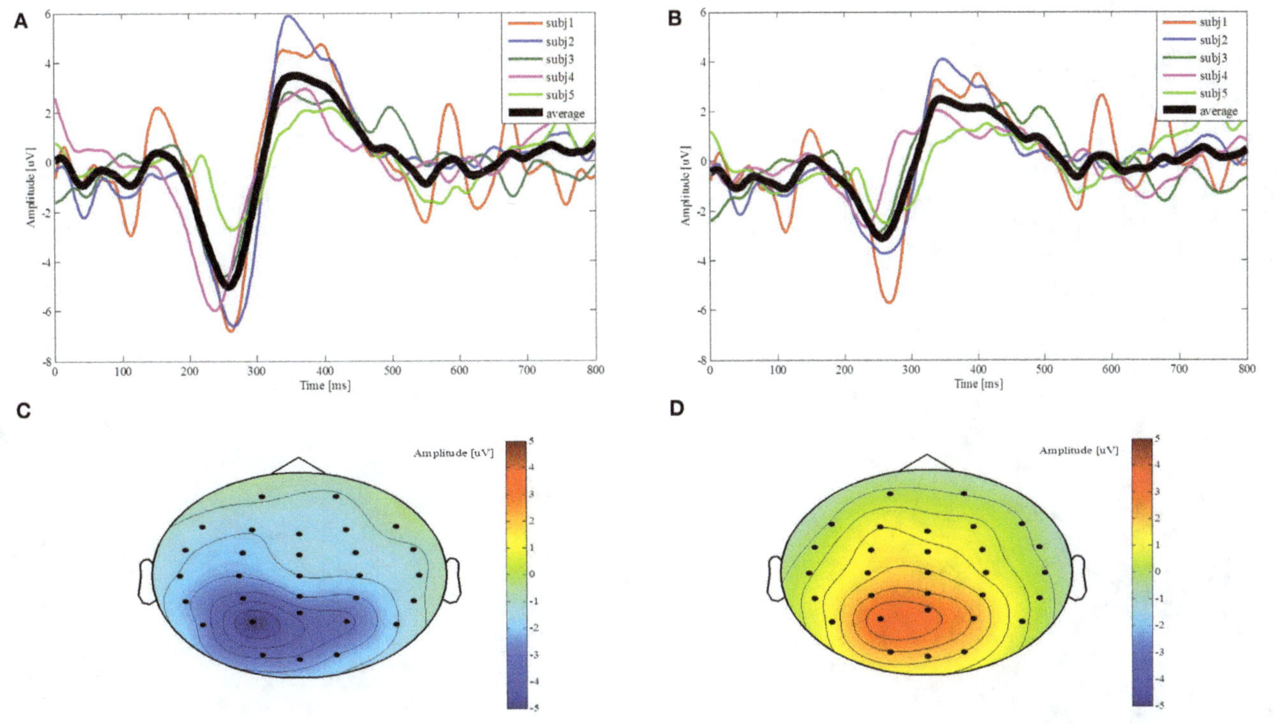

FIGURE 6 | Evoked potentials from channel P3 and CP3 and their topographies along with time points. (A,B) The colorful thin curves represent the five subjects' N200 and P300 potentials from post-stimulus 0–800 ms, respectively, and the black curve represents the average potentials over the five subjects. **(C,D)** The amplitude topographic maps of the average brain signals across five subjects are plotted at 258 ms and 358 ms.

propagate across the scalp, so these electrical potentials may distort the ERPs, but their impact on the ERPs decreases as a distance from the frontal increases. Because the induced N200 potentials mainly appear in the temporal—parietal area that is far from the frontal, the distortion of the N200 potentials induced by using a blue bar scanning visual stimulus images is irrelevant. In this study, therefore, we directly apply the induced N200 potentials to on-line control the humanoid robot.

However, the distortion of the P300 potentials induced by flashing stimulus images may be significant since the P300 potentials mainly appear in the parietal and central areas (Iturrate et al., 2009). Consequently, an additional algorithm has to be designed to remove eye artifacts to ensure high classification accuracy.

OFF-LINE EVALUATION

This subsection evaluates the off-line performance of the N200 model based on the classifier accuracy, which is the ratio between the trials detected correctly over the total trials, the ITR and the PBR.

We averaged the classified accuracy of each subject by the 10-fold cross-validation (Liu et al., 2010). The first step was to determine the candidate channels based on the subject's amplitude topographic map. The second step was to calculate the classified accuracy of each channel and their combinations. The third step was to select the combination that yielded the highest accuracy as the optimal channels for the individual subject, listed in **Table 1**. The three subjects denoted by **N** had no prior BCI experience on the experiments, while the other two subjects

Table 1 | The off-line performance.

Subject	Optimal channels	Accuracy (%)	ITR (bits/min)	PBR (bits/min)
subj1 (Y)	P3, P4, Pz, CP3	98.6	22.22	21.58
subj2 (N)	P3, P4, Pz, CP3	98.6	22.22	21.58
subj3 (N)	P3, P7, CP3	92.9	18.61	15.95
subj4 (Y)	P3, P4, Pz,	97.1	21.19	19.98
subj5 (N)	P3, CPz	81.4	13.28	8.34
Mean	–	93.7	19.50	17.49

denoted by **Y** had prior BCI experience. **Figure 7** depicts the average accuracy for each subject vs. the number of repetitions. The accuracy is clearly increased when increasing the number from 1 to 10. The accuracies of the four subjects reach 100%, and three of them reach 100% with 6 repetitions. The accuracy of subj5 is slightly low. ITR measures the information rate per minute by taking the accuracy and the time needed to classify a visual stimulus described as

$$B = \left[\log_2 N + \log_2 P + (1-P) \times \log_2\left(\frac{1-P}{N-1}\right)\right] \times M$$

where $N = 6$ stands for 6 visual stimuli in the user interface, P is the classifier accuracy, M is the number of outputting commands in a minute (McFarland et al., 2003). The index,

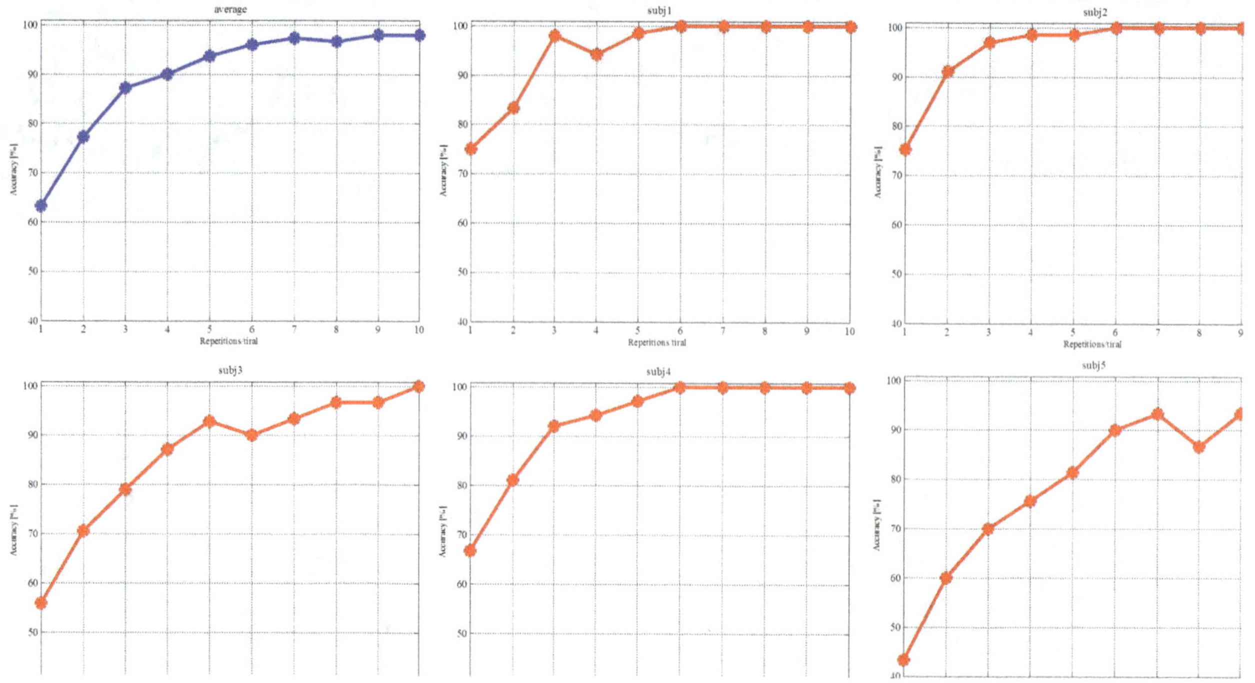

FIGURE 7 | Red curves are the accuracies achieved by the individual subjects and the blue curve is their average accuracy.

PBR, estimates the practical speed of a system, by considering each error classification that needs to be corrected by additional selections (Jin et al., 2012) as below:

$$PBR = B \times [1 - 2 \times (1 - P)]$$

PBR is meaningful only when $P \geq 50\%$. **Table 1** lists the five subjects' accuracies, ITRs and PBRs. For evaluating the off-line ITR, we set both the interval between the repetitions and the one between the trials as 0 ms (Jin et al., 2011), so M is 9.09 ($0.22 \times 6 \times 5 = 6.60$s, $60.00/6.60 \approx 9.09$) when the repetition number is 5. In **Table 1**, each subject's ITR is larger than 10 bits/min. ITR increases when the accuracy is increased. The highest accuracy of 98.57% yields the largest ITR of 22.22 bits/min. PBR is smaller than ITR due to $[1 - 2 \times (1 - P)] \leq 1$. The large accuracy reduces the difference between ITR and PBR. Clearly, a high accuracy allows the subject to correct the error quickly and to realize his/her intention accurately, while a low accuracy needs the subject to spend much time to correct an incorrect command. Improving the accuracy needs to increase the number of repetitions in a trial, i.e., to increase the control cycle, so a trade-off between the accuracy and control cycle speed must be considered according to a task requirement.

CASE STUDIES

In order to validate the developed N200 model, the subjects controlled on-line the NAO humanoid robot to accomplish two popular tasks in robotics research: to navigate the NAO robot to walk with obstacle avoidance and to control the NAO robot to pick up an object. These tasks are challenging because the subjects need live video feedback from a camera embedded in the NAO robot to activate appropriate robot behavior.

The experiments were carried out in a normal office without electromagnetic shielding. The subjects sat in a comfortable chair and 70 cm away from a 22-inch LCD monitor displaying the N200 interface and the live video feedback, as shown in **Figure 8A**. The live video window was placed above the interface window with a distance to reduce mutual influences on subjects' concentrations caused by visual stimuli and live video. During the experiments, the subjects needed to stabilize their heads since the head motion may cause noises. Once a trial began, the subjects relied on live video to observe the robot status and surroundings and focused on a visual stimulus depicting robot behavior whose meaning represented their intention. When a trial was ended, the classification result was transformed to a command to activate an appropriate robot behavior. For the on-line experiments, the interval between repetitions was set 600 ms, therefore the duration of outputting a command with 3 repetitions was 5.76 s; the duration was 9.60 s with 5 repetitions. The interval between trials was set 5 s as the subjects needed this interval to have a short rest and to decide the next behavior. **Figure 8B** shows an example of controlling the NAO robot to shift left with mind. The supplementary material (movie clip) that records the on-line control processes of navigating a humanoid robot in an office environment with an obstacle and picking-up an object is available.

For the navigation task, the subjects controlled the humanoid robot to walk from a start point to a destination by passing an obstacle as shown in **Figure 9A**. Based on the live video from the robot's camera, the subjects used N200 potentials to activate six

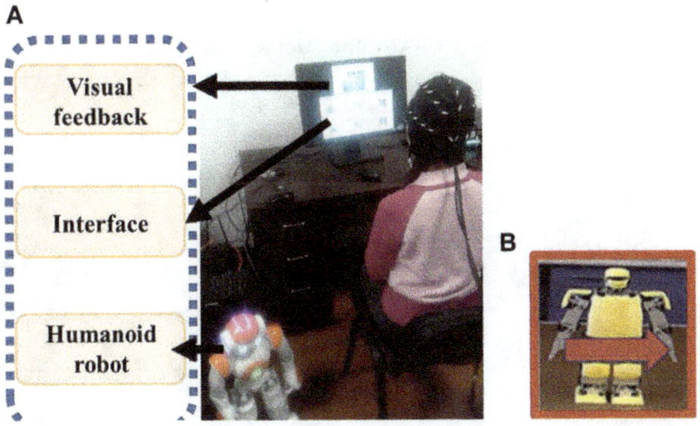

FIGURE 8 | (A) On-line control of the NAO humanoid robot with mind in an office environment **(B)** The visual stimulus of shifting left is classified as a target.

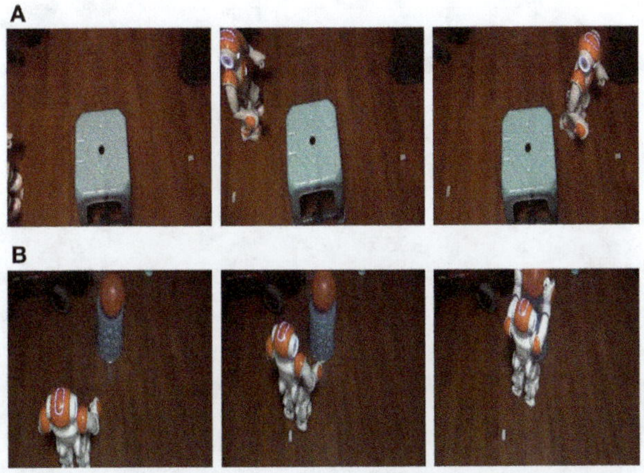

FIGURE 9 | On-line study cases of controlling the humanoid robot using the N200 model. (A) Robot navigation with obstacle avoidance. **(B)** Robot pick-up operation.

types of robot walking behaviors defined by: walking forward for 0.2 m, walking backward for 0.15 m, shifting left for 0.15 m, shifting right for 0.15 m, turning left for 30°, and turning right for 30°. We evaluate their control performance using the following criteria: the total commands for activating robot behaviors, the total time for completing the task, the on-line control success rates, and the number of collisions with an obstacle in the three experiments. The robot may collide with the obstacle when a subject cannot appropriately estimate the distance between the robot and the obstacle from the live video or his/her intention is incorrectly detected. **Table 2** lists the results herein averaged over the three experiments.

For the pick-up operation task, the subjects controlled the humanoid robot to approach a balloon and to pick up this target as shown in **Figure 9B**. The balloon was placed on a round table in the right front of the robot so the subjects had to move the robot to a position close enough to the table and to configure a proper orientation to pick up the balloon. For this task, the subjects used N200 potentials to activate the following defined behaviors: picking-up the target, walking forward for 0.1 m, shifting left/right for 0.1 m, and turning left/right for 15°. A task operation was classified as a failure if the pick-up behavior was activated before the robot reached the proper position. This task operation was repeated until each subject completed three successful experiments. In order to evaluate the on-line control performance, we recorded the total commands for activating robot behaviors in the three successful experiments, the average total time of completing a pick-up operation task, the average on-line success rate averaged over the three successful experiments, and the ratio of the successful experiments over the total ones.

Tables 2, 3 list the experimental results conducted by the five subjects. We compare their on-line control performance using 5 repetitions for a trial as defined in **Table 1** because this repetition number documents that all the subjects achieve their accuracies over 80%. For comparing the on-line control performance, **Tables 2, 3** also list the test results with 3 repetitions of a trial. We address five remarks as follows.

(1) The on-line success rates differ from the off-line accuracies. The experiments of the navigation task documented that subj2, subj3, and subj5's on-line success rates (88.8, 78.4, 73.4%) were lower than their off-line accuracies (98.6, 92.8, 81.4%) when the repetition number was 5; while subj1 and subj4's success rates (100.0, 100.0%) were slightly higher than their off-line accuracies (98.6, 97.1%). The experiments of the pick-up operation task documented that subj1, subj2, and subj4's on-line success rates (95.2, 96.7, 92.3%) were slightly lower than their off-line accuracies (98.6, 98.6, 97.1%), while subj3 and subj5's success rates (100.0, 95.8%) were higher than the off-line accuracies (92.9, 81.4%).
(2) Most of the subjects achieved higher on-line success rates for the pick-up operation task than those for the navigation task. The subjects subj1, subj2, subj3, and subj4 achieved the higher on-line success rates (100.0, 96.3, 95.5, 100.0%) for the pick-up operation task than those (96.4, 84.5, 77.2, 90.9%) for the navigation task when the repetition number is 3. The subjects subj2, subj3, and subj5 achieved the higher on-line success rates (96.7, 100.0, 95.8%) for the pick-up operation task than those (88.8, 78.4, 73.4%) when the repetition number is 5.
(3) A lower success rate results in more total commands and longer total time for completing the operation tasks. For the navigation task, subj2 and subj3's success rates (84.5, 77.2%) with 3 repetitions were lower than the ones (88.8, 78.4%) with 5 repetitions, so their corresponding total commands for three successful experiments (49/3, 75/3) with 3 repetitions were more than ones (34/3, 51/3) with 5 repetitions and their average total times (180.8, 265.3 s) for completing each of the three successful experiments with 3 repetitions are longer than those (163.4, 245.5 s) with 5 repetitions although their duration of 5.76 s for outputting a command with 3 repetitions was shorter than the one of 9.60 s with 5 repetitions. For the pick-up operation task, when subj1, subj3, subj4, and subj5 achieved the higher success rates (100.0, 100.0, 100.0, 95.8%), they generated the fewer commands (19/3, 16/3, 20/3, 19/3). A low success rate increases the possibility

Table 2 | Performance of the navigation task.

Subject	Repetition number	Time/ command	Total time (s)	Total commands	On-line success rate (%)	Collisions
subj1 (Y)	3	5.76	99.8	28/3	96.4	0/3
	5	9.60	144.3	30/3	100.0	0/3
subj2 (N)	3	5.76	180.8	49/3	84.5	1/3
	5	9.60	163.4	34/3	88.8	0/3
subj3 (N)	3	5.76	265.3	75/3	77.2	0/3
	5	9.60	245.6	51/3	78.4	0/3
subj4 (Y)	3	5.76	116.1	33/3	90.9	0/3
	5	9.60	154.3	32/3	100.0	0/3
subj5 (N)	3	5.76	163.4	46/3	78.2	0/3
	5	9.60	229.7	45/3	73.4	4/3

Table 3 | Performance of the pick-up operation task.

Subject	Repetition number	Time/ command	Total time (s)	Total commands	On-line success rate (%) for successful experiments	Successful / total experiments
subj1 (Y)	3	5.76	65.4	19/3	100.0	3/4
	5	9.60	99.3	21/3	95.2	3/3
subj2 (N)	3	5.76	73.7	22/3	96.3	3/3
	5	9.60	105.0	23/3	96.7	3/3
subj3 (N)	3	5.76	70.4	20/3	95.8	3/4
	5	9.60	73.4	16/3	100.0	3/5
subj4 (Y)	3	5.76	69.1	20/3	100.0	3/5
	5	9.60	123.6	26/3	92.3	3/3
subj5 (N)	3	5.76	94.1	27/3	66.7	3/4
	5	9.60	85.0	19/3	95.8	3/5

of incorrectly detecting the subjects' intentions, so outputting additional commands to correct the false ones increases the number of total commands. For the three experiments, subj2 used 34 commands to navigate the NAO robot without collision with the obstacle under the success rate of 88.8%, while subj5 used 45 commands to navigate the NAO robot with 4 collisions with the obstacle under the success rate of 73.4%.

(4) A repetition number of a trial plays an important role in determining a total time for completing an operation task at a high success rate. For completing three successful navigation tasks, subj1, subj4, and subj5 varied slightly their numbers of total commands (from 28 to 30, from 33 to 32, from 46 to 45) when the repetition number increased from 3 to 5. For completing three successful pick-up operation tasks, subj1, subj2, and subj3 varied slightly their numbers of total commands (from 19 to 21, from 22 to 23, from 20 to 16) when the repetition number increased from 3 to 5. For the above cases, changing the repetition number does not affect the number of total commands very much, so the duration of a trial, i.e., the repetition number determines the total time for completing an operation task. Increasing the repetition number from 3 to 5, i.e., growing the duration of a trial from 5.76 to 9.60 s, increases the total times for completing the navigation tasks discussed above from 99.8 to 144.3 s, from 116.1 to 154.3 s, and from 163.4 to 229.7 s, and the total times for completing the pick-up operation tasks from 65.4 s to 99.3 s, from 73.7 to 105.0 s, from 70.4 to 73.4 s, as listed in **Tables 2, 3**.

(5) The experience with the designed experimental procedure is an important factor that impacts the on-line success rates. The subjects subj1 and subj4 with prior experience on the experiments achieved the high on-line average success rates of 97.9 and 95.8%, while the subjects subj2, subj3, and subj5 without prior experience delivered the relatively low success rates of 91.6, 87.9, and 78.5%.

DISCUSSION

THE N200 MODEL

The work (Karakas et al., 2000b) shows that the ERP represents interplay between the oscillations that are mainly in the delta and theta frequencies. We assume that the moving bar scanning over the robot images may impact on event-related oscillations (EROs) in the temporal-parietal area, because the brainwaves acquired from this area deliver the recognizable N200 potentials which may be contributed by the theta oscillation related with orientation and attention (Karakas et al., 2000a,b). We will verify this assumption in our further research.

The interface that we design for inducing the N200 potentials has three advantages. First, the robot images as the visual stimuli are more intuitive and help the subjects understand the meanings of the stimuli better. Second, scanning the static robot images by the blue bar, instead of flashing the robot images in the traditional P300 model, allows the subjects more intensively to concentrate on a target stimulus. The subjects reported that the moving bar could cause less visual fatigue than the flashing images. Third, the proposed visual stimulus mode also induces the P300 potentials, but the amplitudes of the N200 potentials are larger and more recognizable, so we use the N200 potentials to establish the features vector to achieve better classification accuracy.

EFFECTS ON THE ON-LINE SUCCESS RATES

We note that the on-line success rates vary for different operation tasks and their differences depend on the individual subjects. Here, we present the factors that affect the on-line success rates. The on-line success rates achieved in on-line control of the robot are usually lower than classification accuracies in the off-line evaluation. It would be a common fact because the off-line evaluation is an open-loop control, while the on-line task-driven control is a closed-loop control with live video feedback. Different from the off-line control, the on-line telepresence control needs a subject to coordinate his/her attention to both the live video and the visual stimuli, and especially the live video may divert a subject's attention away from the target stimulus, which decreases the on-line success rates (Gergondet et al., 2012). Especially, the poor quality of live videos may significantly deteriorate the subject's control performance. Auditory effect from the surrounding, e.g., the sound of robot's walking steps, may be another factor that distracts the subject's attention. Tidoni et al. (2014) reported that the sound of robot's walking steps delivered synchronously with the robot motion needs less time to control the robot than the asynchronous sound. In general, the success rates of the navigation task with noisy walking steps' sound are lower than those of the pick-up task. The subjects have to make a right decision based on the surrounding information sent by the live video to control the robot behavior. In addition, the subjects may get anxious when the robot falls down or collides with an obstacle caused by an incorrect command.

ANALYSIS OF THE ON-LINE CONTROLLED TASKS

We evaluate the total execution time of completing an on-line controlled task. Because the total time depends on the total commands generated by the induced N200 potentials, quickly and accurately outputting a command shortens the total time. The two factors mainly affect the total number of generated commands. The first factor is the on-line control success rate that indirectly indicates how many incorrect commands are outputted for the on-line control process. Each incorrect command causes an unexpected robot behavior that needs to be corrected by additional control commands. For the navigation task, subj2 and subj3 achieved the success rates with 3 repetitions lower than those with 5 repetitions and for the pick-up operation task subj5 achieved the success rates with 3 repetitions lower than those with 5 repetitions, so they spent more total time to complete their corresponding tasks since they outputted much more additional control commands. The second factor is the individuality of mental activities of planning in real-time to complete an operation task indicated by the following cases: 1. With 5 repetitions, subj5's brain activated fewer control commands than subj2's brain did to accomplish the pick-up operation task; 2. With 3 repetitions, subj3's brain activated fewer control commands than subj2's brain did to complete the pick-up operation task; 3. With 5 repetitions, subj5's brain activated fewer control commands than subj3's brain did to complete the navigation task.

The repetition number of a trial is a very important factor that affects the total time of an on-line task operation. The repetition number determines the duration of outputting a command. The large duration increases the total time. For example, subj1, subj4, and subj5 spent more time with 5 repetitions than with 3 repetitions to accomplish the navigation task, and subj1, subj2, and subj3 spent more time with 5 repetitions than 3 repetitions to complete the pick-up operation task, because each of them outputted the close number of total commands no matter the repetition number is 3 or 5. On the other hand, the large repetition number yields the high success rate. As discussed above, the high success rate reduces the incorrect outputs in the control process. Consequently, the few incorrect commands that need to be rectified shorten the total time. Usually, a high success rate needs the large repetition number to increase the reliability of the control system, but it increases the duration of a trial. How to determine the repetition number is an important issue because a balance between the reliability and the total time needs to be considered.

We used the robot images as the visual stimuli successfully to induce the N200 potentials with recognizable amplitudes. We implemented the proposed N200 model on the Cerebot platform to evaluate its off-line and on-line performances across five subjects. The off-line evaluations show that the average accuracy is 93.71% over the five subjects with 5 repetitions in a trial and two of the five subjects reach their accuracies of 98% with three repetitions. The five subjects participated in the navigation and pick-up operation tasks in an office environment in which the live video feedback provided surrounding information. The success rates affect the total number of commands outputted from the N200 model, the total time for completing an on-line operation task, and the number of collisions caused by the incorrect commands. Therefore achieving a high success rate has a priority using the N200 model to control the humanoid robot. As discussed above, the repetition number of a trial plays a prominent role in achieving the high success rate and shortening the duration of outputting a command. In the future work, we investigate the optimal repetition number according to a variety of on-line operation tasks.

Some research teams applied the steady state visually-evoked potential (e.g., Gergondet et al., 2012; Tidoni et al., 2014) to control a humanoid robot with live video or the motor imagery (e.g., Cohen et al., 2012) to control the robot behavior for a navigation task. In the future work, we will evaluate the performances of these models using the Cerebot platform.

ACKNOWLEDGMENTS

The authors would like to thank Mr. Guoxin Zhao, Mr. Hong Hu, and Ms. Wenxuan Li for their help in conducting the experiments. This work was supported in part by The National Natural Science Foundation of China (No. 61271321, No. 61473207), the Ph.D. Programs Foundation of the Ministry of Education of China (No. 20120032110068) and Tianjin Key Technology Research and Development Program (No. 14ZCZDSF00025).

REFERENCES

Bell, C. J., Shenoy, P., Chalodhorn, R., and Rao, R. P. N. (2008). Control of a humanoid robot by a noninvasive brain-computer interface in humans. *J. Neural Eng.* 5, 214–220. doi: 10.1088/1741-2560/5/2/012

Bian, Z., and Zhang, X. (2000). *Pattern Recognition.* Beijing: Tsinghua University Press.

Choi, B., and Jo, S. (2013). A low-cost EEG system-based hybrid brain-computer interface for humanoid robot navigation and recognition. *PLoS ONE* 8:e74583. doi: 10.1371/journal.pone.0074583

Cohen, O., Druon, S., Lengagne, S., Mendelsohn, A., Malach, R., Kheddar, A., et al. (2012). "fMRI robotic embodiment: a pilot study," in *4th IEEE RAS/EMBS International Conference on Robotics and Biomimetics* (Roma), 314–319.

Farwell, L. A., and Donchin, E. (1988). Talking off the top of your head: toward a mental prosthesis utilizing event-related brain potentials. *Electroencephalogr. Clin. Neurophysiol.* 70, 510–523. doi: 10.1016/0013-4694(88)90149-6

Frensel, S., and Neubert, E. (2010). *Is the P300 speller independent?* arXiv 1006.3688.

Gergondet, P., Petit, D., and Kheddar, A. (2012). "Steering a robot with a brain-computer interface: impact of video feedback on BCI performance," in *21st IEEE International Symposlum on Robot and Human Interactive Communication* (Paris), 271–276.

Guger, C., Daban, S., Sellers, E., Holzner, C., Krausz, G., and Carabalona, R. (2009). How many people are able to control a P300-based brain–computer interface (BCI)? *Neurosci. Lett.* 462, 94–98. doi: 10.1016/j.neulet.2009.06.045

Heinrich, S. P. (2007). A primer on motion visual evoked potentials. *Doc. Ophthalmol.* 114, 83–105. doi: 10.1007/s10633-006-9043-8

Hirai, K., Hirose, M., Haikawa, Y., and Takenaka, T. (1998). "The development of Honda humanoid robot," in *1998 IEEE International Conference on Robotics and Automation* (Leuven), 1321–1326.

Hong, B., Guo., F., Liu, T., and Gao, S. (2009). N200-speller using motion-onset visual response. *Clin. Neurophysiol.* 120, 1658–1666. doi: 10.1016/j.clinph.2009.06.026

Iturrate, I., Antelis, J. M., Kubler, A., and Minguez, J. (2009). A noninvasive brain-actuated wheelchair based on a P300 neurophysiological protocol and automated navigation. *IEEE Trans. Rob.* 25, 614–627. doi: 10.1109/TRO.2009.2020347

Jin, J., Allison, B. Z., Sellers, E. W., Brunner, C., Horki, P., Wang, X., et al. (2011). An adaptive P300-based control system. *J. Neural Eng.* 8:036006. doi: 10.1088/1741-2560/8/3/036006

Jin, J., Allison, B. Z., Wang, X., and Neuper, C. (2012). A combined brain–computer interface based on P300 potentials and motion-onset visual evoked potentials. *J. Neurosci. Methods* 205, 265–276. doi: 10.1016/j.jneumeth.2012.01.004

Joyce, C. A., Gorodnitsky, I. F., and Kutas, M. (2004). Automatic removal of eye movement and blink artifacts from EEG data using blind component separation. *Psychophysiology* 41, 313–325. doi: 10.1111/j.1469-8986.2003.00141.x

Karakas, S., Erzengin, O. U., and Basar, E. (2000a). The genesis of human event-related responses explained through the theory of oscillatory neural assemblies. *Neurosci. Lett.* 285, 45–48. doi: 10.1016/S0304-3940(00)01022-3

Karakas, S., Erzengin, O. U., and Basar, E. (2000b). A new strategy involving multiple cognitive paradigms demonstrates that ERP components are determined by the superposition of oscillatory responses. *Clin. Neurophysiol.* 111, 1719–1732. doi: 10.1016/S1388-2457(00)00418-1

Krusienski, D. J., Sellers, E. W., McFarland, T. M., Vaughan, T. M., and Wolpaw, J. R. (2008). Toward enhanced P300 speller performance. *J. Neurosci. Methods* 167, 15–21. doi: 10.1016/j.jneumeth.2007.07.017

Lebedev, M. A., and Nicolelis, M. A. L. (2006). Brain-machine interfaces: past, present and future. *Trends Neruosci.* 29, 536–546. doi: 10.1016/j.tins.2006.07.004

Liu, T., Goldberg, L., Gao, S., and Hong, B. (2010). An online brain-computer interface using non-flashing visual evoked potentials. *J. Neural Eng.* 7, 1–9. doi: 10.1088/1741-2560/7/3/036003

Li, W., Jaramillo, C., and Li, Y. (2011). "A brain computer interface based humanoid robot control system," in *IASTED International Conference on Robotics* (Pittsburgh, PA), 390–396.

Li, W., Jaramillo, C., and Li, Y. (2012). "Development of mind control system for humanoid robot through a brain computer interface," in *Intelligent System Design and Engineering Application (ISDEA)* (Hainan), 679–682.

Li, M., Li, W., Zhao, J., Meng, Q., Sun, F., and Chen, G. (2013a). "An adaptive P300 model for controlling a humanoid robot with mind," in *IEEE International Conference on Robotics and Biomimetics* (Guangdong), 1390–1395.

Li, M., Li, W., Zhao, J., Meng, Q., Zeng, M., and Chen, G. (2013b). "A P300 model for Cerebot- a mind –controlled humanoid robot," in *2nd International Conference on Robot Intelligent Technology and Applications* (Denver, CO), 495–502.

McFarland, D. J., Sarnacki, W. A., and Wolpaw, J. R. (2003). Brain-computer interface (BCI) operation: optimizing information transfer rates. *Biol. Psychol.* 63, 237–251. doi: 10.1016/S0301-0511(03)00073-5

Mika, S., Ratsch, G., Weston, J., Scholkopf, B., and Mullers, K. R. (1999). Fisher discriminant analysis with kernels. *Neural Netw. Signal Process.* IX, 41–48.

Patel, S. H., and Azzam, P. N. (2005). Characterization of N200 and P300: selected studies of the event-related potential. *Int. J. Med. Sci.* 2, 147–154. doi: 10.7150/ijms.2.147

Polich, J., and Kok, A. (1995). Cognitive and biological determinants of P300: an integrative review. *Biol Psychol.* 41, 103–146. doi: 10.1016/0301-0511(95)05130-9

Renard, Y., Lotte, F., Gibert, G., Congedo, M., Maby, E., Delannoy, V., et al. (2010). OpenViBE: an open-source software platform to design, test, and use brain-computer interfaces in real and virtual environments. *Presence (Camb.)* 19, 35–53. doi: 10.1162/pres.19.1.35

Schaeff, S., Treder, M. S., Venthur, B., and Blankertz, B. (2012). Exploring motion VEPs for gaze-independent communication. *J. Neural Eng.* 9, 045006. doi: 10.1088/1741-2560/9/4/045006

Tidoni, E., Gergondet, P., Kheddar, A., and Aglioti, S. M. (2014). Audio-visual feedback improves the BCI performance in the navigational control of a humanoid robot. *Front. Neurorobot.* 8:20. doi: 10.3389/fnbot.2014.00020

Wei, J. H., and Luo, Y. J. (2010). *Principle and Technique of Event-Related Brain Potentials.* Beijing: Science Press.

Wolpaw, J. R., Birbaumer, N., Heetderks, W. J., McFarland, D. J., Hunter Peckham, P., Schalk,G., et al. (2000). Brain-computer interface technology: a review of the first international meeting. *IEEE Trans. Rehabil. Eng.* 8, 164–173. doi: 10.1109/TRE.2000.847807

Zhao, J., Meng, Q., Li, W., Sun, F., and Chen, G. (2013). "An OpenViBE-based brainwave control system for Cerebot," in *IEEE International Conference on Robotics and Biomimetics* (Guangdong), 1169–1174.

23

Non-invasive brain stimulation for the treatment of brain diseases in childhood and adolescence: state of the art, current limits and future challenges

Carmelo M. Vicario[1]* and Michael A. Nitsche[2]

[1] *School of Psychology, The University of Queensland, St. Lucia, QLD, Australia*
[2] *Clinic for Clinical Neurophysiology, University Medical Center, Göttingen, Germany*

Edited by:
Mikhail Lebedev, Duke University, USA

Reviewed by:
Yoshio Sakurai, Kyoto University, Japan
Estate M. Sokhadze, University of Louisville, USA
Kyongsik Yun, California Institute of Technology, USA

****Correspondence:***
Carmelo M. Vicario, School of Psychology, The University of Queensland, McElwain Building, St. Lucia, QLD 4072, Australia
e-mail: carmelo.vicario@uniroma1.it

In the last decades interest in application of non-invasive brain stimulation for enhancing neural functions is growing continuously. However, the use of such techniques in pediatric populations remains rather limited and mainly confined to the treatment of severe neurological and psychiatric diseases. In this article we provide a complete review of non-invasive brain stimulation studies conducted in pediatric populations. We also provide a brief discussion about the current limitations and future directions in a field of research still very young and full of issues to be explored.

Keywords: pediatric brain stimulation, vascular diseases, epilepsy, ADHD, Tourette, autism, depression, schizophrenia

INTRODUCTION

In the last decades the interest in exploring therapeutic and/or rehabilitative effects generated by non-invasive brain stimulation techniques in neuropsychiatric diseases increased considerably. Although this field of research encompasses numerous stimulation techniques, neuroscientists have primarily focused investigations on the use of two techniques, namely Transcranial Magnetic Stimulation (TMS) and transcranial Direct Current Stimulation (tDCS). In healthy adults, these non-invasive brain stimulation techniques are applied to monitor cortical excitability/dynamics (e.g., single pulse TMS, double pulse TMS), and as neuromodulatory techniques [e.g., repetitive TMS (rTMS), tDCS]. Whereas TMS is primarily used to investigate brain physiology (e.g., task-dependent alterations of cortical maps, excitability, and so on, in health, and disease), the latter techniques are applied to *modify* physiology, and performance. Accordingly, these methods have been adopted to explore, and modulate brain functions such as language (e.g., *rTMS*: Flöel et al., 2008; *tDCS*: Vicario and Rumiati, 2012;), learning, and long-term memory formation [e.g., single pulse *TMS* (spTMS): Vicario et al., 2013a; *tDCS*: Nitsche et al., 2003], working memory (WM) (e.g., *TMS*: Gaudeau-Bosma et al., 2013; *tDCS*: Fregni et al., 2005a) perception (e.g., *TMS*: Hamilton et al., 2013; *tDCS*: Vicario et al., 2013b), and attention (e.g., *TMS*: Lee et al., 2013; *tDCS*: Tanoue et al., 2013), in healthy humans (see Nitsche et al., 2003, 2008; Kuo and Nitsche, 2012 for further examples and Nitsche and Paulus, 2011 for a complete review).

Non-invasive brain stimulation is applied also to rehabilitate cortical functions in neuropsychiatric diseases via induction of neuroplasticity. rTMS has been shown to improve cognitive functions in Parkinson's disease (Pascual-Leone et al., 1994), and improved aphasia (Naeser et al., 2005), motor control after stroke (Takeuchi et al., 2005), epilepsy (see Nitsche and Paulus, 2009 for a review), and depression (Pascual-Leone et al., 1996; O'Reardon et al., 2007), amongst others (Kammer and Spitzer, 2012).

Encouraging clinical effects have been documented also for tDCS, so far in pilot studies. tDCS improves motor and non-motor stroke symptoms (e.g., Fregni et al., 2005b), depression, and might have effects on craving, schizophrenia, and dementia, amongst others (for comprehensive reviews, see, Flöel, 2013; Krause et al., 2013; Kuo et al., 2013). All these results encourage the future therapeutic application of non-invasive brain stimulation techniques also in pediatric populations affected by brain disorders. However, the number of non-invasive brain stimulation studies conducted in childhood is scanty, especially if compared to that available from adult participants.

Two previous reviews (Quintana, 2005; Croarkin et al., 2011) gave an overview of the application of rTMS in children and adolescents. Here, we provide the reader with an updated state of the art of application of non-invasive brain stimulation in general (rTMS and tDCS) in pediatric populations. Moreover, we will discuss current limits and possible future applications of these techniques for the treatment of brain dysfunctions affecting childhood. It is beyond the scope of this review to discuss the mechanisms of how TMS and tDCS alter neural activity and induce brain plasticity in detail. For obtaining this information, some recently published articles provide a complete and exhaustive overview (see for example Stagg and Nitsche, 2011; Freitas et al., 2013; Krause et al., 2013).

NON-INVASIVE BRAIN STIMULATION FOR ENHANCING BRAIN DISORDERS IN CHILDHOOD

VASCULAR DISEASES

Pathophysiologically, stroke is associated with hemispheric dysbalance, i.e., a reduction of the activity of the lesioned brain area and an enhanced activity of the contra-lesional homologous region, which limits re-gain of functions (see Grefkes and Fink, 2011 for a recent review).

Kirton et al. (2008) conducted the first randomized sham-controlled rTMS trial in children (median age 13.25) affected by arterial ischemic stroke. Patients were affected by unilateral hand motor weakness. They received 8 days to 1 Hz rTMS of the contralesional motor cortex, which inhibits regional brain activity (Pascual-Leone et al., 2005) and increases contralateral cortical excitability via reduction of interhemispheric inhibition (Pal et al., 2005). Grip strength increased after real rTMS only, and this effect persisted until day 17 after the start of treatment. Furthermore, rTMS was well tolerated with no relevant side effects.

Valle and colleagues (2007) applied a 5-day course of rTMS upon the affected motor cortex in seventeen children (mean age 9) affected by infantile cerebral palsy and spastic quadriplegia. The study was designed according to the hypothesis that an increase of motor cortex activity would increase its inhibitory influence on spinal excitability, and thus improve spasticity. Patients received five consecutive sessions of rTMS in a randomized, sham controlled, double-blind, parallel, clinical trial design. According to previous works (e.g., Quartarone et al., 2005) showing that 5 Hz rTMS of the primary motor cortex induces an overall increase of excitability of the corticospinal output system, including spinal motoneurons, the authors report a significant reduction of spasticity only in association to this stimulation protocol. Both studies show a potential of rTMS for rehabilitation of motor symptoms originating from vascular injuries in childhood. However, due to the limited number of studies, we are still far from achieving a clear picture of the use of this technique to treat vascular problems in children. No studies for the treatment of vascular disorders in children or adolescents have been conducted with tDCS so far.

EPILEPSY

The pathophysiological substrate of epilepsies and the proneness to develop seizures is an enhanced cortical excitability, leading to paroxysmal depolarization shifts, an enhanced probability of high-frequent and hyper-synchronous activity of neuronal networks (Stafstrom, 2006; Dudek and Sutula, 2007). A reduction of neuronal excitability is the common aim of antiepileptic therapies.

Fregni et al. (2005c), tested the effect of a single 0.5 Hz rTMS session in an open study. Three pediatric patients with focal epilepsy were included. The TMS coil was positioned over the epileptogenic region, or, if this could not be clearly identified, over Cz. rTMS significantly reduced the frequency of epileptiform discharges (ED) for up to 15 and 30 days after rTMS treatment.

The study of Brasil-Neto et al. (2004) included a 6 years old patient. This patient was affected by left fronto-central slow activity. 0.3 Hz rTMS was applied once per day for 3 months. In this case, rTMS treatment was ineffective. Graff-Guerrero et al. (2004) conducted one session of 20 Hz rTMS in two patients (7 and 11 years old) suffering from epilepsia partialis continua (EPC). The patients were first submitted to a single photon emission computed tomography (SPECT) session in order to localize the focal frontal hyperperfused region to define the stimulation site; after rTMS, patients were SPECT-monitored again in order to identify perfusion alterations of the stimulated region. Indeed, cortical perfusion of the stimulated area was reduced in both patients. However, only in one patient epileptic seizures decreased significantly. Morales et al. (2005) conducted a case study involving 2 patients (8 and 16 years old) affected by EPC. One Hertz/six Hertz rTMS were applied in different sessions. No adverse effects occurred, but the treatment resulted in no clinical effects. Kinoshita et al. (2005) treated a 16 years old male suffering from parietal lobe epilepsy with 0.9 Hz rTMS over 5 days. The coil was placed over PCz. No significant improvements have been documented for this patient.

San-Juan et al. (2011) applied cathodal tDCS over the F2 scalp site in a 17 years old patient affected by Rasmussen's encephalitis [4 tDCS sessions of 60 min (on days 0, 7, 30, and 60)]. At follow-up evaluations 6 and 12 months later, seizure frequency was significantly reduced. Additionally, the patient had improved levels of alertness and language. No side effects have been reported. Yook et al. (2011) applied cathodal tDCS applied upon the epileptogenic focus in a 11 year's old patient. The patient was diagnosed with congenital bilateral perisylvian syndrome. Cathodal tDCS was applied over the right temporo-parietal area that showed epileptiform activity in the EEG for 2 weeks. During the two-month period after treatment termination, only six seizures occurred (compared to eight seizures a month before the treatment), and seizure duration decreased. tDCS was repeated for another 2 weeks, 2 months after the first intervention session. For the following two months, only one seizure occurred. No notable side effects of stimulation were observed.

In contrast, in a group of pediatric patients (age range 6–11) showing continuous spikes and slow waves during sleep (CSWS), one session of cathodal tDCS over the peak negativity of the epileptogenic pattern revealed an effect on EEG patterns only in 3 patients (Varga et al., 2011). One reason for this negative result might be that the multifocal/diffuse and poorly defined origin of epileptic activity in CSWS makes it difficult to identify the optimal region for stimulation (Brazzo et al., 2012). Moreover, stimulation was performed with 1 mA in only one session in the latter study, which might have not been sufficient to obtain significant or lasting effects.

More recently, Auvichayapat et al. (2013) enrolled thirty six children (age range 6–15 years) with focal epilepsy in a crossover sham-controlled study. Participants received a single session of cathodal tDCS upon the epileptogenic region. Active tDCS treatment was associated with significant reductions in epileptic discharge frequency immediately and 24 and 48 h after tDCS. Moreover, 4 weeks after treatment, a small (clinically negligible but statistically significant) decrease in seizure frequency was detected. All patients tolerated tDCS well.

These studies deliver some preliminary hints for a possible efficacy of rTMS, and tDCS, to treat epilepsy in children. However, the heterogeneity of the results, possibly due to different stimulation parameters, small numbers, and different etiologies of participants, and the heterogeneous quality of the studies, do not allow to draw definite conclusions.

ADHD

Attention-deficit/hyperactivity disorder (ADHD) is a highly prevalent and impairing disorder, characterized by inattention, hyperactivity, and executive dysfunction. Functional neuroimaging studies have shown functional and abnormalities in cingulate, frontal and parietal cortical regions, including hypoactivation (Bush, 2011). Thus, non-invasive brain stimulation procedures to improve ADHD symptoms are oriented toward excitatory protocols.

Weaver et al. (2008) performed a randomized, sham-controlled, crossover study involving 9 participants affected by ADHD. The age range of the 4 included adolescents was between 15 and 17 years. 10 Hz rTMS over 2 weeks was applied upon the right DLPFC. Clinical global impression and the ADHD-IV scales improved significantly, but similarly for active and sham rTMS. No serious adverse effects did take place. No studies on childhood ADHD have been performed with tDCS so far.

TOURETTE SYNDROME

Tourette's syndrome (TS) is one of the most common neurobehavioral disorders in childhood (see American Academy of Pediatrics, 2000). The pathology is characterized by the presence of tics, which are rapid, stereotyped movements and vocalizations, virtually involving all body segments (Vicario et al., 2010). The neuro-functional profile of childhood TS is characterized by impairment of neural circuits linking the cerebral cortex to the striatum and other sub-cortical regions (Swain et al., 2007; Bush, 2011).

Of interest for the current discussion is the Supplemental Motor Area (SMA). The pre-motor cortex has been reported to be hyperexcitable in patients with TS (George et al., 2001). Therefore, excitability-reducing rTMS to the SMA may be an effective way to treat TS, because this region is extensively connected with regions implicated in motor control (Picard and Strick, 2001).

In an open label 12 weeks cohort pilot study (Kwon et al., 2011), 1Hz rTMS was applied over the SMA for 10 days. At the end of each day subjects completed objective ratings of ADHD, mood, anxiety, tics, and side effects. Statistically significant reductions were seen in the Yale Global TS Severity Scale over the 12 weeks of the study. Le et al. (2013) tested the effect of 1 Hz rTMS upon the SMA in 25 children with TS (aged less than 16 years) for 20 days. Results document a significant improvement of clinical symptoms. Interestingly, the benefits lasted for up to 6 months in 68% of subjects. No studies for TS treatment have been conducted with tDCS. The results provided in these two studies are coherent in terms of therapeutic benefits, stimulation site (SMA) and rTMS frequency (1 Hz). However, an important limit of these studies is the lack of a control group.

AUTISM SPECTRUM DISORDER (ASD)

This syndrome is characterized by a marked decrease in social integration and communication, and affects $\sim$1 in 150 children (Fombonne, 2009). Increased gamma-band responses to several cognitive processes in children with autism spectrum disorder have been described (McFadden et al., 2012). While its precise role is unclear, it is implied in a wide range of processes such as attention (Lakatos et al., 2008), WM (Tallon-Baudry et al., 1998), and language (Tavabi et al., 2011). Non-invasive brain stimulation has been adopted for modulating this physiological parameter and therefore improve the related cognitive abilities.

Baruth et al. (2010) report clinical improvements in pediatric ASD induced via rTMS ($\leq$1 Hz) in a controlled study, the electrophysiological effects of 12 low frequency rTMS sessions, bilaterally applied to the DLPFC were explored in 25 subjects (ages range 9–26) with ASD and 20 age-matched controls. rTMS was administered once per week. The first six treatments were performed over the left, and the remaining six over the right DLPFC. Patients showed significant improvement in discriminatory gamma activity and also significant improvements in behavioral parameters. In another study (Sokhadze et al., 2010) 20 subjects (age range 10–19) with ASD received the same protocol. Performance was tested with the oddball paradigm, which explores attentional shifting (García-Larrea et al., 1992). rTMS minimized early cortical responses to irrelevant stimuli, increased responses to relevant stimuli, reduced the error percentage and repetitive-ritualistic behavior.

Schneider and Hopp (2011) conducted an open tDCS study in children with autism. The purpose was to improve language acquisition in patients with minimal verbal language. In this study the authors selected 10 ASD participants (age range 16–21). Post-anodal tDCS of the Broca area, mean vocabulary scores were significantly higher than the pre-anodal tDCS scores.

The studies are suggestive for therapeutic benefits of non-invasive brain stimulation in autistic children. However, due to the small numbers of studies, in which different protocols had effects on different target functions, statements about optimal protocols are premature.

DEPRESSION

Depression in children and adolescents is associated with significant functional disability in multiple environmental realms (Cosgrove et al., 2013). Depression involves a distributed network of cortical and limbic regions, including the DLPFC (especially the left), and subgenual cingulate gyrus, amongst others (Mayberg, 2007). It has been shown (Fitzgerald et al., 2006) that in depression these areas, and specifically the left-hemispherical ones, may be hypoactive, whereas right-hemispheric hyperactivation might take place, thus constituting an hemispheric dysbalance of activation. The rationale of the brain stimulation studies presented here is to increase the activity of the left DLPFC.

Walter et al. (2001) were the first to report the impact of rTMS on depression in 3 patients younger than 18 years. The patients received daily treatment over 2 weeks of 10 Hz rTMS over the left DLPFC. Two participants improved clinically, but one of them complained about tension headache during two of the treatment sessions. In another case report series, Loo et al.

(2006) tested the effect of 10 Hz rTMS upon the left DLPFC over 6 weeks on two 16-year-old adolescent girls affected by depression and ADHD. No improvements of ADHD symptoms, but a reduction of depression symptoms was reported. Bloch et al. (2008) conducted an open label rTMS study with nine adolescents (16–18 age range) affected by severe treatment-resistant depression. Participants received 14 sessions of 10 Hz rTMS to the left DLPFC. Depression scores of the participants improved significantly. Two of them remained in clinical remission 1 year after therapy (as judged by regular clinical follow-up). Five subjects reported mild headaches. No other adverse effects were reported. More recently, Wall et al. (2011) conducted an open-label trial of adjunctive rTMS in eight adolescents with treatment-resistant depression. These subjects were maintained on a stable dose of a selective serotonin reuptake inhibitor (SSRI). All in all, thirty daily 10 Hz rTMS treatments were given over the left dorsolateral prefrontal cortex. The CDRS-Revised mean scores improved significantly from baseline over the course of 30 treatments and the 6-month follow-up. Pre- and post-treatment neurocognitive testing did not reveal any decline in functioning. These data are preliminary as no control group was included, but this study shows that intensive treatment parameters were well tolerated by adolescent patients. No studies for treatment of depression in children have been conducted with tDCS.

The available studies suggest some therapeutic effect of rTMS for the treatment of childhood depression. A recurring element associated with a successful rTMS therapy is the stimulation of left DLPFC at 10Hz. However, since these are open and/or case report studies, the results of these studies should be interpreted with caution.

SCHIZOPHRENIA

Childhood-onset schizophrenia is a rare and severe form of the disorder (Nicolson and Rapoport, 1999), that is neurobiologically and physiologically continuous with adult onset schizophrenia (David et al., 2011). Hallucinations are, probably, the most dramatic clinical symptom that causes significant problems for the life of patients with schizophrenia.

Physiological abnormalities have been reported in several neural regions including right medial temporal, lateral temporal, inferior frontal cortex, and in the cingulate cortex bilaterally, left DLPFC and left superior temporal gyrus (Vyas and Gogtay, 2012; Hayempour et al., 2013). However, neuroimaging studies have shown relatively less predictive value despite consistent reports of progressive structural brain abnormalities associated with schizophrenia. An increase of left temporoparietal cortex excitability is associated with positive symptoms, specifically auditory hallucinations (AHs) (Silbersweig et al., 1995; Shergill et al., 2000). On the other hand, activity enhancement of the left prefrontal region has been suggested to improve negative symptoms (Heimer et al., 1997), due to its effect on the release of dopamine (Strafella et al., 2001). Therefore, excitability-reducing stimulation is proposed to reduce activity of the left temporoparietal cortex, while excitatory non-invasive brain stimulation has been used to increase left prefrontal region activation for therapeutic application (see Freitas et al., 2009; Demirtas-Tatlidede et al., 2013 for a complete review).

Jardri et al. (2007) report a single case study involving a 11-year-old boy with medication-resistant schizophrenia. An fMRI scan displayed increased auditory cortex activity with concurrent AHs. 10 sessions of 1 Hz rTMS were administered to the left temporoparietal cortex. Verbal AHs decreased by 50%. The improvement obtained with rTMS was maintained by repeating the sessions every 5 weeks. No adverse effects of rTMS were reported. More recently, the same group (Jardri et al., 2012) established a case series of adolescents diagnosed with childhood-onset schizophrenia according to the Schedule for Affective Disorders and Schizophrenia for School-Age Children ($n = 10$, 15.5 years old). All participants had frequent and drug-resistant AHs. The patients received 1 Hz rTMS to the T3-P3 site over 5 days. The authors assessed scalp discomfort clinically and describe only minor discomfort. AHRS scores decreased significantly from baseline to the immediate post-treatment assessment, and from baseline to the 1-month assessment. Furthermore, the Global Assessment of Functioning scores improved significantly immediately and 1 month after the treatment, as compared to baseline values.

For tDCS, one study was recently published with regard to childhood-onset schizophrenia (Mattai et al., 2011). This study aimed to investigate the tolerability of tDCS in this patient group. Twelve participants (12 children, age range 10–17) were assigned to one of two groups: bilateral anodal DLPFC stimulation ($n = 8$) or bilateral cathodal superior temporal gyrus (STG) stimulation ($n = 5$). The stimulation protocol consisted of 20 min per day, per 2 weeks. No subjects reported significant discomfort at the electrode sites. However, four individuals had transient redness of the skin under the electrodes that resolved within about an hour after treatment. Although no significant clinical improvement has been reported, this study is the first to demonstrate that tDCS with the applied parameters is well tolerated in adolescents. Complains of fatigue reported by some patients could be related to unspecific effects, such as medication regimens that frequently include the atypical antipsychotic clozapine.

Taken together, knowledge about the effects of non-invasive brain stimulation in childhood onset schizophrenia is still limited. However, the rTMS case reports provided by Jardri et al. hint for some efficacy in reducing hallucinations. The only available tDCS study is in favor for good tolerability of this stimulation protocol. Systematic studies are needed to explore this field to a larger degree.

DISCUSSION

In this work we reviewed the available literature about the effects of non-invasive brain stimulation in pediatric populations (i.e., younger than 18 years) suffering from neuro-psychiatric diseases. We focused our analysis on studies which have examined the therapeutic efficacy of rTMS and tDCS for rehabilitating neurological functions and ameliorating psychiatric syndromes in children.

In general, the studies provide preliminary evidence in support for a therapeutic potential of non-invasive stimulation techniques in children and adolescents. However, several limitations should be taken into account.

Virtually no double-blinded sham controlled studies are available at present, which makes it difficult to make safe statements

Table 1 | rTMS studies in childhood brain diseases.

Studies	Design		Patients		Stimulation protocol						Outcome	
	Sham controlled	Blinding	Disease	Sample size	rTMS intensity	Stimulation position	Number of sessions/ days	rTMS frequency	Total number of pulses/ session	Duration per session	Effects	Side-effects
VASCULAR DISEASES												
Kirton et al., 2008	Yes	Partially	AIS	10	100% rMT	Controlesional motor cortex	1 session per day/8 days	1 Hz	1200	20 min	Grip strength improvement	None
Valle et al., 2007	Yes	Double blind	CP	17	90% rMT	Motor cortex	1 session per day/5 days	5 Hz	1500	N/A	Reduction of spasticity	None
EPILEPSY												
Brasil-Neto et al., 2004	No	Open	Left front-central slow activity	1	95% rMT	Frontal cortex (Epileptogenic focus)	1 session per day/2 sessions per week/3 months	0.3 Hz	100	N/A	No effects	None
Graff-Guerrero et al., 2004	No	Open	EPC	2	50% of the TMS device power (case 1) 128% rMT (case 2)	Frontal cortex (Epileptogenic focus)	1session/1 day	20 Hz	N/A	N/A	Seizure discharge reduction	None
Fregni et al., 2005a,b,c	No	Open	Cortical mal-formation	3	65% of the TMS device power	Epileptogenic focus vs. Cz	1 session/1 day	0.5 Hz	600	20 min	Seizure discharge reduction	None
Morales et al., 2005	No	Open	EPC	2	N/A	Motor cortex (Epileptogenic focus)	2 sessions/1 day (case 1) 2 session/1 day + 1 session (second day-case 2)	Patient 1: 1–6 Hz Patient 2: 1: 1 Hz-6 Hz-1 Hz	N/A	N/A	No effects	None
Kinoshita et al., 2005	No	Pilot	Extratemporal lobe epilepsy	1	90% rMT	PCz	2 sessions per day/5 days in a week	0.9 Hz	N/A	15 min	No effects	None

(Continued)

Table 1 | Continued

Studies	Design		Patients		Stimulation protocol						Outcome	
	Sham controlled	Blinding	Disease	Sample size	rTMS intensity	Stimulation position	Number of sessions/ days	rTMS frequency	Total number of pulses/ session	Duration per session	Effects	Side-effects
ADHD												
Weaver et al., 2008	Yes	Open	ADHD only	4	100% rMT	Right DLPFC	1 session per day/5 days per week/2 weeks	10 Hz	2000 stimuli	N/A	Improved attention in the Sham + active rTMS condition	None
TOURETTE												
Kwon et al., 2011	No	Open	TS only	2	100% rMT	SMA	10 daily sessions/10 days	1 Hz	1200	N/A	Tics reduction	None
Le et al., 2013	No	Open	TS only	25	100% rMT	SMA	1 session per day/5 days per week/4 weeks	1 Hz	1200	20 min	Tics reduction	None
AUTISM SPECTRUM DISORDERS												
Baruth et al., 2010	Control group	Open	Autistic	22	90% rMT	Bilateral DLPFC	1 session per day/1 day per week/12 weeks	•1 Hz	150	N/A	Reduction of irritability and repetitive behavior	None
Sokhadze et al., 2010	No	Open	Autistic	13	90% rMT	Bilateral DLPF cortices	1 session per day/2 day per week/3 weeks	0.5 Hz	150	N/A	Reduced errors % in the oddball task and ritualistic behaviors	None
DEPRESSION												
Walter et al., 2001	No	Open	Unipolar major depression	3	Between 90 and 110% of the rMT	Left DLPFC	1 session per day/5 days per week/2 weeks	10 Hz	1600	N/A	Improvement in 2 cases on 3	Tension headache reported in one case with improvement
Loo et al., 2006	No	Open	Depression/ ADHD comorbidity	2	110% rMT	Left DLPF cortex	1 session per day/5 days per week/6 weeks	10 Hz	40 trains/5 s per train	N/A	Improvement measured with the CDRS	None

(Continued)

Table 1 | Continued

Studies	Design		Patients		Stimulation protocol						Outcome	
	Sham controlled	Blinding	Disease	Sample size	rTMS intensity	Stimulation position	Number of sessions/ days	rTMS frequency	Total number of pulses/ session	Duration per session	Effects	Side-effects
Wall et al., 2011	No	Open	Depression	8	120% MT	Left DLPF cortex	1 session per day/5 days per week over 6–8 weeks	10 Hz	3000	N/A	Improvement measured with the CDRS	None
Bloch et al., 2008	No	Open	Depression	9	80% MT	Left DLPF cortex	1 session per day over 14 days	10 Hz	20 sessions/2 s per trains	20 min	Improvement measured with the CDRS and BDI	None
SCHIZOPHRENIA												
Jardri et al., 2007	No	Open	Schizophrenia	1	100% rMT	left tem-poroparietal cortex	1 time per day/10 days	1 Hz	1000 stimuli	N/A	The Verbal AHs decreased	None
Jardri et al., 2012	No	Open	Schizophrenia	10	90% rMT	T3-P3	2 times per day/5 days	1 Hz	1200 stimuli	N/A	Improvement measured with the CDRS	Minor discomfort

Shown are studies dedicated to the treatment of Vascular diseases, Epilepsy, ADHD, Tourette, Autism Spectrum Disorder, Depression, Schizophrenia in childhood populations. Study characteristics, details of the stimulation protocols as well as effects of stimulation, including side effects, are shown. AIS, Arterial ischemic stroke; CP, Cerebral Palsy; EPC, Epilepsia partialis continua; ADHD, Attention-deficit/hyperactivity disorder. Stimulation targets areas are described according to the international 10-20 system.

Table 2 | tDCS for the treatment of childhood brain disorders.

Studies	Design		Patients	Stimulation protocol							Outcome	
	Sham controlled	Blinding		Polarity	Therapeutic electrode position	Return electrode position	Current strength (mA)	Electrode size (cm^2)	Duration (min)/sessions	Sample	Effects	Side-effects
EPILEPSY												
San-Juan et al., 2011	No	No	Rasmussen's encephalitis	C	F2	F8	2	12 mm in length × 0.4 mm diameter	60 min/4 sessions (on days 0, 7, 30, and 60)	1	Cathodal tDCS improves epilepsy, linguistic, and motor functions	None
Yook et al. (2011)	No	No	Slow waves/ right hemisphere and intermittent spikes/ temporoparietal area	C	Right temporo-parietal area (between P4-T4)	Left orbit	2	25	20 min/5 days per week/2 weeks	1	Cathodal tDCS reduces seizure attacks and duration	None
Varga et al., 2011	Yes	Partially (patients)	(*n* = 1) SP, GTP (*n* = 1) CP (*n* = 1) SP, CP, GTP (*n* = 1) Atonic (*n* = 1) CP, GTC	C/S	*N* = 1 T7 *N* = 2 FT7 *N* = 3 T7 *N* = 4 TP8 *N* = 5 T7 On the area of peak negativity	On the area of peak positivity (more widespread)	1	25	20 min/2 sessions/1 day	5	Effect on EEG patterns or clinical symptoms only in 3 patients	None
Auvichayapat et al., 2013	Yes	Partially (stati-cian)	(*n* = 18) Idiopathic (*n* = 4) MTS (*n* = 2) FCD (*n* = 3) Others	C/S	Seizure focus	Controlateral shoulder	1	35	20 min (one session)	36	Significant reductions in epileptic discharge frequency immediately and 24 and 48 h after tDCS	None

(Continued)

Table 2 | Continued

Studies	Design		Patients	Stimulation protocol							Outcome	
	Sham controlled	Blinding		Polarity	Therapeutic electrode position	Return electrode position	Current strength (mA)	Electrode size (cm^2)	Duration (min)/sessions	Sample	Effects	Side-effects
AUTISM												
Schneider and Hopp, 2011	No	Partially (stati-cian)	Autism	A	Left DLPFC	Right supraorbital	0.08	25	30 min (one session)	10	Anodal tDCS over left DLPF cortex improved vocabulary score	None
Schizophrenia												
Mattai et al., 2011	Yes	Possibility of open treat-ment	Schizophrenia	C/A/S	Bilateral anodal DLPFC stimula-tion ($N = 8$) Bilateral cathodal superior temporal gyrus (STG) stimula-tion ($n = 5$)	Non-dominant forearm	2	25	20 min/5 days per week/2 weeks	12	None	Tingling ($n = 7$); Itching ($n = 6$)

Shown are studies dedicated to treatment of Vascular diseases, Epilepsy, ADHD, Tourette, Autism Spectrum Disorder, Depression, Schizophrenia in childhood populations. Study characteristics, details of the stimulation protocols as well as effects of stimulation, including side effects, are shown. A, anodal tDCS; C, cathodal tDCS; S, sham tDCS. Stimulation targets areas are described according to the international 10–20 system. Legend: SP, simple partial seizures; GTP, generalized tonic-clonic seizures; CP, complex partial seizures; MTS, Mesial temporal sclerosis; FCD, Focal cortical dysplasia.

about efficacy. Since there seems to be a potential, these studies are urgently needed. Moreover, systematic studies to identify optimal stimulation protocols based on physiology are missing, including comparisons between different protocols, and a systematic evaluation of safety of non-invasive brain stimulation with regard to the developing brain. It is important to note that, although the examined literature does deliver no hint for major adverse effects in children, the evidence currently available is still rather scanty. Studies conducted in adult humans and animal models are probably not transferable one-to-one to children, since anatomy and physiology differs relevantly between these groups (Johnston, 2009). In this regard, it is important to consider that the developing brain is characterized by "sensitive" periods or rather periods during which the effects of the experience on the brain are unusually strong during a limited period in development (Knudsen, 2004). This suggests that, during development, the risk to induce maladaptive neural plasticity due to brain stimulation techniques might be relatively high (Vicario and Nitsche, 2013). Because of this, we suggest that neuroscientists willing to apply non-invasive brain stimulation in children should consider dose-finding studies, and a longitudinal monitoring of neural plasticity triggered by these methods (through neuroimaging and/or electrophysiological techniques), to control for functional and structural changes. In this connection, it will be important to improve knowledge about physiological effects of stimulation in children. This might provide important landmarks for assessing the therapeutic effectiveness of the adopted stimulation protocol as well as the presence of side effects. Moreover, discoveries provided by research in "sensitive" periods at the circuit level might be helpful for this issue as they could supply insights of paramount importance for predicting the trajectories of neural plasticity induced by non-invasive brain stimulation techniques and their related therapeutic results. Worthy of discussion is also the fact that the current state of investigations involving the application of brain stimulation methods in pediatric populations is unbalanced toward TMS (See **Tables 1, 2** for detailed summaries).

No published studies are currently available with regard to the therapeutic efficacy of tDCS in childhood disorders such as stroke and/or brain injury, TS, ADHD, and Depression. Nevertheless, the interest in applying tDCS for treating pediatric populations is growing.

FUTURE DIRECTION OF RESEARCH

The application of non-invasive brain stimulation for the rehabilitation and/or treatment of children might have the potential advantage of promoting improvements superior to those achievable in adulthood, according to the fact that the developing brain is characterized by "sensitive periods" during which the effects of the experience on the brain are unusually strong for a limited period (Knudsen, 2004). Therefore, the improvement of symptoms via non-invasive stimulation treatment in pediatric age might be more stable, and consistent. However, as discussed above, this same "sensitivity" might also be risky in terms of induction of maladaptive neural plasticity.

In order to minimize this risk, future lines of research should address the following, still limited, field of investigations:

- Exploration, also by using animal models, of the physiological effects of non-invasive brain stimulation in children;
- Systematic exploration of childhood clinical populations to clarify the pathophysiology of the respective diseases, which could be objective to non-invasive brain stimulation. This is important for defining optimal protocols.
- Systematic conduction of "dose-finding," sham-controlled, double-blinded studies, which will provide important information not available from the open studies.

These aspects will help to clarify, at several levels of complexity, the potential therapeutic efficacy of non-invasive brain stimulation in children, delivering a realistic basis for clinical application of such stimulation protocols on a large scale.

REFERENCES

American Academy of Pediatrics. (2000). Clinical practice guidelines: diagnosis and evaluation of the child with attention-deficit/hyperactivity disorder. *Pediatrics* 105, 1158–1170. doi: 10.1542/peds.105.5.1158

Auvichayapat, N., Rotenberg, A., Gersner, R., Ngodklang, S., Tiamkao, S., Tassaneeyakul, W., et al. (2013). Transcranial direct current stimulation for treatment of refractory childhood focal epilepsy. *Brain Stimul.* 6, 696–700. doi: 10.1016/j.brs.2013.01.009

Baruth, J. M., Casanova, M. F., El-Baz, A., Horrell, T., Mathai, G., Sears, L., et al. (2010). Low-frequency repetitive transcranial magnetic stimulation (rTMS) modulates evoked-gamma frequency oscillations in autism spectrum disorder (ASD). *J. Neurother.* 14, 179–194. doi: 10.1080/10874208.2010.501500

Bloch, Y., Grisaru, N., Harel, E. V., Beitler, G., Faivel, N., Ratzoni, G., et al. (2008). Repetitive transcranial magnetic stimulation in the treatment of depression in adolescents: an open-label study. *J. ECT* 24, 156–159. doi: 10.1097/YCT.0b013e318156aa49

Brasil-Neto, J. P., de Araújo, D. P., Teixeira, W. A., Araújo, V. P., and Boechat-Barros, R. (2004). Experimental therapy of epilepsy with transcranial magnetic stimulation: lack of additional benefit with prolonged treatment. *Arq. Neuropsiquiatr.* 62, 21–25. doi: 10.1590/S0004-282X2004000100004

Brazzo, D., Pera, M. C., Fasce, M., Papalia, G., Balottin, U., and Veggiotti, P. (2012). Epileptic encephalopathies with status epilepticus during sleep: new techniques for understanding pathophysiology and therapeutic options. *Epilepsy Res. Treat.* 2012, 642–725. doi: 10.1155/2012/642725

Bush, G. (2011). Cingulate, frontal, and parietal cortical dysfunction in attention-deficit/hyperactivity disorder. *Biol. Psychiatry* 69, 1160–1167. doi: 10.1016/j.biopsych.2011.01.022

Cosgrove, V. E., Roybal, D., and Chang, K. D. (2013). Bipolar depression in pediatric populations: epidemiology and management. *Paediatr. Drugs* 15, 83–91. doi: 10.1007/s40272-013-0022-8

Croarkin, P. E., Wall, C. A., and Lee, J. (2011). Applications of transcranial magnetic stimulation (TMS) in child and adolescent psychiatry. *Int. Rev. Psychiatry* 23, 445–453. doi: 10.3109/09540261.2011.623688

David, C. N., Greenstein, D., Clasen, L., Gochman, P., Miller, R., Tossell, J. W., et al. (2011). Childhood onset schizophrenia: high rate of visual hallucinations. *J. Am. Acad. Child Adolesc. Psychiatry* 50, 681.e3–686.e3. doi: 10.1016/j.jaac.2011.03.020

Demirtas-Tatlidede, A., Vahabzadeh-Hagh, A. M., and Pascual-Leone, A. (2013). Can noninvasive brain stimulation enhance cognition in neuropsychiatric disorders? *Neuropharmacology* 64, 566–578. doi: 10.1016/j.neuropharm.2012.06.020

Dudek, F. E., and Sutula, T. P. (2007). Epileptogenesis in the dentate gyrus: a critical perspective. *Prog. Brain Res.* 163, 755–773. doi: 10.1016/S0079-6123(07)63041-6

Fitzgerald, P. B., Oxley, T. J., Laird, A. R., Kulkarni, J., Egan, G. F., and Daskalakis, Z. J. (2006). An analysis of functional neuroimaging studies of dorsolateral prefrontal cortical activity in depression. *Psychiatry Res.* 148, 33–45. doi: 10.1016/j.pscychresns.2006.04.006

Flöel, A. (2013). tDCS-enhanced motor and cognitive function in neurological diseases. *Neuroimage* doi: 10.1016/j.neuroimage.2013.05.098. [Epub ahead of print].

Flöel, A., Rösser, N., Michka, O., Knecht, S., and Breitenstein, C. (2008). Non invasive brain stimulation improves language learning. *J. Cogn. Neurosci.* 8, 1415–1422. doi: 10.1162/jocn.2008.20098

Fombonne, E. (2009). Epidemiology of pervasive developmental disorders. *Pediatr. Res.* 65, 591–598. doi: 10.1203/PDR.0b013e31819e7203

Freitas, C., Farzan, F., and Pascual-Leone, A. (2013). Assessing brain plasticity across the lifespan with transcranial magnetic stimulation: why, how, and what is the ultimate goal? *Front. Neurosci.* 7:42. doi: 10.3389/fnins.2013.00042

Freitas, C., Fregni, F., and Pascual-Leone, A. (2009). Meta-analysis of the effects of repetitive transcranial magnetic stimulation (rTMS) on negative and positive symptoms in schizophrenia. *Schizophr. Res.* 108, 11–24. doi: 10.1016/j.schres.2008.11.027

Fregni, F., Boggio, P. S., Nitsche, M., Bermpohl, F., Antal, A., Feredoes, E., et al. (2005a). Anodal transcranial direct current stimulation of prefrontal cortex enhances working memory. *Exp. Brain Res.* 166, 23–30. doi: 10.1007/s00221-005-2334-6

Fregni, F., Boggio, P. S., Mansur, C. G., Wagner, T., Ferreira, M. J., Lima, M. C., et al. (2005b). Transcranial direct current stimulation of the unaffected hemisphere in stroke patients. *Neuroreport* 16, 1551–1555. doi: 10.1097/01.wnr.000177010.44602.5c

Fregni, F., Thome-Souza, S., Bermpohl, F., Marcolin, M. A., Herzog, A., Pascual-Leone, A., et al. (2005c). Antiepileptic effects of repetitive transcranial magnetic stimulation in patients with cortical malformations: an EEG and clinical study. *Stereotact. Funct. Neurosurg.* 83, 57–62. doi: 10.1159/000086674

García-Larrea, L., Lukaszewicz, A. C., and Mauguière, F. (1992). Revisiting the oddball paradigm. Non-target vs neutral stimuli and the evaluation of ERP attentional effects. *Neuropsychologia* 30, 723–741. doi: 10.1016/0028-3932(92)90042-K

Gaudeau-Bosma, C., Moulier, V., Allard, A. C., Sidhoumi, D., Bouaziz, N., Braha, S., et al. (2013). Effect of two weeks of rTMS on brain activity in healthy subjects during an n-back task: a randomized double blind study. *Brain Stimul.* 6, 569–575. doi: 10.1016/j.brs.2012.10.009

George, M. S., Sallee, F. R., Nahas, Z., Oliver, N. C., and Wassermann, E. M. (2001). Transcranial magnetic stimulation (TMS) as a research tool in Tourette syndrome and related disorders. *Adv. Neurol.* 85, 225–235.

Graff-Guerrero, A., Gonzáles-Olvera, J., Ruiz-García, M., Avila-Ordoñez, U., Vaugier, V., and García-Reyna, J. C. (2004). rTMS reduces focal brain hyperperfusion in two patients with EPC. *Acta Neurol. Scand.* 109, 290–296. doi: 10.1046/j.1600-0404.2003.00222.x

Grefkes, C., and Fink, G. R. (2011). Reorganization of cerebral networks after stroke: new insights from neuroimaging with connectivity approaches. *Brain* 134, 1264–1276. doi: 10.1093/brain/awr033

Hamilton, R. H., Wiener, M., Drebing, D. E., and Coslett, H. B. (2013). Gone in a flash: manipulation of audiovisual temporal integration using transcranial magnetic stimulation. *Front. Psychol.* 4:571. doi: 10.3389/fpsyg.2013.00571

Hayempour, B. J., Newberg, A., and Alavi, A. (2013). Neuromolecular imaging instrumentation demonstrating dysfunctional brain function in schizophrenic patients. *J. Alzheimers Dis. Parkinsonism* 3, pii: 114. doi: 10.4172/2161-0460.1000114

Heimer, L., Harlan, R. E., Alheid, G. F., Garcia, M. M., and de Olmos, J. (1997). Substantia innominata: a notion which impedes clinical-anatomical correlations in neuropsychiatric disorders. *Neuroscience* 76, 957–1006. doi: 10.1016/S0306-4522(96)00405-8

Jardri, R., Bubrovszky, M., Demeulemeester, M., Poulet, E., Januel, D., Cohen, D., et al. (2012). Repetitive transcranial magnetic stimulation to treat early-onset auditory hallucinations. *J. Am. Acad. Child Adolesc. Psychiatry* 51, 947–949. doi: 10.1016/j.jaac.2012.06.010

Jardri, R., Lucas, B., Delevoye-Turrell, Y., Delmaire, C., Delion, P., Thomas, P., et al. (2007). An 11-year-old boy with drug-resistant schizophrenia treated with temporo-parietal rTMS. *Mol. Psychiatry* 12, 320. doi: 10.1038/sj.mp.4001968

Johnston, M. V. (2009). Plasticity in the developing brain: implications for rehabilitation. *Dev. Disabil. Res. Rev.* 15, 94–101. doi: 10.1002/ddrr.64

Kammer, T., and Spitzer, M. (2012). Brain stimulation in psychiatry: methods and magnets, patients and parameters. *Curr. Opin. Psychiatry* 25, 535–541. doi: 10.1097/YCO.0b013e328358df8c

Kinoshita, M., Ikeda, A., Begum, T., Yamamoto, J., Hitomi, T., and Shibasaki, H. (2005). Low-frequency repetitive transcranial magnetic stimulation for seizure suppression in patients with extratemporal lobe epilepsy-a pilot study. *Seizure* 14, 387–392. doi: 10.1016/j.seizure.2005.05.002

Kirton, A., Chen, R., Friefeld, S., Gunraj, C., Pontigon, A. M., and Deveber, G. (2008). Contralesional repetitive transcranial magnetic stimulation for chronic hemiparesis in subcortical paediatric stroke: a randomised trial. *Lancet Neurol.* 7, 507–513. doi: 10.1016/S1474-4422(08)70096-6

Knudsen, E. I. (2004). Sensitive periods in the development of the brain and behavior. *J. Cogn. Neurosci.* 16, 1412–1425. doi: 10.1162/0898929042304796

Krause, B., Márquez-Ruiz, J., and Cohen Kadosh, R. (2013). The effect of transcranial direct current stimulation: a role for cortical excitation/inhibition balance? *Front. Hum. Neurosci.* 7:602. doi: 10.3389/fnhum.2013.00602

Kuo, M. F., and Nitsche, M. A. (2012). Effects of transcranial electrical stimulation on cognition. *Clin. EEG Neurosci.* 43, 192–199. doi: 10.1177/1550059412444975

Kuo, M. F., Paulus, W., and Nitsche, M. A. (2013). Therapeutic effects of non-invasive brain stimulation with direct currents (tDCS) in neuropsychiatric diseases. *Neuroimage* doi: 10.1016/j.neuroimage.2013.05.117. [Epub ahead of print].

Kwon, H. J., Lim, W. S., Lim, M. H., Lee, S. J., Hyun, J. K., Chae, J. H., et al. (2011). 1-Hz low frequency repetitive transcranial magnetic stimulation in children with Tourette's syndrome. *Neurosci. Lett.* 492, 1–4. doi: 10.1016/j.neulet.2011.01.007

Lakatos, P., Karmos, G., Mehta, A. D., Ulbert, I., and Schroeder, C. E. (2008). Entrainment of neuronal oscillations as a mechanism of attentional selection. *Science* 320, 110–113. doi: 10.1126/science.1154735

Le, K., Liu, L., Sun, M., and Xiao, N. (2013). Transcranial magnetic stimulation at 1 Hertz improves clinical symptoms in children with Tourette syndrome for at least 6 months. *J. Clin. Neurosci.* 20, 257–262. doi: 10.1016/j.jocn.2012.01.049

Lee, J., Ku, J., Han, K., Park, J., Lee, H., Kim, K. R., et al. (2013). rTMS over bilateral inferior parietal cortex induces decrement of spatial sustained attention. *Front. Hum. Neurosci.* 7:26. doi: 10.3389/fnhum.2013.00026

Loo, C., McFarquhar, T., and Walter, G. (2006). Transcranial magnetic stimulation in adolescent depression. *Australas. Psychiatry* 14, 81–85. doi: 10.1111/j.1440-1665.2006.02251.x

Mattai, A., Miller, R., Weisinger, B., Greenstein, D., Bakalar, J., Tossell, J., et al. (2011). Tolerability of transcranial direct current stimulation in childhood-onset schizophrenia. *Brain Stimul.* 4, 275–280. doi: 10.1016/j.brs.2011.01.001

Mayberg, H. S. (2007). Defining the neural circuitry of depression: toward a new nosology with therapeutic implications. *Biol. Psychiatry* 61, 729–730. doi: 10.1016/j.biopsych.2007.01.013

McFadden, K. L., Hepburn, S., Winterrowd, E., Schmidt, G. L., and Rojas, D. C. (2012). Abnormalities in gamma-band responses to language stimuli in first-degree relatives of children with autism spectrum disorder: an MEG study. *BMC Psychiatry* 12:213. doi: 10.1186/1471-244X-12-213

Morales, O. G., Henry, M. E., Nobler, M. S., Wassermann, E. M., and Lisanby, S. H. (2005). Electroconvulsive therapy and repetitive transcranial magnetic stimulation in children and adolescents: a review and report of two cases of epilepsia partialis continua. *Child Adolesc. Psychiatr. Clin. N. Am.* 14, 193–210. doi: 10.1016/j.chc.2004.07.010

Naeser, M. A., Martin, P. I., Nicholas, M., Baker, E. H., Seekins, H., Helm-Estabrooks, N., et al. (2005). Improved naming after TMS treatments in a chronic, global aphasia patient–case report. *Neurocase* 11, 182–193. doi: 10.1080/13554790590944663

Nicolson, R., and Rapoport, J. L. (1999). Childhood-onset schizophrenia: rare but worth studying. *Biol. Psychiatry* 46, 1418–1428. doi: 10.1016/S0006-3223(99)00231-0

Nitsche, M. A., Cohen, L. G., Wassermann, E. M., Priori, A., Lang, N., Antal, A., et al. (2008). Transcranial direct current stimulation: state of the art 2008. *Brain Stimul.* 1, 206–223. doi: 10.1016/j.brs.2008.06.004

Nitsche, M. A., and Paulus, W. (2009). Noninvasive brain stimulation protocols in the treatment of epilepsy: current state and perspectives. *Neurotherapeutics* 6, 244–250. doi: 10.1016/j.nurt.2009.01.003

Nitsche, M. A., and Paulus, W. (2011). Transcranial direct current stimulation–update 2011. *Restor. Neurol. Neurosci.* 29, 463–492. doi: 10.3233/RNN-2011-0618

Nitsche, M. A., Schauenburg, A., Lang, N., Liebetanz, D., Exner, C., Paulus, W., et al. (2003). Facilitation of implicit motor learning by weak transcranial direct current stimulation of the primary motor cortex in the human. *J. Cogn. Neurosci.* 15, 619–626. doi: 10.1162/089892903321662994

O'Reardon, J. P., Solvason, H. B., Janicak, P. G., Sampson, S., Isenberg, K. E., Nahas, Z., et al. (2007). Efficacy and safety of transcranial magnetic stimulation in the acute treatment of major depression: a multisite randomized controlled trial. *Biol. Psychiatry* 62, 1208–1216. doi: 10.1016/j.biopsych.2007.01.018

Pal, P. K., Hanajima, R., Gunraj, C. A., Li, J. Y., Wagle-Shukla, A., Morgante, F., et al. (2005). Effect of low-frequency repetitive transcranial magnetic stimulation on interhemispheric inhibition. *J. Neurophysiol.* 94, 1668–1675. doi: 10.1152/jn.01306.2004

Pascual-Leone, A., Amedi, A., Fregni, F., and Merabet, L. B. (2005). The plastic human brain cortex. *Annu. Rev. Neurosci.* 28, 377–401. doi: 10.1146/annurev.neuro.27.070203.144216

Pascual-Leone, A., Rubio, B., Pallardó, F., and Catalá, M. D. (1996). Rapid-rate transcranial magnetic stimulation of left dorsolateral prefrontal cortex in drug-resistant depression. *Lancet* 348, 233–237. doi: 10.1016/S0140-6736(96)01219-6

Pascual-Leone, A., Valls-Solé, J., Brasil-Neto, J. P., Cammarota, A., Grafman, J., and Hallett, M. (1994). Akinesia in Parkinson's disease. II. Effects of subthreshold repetitive transcranial motor cortex stimulation. *Neurology* 44, 892–898. doi: 10.1212/WNL.44.5.892

Picard, N., and Strick, P. L. (2001). Imaging the premotor areas. *Curr. Opin. Neurobiol.* 11, 663–672. doi: 10.1016/S0959-4388(01)00266-5

Quartarone, A., Bagnato, S., Rizzo, V., Morgante, F., Santangelo, A., Battaglia, F., et al. (2005). Distinct changes in cortical and spinal excitability following high-frequency repetitive TMS to the human motor cortex. *Exp. Brain Res.* 161, 114–124. doi: 10.1007/s00221-004-2052-5

Quintana, H. (2005). Transcranial magnetic stimulation in persons younger than the age of 18. *J. ECT.* 21, 88–95. doi: 10.1097/01.yct.0000162556.02720.58

San-Juan, D., Calcáneo, J. D., González-Aragón, M. F., Bermúdez Maldonado, L., Avellán, A. M., Argumosa, E. V., et al. (2011). Transcranial direct current stimulation in adolescent and adult Rasmussen's encephalitis. *Epilepsy Behav.* 20, 126–131. doi: 10.1016/j.yebeh.2010.10.031

Schneider, H. D., and Hopp, J. P. (2011). The use of the Bilingual Aphasia Test for assessment and transcranial direct current stimulation to modulate language acquisition in minimally verbal children with autism. *Clin. Linguist. Phon.* 25, 640–654. doi: 10.3109/02699206.2011.570852

Shergill, S. S., Brammer, M. J., Williams, S. C., Murray, R. M., and McGuire, P. K. (2000). Mapping auditory hallucinations in schizophrenia using functional magnetic resonance imaging. *Arch. Gen. Psychiatry* 57, 1033–1038. doi: 10.1001/archpsyc.57.11.1033

Silbersweig, D. A., Stern, E., Frith, C., Cahill, C., Holmes, A., Grootoonk, S., et al. (1995). A functional neuroanatomy of hallucinations in schizophrenia. *Nature* 378, 176–179. doi: 10.1038/378176a0

Sokhadze, E., Baruth, J., Tasman, A., El-Baz, A., Mansoor, M., Ramaswamy, R., et al. (2010). Low-frequency repetitive transcranial magnetic stimulation (rTMS) affects event-related potential measures of novelty processing in autism. *Appl. Psychophysiol. Biofeedback* 35, 147–161. doi: 10.1007/s10484-009-9121-2

Stafstrom, C. E. (2006). Neonatal seizures: is a novel, mechanism-based treatment finally on the horizon? *Epilepsy Curr.* 6, 130–132. doi: 10.1111/j.1535-7511.2006.00121.x

Stagg, C. J., and Nitsche, M. A. (2011). Physiological basis of transcranial direct current stimulation. *Neuroscientist* 17, 37–53. doi: 10.1177/1073858410386614

Strafella, A. P., Paus, T., Barrett, J., and Dagher, A. (2001). Repetitive transcranial magnetic stimulation of the human prefrontal cortex induces dopamine release in the caudate nucleus. *J. Neurosci.* 21, RC157.

Swain, J. E., Scahill, L., Lombroso, P. J., King, R. A., and Leckman, J. F. (2007). Tourette syndrome and tic disorders: a decade of progress. *J. Am. Acad. Child Adolesc. Psychiatry* 46, 947–968. doi: 10.1097/chi.0b013e318068fbcc

Takeuchi, N., Chuma, T., Matsuo, Y., Watanabe, I., and Ikoma, K. (2005). Repetitive transcranial magnetic stimulation of contralesional primary motor cortex improves hand function after stroke. *Stroke* 36, 2681–2686. doi: 10.1161/01.STR.0000189658.51972.34

Tallon-Baudry, C., Bertrand, O., Peronnet, F., and Pernier, J. (1998). Induced gamma-band activity during the delay of a visual short-term memory task in humans. *J. Neurosci.* 18, 4244–4254.

Tanoue, R. T., Jones, K. T., Peterson, D. J., and Berryhill, M. E. (2013). Differential frontal involvement in shifts of internal and perceptual attention. *Brain Stimul.* 6, 675–682. doi: 10.1016/j.brs.2012.11.003

Tavabi, K., Embick, D., and Roberts, T. P. (2011). Spectral-temporal analysis of cortical oscillations during lexical processing. *Neuroreport* 22, 474–478. doi: 10.1097/WNR.0b013e3283476b84

Valle, A. C., Dionisio, K., Pitskel, N. B., Pascual-Leone, A., Orsati, F., Ferreira, M. J., et al. (2007). Low and high frequency repetitive transcranial magnetic stimulation for the treatment of spasticity. *Dev. Med. Child Neurol.* 49, 534–538. doi: 10.1111/j.1469-8749.2007.00534.x

Varga, E. T., Terney, D., Atkins, M. D., Nikanorova, M., Jeppesen, D. S., and Uldall, P. (2011). Transcranial direct current stimulation in refractory continuous spikes and waves during slow sleep: a controlled study. *Epilepsy Res.* 97, 142–145. doi: 10.1016/j.eplepsyres.2011.07.016

Vicario, C. M., Candidi, M., and Aglioti, S. M. (2013a). Cortico-spinal embodiment of newly acquired, action-related semantic associations. *Brain Stimul.* doi: 10.1016/j.brs.2013.05.010. [Epub ahead of print].

Vicario, C. M., Martino, D., and Koch, G. (2013b). Temporal accuracy and variability in the left and right posterior parietal cortex. *Neuroscience* 245, 121–128. doi: 10.1016/j.neuroscience.2013.04.041

Vicario, C. M., Martino, D., Spata, F., Defazio, G., Giacchè, R., Martino, V., et al. (2010). Time processing in children with Tourette's syndrome. *Brain Cogn.* 73, 28–34. doi: 10.1016/j.bandc.2010.01.008

Vicario, C. M., and Nitsche, M. A. (2013). Transcranial direct current stimulation: a remediation tool for the treatment of childhood congenital dyslexia? *Front. Hum. Neurosci.* 7:139. doi: 10.3389/fnhum.2013.00139

Vicario, C. M., and Rumiati, R. I. (2012). tDCS of the primary motor cortex improves the detection of semantic dissonance. *Neurosci. Lett.* 518, 133–137. doi: 10.1016/j.neulet.2012.04.070

Vyas, N. S., and Gogtay, N. (2012). Treatment of early onset schizophrenia: recent trends, challenges and future considerations. *Front. Psychiatry* 3:29. doi: 10.3389/fpsyt.2012.00029

Wall, C. A., Croarkin, P. E., Sim, L. A., Husain, M. M., Janicak, P. G., Kozel, F. A., et al. (2011). Adjunctive use of repetitive transcranial magnetic stimulation in depressed adolescents: a prospective, open pilot study. *J. Clin. Psychiatry* 72, 1263–1269. doi: 10.4088/JCP.11m07003

Walter, G., Tormos, J. M., Israel, J. A., and Pascual-Leone, A. (2001). Transcranial magnetic stimulation in young persons: a review of known cases. *J. Child Adolesc. Psychopharmacol.* 11, 69–75. doi: 10.1089/104454601750143483

Weaver, L., Mace, W., Akhtar, U., Moss, E., Rostain, A., and O'Reardon, J. (2008). Safety and efficacy of rTMS in treatment of ADHD in adolescents and young persons. *J. ECT* 24, 105–106.

Yook, S. W., Park, S. H., Seo, J. H., Kim, S. J., and Ko, M. H. (2011). Suppression of seizure by cathodal transcranial direct current stimulation in an epileptic patient - a case report -. *Ann. Rehabil. Med.* 35, 579–582. doi: 10.5535/arm.2011.35.4.579

Brain-machine interfacing control of whole-body humanoid motion

Karim Bouyarmane[1]*, Joris Vaillant[2,3], Norikazu Sugimoto[4], François Keith[2,3], Jun-ichiro Furukawa[1,5] and Jun Morimoto[1]

[1] Computational Neuroscience Laboratories, Department of Brain Robot Interface, Advanced Telecommunications Research Institute International (ATR), Kyoto, Japan
[2] Laboratoire d'Informatique de Robotique et de Micro-électronique de Montpellier, CNRS-University of Montpellier 2, Montpellier, France
[3] CNRS-AIST Joint Robotics Laboratory, UMI3218/CRT, National Intitute of Advanced Industrial Science and Technology, Tsukuba, Japan
[4] National Institute of Information and Communications Technology, Osaka, Japan
[5] Graduate School of Frontier Biosciences, Osaka University, Osaka, Japan

Edited by:
Mikhail Lebedev, Duke University, USA

Reviewed by:
Randal A. Koene, Boston University, USA
M. Van Der Meulen, University of Luxembourg, Luxembourg

***Correspondence:**
Karim Bouyarmane, ATR Computational Neuroscience Laboratories, Department of BRI, 2-2-2 Hikaridai, Seika-cho Soraku-gun, Kyoto 619-0288, Japan
e-mail: karim.bouyarmane@lirmm.fr

We propose to tackle in this paper the problem of controlling whole-body humanoid robot behavior through non-invasive brain-machine interfacing (BMI), motivated by the perspective of mapping human motor control strategies to human-like mechanical avatar. Our solution is based on the adequate reduction of the controllable dimensionality of a high-DOF humanoid motion in line with the state-of-the-art possibilities of non-invasive BMI technologies, leaving the complement subspace part of the motion to be planned and executed by an autonomous humanoid whole-body motion planning and control framework. The results are shown in full physics-based simulation of a 36-degree-of-freedom humanoid motion controlled by a user through EEG-extracted brain signals generated with motor imagery task.

Keywords: humanoid whole-body control, brain-machine interfacing, motor imagery, motion planning, semi-autonomous humanoid, contact support planning

1. INTRODUCTION

Due to their design that allows them to be readily used in an environment that was initially arranged to accommodate the human morphology, that makes them more acceptable to the users, and easier to interact with, it is generally admitted that humanoid robots are an appropriate choice as living assistants for the everyday tasks, for instance for the elderly and/or reduced-mobility people. The problem that naturally arises is that of the control of such an assistant and how to communicate the wills and intentions of the user to the robot. This problem is of course general but becomes more challenging when addressing the above-mentioned category of users for which communication capabilities can also be impaired (stroke patients for example). This brings our initial idea of considering brain-machine interfaces (BMI) as the possible communication tool between the human and the humanoid assistant. Notwithstanding, brought along with this reflection was the more general question, non-necessarily application-directed, of a human using its brain motor functions to control a human-like artificial body the same way they control their own human body. This question becomes our main motivation and concern in the present work since solving it would pave the way of the discussed applicative perspectives. We thus propose our solution to it in this paper.

The approach we choose to investigate deals with the following constraints of the problem. First, we only consider easy-and-ready-to-use non-invasive BMI technologies. Among this class of technologies, we aim more specifically at the one that would align best and most intuitively with our expressed desire of mimicking human motor-control function, namely motor-imagery-based BMI, consisting ideally for the human user of imagining a movement of their own body for it to be replicated in the humanoid body, though we do not reach that ideal vision restricting our study for the sake of feasibility demonstration to the use of a generic motor-imagery task (imagining arm movement) that we re-target to the specific motion of the robot at hand (leg motion of the robot). Finally, the control paradigm for the humanoid robot we set as objective in our study is that of low-level joint/link-level control, to keep as general behavior and class of movements as possible for the user to replicate at the robot, without restriction of the class of movements allowed by particular higher-level humanoid motion controllers.

We address the related work and existing proposed solutions for this problem or approaching ones in the next section (Section 2). We then detail our own solution, based on the integration of, for the humanoid motion control part, an autonomous contact-based planning and control framework (Section 3), and for the BMI part, a motor-imagery-task-generated brain-signal classification method (Section 4). The integration of these two originally independent components is discussed in Section 5, 6 presents an example proof-of-concept experiment with a fully physics-simulated humanoid robot. Section 7 concludes the paper with discussion and future work.

2. RELATED WORK AND PROPOSED SOLUTION

Various approaches have been proposed to solve the problem we stated in the introduction of controlling a humanoid robot with

BMI (Bell et al., 2008; Bryan et al., 2011; Chung et al., 2011; Finke et al., 2011; Gergondet et al., 2011; Ma et al., 2013). All approaches, ours included, are based on the integration of a BMI technology with a humanoid controller, and can thus be categorized according to which strategy is followed for each of these two components. See **Figure 1** for an overview.

From the BMI point-of-view, all these works do abide by our posed constraint of using non-invasive BMIs that rely on electroencephalography (EEG), generally utilizing the well-established frameworks of visual-stimulation-based event-related potentials (ERP) such as P300 in Bell et al. (2008), evoked potentials (EP) such as the steady state visually evoked potential (SSVEP) in Bryan et al. (2011); Chung et al. (2011); Gergondet et al. (2011), or hybrid approaches combining electrooculogram (EOG) with ERP such as in Ma et al. (2013), or P300 with motor-imagery-evoked event-related desynchronization (ERD) (Finke et al., 2011; Riechmann et al., 2011). None, however, investigated a solely motor-imagery-based BMI as stated in our motivations of replicating intuitive human motor-control strategies. Hence our first contribution in the integration initiative.

We adapt in this work a motor-imagery decoding scheme that we previously developed for the control of a one-degree-of-freedom robot and for sending standing-up/sitting-down commands to a wearable exoskeleton (Noda et al., 2012). It allows us to generate a three-valued discrete command that we propose to map to a one-dimensional subspace of the multi-dimensional whole-body configuration space motion of the humanoid, and more precisely the motion along a generalized notion of "vertical axis" of the moving end-limb, such as the foot of the swing leg in a biped motion for instance. As we detail in the course of the paper (Section 5), the motivation behind this strategy is to allow the user to assist the autonomous motion that might lead the moving limb to be "blocked" in potential field local minima while trying to avoid collision. The strategy can in future work be developed into a more sophisticated two-dimensional continuous command one as proven possible by recent and ongoing studies on motor-imagery control (Wolpaw and McFarland, 2004; Miller et al., 2010).

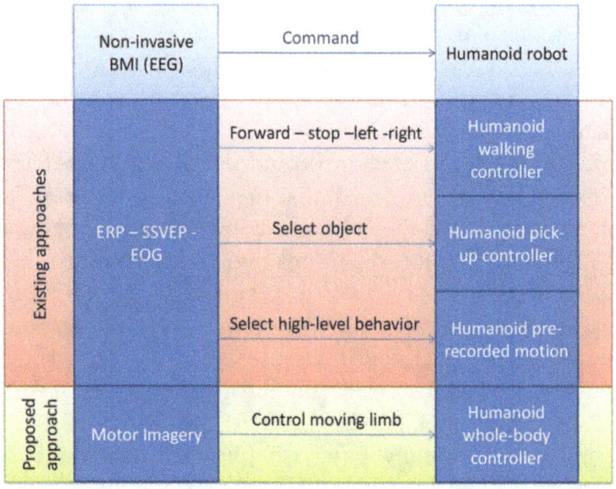

FIGURE 1 | A schematic illustration of the proposed approach vs. the existing ones for controlling a humanoid robot with non-invasive BMI.

From the humanoid controller point-of-view now, the most standard retained solution consists in using available humanoid high level controllers. These can be either walking controllers with the commands "walk forward" "stop" "turn left" "turn right" sent to a walking humanoid, effectively reducing the problem of humanoid motion control to that of walk steering control (Bell et al., 2008; Chung et al., 2011; Finke et al., 2011; Gergondet et al., 2011), or an object selecton/pick-up controller, where the user selects an object in the scene and then the arm reaching/grasping controller of the robot picks up the desired object (Bryan et al., 2011). Finally Ma et al. (2013) use a hybrid control strategy where both walk steering and selecting a high-level behavior among a finite library can be done by switching between EOG and ERP control. With these strategies, a humanoid can be seen as an arm-equipped mobile robot, with wheels instead of legs (as it is actually the case in Bryan et al., 2011 where only the upper body is humanoid), and consequently the considerable amount of work done on BMI wheelchair control, for example, can be readily adapted. However, in doing so, the advantages of using a legged device over a wheeled one are partially lost, and we can no longer claim the need for the humanoid design nor defend the argument of the possibility of using the robot in everyday living environment which would present non-flat structures, such as stairs for example, with which the walking controllers are not efficient to deal.

While we admit that these strategies relying on walking pattern generators can in the long term benefit from the developments in these techniques that would allow them to autonomously cope with unstructured terrain (variable height stairs, rough terrain) (Takanishi and Kato, 1994; Hashimoto et al., 2006; Herdt et al., 2010; Morisawa et al., 2011), and that they can as well use the hierarchical architectures in which they are embedded as it is the case in Chung et al. (2011); Bryan et al. (2011); Ma et al. (2013) for switching, for example, to an appropriate stair-climbing controller when facing stairs, we choose in this work to investigate an entirely different approach that does not incorporate any kind of walking or high-level controller. Instead, we propose to allow the user to perform lower-level joint/link level control of the whole-body motion of humanoid, driven again by the desire of replicating the human low-level motor-control strategies into the humanoid, but also by the belief that a generic-motion generating approach will allow the robot assistant to deal more systematically with unpredictable situations that inevitably occur in everyday living scenarios and for which the discussed hierarchical architectures would not have exhaustively accounted. This is our second contribution. To achieve this goal, we rely on the contact planning paradigm that we previously proposed for fully autonomous robot (Bouyarmane and Kheddar, 2012), adapting it here to the instance of a BMI-controlled robot.

3. HUMANOID CONTROLLER

Our humanoid controller is based on the multi-contact planning paradigm, introduced in Hauser et al. (2008); Bouyarmane and Kheddar (2012). This controller allows for autonomously planning and executing the complex high-degree-of-freedom motion of the humanoid from a high-level objective expressed in terms of a desired contact state to reach. The controller works in two stages: an off-line planning stage and an on-line execution stage.

At the planning stage (Bouyarmane and Kheddar, 2011a), a search algorithm explores all the possible contact transitions that would allow the robot to go from the initial contact state to the desired goal contact state. What we mean by contact transition is either removing one contact from the current contact state (e.g., removing the right foot from a double-support state to transition to a left-foot single-support one) or adding one contact to the current contact state (e.g., bringing the swing right foot in contact with the floor to transition from a left-foot single-support phase to a double support phase). One must however note that a contact is defined as a pairing between any surface designated on the cover of the links of the robot and any surface on the environment, and is not restricted to be established between the soles of the feet and the floor surface. For instance, a contact can be defined between the forearm of the robot and the arm of an armchair, or between the palm of the hand of the robot and the top of a table. This strategy stems from the observation that all motions of humans can be broken down to such a succession of contact transitions, be it cyclic motions such as walking where these transitions occur between the feet and the ground, or more complex maneuvers such as standing up from an armchair were contacts transitions occur between various parts of the body (hands, forearms feet, tights, etc.) and various parts the environment objects (armchair, table floor, etc.). This feature makes our planning paradigm able to cope with situations that are broader than the ones classically tackled by humanoid motion planner that either plan for the motion assuming a given contact state (e.g., planning a reaching motion with the two feet fixed on the ground) (Kuffner et al., 2002; Yamane et al., 2004; Yoshida et al., 2006, 2008), or planning footprint placements assuming a cyclic walking pattern will occur on these footprints (Kuffner et al., 2001; Chestnutt et al., 2003, 2005). This aligns well with our initially expressed objective of controlling whole-body motion of any kind without restriction to a subclass of taxonomically identified motions.

At the above-described contact-transition search stage, every contact state that is being explored is validated by running an inverse-kinematics solver which finds an appropriate whole-body configuration (posture) of the robot that meets the desired contact state, while at the same time satisfying physics constraints to make the posture physically realizable within the mechanical limits of the robots (Bouyarmane and Kheddar, 2010). At the end of the offline-contact planning stage, we are provided with a sequence of feasible contact transitions and associated transition postures, that go from the initial contact state to the the goal.

The second stage of the controller is an on-line real-time low-level controller (Bouyarmane and Kheddar, 2011b) that will successively track each of the intermediate postures fed by the off-line planning stage, until the last element of the planned sequence is reached. The controller is formulated as a multi-objective quadratic program optimization scheme, the objectives being expressed in terms of the moving link of the robot involved in the current contact transition being tracked along the sequence (e.g., the foot if the contact transition is a sole/floor one), the center of mass (CoM) of the robot to keep balance, and the whole configuration of the robot to solve for the redundancies of the high-DOF motion. These objectives are autonomously decided by a finite-state machine (FSM) that encodes the current type of transition among the following two types:

- Removing-contact transition: the motion of the robot is performed on the current contact state, and the step is completed when the contact forces applied on the contact we want to remove vanish. This is done by shifting the weight of the robot away from the being-removed contact, tracking the CoM position of the following configuration in the sequence. There is no end-link motion in this kind of step. The corresponding FSM state is labeled "Shift CoM."
- Adding-contact transition: the motion of the robot is performed on the current contact state, and the motion of the link we want to add as a contact is guided to its desired contact location. There is thus an end-link motion (contact link) in this kind of step. Balance is ensured by also tracking the CoM position of the following configuration in the sequence. The corresponding FSM state is labeled "Move contact link."

As an example, a cyclic walking FSM state transition sequence will look like: Move contact link (left foot) → Shift CoM (on the left foot) → Move contact link (right foot) → Shift CoM (on the right foot) → Move contact link → ... But non-cyclic behaviors are also possible and allowed, for example when standing up from an armchair where contacts between the hands of the robot and arms of chair can be added in succession and removed in succession.

The final output of the quadratic program optimization scheme is a torque command that is sent to the robot at every control iteration, after the execution of which the state of the robot is fed-back to the controller.

4. BMI DECODING

Our aim is for the humanoid system to be controlled by using brain activities in the similar brain regions that are used to control the user's own body. Therefore, we asked a subject to control the simulated humanoid system by using motor imagery of arm movements so that brain activities in motor-related regions such as the primary motor cortex can be used.

As non-invasive brain signal acquisition device we use an electroencephalogram (EEG) system (64 channels and sampling rate of 2048 Hz). The brain signals are decoded and classified using the method that was applied and presented in our previous work (Noda et al., 2012), based on the spectral regularization matrix classifier described in Tomioka and Aihara (2007); Tomioka and Muller (2010). We recall the method here.

The EEG signals, of covariance matrices $\mathbf{C}$ considered as input, are classified into two classes, labeled with the variable k, with the following output probabilities (at sampled time t):

$$P(k_t = +1|\mathbf{C}_t) = \frac{1}{1 + \exp(-a_t)}, \tag{1}$$

$$P(k_t = -1|\mathbf{C}_t) = \frac{\exp(-a_t)}{1 + \exp(-a_t)}, \tag{2}$$

with the logit being modeled as a linear function of $\mathbf{C}$

$$a_t = \mathrm{tr}[\mathbf{W}^\top \mathbf{C}_t] + b\,, \tag{3}$$

and where $\mathbf{W}$ is the parameter matrix to be learned (b is a constant-valued bias).

To learn $\mathbf{W}$ the following minimization problem is solved

$$\min \sum_{t=1}^{n} \ln\left(1 + \exp\left(-k_t a_t\right)\right) + \lambda \|\mathbf{W}\|_1\,, \tag{4}$$

λ being the regularization variable ($\lambda = 14$ in the application below) and

$$\|\mathbf{W}\|_1 = \sum_{i=1}^{r} \sigma_i[\mathbf{W}] \tag{5}$$

being the spectral l_1-norm of $\mathbf{W}$ (r is the rank of $\mathbf{W}$ and $\sigma_i[\mathbf{W}]$ its i-th singular value).

Once the classifier learned, the 7–30 Hz band-pass-filtered measured EEG signals are decoded online, by down-sampling them from 2048 to 128 Hz, and applying Laplace filtering and common average substraction to remove voltage bias. Their covariance matrix, initialized at $\mathbf{C}_t = \mathbf{x}_t^\top \mathbf{x}_t$ for the first time step $t = 1$, where $\mathbf{x}_t \in \mathbb{R}^{1\times 64}$ denotes the filtered EEG signals, are updated at every time step as follows

$$\mathbf{C}_t = \frac{1}{N}\mathbf{x}_t^\top \mathbf{x}_t + \frac{N-1}{N}\mathbf{C}_{t-1}\,, \tag{6}$$

and used to compute the probabilities in Equations (1) and (2).

Finally, the three-valued discrete command c_t that is sent to the robot is selected from these probabilities through the following hysteresis

$$c_t = \begin{cases} +1 & \text{if } P(k_t = +1|\mathbf{C}_t) > P_{\text{thresh}} \text{ and } c_{t-1} \neq +1\,, \\ -1 & \text{if } P(k_t = -1|\mathbf{C}_t) > P_{\text{thresh}} \text{ and } c_{t-1} \neq -1\,, \\ 0 & \text{otherwise}\,, \end{cases} \tag{7}$$

where the threshold is set at $P_{\text{thresh}} = 0.6$.

5. COMPONENT INTEGRATION

The command c_t devised in Equation (7) is sent to the online humanoid whole-body controller via UDP protocol at 128 Hz frequency and used to modify the planned and autonomously executed motion of the humanoid robot as described below and as schematically represented in **Figure 2**.

When the robot is executing a step that requires moving a link to a planned contact location (contact-adding step, executed by the state "Move contact link" of the FSM, see Section 3), then instead of tracking directly the goal contact location, we decompose the motion of the end-link (the contact link, for instance the foot) into two phases:

- Lift-off phase: The link first tracks an intermediate position located at a designated way-point.
- Touch-down phase: The link then tracks its goal location in the planned contact state sequence.

This two-phase decomposition allows the link to avoid unnecessary friction with the environment contact surface and to avoid colliding with environment features such as stairs.

Each of these two phases correspond to a sub-state of the meta-state "Move contact link" of the FSM, namely:

- State "Move contact link to way-point"
- State "Move contact link to goal"

Additionally, in order to avoid stopping the motion of the contact link at the way-point and to ensure a smooth motion throughout the step, we implemented a strategy that makes the transition from the former to the latter sub-state triggered when the contact link crosses a designated threshold plan along the way, before reaching the tracked way-point.

A default position of the intermediate way-point is automatically pre-set by the autonomous framework using the following heuristic (see **Figure 2**, left): Let P_s denote the start position of the contact link (at the beginning of the contact-adding step) and P_g denote its goal position (its location in the following contact state

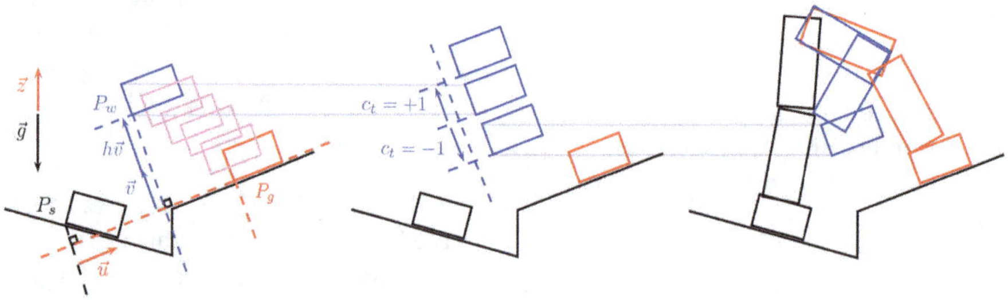

FIGURE 2 | The way-point moving strategy. The rectangles in the left and middle figures represent positions of the moving foot (say the right foot, supposing the left foot is the support foot that is fixed and not represented here). In the right figure the whole leg motion is reconstructed from the foot motion. In all three figures, in black is the initial position of the foot/leg at the beginning of the step, in blue the controlled way-point position of the foot/leg at the middle of the step, and in red is the planned final foot/leg position at the end of the step. The left figure shows how a default position of the way point is initialized autonomously by a translation of the final planned position. $\vec{g}$ is the gravity vector, $\vec{z}$ the vertical unit vector (opposite to $\vec{g}$), $\vec{u}$ is the unit vector from the initial to the goal position along the goal planned-contact surface plane, $\vec{v}$ is the generalized vertical direction unit vector, i.e., the unit vector normal to $\vec{u}$ and in the plane defined by $\vec{u}$ and $\vec{z}$, finally, h is a pre-set default height. The middle figure shows how the way-point position is controlled via the command c_t sent through the motor imagery interface. Finally the left figure shows how the resulting motion of the leg actually looks like with the foot going through the desired way-point that was translated downwards via the command $c_t = -1$.

along the planned sequence). Let $\vec{g}$ denote the gravity vector, $\vec{z}$ the unit vector opposite to $\vec{g}$, i.e., $\vec{z} = -\vec{g}/\|\vec{g}\|$, and $\vec{u}$ the unit vector from $P_{s,g}$ (P_s projected on the goal-contact surface plane) to P_g, i.e., $\vec{u} = \overrightarrow{P_{s,g}P_g}/\|\overrightarrow{P_{s,g}P_g}\|$. Finally let $\vec{v} = \vec{u} \times (\vec{z} \times \vec{u})$ be the unit vector normal to $\vec{u}$ that lies in the plan defined by $\vec{u}$ and $\vec{z}$. The default way-point P_w is defined as

$$P_w = P_g - \frac{1}{2}\overrightarrow{P_{s,g}P_g} + h\vec{v}, \tag{8}$$

where h is the hand-tuned user-defined parameter that specifies the height of the steps. The command c_t in Equation (7) that comes from the BMI decoding system is finally used to modify in real-time this way-point position P_w by modifying its height h (see **Figure 2**, middle). Let δh denote a desired height control resolution, then the modified position of the way-point through the brain command c_t becomes

$$P_w(c_t) = \begin{cases} P_g - \frac{1}{2}\overrightarrow{P_{s,g}P_g} + (h + c_t\,\delta h)\,\vec{v} & \text{if } t = 1, \\ P_w(c_{t-1}) + c_t\,\delta h\,\vec{v} & \text{if } t > 1. \end{cases} \tag{9}$$

The command c_t could have been used in other ways, however we identified two principles that should in our view stand in a BMI low-level control endeavor of humanoid motion such as ours:

- Principle 1: The full detailed motion, that cannot be designed joint-wise by the BMI user, should be autonomously planned and executed from high-level (task-level) command.
- Principle 2: The brain command can then be used to locally correct or bias the autonomously planned and executed motion, and help overcome shortcomings inherent to full autonomy.

The way-point is a key feature to be controlled according to these two principles as it helps surmount the main limitation of the autonomous collision-avoidance constraint expressed in the on-line quadratic-program-formulated controller described in Section 3. This collision-avoidance constraint, that had to be formulated as a linear constraint in the joint acceleration vector of the robot in order to fit within the quadratic-program formulation [adapting to this end the velocity-damper formulation (Faverjon and Tournassoud, 1987)], acts as a repulsive field, with the tracked way-point acting as an attractive field, on the contact link. The resultant field (from the superposition of these two fields) can display local extrema corresponding to equilibrium situations in which the link stops moving though without having completed its tracking task (see **Figure 9**). Manual user intervention, here through the brain command, is then necessary to un-block the motion of the link by adequately moving the tracked way-point. The brain command is thus used here for low-level correction of a naturally limitation-affected full-autonomy strategy.

6. PROOF-OF-CONCEPT EXPERIMENT

The experiment we designed (see **Figure 3** and video that can be downloaded at http://www.cns.atr.jp/~xmorimo/videos/frontiers.wmv) to test the whole framework is described as follows.

An initial and goal configurations (**Figure 4**) are pre-specified manually by the user among a finite number of locations in the environment. In this case the initial configuration is standing in front of a stair and the goal task is to go up on the stair. This selection is for now done manually, but it can later also be selected through a brain command by embedding the strategy described in this work within a hierarchical framework such as the ones suggested in Chung et al. (2011); Bryan et al. (2011), that will switch between the behavior of selecting the high-level goal task and the low-level motion control.

Off-line, the framework autonomously plans the sequence of contact transitions and associated intermediate static postures to reach that goal (**Figure 5**), then the on-line controller is executed.

The user is wearing an EEG cap and is trained with 3 training sessions of approximately 5 min each to learn the parameter of the classifier described in Section 4, through a motor imagery task

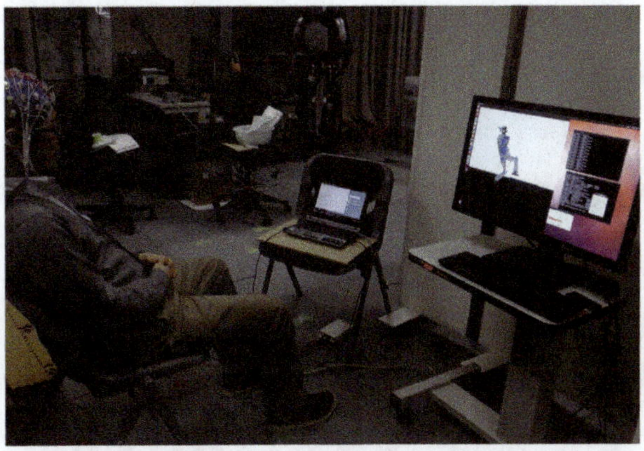

FIGURE 3 | Experiment setup. The user is wearing an EEG cap. The laptop on his left side is used for decoding the motor imagery task signal, the computer on his right runs the real-time physics simulation allowing him to control the position of the moving foot through the visual feedback he gets from the simulator window.

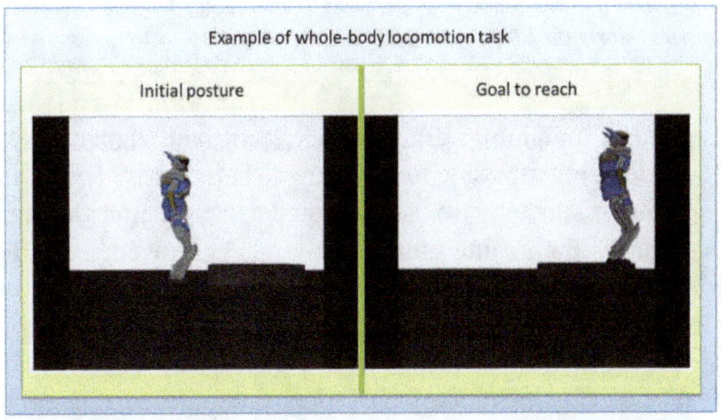

FIGURE 4 | Intial and goal positions for the experiment. Left: initial configuration with the robot standing in front of the stair. **Right**: goal configuration with the robot standing at the extremity up on the srair.

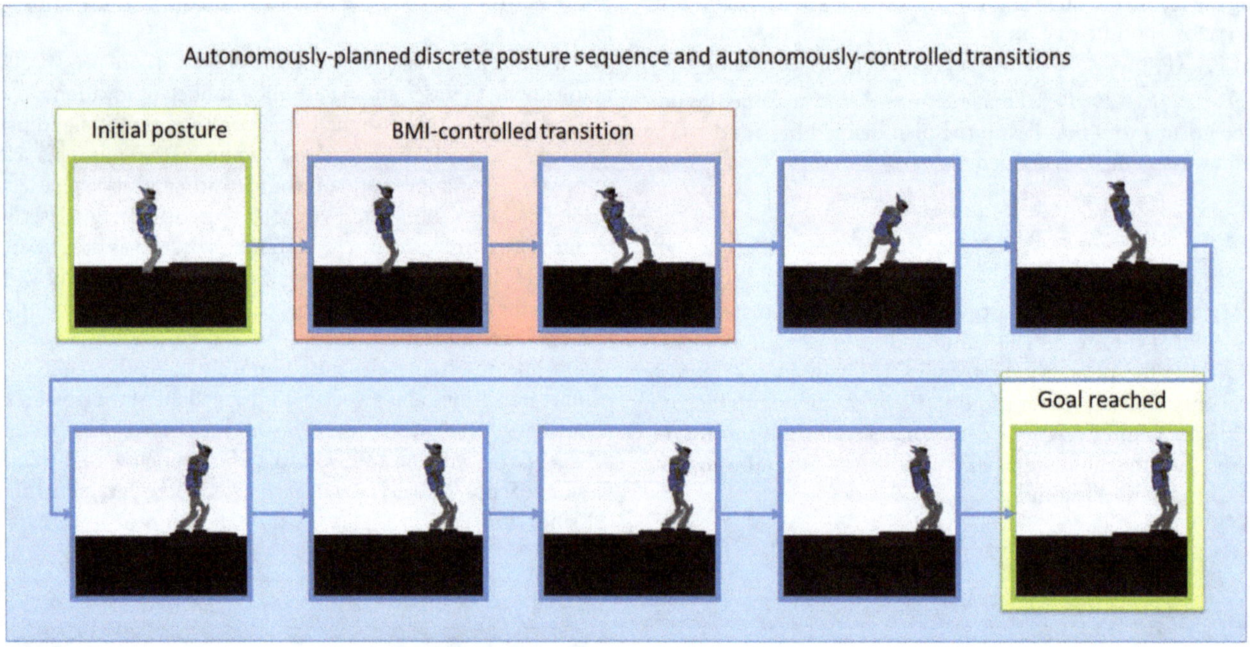

FIGURE 5 | The sequence of static postures planned autonomously. The first posture is the initial posture. The second posture which looks like the first one keeps both feet on the ground but puts all the weight of the robot on the right foot so as to zero the contact forces on the right left to release it for the next posture. The third posture moves the now free left foot and puts it on the stair, but still without any contact force applied on it (all the weith of the robot is still supported by the right foot). the fourth postures keeps both feet at their current locations but shifts all the weight of the robot away from the right foot to put it entirely on the left foot, the right foot becomes free of contact forces, and so on.

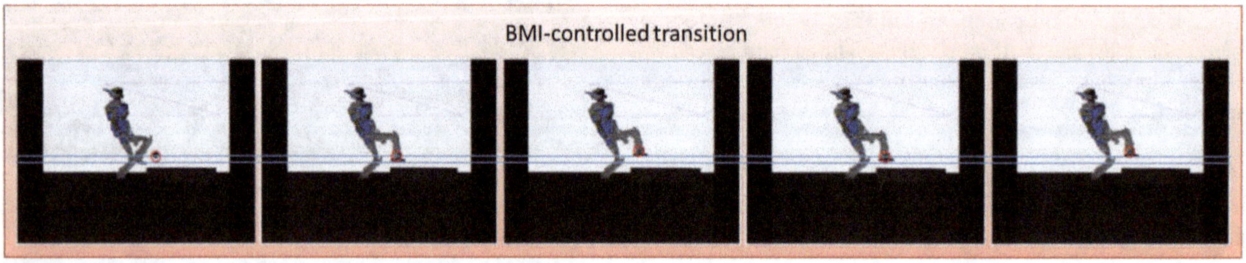

FIGURE 6 | The controlled motion. The figures represent successive snapshots from the real-time controlled motion in the physics simulator. The controlled position of the way point appears in the simulator as a black sphere that we circle here in red for clarity. This position is tracked by the foot (more precisely at the ankle joint) throught the simulation. The two horizontal lines represent the level of the sole of the foot at the two positions sent as a command by the user through the BMI. These lines do not appear in the simulator we add them here only as common visualization reference lines for all the snapshots. In the first two frames the robot tracks the default position of the way point. In the third frame the user decides to move that position up, then down in fourth frame, and finally up again in the fifth frame.

consisting of imagining respectively left arm and right arm circling movements for going up and down. This task is generic and we retained it since it gave us in our experiment better decoding performances than some other tasks (e.g., leg movements). The user has visual feed-back from the simulator on the desktop computer screen (on his right in **Figure 3**) and from a bar-diagram representing in real-time the decoded probability of the motor-imagery task classification on the laptop computer screen (on his left in **Figure 3**). The experiment was successfully completed on the first effective trial, which was the overall third trial (the first two trials were canceled after their respective training sessions since we encountered and fixed some minor implementation bugs before starting the control phase). The subject had prior experience with the same motor-imagery classifier in our previously-cited study (Noda et al., 2012). We only experimented with that one subject as we considered that we reached our aim of testing our framework and providing its proof-of-concept experiment.

The decoding of the BMI command is done in real-time and implemented in Matlab, and the brain command is then sent via UDP protocol to the physics simulator process implemented in C++.

We tested the way-point control strategy in the second step of the motion (the first contact-adding step along the sequence, the highlighted transition in **Figure 5**). **Figure 6** focuses on this controlled part of the motion. The user controlled the position of a black sphere that represents the position of the targeted way-point, that the foot of the robot tracks in real-time, while autonomously keeping balance and avoiding self-collisions, joint limits, and collision with the environment. A total of 8 commands ("up"/"down") were sent during this controlled transition phase, that we voluntarily made last around 300 s (5 min) in order to allow the user to send several commands. We then externally (manually) triggered the FSM transition to the following step along the sequence and left the autonomous controller complete the motion without brain control. That autonomous part was completed in about 16 s. See the accompanying video.

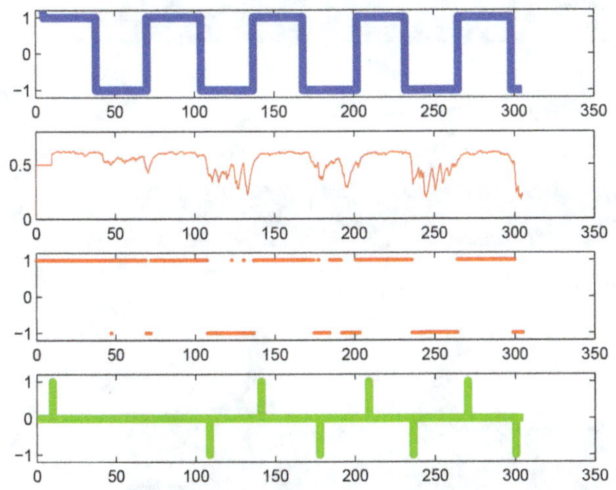

FIGURE 7 | Motor imagery decoding performances. On the horizontal axis is iteration number. From top to bottom: the thick blue line represents the command cue given as an input to the user, the thin red line represents the decoded brain activities [the probability $P(k_t = +1|\mathbf{C}_t)$], the thick red point markers represent the estimated classified label [$P(k_t = +1|\mathbf{C}_t) \geq 0.5$ or < 0.5], finally the thick green line represents the command c_t sent to the robot (based on the threshold $P_{\text{thres}} = 0.6$). Note that this green command does not represent the position of the way-point but the instantaneous rate of change in this position between two successive time steps t and $t + 1$, according to Equation (9), line 2 (i.e., the "derivative" were we talking of a continuous and differentiable function rather than the time-discretized one at hand).

Figure 7 illustrates the decoding performances of the BMI system, while **Figure 8** shows the tracking performance of the humanoid whole-body controller. The table below gives computation time figures executed on a Dell Precision T7600 Workstation equipped with a Xeon processor E5-2687W (3.1 GHz, 20 M). Full details on the physics simulator, including contact modeling and resolution, and collision detection, can be found in Chardonnet et al. (2006); Chardonnet (2012).

Offline planning	2.7 s
Average online control command (QP) (@ 200 Hz)	2.661 ms
Average online simulation step (@ 1 kHz)	0.389 ms
BCI classifier training and learning session	~ 30 min
Average online BCI signal buffering (@ 2048 Hz)	0.137 ms
Avg online BCI classification (@ 128 Hz) no control signal sent ($c_t = 0$)	0.204 ms
Avg BCI classification (@ 128 Hz) control signal sent ($c_t = +1$ or -1)	6.20 ms

From this experiment, we confirmed that the autonomous framework can be coupled with the BMI decoding system in real-time in simulation and that the simulated robot can safely realize the task while receiving and executing the brain command.

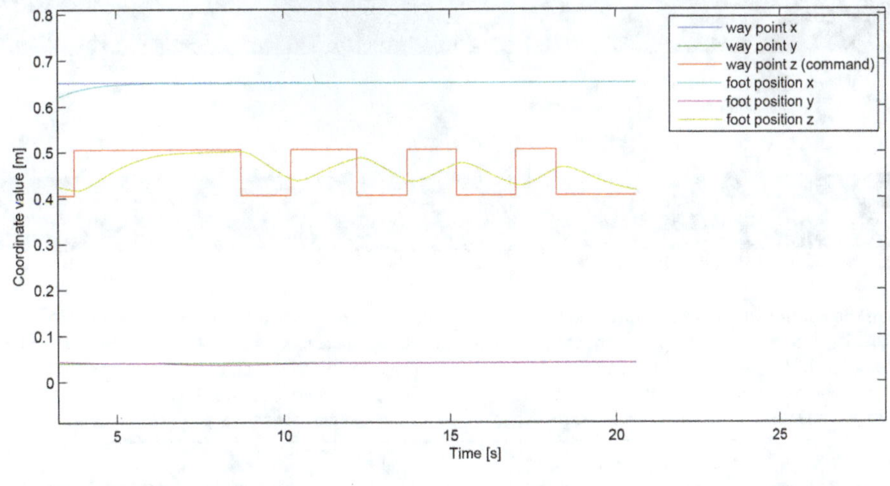

FIGURE 8 | Way-point tracking performance. The user-controlled quantity, that happens to be in the particular case demonstrated here the z-coordinate of the tracked way-point (the "generalized" vertical direction being reduced in this case to the "conventional" vertical direction, meaning $\vec{v} \equiv \vec{z}$ in **Figure 2**, since the goal-contact surface on the stair is horizontal), is represented by the piecewise-constant red curve. The corresponding motion of the foot, that tracks this command-induced way-point position, is shown in yellow curve. the two other coordinates of the foot (x and y) are auonomously maintained by the controller at the corresponding ones of the way-point and stay at their desired values throught the command phase.

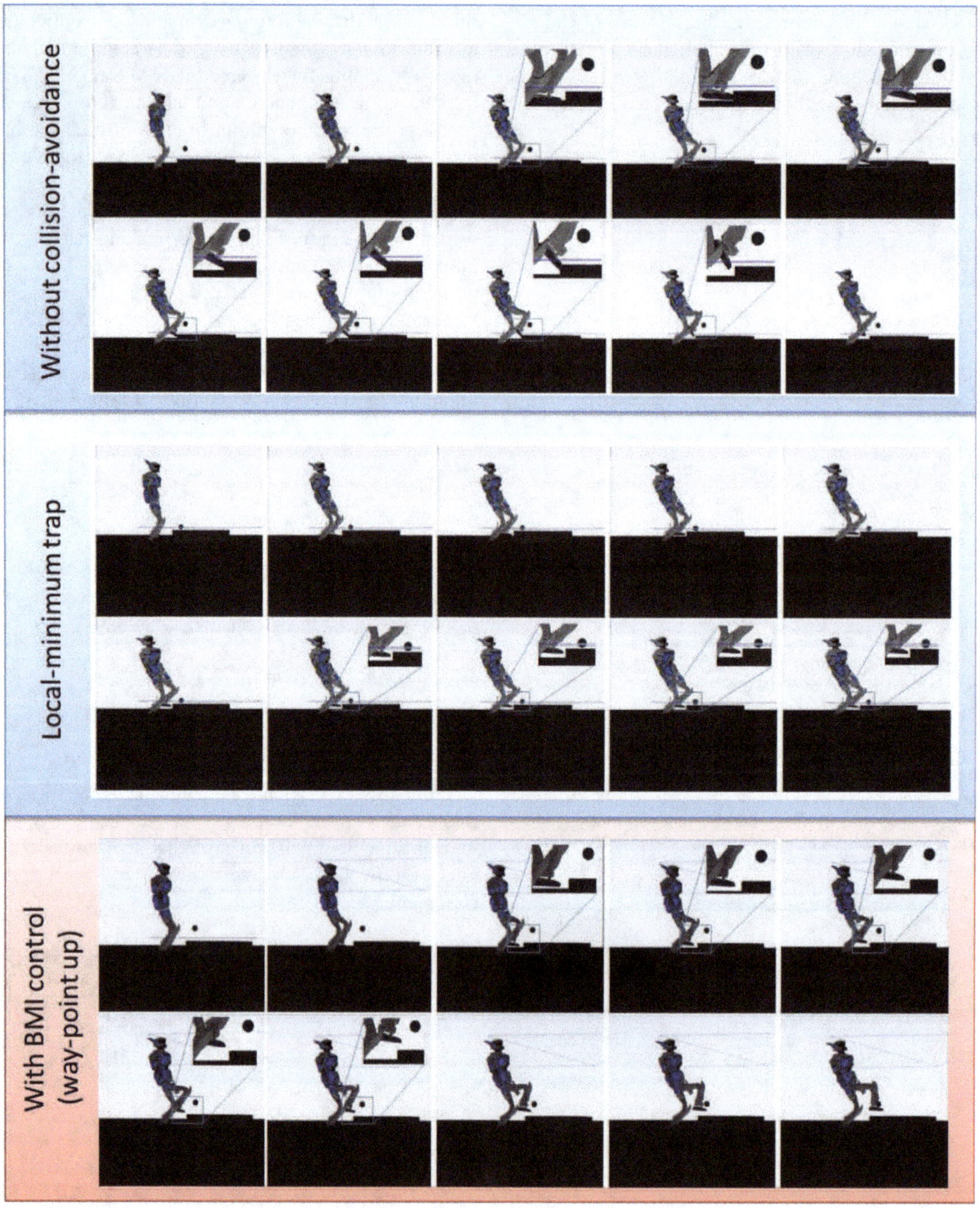

FIGURE 9 | Comparison of the controlled transition motion in three instances. Top: without collision-avoidance constraint, the foot of the robot collides with the stair while targeting its goal, and the simulation stops. **Middle**: with autonomous collision-avoidance constraint that happens to create in this case a local-minimum trap, the robot reaches an equilibrium situation and stays idle for as long as we let the simulation run (infinite time). **Bottom**: The autonomous collision-avoidance strategy combined with the proposed BMI-control approach helps reposition the way-point and overcome the local-minimum problem. The robot safely reaches the goal contact location and the motion along the sequence can be completed.

7. DISCUSSION AND FUTURE WORK

This work demonstrated the technical possibility of real-time online low-level control of whole-body humanoid motion using motor-imagery-based BMI.

We achieved it by coupling an existing EEG decoder and whole-body multi-contact acyclic planning and control framework. In particular, this coupling allowed us to control a one-dimensional feature of the high-DOF whole-body motion, designed as the generalized height of moving link way-point, in a discrete way. Though the motor-imagery task used in our proof-of-concept experiment was a generic one (left-arm vs. right-arm circling movement), we plan in the future to investigate more specific motor-imagery tasks that are in tighter correspondence with the limb of the robot being controlled, along the longer-term user's-mind-into-robot's-body "full embodiment" quest that motivates our study as expressed in our introductory section. Since previous studies reported that imagery of gait and actual gait execution have been found to recruit very similar cerebral networks (Miyai et al., 2001; La Fougère et al., 2010), we may be able to expect that a human can control a humanoid the same way they control their own human body through motor imagery.

We also aim now at continuous control of two-dimensional feature of this whole-body motion, allowing not only the control of the tracked way point but also of a corresponding threshold plan that decides when to trigger the transition between the lift-off and touch-down phases. We believe this can be achieved based on the previous work done for example on motor-imagery two-dimensional cursor control (Wolpaw and McFarland, 2004). Other previous studies also discussed the possibilities of using EEG for such continuous control (Yoshimura et al., 2012). In addition, for the continuous two-dimensional feature control, explicit consideration of individual differences in cerebral recruitment during motor imagery may be necessary (Meulen et al., 2014). As a future study, we may consider using transfer learning approaches (Samek et al., 2013) to cope with this individual difference problem.

Finally, we aim at porting this framework from the simulation environment to the real robot control, so that in future study we may possibly use the proposed framework in a rehabilitation training program to enhance recovery of motor-related nervous system of stroke patients.

ACKNOWLEDGMENTS

This work is supported with a JSPS Postodoctoral Fellowship for Foreign Researchers, ID No. P12707. This study is the result of "Development of BMI Technologies for Clinical Application" carried out under the Strategic Research Program for Brain Sciences by the Ministry of Education, Culture, Sports, Science and Technology of Japan. Part of this research was supported by MIC-SCOPE and a contract with the Ministry of Internal Affairs and Communications entitled "Novel and innovative R&D making use of brain structures." This research was also partially supported by MEXT KAKENHI grant Number 23120004, Strategic International Cooperative Program, Japan Science and Technology Agency (JST) and by JSPS and MIZS: Japan-Slovenia research Cooperative Program Joris Vaillant and François Keith were partially suported by grants from the RoboHow.Cog FP7 www.robohow.eu, Contract N288533. The authors would like to thank Abderrahmane Kheddar for valuable use of the AMELIF dynamics simulation framework.

REFERENCES

Bell, C. J., Shenoy, P., Chalodhorn, R., and Rao, R. P. N. (2008). Control of a humanoid robot by a noninvasive brain-computer interface in humans. *J. Neural Eng.* 5, 214–220. doi: 10.1088/1741-2560/5/2/012

Bouyarmane, K., and Kheddar, A. (2010). "Static multi-contact inverse problem for multiple humanoid robots and manipulated objects," in *10th IEEE-RAS International Conference on Humanoid Robots* (Nashville, TN), 8–13. doi: 10.1109/ICHR.2010.5686317

Bouyarmane, K., and Kheddar, A. (2011a). "Multi-contact stances planning for multiple agents," in *IEEE International Conference on Robotics and Automation* (Shanghai), 5546–5353.

Bouyarmane, K., and Kheddar, A. (2011b). "Using a multi-objective controller to synthesize simulated humanoid robot motion with changing contact configurations," in *IEEE/RSJ International Conference on Intelligent Robots and Systems* (San Fransisco, CA), 4414–4419.

Bouyarmane, K., and Kheddar, A. (2012). Humanoid robot locomotion and manipulation step planning. *Adv. Robot.* 26, 1099–1126. doi: 10.1080/01691864.2012.686345

Bryan, M., Green, J., Chung, M., Chang, L., Scherery, R., Smith, J., et al. (2011). "An adaptive brain-computer interface for humanoid robot control," in *11th IEEE-RAS International Conference on Humanoid Robots* (Bled), 199–204.

Chardonnet, J.-R. (2012). Interactive dynamic simulator for multibody systems. *Int. J. Hum. Robot.* 9, 1250021:1–1250021:24. doi: 10.1142/S0219843612500211

Chardonnet, J.-R., Miossec, S., Kheddar, A., Arisumi, H., Hirukawa, H., Pierrot, F., et al. (2006). "Dynamic simulator for humanoids using constraint-based method with static friction," in *Robotics and Biomimetics, 2006. ROBIO'06. IEEE International Conference on* (Kunming), 1366–1371.

Chestnutt, J., Kuffner, J., Nishiwaki, K., and Kagami, S. (2003). "Planning biped navigation strategies in complex environments," in *IEEE-RAS International Conference on Humanoid Robots* (Munich).

Chestnutt, J., Lau, M., Kuffner, J., Cheung, G., Hodgins, J., and Kanade, T. (2005). "Footstep planning for the ASIMO humanoid robot," in *IEEE International Conference on Robotics and Automation* (Barcelona), 629–634.

Chung, M., Cheung, W., Scherer, R., and Rao, R. P. N. (2011). "A hierarchical architecture for adaptive brain-computer interfacing," in *Proceedings of the Twenty-Second International Joint Conference on Artificial Intelligence Vol. 2* (Barcelona), 1647–1652.

Faverjon, B., and Tournassoud, P. (1987). "Planning of manipulators with a high number of degrees of freedom," in *IEEE International Conference on Robotics and Automation* (Raleigh, NC).

Finke, A., Knoblauch, A., Koesling, H., and Ritter, H. (2011). "A hybrid brain interface for a humanoid robot assistant," in *33rd Annual International Conference of the IEEE Engineering in Medicine and Biology Society (EMBC2011)* (Boston, MA).

Gergondet, P., Druon, S., Kheddar, A., Hintermuller, C., Guger, C., and Slater, M. (2011). "Using brain-computer interface to steer a humanoid robot," in *IEEE International Conference on Robotics and Biomimetics* (Phuket), 192–197.

Hashimoto, K., Sugahara, Y., Kawase, M., Ohta, A., Tanaka, C., Hayashi, A., et al. (2006). "Landing pattern modification method with predictive attitude and compliance control to deal with uneven terrain," in *Proceedings of the IEEE-RSJ International Conference on Intelligent Robots and Systems* (Beijing).

Hauser, K., Bretl, T., Latombe, J.-C., Harada, K., and Wilcox, B. (2008). Motion planning for legged robots on varied terrain. *Int. J. Robot. Res.* 27, 1325–1349. doi: 10.1177/0278364908098447

Herdt, A., Diedam, H., Wieber, P.-B., Dimitrov, D., Mombaur, K., and Diehl, M. (2010). Online walking motion generation with automatic footstep placement. *Adv. Robot.* 24, 719–737. doi: 10.1163/016918610X493552

Kuffner, J., Kagami, S., Nishiwaki, K., Inaba, M., and Inoue, H. (2002). Dynamically-stable motion planning for humanoid robots. *Auton. Robots* 12, 105–118. doi: 10.1023/A:1013219111657

Kuffner, J., Nishiwaki, K., Kagami, S., Inaba, M., and Inoue, H. (2001). "Footstep planning among obstacles for biped robots," in *IEEE/RSJ International Conference on Intelligent Robots and Systems - Vol. 1* (Maui, HI), 500–505.

La Fougère, C., Zwergal, A., Rominger, A., Förster, S., Fesl, G., Dieterich, M., et al. (2010). Real versus imagined locomotion: an intraindividual [18F]-FDG PET - fMRI comparison. *Neuroimage* 50, 1589–1598. doi: 10.1016/j.neuroimage.2009.12.060

Ma, J., Zhang, Y., Nam, Y., Cichocki, A., and Matsuno, F. (2013). "EOG/ERP hybrid human-machine interface for robot control," in *IEEE-RAS International Conference on Intelligent Robots and Systems* (Tokyo), 859–864.

Meulen, M. V. D., Allali, G., Rieger, S., Assal, F., and Vuilleumier, P. (2014). The influence of individual motor imagery ability on cerebral recruitment during gait imagery. *Hum. Brain Mapp.* 35, 455–470. doi: 10.1002/hbm.22192

Miller, K. J., Schalk, G., Fetza, E. E., den Nijs, M., Ojemanne, J., and Rao, R. (2010). Cortical activity during motor execution, motor imagery, and imagery-based online feedback. *Proc. Natl. Acad. Sci. U.S.A.* 107, 4430–4435. doi: 10.1073/pnas.0913697107

Miyai, I., Tanabe, H., Sase, I., Eda, H., Oda, I., Konishi, I., et al. (2001). Cortical mapping of gait in humans: a near-infrared spectroscopic topography study. *Neuroimage* 14, 1186–1192. doi: 10.1006/nimg.2001.0905

Morisawa, M., Kanehiro, F., Kaneko, K., Kajita, S., and Yokoi, K. (2011). "Reactive biped walking control for a collision of a swinging foot on uneven terrain," in *Proceedings of the IEEE-RAS International Conference on Humanoid Robots* (Bled).

Noda, T., Sugimoto, N., Furukawa, J., Sato, M., Hyon, S., and Morimoto, J. (2012). "Brain-controlled exoskeleton robot for bmi rehabilitation," in *12th IEEE-RAS International Conference on Humanoid Robots* (Osaka), 21–27.

Riechmann, H., Hachmeister, N., Ritter, H., and Finke, A. (2011). "Asynchronous, parallel on-line classification of P300 and ERD for an efficient hybrid BCI," in *5th IEEE EMBS Conference on Neural Engineering (NER2011)* (Cancun).

Samek, W., Meinecke, F. C., and Muller, K.-R. (2013). Transferring subspaces between subjects in brain-computer interfacing. *IEEE Trans. Biomed. Eng.* 60, 2289–2298. doi: 10.1109/TBME.2013.2253608

Takanishi, A., and Kato, I. (1994). "Development of a biped walking robot adapting to a horizontally uneven surface," in *Proceedings of the IEEE-RSJ International Conference on Intelligent Robots and Systems* (Munich).

Tomioka, R., and Aihara, K. (2007). "Classifying matrices with a spectral regularization," in *24th International Conference on Machine Learning* (New York, NY), 895–902.

Tomioka, R., and Muller, K. (2010). A regularized discriminative framework for EEG analysis with application to brain-computer interface. *Neuroimage* 49, 415–432. doi: 10.1016/j.neuroimage.2009.07.045

Wolpaw, J. R., and McFarland, D. J. (2004). Control of a two-dimensional movement signal by a noninvasive brain-computer interface in humans. *Proc. Natl. Acad. Sci. U.S.A.* 101, 17849–17854. doi: 10.1073/pnas.0403504101

Yamane, K., Kuffner, J., and Hodgins, J. K. (2004). Synthesizing animations of human manipulation tasks. *ACM Trans. Graph.* 23, 532–539. doi: 10.1145/1015706.1015756

Yoshida, E., Kanoun, O., Esteves, C., and Laumond, J. P. (2006). "Task-driven support polygon reshaping for humanoids," in *6th IEEE-RAS International Conference on Humanoid Robots* (Genova), 208–213.

Yoshida, E., Laumond, J.-P., Esteves, C., Kanoun, O., Sakaguchi, T., and Yokoi, K. (2008). "Whole-body locomotion, manipulation and reaching for humanoids," in *Motion in Games*, Volume 5277 of *LNCS*, eds A. Egges, A. Kamphuis, and M. Overmars (Berlin; Heidelberg: Springer), 210–221.

Yoshimura, N., Dasalla, C., Hanakawa, T., Sato, M., and Koike, Y. (2012). Reconstuction of flexor and extensor muscle activity from electroencephalography cortical currents. *Neuroimage* 59, 1324–1337. doi: 10.1016/j.neuroimage.2011.08.029

Permissions

All chapters in this book were first published in ABFFFC, by Frontiers; hereby published with permission under the Creative Commons Attribution License or equivalent. Every chapter published in this book has been scrutinized by our experts. Their significance has been extensively debated. The topics covered herein carry significant findings which will fuel the growth of the discipline. They may even be implemented as practical applications or may be referred to as a beginning point for another development.

The contributors of this book come from diverse backgrounds, making this book a truly international effort. This book will bring forth new frontiers with its revolutionizing research information and detailed analysis of the nascent developments around the world.

We would like to thank all the contributing authors for lending their expertise to make the book truly unique.

They have played a crucial role in the development of this book. Without their invaluable contributions this book wouldn't have been possible. They have made vital efforts to compile up to date information on the varied aspects of this subject to make this book a valuable addition to the collection of many professionals and students.

This book was conceptualized with the vision of imparting up-to-date information and advanced data in this field. To ensure the same, a matchless editorial board was set up. Every individual on the board went through rigorous rounds of assessment to prove their worth. After which they invested a large part of their time researching and compiling the most relevant data for our readers.

The editorial board has been involved in producing this book since its inception. They have spent rigorous hours researching and exploring the diverse topics which have resulted in the successful publishing of this book. They have passed on their knowledge of decades through this book. To expedite this challenging task, the publisher supported the team at every step. A small team of assistant editors was also appointed to further simplify the editing procedure and attain best results for the readers.

Apart from the editorial board, the designing team has also invested a significant amount of their time in understanding the subject and creating the most relevant covers. They scrutinized every image to scout for the most suitable representation of the subject and create an appropriate cover for the book.

The publishing team has been an ardent support to the editorial, designing and production team. Their endless efforts to recruit the best for this project, has resulted in the accomplishment of this book. They are a veteran in the field of academics and their pool of knowledge is as vast as their experience in printing. Their expertise and guidance has proved useful at every step. Their uncompromising quality standards have made this book an exceptional effort. Their encouragement from time to time has been an inspiration for everyone.

The publisher and the editorial board hope that this book will prove to be a valuable piece of knowledge for researchers, students, practitioners and scholars across the globe.

List of Contributors

Beatrix Krause and Roi Cohen Kadosh
Department of Experimental Psychology, University of Oxford, Oxford, UK

Dong Song, Madhuri Harway, Vasilis Z. Marmarelis and Theodore W. Berger
Department of Biomedical Engineering, University of Southern California, Los Angeles, CA, USA

Robert E. Hampson and Sam A. Deadwyler
Department of Physiology and Pharmacology, School of Medicine, Wake Forest University, Winston-Salem, NC, USA

Elisabeth Hildt
Center for the Study of Ethics in the Professions, Illinois Institute of Technology, Chicago, IL, USA

Tal Dotan Ben-Soussan
The Leslie and Susan Gonda (Goldschmied) Multidisciplinary Brain Research Center, Bar-Ilan University, Ramat-Gan, Israel
Research Institute for Neuroscience, Education and Didactics, Cognitive Neurophysiology Laboratory, Patrizio Paoletti Foundation, Assisi, Italy

Keren Avirame
The Leslie and Susan Gonda (Goldschmied) Multidisciplinary Brain Research Center, Bar-Ilan University, Ramat-Gan, Israel
Department of Neurology, Charité - Universitätsmedizin, Berlin, Germany

Joseph Glicksohn
The Leslie and Susan Gonda (Goldschmied) Multidisciplinary Brain Research Center, Bar-Ilan University, Ramat-Gan, Israel
Department of Criminology, Bar-Ilan University, Ramat-Gan, Israel

Abraham Goldstein
The Leslie and Susan Gonda (Goldschmied) Multidisciplinary Brain Research Center, Bar-Ilan University, Ramat-Gan, Israel
Department of Psychology, Bar-Ilan University, Ramat-Gan, Israel

Yuval Harpaz
The Leslie and Susan Gonda (Goldschmied) Multidisciplinary Brain Research Center, Bar-Ilan University, Ramat-Gan, Israel

Michal Ben-Shachar
The Leslie and Susan Gonda (Goldschmied) Multidisciplinary Brain Research Center, Bar-Ilan University, Ramat-Gan, Israel
Department of English, Linguistics Division, Bar-Ilan University, Israel

Gytis Baranauskas
Neurophysiology Laboratory, Neuroscience Institute, Lithuanian University of Health Sciences, Kaunas, Lithuania

Jun Il Kang
École d'optométrie, Université de Montréal, Montréal, QC, Canada
Département de Neuroscience, Université de Montréal, Montréal, QC, Canada

Frédéric Huppé-Gourgues and Elvire Vaucher
École d'optométrie, Université de Montréal, Montréal, QC, Canada

Hannah Maslen
Oxford Martin School, University of Oxford, Oxford, UK

Nadira Faulmüller
Department of Experimental Psychology, University of Oxford, Oxford, UK
Department Values, Technology and Innovation, Delft University of Technology, Delft, Netherlands

Julian Savulescu
Oxford Uehiro Centre for Practical Ethics, University of Oxford, Oxford, UK

Susanne Diekelmann
Institute of Medical Psychology and Behavioral Neurobiology, University Tübingen, Tübingen, Germany

Mirko D. Garasic
The Federmann School of Public Policy and Government Campus, The Hebrew University of Jerusalem, Jerusalem, Israel

Andrea Lavazza
Centro Universitario Internazionale, Arezzo, Italy

Filippo Santoni de Sio
Department Values, Technology and Innovation, Faculty Technology, Policy and Management, Delft University of Technology, Delft, Netherlands

Nadira Faulmüller
Department Values, Technology and Innovation, Faculty Technology, Policy and Management, Delft University of Technology, Delft, Netherlands
Department of Experimental Psychology, University of Oxford, Oxford, UK

Nicole A Vincent
Department Values, Technology and Innovation, Faculty Technology, Policy and Management, Delft University of Technology, Delft, Netherlands
Department of Philosophy, Georgia State University, Atlanta, GA, USA

Guilherme Wood, Silvia Erika Kober, Matthias Witte and Christa Neuper
Department of Psychology, Karl-Franzens-University Graz, Graz, Austria
BioTechMed, Graz, Austria

Raymond van de Berg and Herman Kingma
Division of Balance Disorders, Department of Otorhinolaryngology and Head and Neck Surgery, Faculty of Health Medicine and Life Sciences, School for Mental Health and Neuroscience, Maastricht University Medical Center, Maastricht, Netherlands
Faculty of Physics, Tomsk State University, Tomsk, Russia

Nils Guinand, Maurizio Ranieri, Samuel Cavuscens, Jean-Philippe Guyot and Angelica Perez-Fornos
Service of Otorhinolaryngology and Head and Neck Surgery, Department of Clinical Neurosciences, Geneva University Hospitals, Geneva, Switzerland

T. A. Khoa Nguyen
Translational Neural Engineering Lab, Center for Neuroprosthetics, Interfaculty Institute of Bioengineering, École Polytechnique Fédérale de Lausanne, Lausanne, Switzerland

Robert Stokroos
Division of Balance Disorders, Department of Otorhinolaryngology and Head and Neck Surgery, Faculty of Health Medicine and Life Sciences, School for Mental Health and Neuroscience, Maastricht University Medical Center, Maastricht, Netherlands

Elena Rusconi
Department of Security and Crime Science, University College London, London, UK
Division of Psychology, Abertay University, Dundee, UK
Department of Neurosciences, University of Parma, Parma, Italy

Timothy Mitchener-Nissen
Department of Science and Technology Studies, University College London, London, UK

Yoshio Sakurai
Department of Psychology, Graduate School of Letters, Kyoto University, Kyoto, Japan

Jörn M. Horschig and Ali Bahramisharif
Radboud University Nijmegen, Donders Institute for Brain, Behaviour and Cognition, Nijmegen, Netherlands

Johanna M. Zumer
Radboud University Nijmegen, Donders Institute for Brain, Behaviour and Cognition, Nijmegen, Netherlands
School of Psychology, University of Birmingham, Birmingham, UK

Cheryl A. Frye
Department of Psychology, The University at Albany-SUNY, Albany, NY, USA
Department of Biological Sciences, The University at Albany-SUNY, Albany, NY, USA
The Center for Neuroscience Research, The University at Albany-SUNY, Albany, NY, USA
The Center for Life Sciences Research, The University at Albany-SUNY, Albany, NY, USA
Department of Chemistry and Biochemistry, The University of Alaska-Fairbanks, Fairbanks, AK, USA
Institute of Arctic Biology, The University of Alaska-Fairbanks, Fairbanks, AK, USA
IDeA Network of Biomedical Excellence (INBRE), The University of Alaska-Fairbanks, Fairbanks, AK, USA

Carolyn J. Koonce
Department of Psychology, The University at Albany-SUNY, Albany, NY, USA
Institute of Arctic Biology, The University of Alaska-Fairbanks, Fairbanks, AK, USA
IDeA Network of Biomedical Excellence (INBRE), The University of Alaska-Fairbanks, Fairbanks, AK, USA

Alicia A. Walf
Department of Psychology, The University at Albany-SUNY, Albany, NY, USA
Institute of Arctic Biology, The University of Alaska-Fairbanks, Fairbanks, AK, USA
IDeA Network of Biomedical Excellence (INBRE), The University of Alaska-Fairbanks, Fairbanks, AK, USA

Hikaru Takeuchi, Hiroshi Hashizume and Yuko Sassa
Division of Developmental Cognitive Neuroscience, Institute of Development, Aging and Cancer, Tohoku University, Sendai, Japan

Yasuyuki Taki
Division of Developmental Cognitive Neuroscience, Institute of Development, Aging and Cancer, Tohoku University, Sendai, Japan
Division of Medical Image Analysis, Department of Community Medical Supports, Tohoku Medical Megabank Organization, Tohoku University, Sendai, Japan
Department of Radiology and Nuclear Medicine, Institute of Development, Aging and Cancer, Tohoku University, Sendai, Japan

Rui Nouchi, Atsushi Sekiguchi and Yuka Kotozaki
Department of Advanced Brain Science, Smart Ageing International Research Center, Institute of Development, Aging and Cancer, Tohoku University, Sendai, Japan

Seishu Nakagawa and Carlos Makoto Miyauchi
Department of Functional Brain Imaging, Institute of Development, Aging and Cancer, Tohoku University, Sendai, Japan

Ryuta Kawashima
Division of Developmental Cognitive Neuroscience, Institute of Development, Aging and Cancer, Tohoku University, Sendai, Japan
Division of Medical Image Analysis, Department of Community Medical Supports, Tohoku Medical Megabank Organization, Tohoku University, Sendai, Japan
Department of Advanced Brain Science, Smart Ageing International Research Center, Institute of Development, Aging and Cancer, Tohoku University, Sendai, Japan

Jean-Louis Honeine
Department of Public Health, Experimental and Forensic Medicine, University of Pavia, Pavia, Italy

Marco Schieppati
Department of Public Health, Experimental and Forensic Medicine, University of Pavia, Pavia, Italy
Centro Studi Attività Motorie (CSAM), Fondazione Salvatore Maugeri (IRCSS), Scientific Institute of Pavia, Pavia, Italy

Kimberly R. Urban
Department of Psychology, University of Delaware, Newark, DE, USA

Wen-Jun Gao
Department of Neurobiology and Anatomy, Drexel University College of Medicine, Philadelphia, PA, USA

Michael A. Nitsche
Clinic for Clinical Neurophysiology, University Medical Center, Göttingen, Germany

Riccardo Bravi, Eros Quarta, Erez J. Cohen and Diego Minciacchi
Department of Experimental and Clinical Medicine, University of Florence, Florence, Italy

Anna Gottard
Department of Statistics, Informatics, Applications, University of Florence, Florence, Italy

Soojin Lee, Diana J. Kim and Martin J. McKeown
Pacific Parkinson's Research Centre, Department of Medicine, University of British Columbia, Vancouver, BC, Canada

Daniel Svenkeson, Gabriel Parras and Meeko Mitsuko K. Oishi
Department of Electrical and Computer Engineering, University of New Mexico, Albuquerque, NM, USA

Wei Li
Department of Computer and Electrical Engineering and Computer Science, California State University, Bakersfield, CA, USA
School of Electrical Engineering and Automation, Tianjin University, Tianjin, China

Mengfan Li and Jing Zhao
School of Electrical Engineering and Automation, Tianjin University, Tianjin, China

Carmelo M. Vicario
School of Psychology, The University of Queensland, St. Lucia, QLD, Australia

Karim Bouyarmane and Jun Morimoto
Computational Neuroscience Laboratories, Department of Brain Robot Interface, Advanced Telecommunications Research Institute International (ATR), Kyoto, Japan

Joris Vaillant and François Keith
Laboratoire d'Informatique de Robotique et de Micro-électronique de Montpellier, CNRS-University of Montpellier 2, Montpellier, France
CNRS-AIST Joint Robotics Laboratory, UMI3218/CRT, National Intitute of Advanced Industrial Science and Technology, Tsukuba, Japan

Norikazu Sugimoto
National Institute of Information and Communications Technology, Osaka, Japan

Jun-ichiro Furukawa
Computational Neuroscience Laboratories, Department of Brain Robot Interface, Advanced Telecommunications Research Institute International (ATR), Kyoto, Japan
Graduate School of Frontier Biosciences, Osaka University, Osaka, Japan

Index

www.ingramcontent.com/pod-product-compliance
Lightning Source LLC
LaVergne TN
LVHW080926210926
848485LV00004B/736